C000133124

Medicolegal Reporting in Orthopaedic Trauma

To Denise, Judith, Caroline, Jonathan, Matthew, Stephen and Paul for the hours that we didn't spend together.

Medicolegal Reporting in Orthopaedic Trauma

Edited by

Michael A. Foy FRCS
Consultant Orthopaedic Surgeon,
Princess Alexandra Hospital,
RAF Wroughton, UK

Phillip S. Fagg MB BS FRCS
Consultant Orthopaedic Surgeon,
Princess of Wales RAF Hospital,
Ely, UK

CHURCHILL LIVINGSTONE
EDINBURGH LONDON MELBOURNE AND NEW YORK 1990

CHURCHILL LIVINGSTONE
Medical Division of Longman Group UK Limited

Distributed in the United States of America by Churchill
Livingstone Inc., 1560 Broadway, New York, N.Y. 10036,
and by associated companies, branches and representatives
throughout the world.

© Longman Group UK Limited 1990

All rights reserved; no part of this publication may be
reproduced, stored in a retrieval system, or transmitted in
any form or by any means, electronic, mechanical,
photocopying, recording or otherwise, without either the
prior written permission of the publishers (Churchill
Livingstone, Robert Stevenson House, 1–3 Baxter's Place,
Leith Walk, Edinburgh EH1 3AF) or a licence permitting
restricted copying in the United Kingdom issued by the
Copyright Licensing Agency Ltd, 33–34 Alfred Place,
London WC1E 7DP.

First published 1990

ISBN 0-443-03918-6

British Library Cataloguing in Publication Data
Medicolegal reporting in orthopaedic trauma.
  1. Great Britain. Personal injuries & death. Damages.
Law
I. Foy, Michael A.   II. Fagg, Phillip S.
344.1063′23

Library of Congress Cataloging in Publication Data
Medicolegal reporting in orthopaedic trauma/edited by
Michael A. Foy and Phillip S. Fagg.
     p. cm.
   Includes bibliographies and index.
   1. Wounds and injuries — Reporting — Great
Britain. 2. Fractures — Reporting — Great Britain. 3.
Medical jurisprudence — Great Britain. 4. Malpractice —
handbooks.   I. Foy, Michael A.   II. Fagg, Phillip S.
III. Title: Orthopaedic trauma.
[DNLM: 1. Insurance, Liability — handbooks. 2.
Medical Records — handbooks.
3. Orthopaedics — handbooks. 4. Wounds and Injuries —
handbooks.   WE 39 M489]
RD939.G7M43   1990
614′.1 — dc20
DNLM/DLC
for Library of Congress

Produced by Longman Group (FE) Ltd
Printed in Hong Kong

Preface

There is an increasing tendency for people to seek some form of compensation following personal injury. This is reflected in an increasing demand for medicolegal reports. These reports require details, not only of the injuries sustained, but also of the rate of recovery and the prognosis.

All too often the busy orthopaedic surgeon resorts to a 'best guess' philosophy to answer these questions, as he rarely has the time to research the literature on the specific injury he is being asked to report on. Our aim in preparing this book has been to provide a ready source of those answers that the orthopaedic surgeon (and solicitor) require without the need to spend hours in a library. We have attempted to cull from the world literature the relevant data and present it in an easy-to-read format. Despite extensive reading of published papers we may well have missed some important works and therefore the percentages and recovery times we quote are only guidelines.

Authors adopt different criteria both in classifying fracture patterns and in categorizing results of treatment after musculoskeletal injuries. We accept that direct comparison is not always possible, but we have tried to compare 'like with like'. We defend our actions in comparing different authors' works by stressing that it is our intention to provide prognostic guidelines only. Different methods of treatment are compared, but we have not intended to recommend one method of treatment over another. We merely report what has been written in the past. At the end of the day, the correct treatment for any patient is that which the treating surgeon feels is most appropriate, and which gives the best results in his own hands.

We have tried to present the material in an easy-to-read fashion, so that relevant details can be obtained quickly. Many references are given to allow further reading if required.

We hope that this book will go some way toward filling the void which exists in the orthopaedic literature on the important subject of personal injury litigation.

Wroughton and   M.A.F.
Ely, 1990   P.S.F.

Acknowledgements

The editors would like to thank the following friends, colleagues and mentors who have provided constructive criticism and assistance in the preparation of this text; Mr John Crawford-Adams, Air Commodore Tony Merrifield, Professor Marvin Tile, Professor Angus Wallace, Mr Chris Colton, Mr John Webb, Mr George Milligan, Mr Ian Forster, Miss Heather Prince, Group Captain Tom Bucher, Wing Commander Brian Morgans, Squadron Leader Cormack O'Connell and Major Nigel Hobbs.

We have received invaluable secretarial support from Penny Harvey, Judith Fagg, Kate Marshall, Shirley Blythe and Denise Foy. We are grateful for their tireless, good humoured assistance, without which the preparation of this manuscript would not have been possible. Our thanks also go to Lyndon Cochrane for the artwork in chapters 13 and 15.

Finally, we would like to thank the staff at Churchill Livingstone for their support during this project, particularly Elif Fincanci-Smith, Ann Kelsall and Peter Richardson.

M. A. F.
P. S. F.

Contributors

George L. W. Bonney MS FRCS
Honorary Consulting Orthopaedic Surgeon, St Mary's Hospital, London, UK

Roger N. Bloor MRCS LRCP MRCPsych MPsyMed
Consultant Psychiatrist, City General Hospital, Stoke on Trent, UK

Timothy D. Bunker MCh MB BS(Hons) BSc(Hons) FRCS FRCSEd
Senior Registrar, University Hospital, Nottingham, UK

T. J. Dowling Jr MD
Smithtown, New York, USA

Stephen I. Esses BSc MD MSc FRCSC
Assistant Professor, Dewar Spine Unit, Toronto General Hospital, Toronto, Ontario, Canada

Phillip S. Fagg MB BS FRCS
Consultant Orthopaedic Surgeon, Royal Air Force Hospital, Ely, UK

Michael A. Foy FRCS
Consultant Orthopaedic Surgeon, Princess Alexandra Hospital, RAF Wroughton, UK

Lindsay A. Frankland
Research Secretary, The National Spinal Injuries Centre, Stoke Mandeville Hospital, Aylesbury, UK

J. P. Jackson MB BS FRCS(Eng)
Surgeon Emeritus, Queens Medical Centre, Nottingham and Harlow Wood Orthopaedic Hospital, Mansfield; Clinical Teacher, University of Nottingham, Nottingham, UK

Bryan Jennett MD FRCS
Professor of Neurosurgery, Institute of Neurological Sciences, Southern General Hospital, Glasgow, UK

M. A. M. S. Leigh
Hempsons Solicitors, 33 Henrietta Street, London, UK

Peter G. Lunn MB FRCS FRCS(Ed)
Consultant Orthopaedic and Hand Surgeon, Derbyshire Royal Infirmary,
Derby, UK

John R. Silver MB BS FRCP(Ed and Lond)
Consultant in Spinal Injuries, The National Spinal Injuries Centre, Stoke
Mandeville Hospital, Aylesbury, UK

Thomas G. Wadsworth MChOrth FRCS FRCSE FACS
Consultant Orthopaedic Surgeon, St Bartholomew's and Homerton
Hospital, London; Member of Council, British Society for Surgery of the
Hand; Examiner for Part I and II FRCS Edinburgh and Section
Chairman Primary FRCS Eng, UK

Martyn W. Ward OBE MB BS FRCS(Ed)
Consultant Orthopaedic Surgeon, Royal Air Force Hospital, Wegberg,
BFPO 40

David A. White MBBCh(Wales) DRCOG FFARCS(Eng)
Consultant in Anaesthesia and Intensive Care, Princess of Wales, RAF
Hospital, Ely, UK

Contents

SECTION 1
Preparation of medicolegal reports

1. The orthopaedic surgeon's viewpoint   3
   G. Bonney

2. The legal viewpoint   15
   M. A. M. S. Leigh

SECTION 2
Results following upper limb fractures

3. The shoulder   29
   P. S. Fagg

4. The humerus   87
   P. S. Fagg

5. The elbow   107
   T. G. Wadsworth

6. The forearm   137
   P. S. Fagg

7. The wrist   161
   P. S. Fagg

8. The hand   221
   P. G. Lunn

SECTION 3
Results following lower limb fractures

9. The hip   237
   M. A. Foy

10. The femur   267
M. A. Foy

11. The knee   291
T. D. Bunker

12. The tibia and fibula   323
M. A. Foy

13. The ankle   339
M. A. Foy

14. The foot   357
M. A. Foy

SECTION 4
Results following fractures of the axial skeleton

15. The pelvis   387
M. A. Foy

16. The spine   407
S. I. Esses and T. J. Dowling

17. Traumatic spinal cord injury   417
J. R. Silver and L. A. Frankland

18. Head injury   431
B. Jennett

SECTION 5
Miscellaneous topics

19. Repetitive stress injury   447
J. P. Jackson

20. The psychological effects of trauma   457
R. N. Bloor

21. The metabolic consequences of polytrauma   469
D. A. White

22. Post-traumatic reflex sympathetic dystrophy   487
M. W. Ward

Appendix   497

Index   501

Preparation of medicolegal reports

1. The orthopaedic surgeon's viewpoint

G. Bonney

INTRODUCTION

The concept of a system of restitution for damage or injury is very old. We read in Deuteronomy 19, 21: 'Life for life, eye for eye, tooth for tooth, hand for hand, foot for foot'. In Great Britain, our Saxon ancestors developed a system of regulated penalties and payments in compensation for injuries, including mortal injury. These concepts have over the years been refined into a system of compensation — usually by money — for damage or injury. The clinician's part in these procedures is in the assessment of the degree and effects of that damage and in establishing its cause or causes. He will then advise the injured person's legal representative about these matters, or will indicate to an insurance company the extent of damage.

Formerly, only the very rich could afford to seek compensation through legal action. The introduction of Legal Aid has changed all that; now, both very rich and rather poor can proceed in this way. The rise of the insurance companies and the introduction of compulsory third party insurance for motorists have greatly increased the injured person's chance of obtaining compensation. The various acts controlling conditions of work have conferred on the worker advantages hardly imaginable as recently as 100 years ago. The spread of superficial education has increased the public perception of the fallibility of professional advisers, so that claims for damage from alleged negligence are now common.

Doctors are well aware of this last tendency; the subscription rate of one British defence organization has increased from less than £1 in 1942 to more than £1000 in 1988 — an increase far in excess of the rate of inflation. The sums awarded by way of compensation have risen too; less than 10 years ago an award of £10 000 was deemed large. Now, awards of £1 000 000 and over are hardly the subject of comment. With this increase in the value and frequency of claims, the reporting clinician's responsibility increases steadily.

The clinician will be asked — usually by solicitors or by an insurance company — to provide information on causation, degree of damage and effects of damage. Most commonly, the damage has been caused by industrial or road traffic accident or by (alleged) negligence. The information is required to enable the client's legal adviser to formulate the claim and to make proposals about the monetary value of the suffering and disability. With this information the adviser will be able to make proposals for settlement, to negotiate, and if negotiation fails, to bring the matter to the arbitrament of the court.

The reporting clinician should always remember that he has a duty to both parties to report as accurately as possible, so that there may be no unnecessary delay in reaching settlement. Delay is harmful not only to the patient (Wynn Parry 1981) but also to insurers: prolonged disability with establishment of an unalterable pattern of symptoms may lead to a large increase in the size of the claim. It is often difficult to convince lawyers of this fact, which is so simple and so well known to clinicians; the effect of their training is to incline them to the supposedly superior claims of procrastination.

As is widely known, an adversarial system of examining the merits of cases is operated in most parts of the UK. Thus, the plaintiff's case is put and is supported by evidence; then, the defendant's case is similarly put and supported. It follows that a clinician may be approached by those acting for either side. In these circumstances of adversarial proceeding the clinician must keep a cool head and maintain an impartial posture. The temptation is great to give the report a bias in favour of the paymaster's client, in the not unreasonable belief that if this is not done the invitation to report will not be repeated. This temptation should be resisted; the profession of medicine is too august to be sullied by such paltry dealings. Nor should the reporting clinician make a judgement; that is for the judge — as indeed the word suggests. The clinician should display the facts and the evidence as presented, and may then hazard an opinion on the medical aspects of the case.

Reporting clinicians should be aware that at a certain stage in the proceedings reports will be disclosed to the other party. This is now the case in actions for alleged medical negligence as well as in those for compensation for accidental injury. This useful check on hyperbole is to some extent marred by the growing practice of producing two reports — one for disclosure, and one giving a frank expression of opinion. Lawyers have not been blameless here. The clinician should at all times aim to produce a report which is fair and balanced and which can be disclosed with one object alone — that of clarifying the case so that, within the limits of human fallibility, justice may be done. Practitioners should not forget that in the preparation of reports they are as much exposed to allegations of negligence as they are in clinical practice.

PREPARATION OF THE REPORT

It is a good plan to ask solicitors to make available as much as possible of the relevant documentation — the hospital record, the general practitioner's notes, radiographs, films produced by other imaging techniques. Hospital authorities are obliged to disclose documents concerning a claimant's treatment, but from time to time, encouraged by their legal advisers, they display a marked reluctance to do so. Such behaviour is of course self-defeating; reluctance to release documents is very likely to create the impression that there is something to hide.

Usually, the clinician is asked to see the claimant and to formulate a report having heard his story and having read the relevant documents. Occasionally — and of course unavoidably when the injured person has lost his life — the report has to be based on the perusal of documents. So in most cases the next step is to see the claimant. It goes without saying that in the case of persons less than 16 years old, the parent or guardian of the patient should be present on this occasion. It is generally helpful if a spouse or other partner is present at the meeting; rarely, the services of an interpreter will be required.

The claimant should be told the purpose of the examination and the identity of the person or firm to whom the report is to be made. When the report is to be made to the claimant's solicitor or insurance company there is no need for formal consent to be obtained. Formerly it was thought necessary to obtain consent when a report was to be made to an 'opposing' party. Now, however, with the present rules of disclosure and with increased frankness on the part of solicitors, such consent is rarely necessary so long as the claimant is made aware of the nature of the proceedings. It is however necessary to be very careful in making reports to employers. Consent to such reporting should regularly be obtained; some employers' attitudes to employees are entirely benevolent, but others are seeking excuses for relieving employees of their posts.

History

The patient's name, age, sex, address and occupation should be recorded, together with the date of the examination. The patient's present and former occupations should be recorded. Here it is convenient to record the period over which the claimant had pursued his occupation at the time of the accidental injury which forms the subject of the report. It is also a good plan to introduce at this stage a note of the claimant's civil state and of home circumstances.

Now the event that gave rise to the claim or complaint is discussed. In the case of drivers or passengers involved in road traffic accidents it is especially important to determine whether the claimant was wearing a seat belt and whether the seat was fitted with a head restraint. The circumstances of the collision should be examined, with particular reference to the claimant's recollection of the event: 'I remember this car coming at me; the next thing I remember is waking up in hospital'. The story of treatment and of convalescence will give some measure of the degree of distress and inconvenience suffered by the claimant. Often it is possible to record quite accurately the amount of time lost from work; frequently, it has to be recorded that the accident has marked the end of the claimant's working life.

Once the story has been brought up to the present time, the claimant's past medical history should be recorded. In particular, in the case of spinal or paraspinal injury, it is necessary to determine whether there has previously been any complaint of back or neck pain. Some patients find it difficult to be altogether frank about such matters; others have genuinely forgotten. A history of past injury should be recorded.

In passing to the claimant's present condition the clinician must bear in mind that he must judge whether that condition is effectively final, or whether improvement or deterioration can be expected. First, symptoms should be recorded. These are likely to be new symptoms; they may however represent a continuation or exacerbation of symptoms present before the accident. Pain in particular should be described: site, severity, periodicity, modes of relief, modes of exacerbation, radiation, presence at night, presence at the time of the examination. Pain is of course a common and important symptom of derangement of function; it is surprising that so few clinicians have shown interest in its mechanism, character and significance. It is also a symptom whose significance is difficult to determine. Different people at different times respond differently to the same painful stimulus; the response of the same tissue to a stimulus may be changed by changes in that tissue. Most important for reporting clinicians is the fact that for one reason or another a claimant may exaggerate or even invent a pain.

Pain, dysaesthesia and hyperaesthesia are symptoms common after injury to the nervous system. When there has been injury to the spinal cord or cauda equina, particular inquiry must be made concerning the function of the bladder and bowels, spasms of limbs and defect of skin nutrition (see Chapter 17). Deformity, scarring and wasting may form the subject of complaints and should be noted.

Many adult claimants now lay particular stress on disturbance of sexual function resulting from accidental injury. Adult males lead the field; nowadays scarcely any injury which is the subject of litigation does not give rise to a complaint of marring of 'sex life'. Most commonly, this marring is traced to pain consequent on physical performance; sometimes — as in the case of a lesion of the cauda equina — there is true physical dysfunction. The examiner must record what the claimant reports, however remarkable it may appear to one with conventional views and practices; the clinician will later have to form a view about this persistent symptom.

Lastly it is very important to record whether symptoms are advancing or steady or receding.

The next step is to record as accurately as possible the effects of symptoms on the claimant's life: on ability to work; on ability in recreation in comparison with the former state, and on activity in and around the home.

Loss of employment is, for a working person, one of the most serious consequences of accidental injury. This is especially so in the UK where there are currently more than 2.5 million unemployed. Loss of employment at 40 years of age means, for a person without special education or special skills, a permanent place on the dole. The consequences of such an event are very serious for the injured person and his family.

Loss of facility in recreation is a common, though to most people, less important sequel of accidental injury. A few people find themselves so dedicated to a particular sport that loss of this facility creates great hardship; others are more easily reconciled to such disability.

Impairment of ability in daily life and in the home may be a problem. The home improvement enthusiast, the keen gardener, the avid motor mechanic — all may have difficulty continuing these activities. Inquiry should be made about problems with ordinary activities, such as eating, dressing, bathing, using the lavatory, driving a car and using public transport. It is salutary for the practitioner to travel by public transport from time to time and to learn the hazards and discomfort of this medium in the Britain of the 1990s.

In the cases of young people of school age, loss of schooling and ability to attend school and take part in physical education must be recorded.

Examination

The claimant's height, weight and blood pressure should always be recorded. When circumstances permit, the urine should be examined. It is demeaning to the profession that persons professing scientific knowledge and a general education should record: 'This man would seem to be somewhat overweight . . .' when it is possible without difficulty to record the facts on which this view is based. Stance and gait should be described. Some examiners place great stress on the performance of athletic activities such as squatting, rising unsupported on one lower limb, or sinking on the bended knee in a parody of a curtsey. The examiner must decide whether observation of such activities gives a useful measure of the degree of disability.

Lengths and circumferences of limbs and lengths and character of scars should be recorded, although the value of exact measurements is doubtful. Deformity, range of active and passive movements of joints and power and dexterity should also be recorded.

Nerve lesions

Our methods of examining and recording motor power leave much to be desired. Frequently it is the progressive diminution of power in repeated contractions which produces disability: the finding of 'normal' power in a single effort does not give an accurate measure of functional capacity. Again, methods of examining and recording dexterity are defective. In order to get a true measure of the degree of disability, it is necessary to see the patient in his own environment over a period of several hours. Alternatively a functional assessment may be carried out in a prepared environment.

Methods of testing and recording sensibility are equally defective, especially in the case of the hand, where without adequately refined sensibility there may be severe impairment of function. We can do our best with superficial sensibility and two-point discrimination and tests of stereogenesis, but the measurement is certain to be less than adequate.

Arterial and venous damage

The after-effects of damage to a main artery may be felt in episodic ischaemia of muscle (claudication) and in defective nutrition of the skin. Thus, activity may be limited by pain or the limb may react severely to cold. Very severe ischaemia may of course have resulted in the loss of a limb: under such circumstances the condition of the stump must be recorded. The consequences of venous damage are less severe, but ulceration and swelling are disabling sequelae.

Radiological and other examinations

The results of radiological examination should be recorded. It will often be necessary to insist on a new examination if there has been a long interval between the clinical and the last radiological examinations. In some cases the results of special investigations, such as myelography, computerized tomography or even magnetic resonance imaging may be available. In the case of nerve injury, the results of electrophysiological examination may aid in the determination of the site and depth of the lesion and its prognosis.

It may sometimes be necessary to consider or request examinations of body fluids. Injured patients are not necessarily healthy before injury; the accident may have been determined by the effects of an existing condition such as diabetes, alcoholism, hypothyroidism or senility.

THE COMMENT AND THE PROGNOSIS

It is nearly always possible to record what the patient has lost or suffered because of injury. Thus; initial pain, hospitalization, operations, convalescence, period off work, residual permanent disability, loss of expectation of life. The last two are often the subject of debate, with the claimant insisting on his own assessment of the degree of disability, while the insurers insist on a lesser degree. When the examiner thinks that the claimant's assessment of the degree of disability is exaggerated, he should record as exactly as possible the patient's own assessment. The clinician's general view on the extent to which this assessment is supported by evidence should then be recorded. The true malingerer — the claimant who invents or greatly exaggerates the severity of symptoms — is rare. On the other hand, few of us, damaged through someone else's fault, are likely to discount persistent symptoms if even moderate sums of tax-free money are at stake. In most circumstances, large sums are at stake when employment has been lost and a claim for some years' loss of earning is made. Insurers owe it to their shareholders to be circumspect about paying out large amounts of money. We can expect such claims to be contested keenly — to the doors of the court and even into the court itself.

In some cases the prognosis is easy: there is little disability, and what there is, will not get worse; or, there is serious disability certain to increase with time. In many cases, however, we are asked to envisage a future course and to compare it with a hypothetical situation on the premise that the injury had not occurred. This invitation for the disciple of Asclepius to poach on the preserves of the Delphic Apollo cannot often be disregarded.

To take an example: a patient's neck is injured; there is persistent pain; radiographs show marked degenerative changes, evidently of long standing, though there were only slight or no symptoms before the accident. We are commonly asked in such cases to estimate the length of the period by which the onset of symptoms has been advanced. Such estimations are for the most part guesswork, and should be recorded as such.

Serious errors in the estimation of prognosis commonly arise from an over-optimistic approach by the examiner, especially if he is the clinician who has been responsible for the patient's treatment. Failure to enter reservations, with consequent premature settlement for a sum shown later to be too small, *may lead to process for negligence against the reporting clinician*. Such process was not uncommon in days when fracture through the femoral neck was treated by internal fixation. The examiner would indicate a final state and the case would be settled. Later the prognosis would be falsified by the development of avascular necrosis with consequent increase of disability. Many orthopaedic surgeons have of course guarded against this disagreeable consequence by the early removal of the femoral head, whose fate after such process can no longer remain in doubt.

The problem of late arthritis

It is clear that when a joint surface has been breached by the extension of a fracture into it there is a danger of the later development of arthritis. In some cases the damage is so severe that the outcome cannot be in doubt. In others, the damage is less severe, or skilled operation has succeeded in replacing accurately the pieces of the joint surface. It is usually possible when making a forecast of the late outcome to indicate the likelihood of arthritis. It is however more difficult to estimate the amount of trouble that the arthritis will cause the claimant. Arthritis in joints which do not bear the weight of the body may not be any problem in the case of one who does not work with his hands. It may interfere with the stockbroker's golf, but it is hardly likely to interfere with his capacity to make a living. On the other hand, arthritis of the wrist may mean the end of working life for a fitter. In the case of joints which bear the weight of the body, the trouble caused by arthritis is certain to be much more serious and more widespread throughout the classes of society. A barrister has to stand and walk: the consequences of arthritis of the knee are as severe as they would be for a police officer. Arthritis of the hip is a heavy burden to anyone in almost any occupation or any class of society.

It is hard to know how much may be expected from surgical replacement of pieces of articular cartilage. Enthusiastic surgeons must feel that a radiologically accurate replacement must be followed by a risk of arthritis less than would occur if replacement was less accurate. The thinking may be inexact: cartilage damaged in this way may be doomed to premature degeneration irrespective of the accuracy of replacement.

It is almost certainly correct when making such prognoses to err on the side of caution. Even when there is no radiological evidence of a breach of the joint surface, fractures near a joint may have caused damage to the joint which will result in the later development of arthritis. The likelihood of later trouble is almost certainly greater when the plane of a weight-bearing joint has been left out of true because of malunion of a fracture.

In some cases the occupation of the claimant makes it unlikely that he will return to the original work after an injury sustained in the course of employment. Thus, those who work from ladders may fall and fracture their calcanei. The consequences of such a fracture are such that they often prohibit return to work from ladders. In general, workers whose occupations involve a certain degree of physical hazard find it difficult to return to such work after injury. It may simply be impractical; very often an employer is unwilling to run the risk of allowing a partly disabled employee to undertake work which may involve physical hazard.

Accidental injury in children

It is of course particularly difficult to give an accurate prognosis in the case of the severely injured child. The clinician should not be in any hurry to indicate a final state, though repeated examinations and interviews with lawyers may be so distressing for a child as to produce permanent effects. In the author's experience, children resist these traumas better than do their seniors. Perhaps they do not, as their seniors often do, see the events as critical for their future.

In particular the clinician must be aware of the possibility of retardation or even acceleration of growth and of cosmetic deformity. In the case of fractures involving the elbow, defects of growth are particularly troublesome. It is unwise to consider that corrective operation will produce a permanent improvement in appearance. Often it is right to wait until the growth period is nearing its end.

Regrettably, some parents seek to magnify the effects on their children of accidental injury, some going so far as to indicate in front of the child a degree of incapacity quite beyond that warranted by physical evidence. The effect on the child of this hyperbole may be severe. Clinicians should learn to guard against this tendency; the examiner reporting for the infant plaintiff should not seek to encourage a parent in this attempt to cripple a child with unwise words, even if such restraint leads to the clinician's dismissal from the case.

Impairment of puerperal function

The orthopaedic examiner should not forget that severe pelvic injury may distort the bony pelvis to an extent sufficient to impair puerperal function. Distortion may be sufficient to make difficult or even prevent delivery through the vagina. In days when natural childbirth is strongly commended, such impairment may cause the patient serious concern. It is however unwise for the orthopaedic examiner to give an unaided view on this matter; there should be no hesitation in recommending that the advice of an obstetrician should be sought.

Life expectancy

Estimation of loss of life expectancy is difficult, except in cases where injury has produced clear derangement of functions vital to life. When a patient has suffered damage to the spinal cord with permanent paraparesis or paraplegia, the derangement of bladder function is likely to lead to impairment of renal efficiency. This may limit life expectancy (see Chapter 17). Again when there has been serious damage to the thoracic cage, there may well be impairment of respiratory function with the inevitable consequence of increased liability to respiratory diseases. More difficult is the case of serious injury associated with considerable loss of blood and grave shock. In such cases it is reasonable to assume that the effect on the system must have some effect on life expectancy, though it may be hard to define exact reasons for this belief. The orthopaedic examiner may find it more prudent to refer such questions to other specialists, even at the risk of irritating those instructing him.

Reporting clinicians from time to time find themselves confronted with a claimant whose disability can, in their view, be improved by operation. The debate about the advisability of operating on a patient for a condition when litigation is in process about that condition is likely to be continued. It is the author's view that unless the condition threatens life or is *certain* to deteriorate gravely, it is best to defer all operative treatment until the claim has been settled. Claimants and lawyers are likely to dispute that view, pointing out, reasonably enough, that it can hardly be thought that finality has been reached until the results of operative treatment are known. Although it is superficially easy for the independent examiner to recommend a line of treatment for which he will not be responsible, the temptation should be resisted. At least, any such recommendation should be hedged with caution. This is especially so in the case of persistent cervical pain after whiplash injury. Some enthusiastic surgeons have believed or affected to believe that operation has a place in such cases. It is in fact extremely rare that this is so: in few cases does operation offer any hope of relief.

THE NEGLIGENCE ISSUE

Sometimes in reporting the consequences of accidental injury clinicians become aware that a significant contribution to permanent disability, pain and suffering or to time off work has been made by inadequate care on the part of those in charge of treatment. Should they indicate as much in a report? The answer is not as easy as it may appear. The suggestion of 'negligence' is certain to lead insurers to repudiate liability altogether; the hint to the claimant may lead him into a prolonged struggle against 'accepted medical opinion', with the consequences of years out of work and of corroding thought about what he might have missed. It is no light matter in such cases to hint at 'medical negligence' as a contributory factory, although some advisers to insurance companies may find such hints convenient sources of relief to their paymasters. It is best to indicate the circumstances to the best of one's knowledge, and to indicate that if insurers wish to pursue the question of attributability to want of care, they should seek a further opinion.

CONCLUSIONS

All clinicians should bear in mind when writing a report that they may have to speak in court to support that report under cross-examination by a person trained in the arts of public speaking, obfuscation and confusion of purpose. The report should be written as plainly as possible. Loose and imprecise terms should be avoided; the excesses of partisanship should be eschewed. It is not necessary to employ the language of the law; it is not necessary to use eight words when one will do. It will come as a relief to most expert witnesses to find that judges expect no more than plain speaking and honest accounts, and that senior counsel are in most cases similarly motivated. From time to time reliance may have to be placed on the written word of an article in a learned journal. It is obviously better to rely on articles written by oneself if they are available. However, in the majority of personal injury cases this situation will not exist and articles written by other clinicians will be used.

It comes as a shock to those with little experience of British law to realize the importance of adversarial proceeding. The excesses of this practice have to some extent been mitigated by the change of regulations regarding disclosure of reports; but counsel still have to earn their living by exaggeration of the strength of their clients' cases. We must all hope that public realization of the folly of these proceedings will in years to come produce a system of settling disputes better suited to the modern age and more likely to produce equitable results.

REFERENCE

Wynn Parry C B 1981 Rehabilitation of the hand, 4th edn. Butterworth, London, p 389

2. The legal viewpoint

M. A. M. S. Leigh

INTRODUCTION

At the back of every lawyer's mind while instructing an expert to prepare a report in the course of litigation is the knowledge that the report will have to be disclosed to the other side if it is to be used at trial. The lawyer is anxious, therefore, to ensure that the report will present the client's case in its best light and there is a temptation to play down any potential weaknesses. As a result there used to be a trend for lawyers to become increasingly involved in the preparation of reports until the so-called 'expert' report assumed the colour of a special pleading rather than an impartial opinion. The apogee of this practice was in the mid 1970s when the House of Lords dealt with the case of *Whitehouse* v. *Jordan* [1981] 1 ALL ER 267. There a joint report was prepared on the plaintiff's behalf by two eminent obstetricians. It was prepared after a long conference between the doctors and counsel, and although it appeared otherwise, the final report was actually settled by counsel. The result was disastrous. The joint report did not stand up against the defendants' reports and, after rigorous cross-examination, the experts were forced to recant from crucial parts of their report. On the subject of medical reports Lord Wilberforce said:

> While some degree of consultation between experts and legal advisers is entirely proper, it is necessary that expert evidence presented to the Court should be and should be seen to be, the independent product of the expert, uninfluenced as to form or content by the exigencies of litigation.
> (*Whitehouse* v. *Jordan* [1981] 1 ALL ER 267)

It is now clear that a lawyer must not exert undue influence over an expert in the preparation of reports and must endeavour to limit his role to what is considered a proper level of consultation.

Having seen the lawyers' role in the preparation of reports curtailed, it should not be forgotten that an expert's report is an important document which will play a crucial role in the course of litigation. There are two types of medical report: those dealing with liability and those describing the plaintiff's present condition and prognosis. The first category is used predominantly to establish liability in medical negligence cases and as such is outside the scope of this book. This chapter is concerned with reports as to condition and prognosis which are common to all types of personal injury litigation.

PURPOSE OF MEDICOLEGAL REPORTS: ASSESSMENT AND COMPOSITION OF DAMAGES

The purpose of a report as to condition and prognosis is usually to assist the court to quantify the plaintiff's claim in the event that the defendant is found to have been negligent. In most cases a victim of personal injury will be able to obtain compensation for two types of damages — pecuniary and non-pecuniary. Broadly speaking, pecuniary damages are those which can be translated into monetary terms whilst non-pecuniary damage covers immeasurable elements such as pain and suffering. In legal terms a pecuniary loss is called 'special damage' and a non-pecuniary loss is 'general damage'.

The underlying principle in awarding special damages is *restituto integrum*. In the words of Lord Blackburn in 1880, the court should award 'that sum of money which will put the party who has been injured, or who has suffered, in the same position as he would have been in if he had not sustained the wrong for which he is now getting his compensation or reparation' (*Livingstone* v. *Reywards Coal Co.* [1880] 5 App Cas 25). It is not possible to calculate non-pecuniary damages on the same basis since the value of the loss of a leg cannot be quantified, so the better view would be to consider this as 'fair' compensation for the injury the plaintiff has suffered as a result of the defendant's negligence.

Examples of damages which may be awarded are as follows:

Medical and other expenses

A successful plaintiff may be able to recover, as part of his special damages, any medical or other expenses which have been reasonably incurred as a result of the injury. Any prospective expenses will be awarded as part of the general damages. The expenses will have been 'reasonably incurred' if they were not too excessive and were reasonably necessary to improve the quality of the plaintiff's life. He should thus be able to recover the cost of any special equipment needed as a result of the injuries, the cost of adapting his house and of any special attendances which might be required at home. The capital cost of acquiring accommodation is not, however, recoverable although the cost of mortgage interest is. Thus reports should describe the needs of the patient in each of these respects and the reasonableness of solutions proposed (see particularly Chapter 17).

In the case of medical expenses the plaintiff is entitled to seek private treatment and, to the extent that he wishes to do so, he is able to recover such sums as he would have to bear if he received private care (Law Reform (Personal Injuries) Act 1948 s. 2(4)). If his care requires him to stay in a special hospital or institution, the cost will be recoverable. Similarly, the expert should describe the likely future course of the plaintiff's condition and any operations which might be necessary.

Third party expenses

If a third party incurs financial loss as a result of the plaintiff's injury such sums are recoverable from the defendant. Thus, if a third party has to give up work in order to care for the plaintiff he should be able to recover damages in respect of reasonable loss of earnings. Similarly, if the third party has incurred expense in providing the plaintiff with medical or nursing care or equipment, the sums are recoverable as special damages. In addition a third party may be entitled to recover such expenses as were incurred in visiting the plaintiff in hospital. *The medical expert's role is not to list the equipment or the visits, but to describe the needs of the patient so that a judge can assess whether the sums claimed are reasonable.* The expert may help tell the court whether the expenditure claimed is reasonable: doctors are wise to err on the side of explicitness in expressing medical opinions for the laity.

Loss of earnings

The plaintiff will be awarded damages in respect of any loss of earnings incurred, together with compensation for the loss of any benefits such as a company car if this results from the accident. Such damages will be calculated from the date of the cause of action to the date of trial and will form part of the plaintiff's special damages. Thus if the plaintiff claims for the loss of employment, the expert should assess the extent to which the injury is responsible and is a handicap in the labour market.

Prospective loss of earnings will be calculated separately. The plaintiff may be prevented from working in the future for a number of reasons totally unconnected with the accident. In addition his future earning power will not be obvious as it will depend on a number of factors such as future employment prospects and redundancy. For these reasons future loss of earnings is not calculated on a straight mathematical basis. Instead a reasonable figure for the plaintiff's net annual loss (the multiplicand) is multiplied by a figure (the multiplier) to reflect the number of years the loss is expected to last, discounted to allow for the interest the money will earn. The multiplier will reflect the age, sex and life expectancy of the plaintiff. *A report should always say if and by how much a plaintiff's life expectancy has been diminished.*

Loss of earning capacity

The plaintiff is entitled to receive compensation if he is placed at a disadvantage in the labour market as a result of the defendant's negligence. This is so even if the plaintiff is at present in employment: probable difficulties in finding another job in the event of losing this one have a bearing on damages.

Pain and suffering

Damages are recoverable in respect of pain and suffering, both actual and prospective, which are directly attributable to the plaintiff's injuries. Damages recoverable under these headings include the pain and suffering attendant on any operation which is necessary as a result of the defendant's negligence. The court will be helped by the clinician's description and assessment of the pain and discomfort involved, and the experiences the plaintiff has already suffered.

Loss of amenity

A plaintiff will be entitled to compensation under this heading in respect of loss of enjoyment of life consequent to the injury. The court tries to assess the damages according to the severity of the injury, and thus the plaintiff who has lost a finger will receive a smaller amount of compensation under this head than a plaintiff who has lost an arm. The amount of an individual award is necessarily conventional, if not arbitrary. The law assesses such awards on the basis of precedents so that the amount of an award is derived from the judge's understanding of what has been awarded in previous cases involving similar injuries. It is relatively easy, therefore, for a lawyer to predict the probable level of damages in any particular case. This figure may then be adjusted according to the plaintiff's pre-accident circumstances. If, for example, the plaintiff was an enthusiastic sportsman and as a result of the injury is no longer able to participate in the sport, his damages under this heading will be increased to reflect the diminution in his enjoyment of life. Similarly, if a plaintiff is disfigured by the accident and as a result his professional prospects or social life are impaired, he will be entitled to recover increased damages. All of these things should be described in appropriate cases because the medical expert has a vital role to play in describing to a judge what the effect of a given injury has been to a specific individual.

PRESENTATION OF MEDICOLEGAL REPORTS

Background information

A medical report may be commissioned by either party to an action at any time during the course of litigation or by a potential litigant exploring his case before deciding to issue proceedings. The expert will usually be approached by a solicitor who will give a brief explanation of the case, and ask the expert whether he would be prepared to give an opinion.

In many cases the expert consulted by the patient's solicitor will have actually treated the patient and will therefore have access to the notes and documents. In other cases the instructing solicitor will arrange for a full set of papers to be sent to the clinician. These should usually include a copy of the plaintiff's medical records and X-rays together with a detailed account of the circumstances giving rise to the injury. If proceedings have already begun the solicitor will inform the expert how far they have got, sending copies of the relevant pleadings.

Major personal injury actions are commenced in the High Court, although the county courts have jurisdiction to hear cases where the total damages claimed do not exceed £5000. Pleadings in both courts serve the same broad purpose although their form may differ. In a High Court action an expert might expect to receive the following pleadings: writ, statement of claim, defence and request for further and better particulars.

Writ

Legal proceedings in the High Court are begun when the writ is served on the defendant. The writ is a formal document which notifies the defendant that the plaintiff intends to pursue a claim against him. The writ must be issued at the court within 3 years of the date of the cause of action, or within 3 years of the plaintiff realizing that his injuries were caused by the defendant's negligence. If there is a medical reason why the plaintiff would not have known of his cause of action, then this may usefully be described in the report. If the plaintiff is a minor at the relevant date, the 3-year period does not begin until he is 18. Once issued, the writ must be served on the defendant within 12 months unless the court authorizes an extension of time for service.

The county court equivalent to a writ is a summons.

Statement of claim

The writ may be endorsed with a statement of claim or this document may be served separately. This sets out the details of the plaintiff's claim against the defendant, and lists the alleged acts of negligence which caused the plaintiff's damage. It will also itemize the plaintiff's injuries and claim damages together with interest.

The county court equivalent to this document is the particulars of claim.

The expert should still take his own history of the injury, and should note any discrepancy with the pleadings.

Defence

The defence contains the defendant's response to the allegations made against him. He can either admit, deny or not admit any of the allegations made against him. If the defendant does not admit a fact he is neither admitting nor denying it but merely inviting the plaintiff to prove the point. If he denies an allegation he gives notice that the alleged fact is in issue.

The defence may be a detailed pleading of the defendant's case which clearly identifies the ground on which the case is to be fought, or it may be a simple blanket denial of the allegations.

Request for further and better particulars

Although not strictly speaking a pleading, either party to a claim can ask for further and better particulars of their opponent's pleadings or raise interrogatories on what is pleaded. Where the expert would be assisted by more information he should say so since those instructing him may be able to obtain it.

Format of the report

Following the decision of the House of Lords in *Whitehouse* v. *Jordan* [1981] 1 ALL ER 267 the form and content of an expert's report must be left to his own discretion. The following format is thus intended to act as a general guide only (see also Appendix).

Heading

The heading of the report should begin with the title of the report, making clear that it is a report on condition and prognosis, giving the date of the examination and where it took place. The information and documents available to the expert should be specified and any restrictions or adverse circumstances spelled out.

Particulars of patient

This part of the report should state the name, age, and pre-accident occupation of the plaintiff. If an injury to the upper limbs has been sustained, it is important to state the handedness of the patient. The report should also include a brief account of the plaintiff's relevant previous medical history.

History of present injury

1. Date of accident.
2. Note of how the accident occurred. This record should be kept as brief as possible. It should merely set the scene rather than providing

a definitive account of what occurred. It is not the medical expert's role to give an opinion on the non-medical circumstances giving rise to the injury.

3. Comment on the management of the plaintiff's case to date. This should include a description of the type of treatment which the plaintiff has received, together with the number of attendances and operations undergone. If the treatment has been unpleasant or uncomfortable, the expert should mention this and explain why.

Present condition

This should explain the expert's findings on examination:

1. The patient's appearance and demeanour.
2. The type of examination undertaken and its results.
3. Whether any investigations were carried out, and if so, the results.
4. Interpretation of X-rays.

If the injury is disfiguring the expert may illustrate the report with photographs.

Present complaint

The expert will ask the plaintiff whether he experiences any residual pain as a result of the injury. If he does, the clinician should state whether the pain is continuous or whether it is brought on in certain circumstances. He should also describe the type of pain and its severity as well as any analgesia necessary. The plaintiff may complain of a restriction of mobility or difficulty in adjusting to his post-accident lifestyle. He may have problems adapting to special aids. If the plaintiff mentions marital or social problems arising from the injury, these should be included in the report. The expert should also bear in mind the possibility of psychological trauma and its likely significance in the present case. The whole should add up to an accurate assessment of the cause of the plaintiff's injury and present disabilities.

The prognosis

1. Whether any further treatment is required and if so, its nature, extent, likely duration and gravity.
2. Whether the plaintiff will need to take any more time off work. If so, how much and whether it is likely to interfere with earning capacity.
3. The risks or complications associated with the particular injury or course of treatment.
4. Whether the plaintiff is able to go back to his pre-accident work. If not, what other type of work would he be suited for?

5. Whether the plaintiff is still able to enjoy his pre-accident hobbies and pastimes.
6. The plaintiff's cosmetic appearance and whether it is likely to improve or deteriorate.
7. The plaintiff's psychological state and its likely prognosis.
8. Whether there are any other problems arising from the injury and the likely duration of these problems.
9. If the plaintiff's injuries are so serious that his life expectancy is reduced, a report should include an estimate of how long the plaintiff is likely to live. This is usually an unanswerable question which the expert should approach by imagining 100 patients in the position of the plaintiff; what is required is the date when, doing the best he can, he thinks it most likely that the 50th patient would die.
10. Whether the plaintiff has any special needs, i.e. special care and attendance, housing, transport and special equipment.
11. Whether the plaintiff will be likely to benefit from paramedical help such as physiotherapy, speech therapy, occupational therapy or social workers.
12. Whether in the clinician's opinion the plaintiff should qualify for benefits such as mobility or attendance allowance.

Conclusion

The report should be signed by its author together with details of his qualifications and specialist knowledge.

Any medical report should be written in clear and unambiguous terms. The expert should explain his findings as fully as possible, bearing in mind that the report will be read by lay people.

Use of published works and statistics

There has been a recent development in the practice relating to medical negligence actions which is likely to spread to other personal injury actions, whereby the parties are required to exchange lists of written material, published or unpublished upon which the expert medical witnesses intend to rely in support of their opinions (*Naylor* v. *Preston Area Health Authority et al* (1987) 2 ALL ER 353). It is hoped that this direction will prevent a party from surprising his opponent at the trial by relying on specific medical or scientific literature in support of his case without affording the opposing party the opportunity of considering the supportive material before trial. It is not intended that a medical expert should conduct a thorough search of medical literature to find any printed material to support his opinion. Rather, it is hoped that there will be disclosure of the printed material on which the expert has particularly relied when making his report. It is good practice, therefore, for an expert to refer in his report to any published opinions or literature which he has used in the preparation of his report or which he thinks will assist the court.

GIVING EVIDENCE IN COURT

The majority of personal injury actions will be settled before the matter comes to court. An action can be settled at any stage in the proceedings and it is not uncommon for the settlement to take place 'at the door of the court'. In a minority of cases, however, a settlement is not possible and the parties must try to prove their cases in court.

Every doctor asked to prepare a report should assume that he will be required to give evidence. He should thus ensure that he is able to rearrange his commitments, sometimes at short notice, in order to give this evidence. In most cases a clinician may be given a long period of notice of the trial date. In the High Court in London, at the time of writing, the present waiting time for a 3-day hearing is approximately 2 years. This time is considerably shorter in the case of trials outside London. As both parties expect to call expert evidence it is the normal practice in personal injury cases to request a fixture. This means that the trial is fixed to take place on a certain date or dates as opposed to floating in a list and slotted in when a vacancy arises, often at very short notice. An expert should expect, as a matter of courtesy, to be asked by his instructing solicitors for a list of dates when it would not be convenient for him to attend court before the trial date is fixed.

At some stage in the proceedings the expert's report will have been disclosed to the other side. If the report can be agreed the other side will not need to produce their own expert evidence and it may not be necessary for the original expert to give oral evidence as his report could be read in open court.

If the reports are not agreed the expert will be shown the report of his counterpart and asked to comment. If it seems that the parties are not too far apart it may still be possible to agree one report. If not, the expert must be equipped to deal with any opposing findings in his opponent's report.

As the date of trial draws nearer, the expert is likely to be asked to attend a conference with the counsel who will be arguing the case in court. This will give counsel the opportunity to question the expert in detail on his report and discover whether there are any areas of vulnerability. The expert must also be prepared to educate counsel if necessary about the medical aspects of the case by explaining the report in lay terms. In civil cases there is normally no reason why the expert should not sit through the entire case and hear all the evidence, including that of his opponent. This is particularly important when acting for a defendant as it will give the clinician time to consider the weight of his opponent's evidence, but it is also helpful for a plaintiff's expert as he will be on hand to advise counsel about the medical points raised.

When called to give evidence the expert may take into the witness box a copy of his report and all the papers on which he relies. He will be asked to swear an oath in a form suitable for his religion or, if he so chooses, simply to affirm that the evidence he gives will be the truth.

The expert will then be examined in chief by the barrister instructed by the solicitors who instructed him. This means that the barrister will guide the expert through his report and raise any supplemental points which have come out during the course of the trial. The expert should think carefully about the evidence he is to give and should try to stick as closely as possible to his original report. It is usually counterproductive if an expert surprises his counsel by coming up with a new idea in the box.

When the evidence in chief has been completed the counsel will sit down and the barrister for the other party will rise to his feet. He will then conduct a cross-examination challenging those points of the evidence which do not fit in with his client's case and putting forward an alternative view. This examination is rarely acrimonious but counsel will be trying very hard to get the expert to tone down his evidence. An expert must be aware of this and avoid falling into any carefully laid traps. He should take time to consider his replies and think very carefully before conceding any issue. The line of attack should not take the expert too much by surprise as he will have seen the report of his opponent beforehand and this will form the basis of the cross-examination.

When the cross-examination is completed the expert may be re-examined by his own barrister. This gives the barrister the opportunity to cover points raised in cross-examination and not dealt with in the examination in chief. It also gives counsel the chance to set the record straight on any issue which has become clouded.

When the re-examination is ended the expert may step down from the witness box. The judge will usually order that each witness is free to leave the court as soon as his evidence is completed.

The question of an expert's fee should not be overlooked. The expert is entitled to charge for time spent reconsidering the papers and preparing any supplemental reports which may be necessary. He is also entitled to charge for time and expenses incurred in attending the trial. These are matters which should be discussed with and recovered from his instructing solicitors.

A witness can be compelled to attend court in order to give evidence by a subpoena. This is an order of the court requiring the witness to attend on a specified day and remain in the court until such time as the case is completed. Failure to comply with this order is contempt of court punishable by a fine and/or imprisonment. In most cases an expert will be happy to attend court voluntarily and it will not be necessary for solicitors to issue a subpoena. In some cases, however, the expert may require a subpoena before his employers will allow him the time off to attend court. In these cases a subpoena will be issued and served on the doctor.

Results following upper limb fractures

Results following upper limb fractures

3. The shoulder

P. S. Fagg

STERNOCLAVICULAR JOINT

Introduction

Sternoclavicular joint injuries are not common. Rowe & Marble (1958) found 10 injuries to the sternoclavicular joint in their analysis of 1603 shoulder-girdle injuries (0.6%), Brown (1927) indicated that 10% of all dislocations occur at the clavicle but only 1% occur at the sternal end. Both Cave (1961) and Rowe & Marble (1958) found only one case of posterior dislocation of the sternoclavicular joint in 1660 shoulder-girdle injuries (0.06%).

Injuries of the sternoclavicular joint may be classified as follows:

Grade I: minor sprains and contusions.
Grade II: subluxations, usually anterior.
Grade III: complete dislocations, anterior or retrosternal.
Grade IV: recurrent dislocation.

Results of treatment

Grade I and II injuries

A grade I injury or sprain of the sternoclavicular joint results from a mild medially directed force applied to the lateral aspect of the involved shoulder or from the shoulder being suddenly forced forward. The ligaments remain intact. Treatment is symptomatic with a forearm sling and no long-term sequelae are expected.

In the grade II injury or subluxation of the sternoclavicular joint there is rupture of the sternoclavicular ligaments but the continuity of the costoclavicular ligaments is maintained. There is little in the literature on the prognosis for these injuries. In 1980 Neviaser suggested that the prognosis was good following treatment. Whilst this is generally true, Pierce (1979) described four cases of internal derangement of the intra-articular disc as a result of indirect trauma unassociated with frank

29

dislocation. These patients complained of persistent tenderness, swelling and a clicking sensation over the joint. Surgery was required in each case and, in one patient who underwent surgery 8 years after the initial injury, some degenerative changes were present in the joint. All these patients became asymptomatic with a full range of motion after surgery.

Grade III injuries: anterior dislocation

Anterior dislocations of the sternoclavicular joint are approximately 10 times more common than posterior dislocations. Not all of these dislocations are due to ligamentous and meniscal damage alone. In 1967 Omer found an intra-articular subchondral clavicular fracture in all four of his patients who underwent clavicular osteotomy for the surgical reduction of their dislocation. All four patients had a stable reduction without recurrent dislocation, although one patient developed arthritic symptoms 2 years after the injury. Denham & Dingley (1967) described epiphyseal separation of the medial end of the clavicle in three patients. In all three cases reduction was stable. They pointed out that the medial epiphysis of the clavicle was only a few millimetres thick, did not ossify until age 18 and may not unite with the metaphysis until the age of 22–25 years.

The treatment of acute anterior dislocation of the sternoclavicular joint is by closed or open procedures. When reviewing the cases of 15 military hospitals, Omer (1967) found that elective surgery was required in 23 of 82 cases (28%). Reviewing 60 anterior dislocations from the Mayo Clinic in 1968, Nettles & Linscheid found that only 13 required surgery (21.6%). Eleven of these cases were for chronic recurrent dislocation.

Many surgical procedures have been advocated for what is in effect a relatively rare condition. These procedures include the use of fascial loops, subclavius tenodesis, clavicular osteotomy or use of the sternomastoid muscle to reinforce the anterior capsule. There are insufficient cases reported to appraise fully the benefits of each particular procedure.

Transfixing pins running from the clavicle to the sternum have been used to reinforce some of the above procedures. In 1961 Brown reported a 30% complication rate in 10 cases of transfixing wires. These complications included wire breakage and penetration of the pulmonary artery. However, despite these grave complications he felt that in view of the stable reduction achieved, the method was justified. Further cases of perforation of the major vessels have been reported (Pate & Wilhite 1969, Clark et al 1974).

Whilst the functional results following open reduction are generally good, recurrent dislocation is not uncommon. Recurrent dislocation has been reported to occur in 21–33% of patients (Nettles & Linscheid 1968, Salvatore 1968).

Recurrent anterior dislocation may cause little functional disability, but may cause cosmetic problems, especially in young women. A total of 60–79% of patients with recurrent anterior dislocation had no pain, limitation of movement or functional disability (Nettles & Linscheid 1968, Savastano & Stutz 1978). Troublesome disability seems to be more common in men performing heavy labour or vigorous athletic activity (Lunseth et al 1975). Occasionally habitual dislocation is seen, especially in young adolescent girls, occurring spontaneously or as the result of only minor trauma. Booth & Roper (1979) described four such patients in whom pain, discomfort or apprehension during use necessitated operative repair.

Grade III injuries: retrosternal dislocation

Retrosternal dislocations of the sternoclavicular joint are approximately 10 times less common than anterior dislocations. The diagnosis is often not immediately apparent although the symptoms are often severe. Serious complications are often quoted but reported cases are not common. Death has occurred due to laceration of the trachea or haemothorax (Kennedy 1949). Injury to the mammary vessels, subclavian vessels, brachial plexus and rupture of the thoracic duct may also occur (Peacock et al 1970, Buckerfield & Castle 1984).

Almost all authorities believe that reduction of the dislocation is essential because of damage to the underlying major vessels from prolonged dislocation. Obstruction of the subclavian vessels has been reported to occur up to 10 years after retrosternal dislocation (Howard & Shafer 1965, Mehta et al 1973).

However, not all cases of chronic retrosternal dislocation are necessarily symptomatic. Savastano & Stutz (1978) reported one patient who redislocated almost immediately after closed reduction and who was asymptomatic 23 years later, and another who was asymptomatic 21 months post-injury. In 1957 Stein reported a patient who had recurrent posterior dislocation of his sternoclavicular joint 3 years after open reduction. He described a popping sensation on certain movements of the shoulder girdle.

Open and closed techniques of reduction of retrosternal dislocations are reported. Whereas Buckerfield & Castle reported a 100% success rate with the closed reduction of seven cases and, similarly, Ferry et al (1957) complete success in six cases, many other authors have resorted to open reduction due to the failure of closed methods (Paterson 1961, Simurda 1968, Selesnick et al 1984).

Unlike anterior dislocations, retrosternal dislocations are generally stable once reduced. Only Mehta et al (1973) and Savastano & Stutz (1978) have reported recurrences, with one case of recurrent subluxation and one case of recurrent dislocation, respectively.

Most cases once reduced appear to have normal function. In 1963 McKenzie reported that both of her cases of retrosternal dislocation treated by closed reduction had some thickening of the medial end of the clavicle. This thickening is variably reported by other authors (Ferry et al (1957) noted it in 33% of patients) and it is probably overlooked in some reports. In 1968 Heinig estimated that approximately one-half of his patients with stable reductions and full function were mildly symptomatic with some crepitation on abduction and external rotation of the involved shoulder and with mild discomfort on excessive use of the involved extremity.

Sternoclavicular injuries in children

Sternoclavicular injuries are occasionally reported in children. Nettles & Linscheid (1968) reported two cases of anterior dislocation and one of retrosternal dislocation in newborn babies after difficult labours, but they make no specific comment as to their treatment or outcome.

Wheeler et al (1979) reported a 7-month-old white girl treated by closed reduction with full function at 10 weeks. Stein (1957) reported a 6-year-old coloured child reduced by closed reduction, and Selesnick et al (1984) reported on two black children aged 6 and 8 years, one requiring open and the other closed reduction; both had normal function at follow-up.

Traumatic floating clavicle

Panclavicular dislocation of the clavicle has been reported occasionally (Beckman 1923, Gearen & Petty 1982, Jain 1984). Operative treatment is reported as technically difficult and conservative treatment may provide satisfactory function (Jain 1984).

Summary

1. Sternoclavicular joint injuries account for 0.6% of all shoulder-girdle injuries.
2. Grade I sprains and grade II subluxations have a good prognosis.
3. Occasionally, indirect injury to the sternoclavicular joint will result in internal derangement of the intra-articular disc.
4. Epiphyseal injuries may occur at the sternoclavicular joint at up to 25 years of age and may mimic true dislocations.
5. Anterior dislocation of the sternoclavicular joint may occur spontaneously or after minimal trauma in adolescent girls with habitual dislocation.
6. Kirschner wires used as transfixing pins to stabilize operative repair have a 30% serious complication rate including penetration of mediastinal structures.
7. There is a 20–30% recurrent dislocation rate following operative or closed reduction of anterior sternoclavicular dislocation.

8. Recurrent or persistent anterior dislocation of the sternoclavicular joint produces a cosmetic deformity.
9. In 60–66% of recurrent anterior dislocations there are minimal symptoms. Heavy labourers and keen sportsmen are most likely to be troubled by symptoms.
10. Retrosternal dislocations occasionally cause immediate damage to adjacent major vessels with occasional fatal results.
11. Late complications to adjacent major vessels from unreduced retrosternal dislocations may occur many years after the initial injury.
12. Recurrent dislocation after open or closed reduction occurred in 21–33% of patients.
13. Thickening of the medial end of the clavicle may occur following open or closed reduction.
14. Approximately 50% of patients with stable reductions may have mild symptoms despite full function.
15. Dislocation of the sternoclavicular joint may occur in infants following difficult labour, but normal function is invariably reported after treatment.

ACROMIOCLAVICULAR JOINT

Tossy et al (1963) classified acromioclavicular injuries into three grades. Grade 1 injuries include strains and contusions of the acromioclavicular joint with no gross deformity. Grade 2 injuries are due to rupture of the capsule and acromioclavicular ligament with an intact coracoclavicular ligament, whilst grade 3 injuries are due to rupture of the acromioclavicular and coracoclavicular ligaments. In addition, posterior and inferior dislocations can occur.

The incidence of complete acromioclavicular dislocations is estimated at 3 or 4 per 100 000 population per annum (Larsen et al 1986). Rowe & Marble (1958) found 52 acromioclavicular injuries in 1603 shoulder-girdle injuries (3.25%).

The incidence of injury in the three grades as noted from four papers is shown in Table 3.1. The figure of 25% for grade 1 injuries is probably artificially low as many of these patients may not report to a doctor or hospital with their injury.

Table 3.1 The incidence of acromioclavicular joint injuries classified by grade

Reference	Grade 1	Grade 2	Grade 3	Total
Rowe & Marble (1958)	8	17	27	52
Weaver & Dunn (1972)	16	16	15	47
Tossy et al (1963)	12	6	23	41
Allman (1967)	29	55	36	120
Total	65 (25%)	94 (36%)	101 (39%)	260

Results of treatment

Grade 1 and 2 injuries

There are few reports documenting the results of grade 1 and 2 injuries (Table 3.2). Overall 94% achieve an excellent or good result. All the poor results tend to occur in elderly patients. Arner et al (1957) found arthritis of the acromioclavicular joint present in all of the poor results in their paper. They did not find the degree of arthritis to be correlated with the end functional result. This point will be discussed later.

Table 3.2   Results of grade 1 and 2 acromioclavicular injuries

Reference	Excellent	Good	Poor	Total
Arner et al (1957)	18	3	1	22
Lazcano et al (1961)	25	6	4	35
Bjerneld et al (1983)	24	13	0	37
Total	67 (71%)	22 (23%)	5 (6%)	94

Acute superior dislocation (grade 3 injuries)

Controversy rages over whether grade 3 acromioclavicular injuries should be treated operatively or non-operatively. Numerous operations and orthoses have been designed and reported upon. It is not the purpose of this book to promulgate any particular treatment regime but to give an overview of the results as reported in the English literature.

Conservative treatment. The results of conservative treatment vary from series to series (Table 3.3). Direct comparisons are difficult as authors report their results in different ways. However those factors which appear

Table 3.3   Results of conservative treatment of grade 3 acromioclavicular dislocations

	Number	Reference
No or minimal pain	35 of 35 cases	Glick et al (1977)
	30 of 33 cases	Bjerneld et al (1983)
	18 of 20 cases	Anzel & Streitz (1973)
	4 of 17 cases	Dawe (1980)
Total	87 of 105 cases (82%)	
Return to sport	32 of 35 cases	Glick et al (1977)
	12 of 17 cases	Dawe (1980)
Total	44 of 52 cases (85%)	
Return to original work	30 of 33 cases	Bjerneld et al (1983)
	14 of 17 cases	Dawe (1980)
Total	44 of 50 cases (88%)	
Full range of movement	35 of 35 cases	Glick et al (1977)
	13 of 17 cases	Jacobs & Wade (1966)
Total	48 of 52 cases (92%)	

to be reported in comparable fashion are listed. All untreated grade 3 dislocations have a prominent lateral end of clavicle but this prominence was considered significant in only 3 of 17 patients (18%) in Dawe's series (1980) and 3 of 35 patients (9%) reported by Glick et al (1977). Calcification of the coracoclavicular ligament was seen in 8 of 17 patients (47%) in Jacobs & Wade's (1966) series and 21 of 33 patients (64%) in the (1983) series of Bjerneld et al. The question of the significance of soft tissue calcification in this injury will be discussed later.

Table 3.4 Comparison of results between conservatively and surgically treated groups

Reference	Rating	Conservative	Operative
Baker & Stryker (1965)	excellent/good	4 of 7 cases	18 of 25 cases
Arner et al (1957)	excellent/good	15 of 17 cases	13 of 16 cases
Rosenørm & Pederson (1974)	good/fair	12 of 13 cases	9 of 11 cases
Powers & Bach (1974)	good	24 of 28 cases	12 of 18 cases
Imatani et al (1975)	satisfactory	7 of 12 cases	5 of 11 cases
Galpin et al (1985)	pain-free	15 of 21 cases	12 of 16 cases
Jacobs & Wade (1966)	asymptomatic	21 of 43 cases	23 of 51 cases
Larsen et al (1986)	excellent/good	39 of 43 cases	38 of 41 cases

Aggregated total of satisfactory results:
> 137 of 184 cases (74.5%) — conservative treatment
> 130 of 189 cases (69%) — operative treatment

Comparison of conservative and operative treatment. A number of papers make comparisons between different conservative and operative treatments, although there is no uniform method of presenting results (Table 3.4). These papers suggest that the percentage of satisfactory results is marginally better with conservative treatment. The results of the paper of Larsen et al (1986) provided a 13-month follow-up. Their figures for excellent/good results at 3 months suggest that conservatively treated patients achieve this result more quickly. Certainly Galpin et al (1985) reported that their conservatively treated patients returned to work at an average of 2.6 weeks post-injury as compared with 6.8 weeks for their operative group. Similarly their conservative group of patients returned to sport at 1.7 months compared with 2.2 months for their operative group. Rosenørm and Pederson (1974) also found that their conservatively treated group of patients returned to work earlier than their operative group (at 6 compared with 9 weeks). Table 3.5 compares other factors in this group of patients. Conservatively treated groups had a higher percentage of patients with a full range of motion (90%) and full strength (91%) as compared with the operative group (79 and 88% respectively). The degree of calcification in the coracoclavicular ligament was higher in the operative group (72 compared with 55%). As would be expected, almost 100% of

Table 3.5 Comparison of results between conservatively and surgically treated groups

Reference	Conservative	Operative
Full range of motion		
Jacobs & Wade (1966)	34 of 43 cases	35 of 51 cases
Larsen et al (1986)	43 of 43 cases	38 of 41 cases
Total	77 of 86 (90%)	73 of 92 (79%)
Full strength		
Galpin et al (1985)	15 of 21 cases	12 of 16 cases
Larsen et al (1986)	43 of 43 cases	38 of 41 cases
Total	58 of 64 (91%)	50 of 57 (88%)
Calcification of coracoclavicular ligament		
Arner et al (1957)	8 of 17 cases	14 of 16 cases
Larsen et al (1986)	25 of 43 cases	27 of 41 cases
Total	33 of 60 (55%)	41 of 57 (72%)
Prominent lateral end of clavicle		
Arner et al (1957)	9 of 17 cases	4 of 16 cases
Galpin et al (1985)	21 of 21 cases	3 of 16 cases
Jacobs & Wade (1966)	39 of 43 cases	22 of 51 cases
Larsen et al (1986)	43 of 43 cases	2 of 41 cases
Total	112 of 124 (97%)	31 of 124 (25%)

conservatively treated patients had a prominence of the lateral end of the clavicle. However, a surprisingly high number (25%) of the operated group also had some deformity.

Operative treatment. Numerous operative techniques are reported for grade 3 acromioclavicular injuries. Table 3.6 shows only the larger reported series, but it must be stressed that many different techniques are reported in these papers.

Excision of the outer end of the clavicle is often used in treating the symptomatic chronically dislocated acromioclavicular joint. In 1964

Table 3.6 Results of operative treatment of grade 3 acromioclavicular dislocations

Reference	Number of good/ excellent cases*	Total	% good/excellent
Roscoe & Simmons (1984)	151[†]	168	90
Bargren et al (1978)	43	63	68
Kawabe et al (1984)	40	41	98
Deterbeck & Barnhart (1976)	25	30	83
Berson et al (1978)	28	29	97
Kennedy & Cameron (1954)	22	27	82
Alldredge (1965)	22	24	92
Kappakas & McMaster (1978)	18	20	90
Aggregated total	349	402	87

*Individual authors' assessment.
[†]This figure is calculated from figures given in the article.

Gillespie reported his results following excision of the outer end of the clavicle in 30 patients. Five patients had to change to lighter employment. Overall, 13 patients were felt to have an unsatisfactory result. It was found that advancing age influenced the results unfavourably, and 70% of patients aged 50 years or more had unsatisfactory results.

Complications of acromioclavicular dislocations. The main complications of acromioclavicular dislocations are calcification in the coracoclavicular space, post-traumatic arthritis of the acromioclavicular joint and osteolysis of the distal end of the clavicle.

Calcification of the coracoclavicular space. Calcification of the coronoid and trapezoid ligaments is relatively common after dislocation of the acromioclavicular joint in those cases treated both conservatively and surgically (Table 3.7). The incidence appears to be higher in those cases treated operatively (53%) than in those treated conservatively (39%). This is a consistent finding in papers which compare the two groups. The incidence is higher in complete dislocations when compared with grade 2 injuries. Jacobs & Wade (1966) found that 2 of 26 patients (8%) with partial separation had calcification whereas it occurred in 8 of 17 (47%) of grade 3 injuries. Similar results were reported by Bjerneld et al (1983) who found that 8% of 37 patients with partial separation and 64% of 33 patients with complete separations had calcification of the coracoclavicular space.

Table 3.7   Incidence of calcification after acromioclavicular dislocation

Reference	Incidence	
	Non-operative	Operative
Alldredge (1965)		12 of 24 cases
Larsen et al (1986)	25 of 43 cases	27 of 41 cases
Jacobs & Wade (1966)	10 of 43 cases	
Kawabe et al (1984)		11 of 41 cases
Bjerneld et al (1983)	24 of 70 cases	
Arner et al (1957)	8 of 17 cases	14 of 16 cases
Aggregated total	67 of 173 (39%)	64 of 122 (53%)

Moseley & Templeton (1969) felt that the poor results in their series of acromioclavicular dislocations were related to excessive calcification in the coracoclavicular ligament, but the majority of authors found that it did not influence the final clinical outcome. Larsen et al (1986) found that only 2 of their 52 cases (3.8%) with coracoclavicular calcification had a fair or poor result. Excessive calcification may cause slight restriction of abduction in the affected shoulder.

Post-traumatic arthritis. Degenerative arthritis of the acromioclavicular joint may occur without a clear history of trauma, as occurred in 56 (67%) of the 83 patients reported by Worcester & Green in 1968. They pointed out that the degenerative changes began during the second decade.

Zlotsky & Ballard (1966) stated that symptomatic arthritis after acromioclavicular injuries in athletes developed surprisingly early, usually within 3 months. The incidence of post-traumatic arthritis reported in the literature is shown in Table 3.8. Arner et al (1957) found no positive correlation between the presence of arthritis and symptoms, and none of Neviaser's cases (1952) were symptomatic. However, Jacobs & Wade (1966) found that 65% of their patients with traumatic arthritis were symptomatic.

Table 3.8 Incidence of post-traumatic arthritis after acromioclavicular injuries

Reference	Conservative	Operative
Jacobs & Wade (1966)	5 of 43 cases	12 of 35 cases
Berson et al (1978)		0 of 29 cases
Arner et al (1957)	20 of 39 cases	10 of 17 cases
Neviaser (1952)		5 of 14 cases
Aggregated total	25 of 82 (30%)	27 of 95 (28%)

Osteolysis of the distal end of the clavicle. Osteolysis of the lateral end of the clavicle has been described following dislocation or subluxation of the acromioclavicular joint. However, the incidence remains unknown. The changes may occur very early after trauma. Stahl (1954) described two cases, one of which showed early radiographic changes at 3 weeks. Levine et al (1976) stated that the onset may occur several years after the injury.

Jacobs (1964) described the symptoms as pain and a .sense of weakness during abduction and flexion of the arm and he stated that these symptoms may persist for up to 2 years. He also stated that the symptoms may recur after further trivial trauma. Not all cases however are due to trauma. In 1982 Cahill reported on 46 male athletes with osteolysis of the distal part of the clavicle. None of them had a history of acute injury to the acromioclavicular area but all were athletes and 45 lifted weights as part of their training. Twenty-one of his patients underwent excision of the distal end of the clavicle, with relief of symptoms in the 19 patients followed up. He states that no case has been reported in a woman.

Other dislocations

Posterior dislocation of the acromioclavicular joint has occasionally been described. Interposition of soft tissues such as meniscus and capsule prevents correction of the posterior displacement, and operative reduction is invariably required (Malcapi et al 1978). Patterson (1967) reported a case of inferior dislocation of the distal end of the clavicle which required open reduction. Hastings & Horne (1977) reported two cases of anterior dislocation of the acromioclavicular joint. Their acute management was by conservative means. These are rare types of dislocation.

Summary

1. Acromioclavicular joint injuries comprise 3.25% of shoulder-girdle injuries.
2. In all, 25% are grade 1, 36% grade 2 and 39% grade 3 injuries.
3. A total of 94% of grade 1 and 2 injuries had excellent/good results. Poor results tended to occur in elderly patients.
4. Some 82% of grade 3 acromioclavicular injuries treated conservatively had minimal or no pain and 92% had no restriction of movement.
5. Of grade 3 injuries, 85% returned to their previous sport and 88% to their original work.
6. The prominent lateral end of clavicle was a cosmetic problem in 9–18% of patients with grade 3 injuries treated conservatively.
7. Conservatively or operatively treated patients had excellent/good results in 70–75% of cases.
8. Conservatively treated grade 3 patients returned to work earlier, and resumed sport sooner than operated patients. They also had a better return to full power and a better range of motion.
9. Deformity of the lateral end of the clavicle is inevitable after the conservative treatment of grade 3 injuries and occurred in 25% of those treated surgically.
10. Calcification of the coracoclavicular ligament occurred in 39% of conservatively treated patients and 53% of operated cases.
11. In all, 8% of grade 2 injuries have calcification as compared with 47–64% of grade 3 injuries.
12. Calcification has an adverse affect on the result in 4% of cases.
13. Post-traumatic arthritis occurred in 28–30% of acromioclavicular dislocations. Its effect on the overall result is uncertain.
14. The incidence of osteolysis of the lateral end of the clavicle is uncertain. It may occur within 3 weeks or after several years. Symptoms usually settle within 2 years.

CLAVICLE

The clavicle is the most commonly fractured bone, comprising 5–10% of all fractures (Moore 1951). Allman (1967) divided fractures of the clavicle into three groups:

Group I: Fractures of the middle third.
Group II: Fractures lateral to the coracoclavicular ligament.
Group III: Fractures of the proximal end of the clavicle.

Neer (1968) further subdivided group II fractures into type I — coracoclavicular ligaments intact — and type II — with these ligaments detached from the medial segment.

Rowe (1968) reviewed 690 fractures of the clavicle and found that 82% involved the middle third, 12% the lateral third and 6% the medial third.

Conservative treatment

Middle third fractures

Although middle third fractures of the clavicle are by far the commonest type, there are few papers which discuss the results of conservative treatment. Rowe (1968) stated that the usual healing period of a fracture of the middle third of the clavicle was 4–6 weeks in young adults and 6 weeks or more in older people. Kessel (1982) stated that full functional recovery was achieved by 4 months. However, as the clavicle is a subcutaneous bone, a healed fracture of the middle third may well produce an obvious bony swelling which may be a source of cosmetic embarrassment, especially to females, and may cause irritation to people who carry packs and webbing (such as in the armed services). The average incidence of non-union quoted in the literature (Table 3.9) is 0.9%.

Table 3.9 Incidence of non-union after conservative treatment of fractures of the middle third of the clavicle

Reference	Total number of patients	Number of non-union	Incidence
Neer (1960)	2235	3	0.1%
Rowe (1968)	680		0.8%
Taylor (1969)		no figures quoted	0.9%
Fowler (1966)		no figures quoted	0.5%
Marsh & Hazarion (1970)		no figures quoted	1.9%
Annersten (1948)*	350		1.3%

*Quoted by Johnson & Collins (1963).

Lateral third fractures

Both Allman (1967) and Neer (1968) agreed that the type I fracture of the lateral third of the clavicle healed promptly with minimal treatment. Only rarely, when the fracture enters and distorts the joint surface, do symptoms persist. These symptoms are due to traumatic arthritis of the acromioclavicular joint. Neer found only 2 out of 75 patients (2.6%) with persistent symptomatology after this type of fracture. These symptoms were eliminated by late excision of the outer end of the clavicle (leaving the coracoclavicular ligaments intact).

In 1985 Kavanagh et al reported on 30 patients with type II fractures. Fifteen were treated non-operatively and 15 surgically. Neer (1968) reported on 23 similar patients: 12 treated conservatively, 4 with excision of the outer end of the clavicle and 7 by surgical stabilization. The results

Table 3.10 Healing in type II fractures of the lateral third of the clavicle

Reference	Total number of patients	Delayed union	Non-union
Conservative treatment			
Neer (1968)	12	8 (66%)	4 (33%)
Kavanagh et al (1985)	15	6 (40%)	6 (40%)
Total	27	14 (52%)	10 (37%)
Excise outer end of clavicle			
Neer (1968)	4	only one achieved satisfactory result	
Open reduction and transacromial wire fixation			
Neer (1968)	7	0	0
Kavanagh et al (1985)	15	0	0

All patients in both series healed in 6–10 weeks.

are given in Table 3.10 and show a high incidence of delayed union and non-union (52 and 37% respectively) in the patients treated conservatively. Neer pointed out that the eventual functional results in the conservative group were satisfactory in 7 out of 12 patients, although when union occurred it was with excessive callus and posterior angulation, and it never occurred before 16 weeks.

Medial third fractures

Medial third fractures are not reported in detail and, according to Allman (1967), heal well with minimal treatment.

Primary operative treatment

A number of papers report the results of primary internal fixation of clavicular fractures. Some of these papers, it will be seen, report 100% union rates with their surgical techniques, but it should be stressed that none of the authors advocated routine internal fixation. They suggest that it should be reserved for complicated fractures or those with skin or neurovascular complications. Neer (1960) reported an incidence of non-union of 4.6% following primary open reduction and internal fixation, and Rowe's (1968) non-union rate after surgery was 3.7%. Their non-union rates for conservatively treated fractures of the middle third of the clavicle were 0.1 and 0.8% respectively.

Table 3.11 shows the results of internal fixation via intramedullary techniques or ASIF plates as reported in the literature. Only one of these papers gave less than a 100% union rate. In the largest series, Paffen & Jansen (1978) had a 6.8% non-union rate. Zenni et al (1981) found that six patients (24% of their series) had minor aching pain at the fracture site during changes in the weather. The time to union ranged between $5\frac{1}{2}$ and 12 weeks for normal healing and return to full function occurred in $7\frac{1}{2}$–11 weeks.

Table 3.11 The results of primary internal fixation of clavicular fractures

Reference	Number of patients	Union	Average time to union	Time to full function
Intramedullary techniques				
Neviaser et al (1975)	7	7		All (no time specified)
Moore (1951)	21	21*	10 weeks	Not specified
Bonnet (1975)	25	25		
Zenni et al (1981)	25	25	12 weeks	
Paffen & Jansen (1978)	73	68	5½–9 weeks	
Plating techniques				
Khan & Lucas (1978)	19	19		

*It is not clear from this paper whether all 21 patients were followed up to union but no failure of union is mentioned for fresh fractures.

The treatment of non-union

Most clavicular non-unions occur in the middle third of the bone. The proportion of non-unions occurring in the middle third is reported at between 68 (Johnson & Collins 1963) and 95% (Sakellarides 1961). The incidence of the various symptoms, when reported, is given in Table 3.12. As may be seen from this table, not all clavicular non-unions are asymptomatic. The incidence varies between 0 (Ghormley et al 1941) and 40.5% (Johnson & Collins 1963). This wide variation may well be due to the authors' interpretation of 'minimal symptoms'. Taking the five reported papers as a whole, the incidence of clavicular non-unions with no or minimal symptoms is 25%. Significant pain from clavicular non-union occurs in 65% of patients.

Table 3.12 The symptoms of clavicular non-union

	Taylor (1969)	Wilkins & Johnston (1983)	Sakellarides (1961)	Ghormley et al (1941)	Johnson & Collins (1963)
Number of patients	31	33	20	17	69
No or minimal symptoms	3 (9.6%)	11 (33%)	2 (10%)	0	28 (40.5%)
Pain	28 (90%)	24 (73%)	18 (90%)	8 (47%)	33 (48%)
Crepitation		9		13	
Paraesthesiae		2	5	3	10
Cosmetic		5		5	2
Severe weakness		4			7
Loss of movement			7	3	3

The surgical treatment of non-union varies from the use of intramedullary fixation to external compression plates. All authors agree on the necessity for additional bone grafting. Tregonning & MacNab (1976) claimed equal rates of union (80%) with either ASIF plates or intramedullary pins combined with bone graft. Taylor (1967) had 2 cases of non-union in the 15 patients he followed up. All of these patients had undergone intramedullary fixation with or without bone graft. The author stressed the importance of the graft but made no mention of whether the failures occurred in grafted or non-grafted cases. Manske & Szabo (1985) had 100% union in 10 patients with compression plating and iliac bone grafting, as did Sakellarides (1961) with 7 patients treated by intramedullary fixation and bone grafting. Manske & Szabo (1985) found the average time to radiographic union to be 19 weeks, with symptomatic recovery occurring at 10 weeks. Pyper (1978) found that full function returned in his 3 plated and grafted cases at or before 10 weeks. Neer (1960) reported that whilst all of his hypertrophic non-unions united with intramedullary fixation and bone graft at 12 weeks, 3 of his 6 atrophic non-unions failed to unite. Conversely, however, 8 of the 10 cases in Manske & Szabo's (1985) paper had atrophic non-union yet all united with compression plate and bone graft.

Other complications

The most commonly reported complication of clavicular fractures, other than non-union, is compression of the neurovascular bundle. Early complications involving the subclavian artery, vein and brachial plexus are invariably due to direct trauma. The prognosis depends upon the success of the vascular repair or upon the relief of compression to these vessels achieved by internal fixation of the fracture. The results of the vascular repair are outside the scope of this book and the results of internal fixation of fresh clavicular fractures have previously been discussed.

Many authors, however, point out that compression can occur as a late event due to malunion or non-union. It is impossible to predict the frequency of this late complication other than to state that it is a rare complication. Howard & Schafer (1965) reported, amongst their cases, a patient with a brachial plexus compression injury occurring 2 years after the original fracture. Penn (1964) stated that vascular complications have manifest themselves 20–48 years after the clavicular injury. Penn also quoted a case of chylothorax from a thoracic duct injury occurring $6\frac{1}{2}$ years after the original fracture.

Pulmonary complications can also occur as an early complication of clavicular fractures. In his series of 690 clavicular fractures, Rowe (1968) reported that pneumothorax occurred in 3%, haemothorax in 1% and refracture of the clavicle in 2% of patients.

Fractures in childhood and adolescence

Fractures of the clavicle during childbirth are well documented and these fractures heal with no problems in 2–3 weeks. Fractures in children from 2 to 12 years of age unite in 2–4 weeks. The prognosis for children who have had a fracture of the clavicle, excluding those complicated by a neurovascular injury, is excellent. Non-union is rarely reported (Nogi et al 1975) and its differentiation from congenital pseudarthrosis is important. Wall (1970) stressed that no callus is seen in cases of congenital pseudarthrosis.

Epiphyseal separation of the medial end of the clavicle may simulate sternoclavicular dislocation. Whilst some authors (Brooks & Henning 1972) report good functional results after the open reduction and smooth Kirschner wire fixation of these injuries, others (Rockwood 1984b) recommend conservative treatment, as they claim that remodelling from the periosteum and the remaining epiphysis occurs quite rapidly, with no long-term disability.

Similarly, Rockwood (1984b) recommended the conservative treatment for epiphyseal separation of the lateral end of the clavicle simulating acromioclavicular dislocation, as he felt that rapid remodelling occurred. However Ogden (1984), whilst reporting excellent results with either conservative or surgical treatment, did report partial duplication of the clavicle which caused a painful, tender, palpable lump requiring resection of the original clavicle back to the beginning of the duplication.

Summary

1. Middle third fractures heal in 4–6 weeks with full function returning by 4 months.
2. The non-union rate in conservatively treated middle third fractures is 0.9%.
3. Type I lateral third fractures heal well with a 2–3% incidence of persistent symptoms from damage to the acromioclavicular joint.
4. Type II lateral third fractures treated conservatively have a 37% non-union rate and 52% delayed union beyond 16 weeks, although function is eventually satisfactory if healing occurs.
5. The non-union rate for internal fixation of fresh clavicular fractures is 4–7%. The time to union is $5\frac{1}{2}$–12 weeks, and full function occurs in $7\frac{1}{2}$–11 weeks.
6. A total of 24% of surgically treated patients may experience minor aching pain at the fracture site with weather changes.
7. Approximately 25% of clavicular non-unions are asymptomatic, and significant pain occurs in 65%.
8. The incidence of union in the surgically treated and bone-grafted clavicular non-union is 80–100%.
9. The average time to radiographic union is 12–19 weeks, and full function returns in an average of 10 weeks.

10. Late brachial plexus lesions have been reported 2 years after the initial injury, and late vascular lesions have occurred 48 years later.
11. Refracture of the clavicle is reported in 2% of cases.
12. Fracture of the clavicle in children heals with no problem. Non-union is very rare and must be differentiated from congenital pseudarthrosis.
13. Fracture separation of the medial clavicular epiphysis may be treated conservatively with excellent results.
14. Untreated fracture separation of the lateral clavicular epiphysis usually heals with excellent results and rapid remodelling. However reduplication of the clavicle may occur, causing a tender lump which requires excision.

FRACTURES OF THE SCAPULA

Scapular fractures are relatively rare, constituting 1% of all fractures (Zdravkovic & Damholt 1974) and 3.4% of shoulder-girdle injuries (Rowe 1963). Fractures of the scapula are often classified according to anatomical sites (Hardegger et al 1984) but from a prognostic point of view are best classified into three types (DeCoulx, as quoted by Zdravkovic & Damholt 1974):

Type I: Fractures of the body.
Type II: Fractures of the apophysis (acromion, spine and coracoid process).
Type III: Fractures through the superior lateral angle (glenoid rim, glenoid fossa, anatomical neck and surgical neck).

Patients with scapular fractures often have other injuries, some serious, which may have significant effects on the functional outcome of the injury. Thus the subclavian artery (Halpern et al 1979) and brachial plexus (Oreck et al 1984) may be injured in association with scapular fractures.

Whilst Hardegger et al (1984) found only 21.6% associated injuries in their series of 37 patients undergoing internal fixation for scapular fractures, Rowe (1963) found that 75% of his 54 patients had other injuries and Wilber & Evans (1977) had an 82.5% incidence in their 40 patients.

McLennan & Ungersma (1982) reported a 53% incidence (16 of 30 patients) of pneumothorax occurring in association with scapular fractures. Six occurred on presentation and 10 were delayed for 1–3 days. Only 2 of these 16 pneumothoraces were associated with rib fractures.

Type I: fractures of the body

Fractures of the scapular body can usually be treated conservatively. The muscles covering the body prevent significant displacement of the fragments. Wilber & Evans (1977) found that all 27 patients with isolated fractures of the body of the scapula recovered full glenohumeral motion regardless of the type of treatment. In 1937 Findlay stated that these fractures required up to 5 weeks of treatment with slings and physiotherapy. Neviaser (as quoted by Rowe 1963) mentioned the condition of so-called pseudorupture of the rotator cuff. Haemorrhage into the muscle bellies of supraspinatus, infraspinatus and subscapularis muscles produces signs typical of a rotator cuff rupture. As the haematoma formation absorbs, rotator cuff power returns.

Type II: fractures of the apophysis

Acromion

Fractures of the acromion with minimal displacement may be treated conservatively and, according to Findlay (1937), union will occur in 3–4 weeks. Although reported cases are sparse, function would appear to return to normal.

Displaced acromial fractures can compromise the function of the rotator cuff and painful non-union can develop. Few documented cases have been reported. Paralysis of the deltoid, secondary to axillary nerve damage, in association with a fractured acromion (plus associated acromioclavicular joint separation) has been reported by McGahan & Rab (1980). The neural injury went unrecognized for 2 months.

Scapular spine

There has been little written concerning fractures of the scapular spine. They appear to heal well with conservative treatment, unless severely displaced. The three cases reported by Wilber & Evans in 1977 all regained full glenohumeral movement.

Coracoid process

Fractures of the coracoid process are well documented. They may occur in isolation (Froimson 1978), in association with acromioclavicular dislocation (Bernard et al 1983), with avulsion fractures of the superior border of the scapula (Ishizuki et al 1981) and in association with dislocation of the shoulder (Garcia-Elias & Salo 1985).

When the fracture occurs in isolation and is minimally displaced conservative treatment is indicated. In the 10 patients reported by Froimson (1978) and Zilberman & Rejovitzky (1981) the fractures united in 2–4 months. Patients were able to resume full work from 6 weeks to 3 months after the injury, and a full range of movement was restored by 4 months. Two (20%) of these patients had slight pain after heavy work and one had minimal limitation of abduction and internal rotation at 4 months.

Three cases of non-union have been reported (Findlay 1931, Benton & Nelson 1971, De Rosa & Kettelkamp 1977). Two patients had the ununited fragment excised: one had a poor functional result, and one had some residual weakness of abduction and a vague discomfort in the posterior aspect of the shoulder. The third case had a screw fixation with a full return of function.

Fractures of the coracoid process occurring in association with acromioclavicular dislocations appear to heal well with conservative treatment. Full function is reported to return within 6 weeks (Bernard et al 1983). Persistent symptoms have only been reported in association with the internal fixation of the acromioclavicular dislocation. Wilber & Evans (1977) reported a poor functional result with moderate persistent pain and over 25% loss of abduction and flexion in their only patient. Other authors have reported full return of function (Smith 1975, Montgomery & Loyd 1977). Three of the four patients reported by Ishizuki et al (1981) with coracoid process fractures in association with avulsion fractures of the superior border of the scapula and acromioclavicular dislocations had an almost full return of function at 3 months. The result of the fourth patient is not recorded.

A case of a coracoid fracture in association with a subglenoid dislocation of the shoulder was reported by Benchetit & Friedman in 1979. Full function returned by 8 weeks after conservative management. The case reported by Garcia-Elias and Salo (1985) required excision of the coracoid process fragment after 10 weeks because of persistent symptoms. Six weeks post-operatively the patient's symptoms had disappeared.

Type III: fractures through the superior lateral angle

In 1977 Wilber & Evans reported the results of 8 patients with fractures of the neck of the scapula treated conservatively. All 8 regained a full range of motion. In contrast, their 6 patients with glenoid fractures all had some loss of mobility. Three of these patients were seen 1–12 years after the injury. Two patients had slight pain and less than 25% loss of abduction and flexion — a fair result according to the authors — and the third patient had moderate pain and greater than 25% loss of abduction and flexion — a poor result.

Zdravkovic & Damholt (1974) reviewed 40 patients with fractures through the superior lateral angle. Only 7 of these patients had their fractures extending into the glenoid cavity. A total of 28 patients were followed up: 17 (61%) had mild degenerative changes in the glenohumeral joint and 1 (3.6%) had severe changes. However, only 9 patients (32%) had symptoms, of whom 4 (14%) had pain at rest. Ten (35.7%) had grating from the glenohumeral joint on movement but all had full strength. Abduction with unrestricted scapulothoracic movement was limited in 8 patients (28.6%) by an average of 30°. However, abduction with a fixed scapula was restricted in more patients although the precise figure is not clear from this paper.

Only three glenoid fractures were reviewed in the long term. All were asymptomatic but only one had a full range of motion.

Summary

1. Scapular fractures constituted 1% of all fractures and 3.4% of shoulder-girdle injuries.
2. Other injuries were seen in association with 75–82.5% of scapular fractures — some of these injuries had profound effects on the late functional result.
3. Pneumothorax was reported to occur in 53% of scapular fractures.
4. Fractures of the body of the scapula invariably resulted in full return of function.
5. Undisplaced fractures of the acromion heal in 3–4 weeks with full return of function, but displaced fractures may cause persistent symptoms.
6. Fractures of the scapular spine should recover full function.
7. Coracoid process fractures should return to full function with conservative measures within 6 weeks to 4 months. Painful non-unions are reported.
8. Some 32% of patients with fractures of the superior lateral angle had persistent symptoms, of whom 14% had pain at rest. Degenerative change occurred in 61%.
9. Abduction (with unrestricted scapulothoracic movement) was reduced in about 30% of patients, by an average of 30° in those cases with a fracture of the superolateral angle.

RUPTURE OF THE BICEPS BRACHII MUSCLE OR ITS TENDONS

Rupture of the biceps brachii may occur at four sites:

1. At the long head of biceps.
2. At the short head of biceps.
3. Through the muscle belly.
4. At the distal tendon.

Of the 102 cases reported by Gilcrest (1934), 77 (75.5%) occurred in the long head of biceps, 2 (2%) were found in the short head, 17 (16.5%) through the muscle and 6 cases (6%) through the distal tendon. Waugh et al (1949) found that 10% of the ruptures in their series occurred in the distal tendon whereas Cassels & Hamilton (1967) found the incidence of distal rupture to be 26.5%.

In many cases of rupture of the long head of biceps the event occurred after relatively trivial injury secondary to degenerative changes in the bicipital groove. However, acute rupture can occur in the young athlete, usually due to a very forceful muscular contraction during athletic activity. Soto-Hall & Stroot (1960) found that after recent rupture, the power of flexion of the elbow was about 20% less than that of the opposite side, and the power of shoulder abduction with the arm in external rotation was about 17% less than the opposite side. However, in late ruptures no appreciable weakness was noted. Cassels & Hamilton (1967) found that 1 year after injury, weight-lifting ability was equal to the uninjured side and loss of supination was not present. These patients returned to work at an average of 4 weeks after injury.

After traumatic closed transection of the muscle of biceps brachii in military parachutists, Heckman & Levine (1978) found that in 28 untreated cases, 25 patients (89%) had weakness of the arm and easy fatiguability with activities requiring rapid, repetitive elbow flexion and 12 patients (43%) had pain in the area of the defect. The range of elbow flexion in these young fit men was excellent but the maximum flexion power at 90° of elbow flexion was only 53% of normal. This maximum flexion power was increased to 76.5% in the 9 cases reviewed following early surgical repair, and increased to 77% in the 10 cases treated by aspiration of the haematoma and plaster immobilization.

The treatment of distal avulsion of the biceps tendon remains controversial. Cassels & Hamilton (1967) had 10 cases of distal avulsion in their series of 100 patients, and at 1 year weight-lifting ability and supination equalled the uninjured side. Smith (1963) reported 2 cases treated along conservative lines. However, both had some weakness on sustained effort and one patient had slight loss of the power of supination. Norman (1985) reported on 15 cases of distal rupture. One patient was reviewed 11 years after conservative treatment and had a severe loss of flexion power and of supination of the forearm but a full range of motion.

Most authors advocate surgical repair of these distal lesions as there is rarely any underlying problem of degenerative change and the injury tends to occur in younger, more athletic patients (Kessel 1982).

In Norman's (1985) series of 14 cases treated surgically, 3 (21.5%) were considered excellent (power and range of motion fully restored), 10 (71.5%) good (minimal amount of residual impairment), and 1 (7%) fair (disability interfering with certain activities). However, Froncioni & Lenczner (1985) reported 6 patients treated by operation and 2 treated conservatively. They found flexion and supination strength to be similar in the two groups, although the conservatively treated patients had more pain and deformity.

Out of 16 patients, Boucher & Morton (1968) reported good results in the 3 patients treated conservatively. Of their surgical cases 8 (61.5%) were excellent, 3 (23%) were good and 2 (15.5%) were rated as poor.

A few cases of isolated rupture of the short head of biceps have been reported (Postacchini & Ricciardi-Pollini 1977).

Summary

1. Rupture of the long head of biceps usually occurs secondary to degenerative changes. At 1-year follow-up no appreciable weakness was reported in the injured side as compared with the uninjured limb. However, this may not be true in the younger, athletic patient.
2. Untreated closed rupture of the biceps brachii muscle in young men resulted in weakness and easy fatiguability in 89% of cases and residual pain in 43%. The range of elbow flexion remained good but maximum flexion power at 90° of elbow flexion was 53% of normal. This was increased to 77% in surgically repaired lesions or those treated with closed reduction and plaster immobilization.
3. Distal avulsions of the biceps tendon treated surgically achieved good or excellent results in 85–90% of cases. However, similar results may be achieved by conservative methods of treatment according to some authors.

ROTATOR CUFF TEARS

Rotator cuff tears usually fall into one of four categories (Kessel 1982):

1. Due to a fracture of the greater tuberosity as the result of a single major injury. This type will be dealt with in a later section of this chapter.
2. Acute massive avulsion without fracture. This also occurs as the result of a single major injury with or without anterior dislocation of the shoulder. It tends to occur in the younger, athletic patient. It can result from direct trauma to the shoulder after a fall or indirect trauma transmitted up the outstretched arm. Bateman (1973) stated that subscapularis rupture can occur due to repetitive throwing actions.
3. Acute-on-chronic rupture.
4. Chronic rupture.

The last two categories are seen more typically in the elderly patient. The rotator cuff is vulnerable to degenerative changes secondary to poor vascularity. Attrition of the avascular part near the insertion of the cuff over a long period of time may result in rotator cuff tears occurring with minimal trauma.

Acute-on-chronic and chronic ruptures are less likely to be involved in medicolegal action than the acute type. They will however be mentioned later for completeness.

Acute tears

Acute rotator cuff tears tend to occur after severe trauma through relatively healthy tendinous tissue or as the result of acute anterior dislocation of the shoulder. In 1969 Reeves reported the results of arthrograms performed on 47 patients with acute anterior dislocation of the shoulder. A total of 26 of the patients had an associated capsular rupture; Reeves found this to be the predominant injury sustained at the time of dislocation in patients over 50 years of age. When the arthrogram was repeated 7–10 days later, 5 patients showed rotator cuff defects.

The requirement for surgery in the acute group remains controversial. Wolfgang (1978) stated: 'In my experience, the athletic rotator cuff patient has a very excellent prognosis with conservative management, and I have not seen a need for early surgical repair'. However, Wallace & Wiley (1986) reported the long-term results of the conservative management of 36 manual workers with 37 acute shoulder injuries. In all, 28 were stated to have definite full-thickness tears. After a mean follow-up of 5 years 30 patients (81%) had significant pain; 28 patients (76%) stated that they were the same or worse than at the 6-months review. All the patients had a diminished range of motion, there was a marked reduction of power (by more than 60% measured on Cybex equipment), and only 13 of 24 patients (54%) who were under 65 years old were able to work.

In 1975 Nixon & DiStefano stated that surgery was indicated in the young adult with a complete avulsion of the cuff. Bassett & Cofield (1983) reported the results of 37 acute rotator cuff repairs performed within 3 months of injury. Pain relief was good despite any delay in surgery from the time of injury but the range of active abduction achieved post-operatively was diminished by such a delay. Thus an average 168° of abduction was obtained in the 12 cases repaired within 3 weeks of injury, decreasing to 129° in the 19 cases repaired after 6 weeks. They found no correlation between the result and the size of the defect. Thirteen patients (35%) had no pain and the remaining 24 (64%) had slight pain. Only 4 patients (11%) did not feel that surgery had achieved any improvement.

Tibone et al (1986) reported 10 good results (67%) in 15 athletes treated by surgery for their complete rotator cuff tears.

Chronic tears

Chronic tears are not necessarily symptomatic. On reviewing rotator cuff tears Cofield (1985) stated that between 5 and 32% of cadavers studied had complete rotator cuff tears with no history of pre-existing shoulder symptoms. Early studies had suggested that 80–90% of shoulders would improve without surgery although often these studies had not utilized arthrography in the diagnosis. Takagishi (1978) reviewed the conservative treatment of 39 patients with arthrographically proven rotator cuff tears. Overall, 17 patients (44%) achieved satisfactory recovery — 16 (76%) of 21 patients will small tears, and only 1 (5%) of 18 patients with large tears.

There are many reports of the surgical treatment of these chronic tears utilizing a variety of methods. Unfortunately there is no standard method of classifying the size of the rupture or the quality of functional recovery. The results of a few of the larger series reporting pain relief are shown in Table 3.13 and those showing functional improvement in Table 3.14.

Table 3.13   Pain relief following repair of ruptured rotator cuffs

Reference	Number of cases	Satisfactory pain relief	%
Hawkins et al (1985)	100	86	86
Cofield & Lanzer (1985)	88	86	98
Weiner & MacNab (1970)	71	55	77
Packer et al (1983)	63	40	63
Post et al (1983)	59	56	95
Total	381	323	85

Table 3.14   Satisfactory function following rotator cuff repair

Reference	Number of cases	Satisfactory function	%
Hawkins et al (1985)	100	92	92
Watson (1985)	89	62	70
Cofield & Lanzer (1985)	88	73	83
Weiner & MacNab (1970)	71	51	72
Wolfgang (1978)	65	45	69
Total	413	323	78

The definition of satisfactory pain relief differs from paper to paper and may to some extent reflect the authors' satisfaction with their results rather than patient satisfaction. However, taking the five larger series specifying the percentage of patients with satisfactory pain relief, we can conclude that on average 85% of patients with chronic rotator cuff ruptures treated surgically will have satisfactory pain relief.

The criteria for the assessment of functional improvement also differ widely. However, from Table 3.14 it can be seen that on average 78% of patients will achieve a satisfactory functional outcome. This functional grading accepts that some residual disability will persist, especially in prolonged use of the arms above shoulder level.

There is no agreement on the results of surgery in relation to the size of the defect, or to the timing of surgery. Hawkins et al (1985) found that the size of the tear did not significantly affect the results, although they did state that patients with a smaller tear tended to fare slightly better. Weiner & MacNab (1970) however found that the results in massive tears were generally unsatisfactory. In 1978 Wolfgang reported that any delay between rupture and surgery had no bearing on the final result, whereas Heikel (1968) found that a delay of more than 6 months tended to give a poorer result. Watson (1985) felt that the age of the patient was an important factor. He found that maximal improvement occurred up to 2 years post-operatively but that with longer follow-up patients over 60 years of age tended to deteriorate.

Hawkins et al (1985) stated that it was their impression that patients involved in litigation achieved worse results than other patients. Patients receiving compensation took twice as long to return to work.

The results of a second attempt at surgical repair for a failed initial rotator cuff repair are not very good, according to De Orio & Cofield (1984). Satisfactory pain relief was achieved in only 37% of patients and a good overall result was achieved in only 17%.

Summary

1. The conservative treatment of acute rotator cuff injuries in manual workers resulted in 81% of patients having significant residual pain, loss of motion and a 60% reduction in strength.
2. A total of 67–89% of patients with acute tears had a satisfactory result from surgery.
3. The earlier after rupture the surgery was performed, the better was the final range of movement obtained, although pain relief was less dependent on early surgery.
4. Some 44% of patients with chronic rotator cuff tears achieved satisfactory results with conservative treatment.
5. A total of 85% of surgically treated patients with chronic tears had satisfactory pain relief, and 78% achieved a satisfactory functional result.
6. Improvement after surgery continued to occur over 2 years. However in patients over the age of 60 there may be some deterioration of the initial functional recovery obtained after surgery.
7. Revision surgery gave good results in 17% of patients and satisfactory pain relief in 37%.

ANTERIOR DISLOCATION AND SUBLUXATION OF THE GLENOHUMERAL JOINT

Incidence and classification

Despite the frequency with which anterior dislocations of the shoulder occur, there are very few data concerning the incidence of shoulder dislocations in the general population. In a small random sample in Sweden, Hovelius (1982) found that 1.7% of people between the ages of 18 and 70 had reported such an occurrence.

In 1984 Simonet et al reported the overall incidence of initial traumatic shoulder dislocations in Olmsted County, Minnesota, USA as 7.5/100 000 person-years. No data have been found to indicate the incidence of anterior shoulder dislocation in the UK (Simonet et al 1984a).

In 1980 Rowe suggested the following classification of anterior shoulder dislocations:

1. Traumatic anterior dislocation
   a. Primary anterior dislocation
   b. Transient anterior dislocation
   c. Recurrent anterior dislocation
   d. Chronic anterior dislocation
2. Atraumatic anterior dislocation
   a. Primary and recurrent anterior dislocation
   b. Recurrent voluntary anterior dislocation

To this list should be added congenital or developmental dislocations. Only the first group, primary anterior dislocation, which is likely to result in medicolegal action, will be considered further here.

Primary anterior dislocation

Many factors play a part in determining the prognosis after primary anterior dislocation of the shoulder: the age of the patient is probably the most important.

Rockwood (1984a) stated that a full range of movement and normal muscle strength will return after 4–6 months in patients immobilized for 4 weeks. Aronen & Regan (1984) treated 20 young American midshipmen for 3 weeks with a sling, followed by an intensive rehabilitation programme and reported that their patients were back to full unrestricted activity at 3 months. Recovery time will be longer in older people, who have an increased incidence of rotator cuff tear associated with their primary dislocation.

In 1986 Hawkins et al reported the results of 39 patients, all over the age of 40, followed prospectively from the time of primary anterior dislocation of the shoulder for an average of 32 months. Thirty patients still experienced discomfort at final follow-up; 15 were experiencing occasional pain and 15 nocturnal pain. Fifteen patients were impaired in overhead work; 66% of the 39 patients had significant impairment of active motion with less than 120° of forward elevation and less than 30° of external rotation.

Kiviluoto et al (1980) found that 42 patients of a total of 226 (19%) had some residual stiffness of the affected shoulder 1 year after treatment. Only 1 in 4 patients were aged under 30 in this series. Only 1 (4%) of the 26 patients under the age of 30 had residual stiffness compared with 40 (26%)

of the 154 patients aged over 30, after a comparable period of immobilization of 1 week. The other patients in this series had different periods of immobilization.

Studying this same group of patients, Pasila et al (1980) found that 38 patients (25%) of those over 50 years of age failed to attain normal mobility of the shoulder after 1 year. The corresponding figures for those aged under 50 years was 4 of 99 patients (4%). The median time to recovery of normal mobility in these patients was 3 weeks after 1 week's immobilization, increasing to 5 weeks after 3 weeks' immobilization. This recovery period increased to 7 weeks in those patients over 50 years of age regaining normal mobility.

If the dislocation had been present for longer than 12 hours, the median period for recovery of normal mobility was 4–5 months, as compared with 30 days for the study group taken as a whole.

Recovery time was also related to the degree of violence initiating the dislocation. Shoulders dislocating as the result of torsion recovered full mobility in a mean period of 24 days as compared with the 60 days required after a fall from a height.

In this group Pasila et al (1980) also found that of 108 patients attaining normal mobility within 1 month, 25 (23%) redislocated. Residual stiffness present after 1 year tended to be permanent, and only 4 of 42 patients (9.5%) with this problem improved their mobility after 1 year.

Kazár & Relovszky (1969) evaluated 408 cases of acute anterior dislocation after treatment by immobilization (of which the duration varied from patient to patient). They also noted the detrimental effect that the age of the patient had on the recovery of function. In their under-30 age group 1 patient out of 48 (2%) had at least 90° limitation of movement as compared with 16 of 110 patients (14.5%) aged 31 to 50, and 94 of 250 (37.6%) aged over 50 years.

In 1956 Rowe reported the functional recovery in those patients whose dislocation did not recur. Of 110 shoulders, 69 (63%) were normal as regards function and comfort. Some 24 (22%) had mild limitation of activity whilst 14 (13%) had moderate limitation of activity (inability or unease at work or in sport when using the arm in an elevated or overhead position). Three patients (3%) had marked limitation of usefulness and function. Rowe felt that the moderate and poor results were associated with those patients with associated rotator cuff tears.

Factors related to recurrence of dislocation

Many published series quote recurrence rates following anterior dislocation but the many variable factors between each series makes a direct comparison of doubtful value. However the recurrence rates in the larger series are shown in Table 3.15. The highest incidence occurred in Henry & Genung's (1982) series with 88% having recurrent dislocation. The

Table 3.15   Incidence of recurrent dislocation after primary anterior dislocation

Reference	Total primary anterior dislocation	Recurrence	%
Kazár & Relovszky (1969)	566	48	8.5
Rowe (1956)	398	151*	38
Rowe & Sakellarides (1961)	324	136	42
Hovelius (1987)	256	112	44
Kiviluoto et al (1980)	226	30	13
Henry & Genung (1982)	121	107	88
Total	1891	584	31

*Figure estimated from data given in paper.

average age of this group was 19 years. The lowest incidence was in Kazár & Relovszky's series (1969) with an 8.5% recurrence rate. In this series 79% of patients were aged over 40 years.

The length of follow-up is important when considering the incidence of recurrent dislocation. Hovelius (1987) noted 77 recurrences (30%) out of 257 primary dislocations occurring 2 years after injury and in the same group of patients the incidence was 112 (44%) of 256 patients at 5 years. In Rowe's (1956) series, out of 151 recurrences 70.5% had recurred by 2 years, a further 19% by 2–5 years, 6% by 5–10 years and 4.5% did not recur until more than 10 years after the initial dislocation.

The various factors that affect the prognosis relating to the recurrence of dislocation are:

1. The age of the patient.
2. The length of immobilization.
3. The severity of the initial trauma.
4. The sex of the patient.
5. The presence of associated fractures.
6. The effect of rehabilitation.

The age of the patient

The age of the patient at the time of initial dislocation appears to play an important part in whether there will be recurrence of the dislocation. Table 3.16 records the variation in recurrence rates as compared with age in the major series reviewed. Again, although the figures vary from series to series, patients under the age of 20 have a significantly higher risk of redislocation (46–94%) compared with those aged over 40 (4.5–14.5%).

The length of immobilization

Table 3.17 records the recurrence rate compared to the length of immobilization. Thus it appears that in those papers reviewing treatment

Table 3.16 The incidence of recurrent dislocation as compared with age at the time of primary dislocation

Reference	<20 years			20–40 years			40+ years		
	n	Recur	%	n	Recur	%	n	Recur	%
Hovelius (1987)*	102	68	67	154	47	30.5			
Rowe (1956)	57	47[†]	83	77	49[†]	63	220[‡]	26[†]	12
Rowe and Sakellarides (1961)	53	50	94	80	59	74	186	27	14.5
Kazár & Relovszky (1969)	28	13	46	97	15	15.5	441	20	4.5
Kiviluoto et al (1980)	18	10	55.5	65	11	17	143	9	6
Simonet & Cofield (1984)	32	27	84	43	21	49	41	4	10

*Age range 0–22 and 23–40 years.
[†]Figures estimated from data in text.
[‡]Figures for 50 years and over.

Table 3.17 Incidence of recurrence compared with length of immobilization

Reference	Immobilization time											
	None			1 week			2–3 weeks			3–6 weeks		
	Recur	n	%	Recur	n	%	Recur	n	%	Recur	n	%
Hovelius et al (1983)*	46	104	44							51	112	45.5
Rowe (1956)	52	63	82.5	29	46	63	41	98	42	35	66	53
Rowe & Sakellarides (1961)	46	66	70				61[†]	176	35	26	76	34
Kiviluoto et al (1980)				13	26	50	6	27	22			

*Patients less than 40 years old.
[†]Group immobilized from 1 to 3 weeks.

of the general population (Rowe 1956, Rowe & Sakellarides 1961, Kiviluoto et al 1980) the figures for recurrent dislocation were improved by a period of up to 3 weeks' immobilization, whereas immobilization beyond 3 weeks was of questionable value. On the other hand, Hovelius et al (1983) suggested that, in a group excluding patients over 40 years of age, immobilization had no effect on the incidence of recurrence of dislocation. This conclusion was supported by Henry & Genung (1982). In 59 of their patients who were not immobilized, 50 (85%) redislocated their shoulders. Of the group who were immobilized (length of immobilization was not stated) 56 of the 62 patients (90%) developed recurrent dislocation. In contrast, Watson-Jones claimed that recurrence never occurred if a shoulder was immobilized for 3–4 weeks (Kessel 1982).

The severity of the initial trauma

In their series of 257 primary anterior dislocations in the under-40 age group, Hovelius et al (1982) reported that the severity of the initiating trauma had no influence on the rate of recurrence of the dislocation. Rowe (1956) suggested that the recurrence rate when compared with the type of initiating trauma was significant but cautioned that this must also be interpreted with respect to the age of the patient. Rowe & Sakellarides (1961), Kazár and Relovszky (1969), and Kiviluoto et al (1980) all suggested that there was a decreasing incidence of recurrent dislocation with increasing severity of initiating trauma. Again direct comparison between these series is difficult.

The sex of the patient

There is some controversy as to whether the sex of the patient has any bearing on the likelihood of recurrent dislocation. Rowe (1956) found that the incidence of recurrence was twice as common in males as in females. However, both Hovelius et al (1982) and Simonet & Cofield (1984) reported that the incidence of recurrence was not increased in either sex when the patients were age-matched.

The presence of associated fractures

The presence of a fractured greater tuberosity decreases the likelihood of recurrent dislocation. Hovelis (1987) reported that only 1 of his 32 patients (3%) with this fracture had a recurrence of dislocation, compared with recurrence in 74 of 192 patients (38.5%) without this fracture. Rowe (1956) found that recurrence occurred in 3 of 44 patients (6.8%) with fracture of the greater tuberosity as compared with a recurrence rate of 38% in his study group as a whole. When Rowe & Sakellarides (1961) increased the number of patients in Rowe's 1956 series, the incidence fell to 3 recurrences in 66 patients (4.5%).

Humeral head defects may be seen in shoulders with no history of dislocation. In 1956 Rowe examined the radiographs of 200 patients with no history of dislocation and found humeral head defects in 10%. Of his patients with primary dislocations, 38% had evidence of these defects, as compared with 57% of patients with recurrent dislocation. Hovelius (1987) found that the rate of recurrence in his patients aged under 22 years was not related to the presence or absence of a humeral head defect, but that in the middle and older age groups the incidence of recurrence was significantly greater when a defect was present.

In 1983 Hovelius et al reported that 8% of their patients with an anterior dislocation had a fracture of the glenoid rim, although they felt that the real incidence was higher. The found that the incidence increased with the age of the patient but that it bore no relation to the incidence of later redislocation.

This was contrary to Rowe's (1956) findings; Rowe's incidence of glenoid rim fracture was 5.4%, but 13 of 21 patients (62%) with this associated fracture had a recurrence of dislocation.

Aston & Gregory (1973) described 3 shoulders in which large fractures of the glenoid played a definite part in destabilizing the shoulder. In 2 of the 3 patients the fragments were reattached but additional repair was performed. The shoulders were stable; however, length of follow-up was not mentioned.

The effect of rehabilitation

In 20 midshipmen with an average age of 19.2 years Aronen & Regan (1984) reported a recurrence of dislocation or subluxation in 25% after 3 weeks' immobilization and an intensive rehabilitation programme.

Yoneda et al (1982) reported on 104 male patients with an average age of 21.5 years whose shoulders were immobilized for 5 weeks followed by 6 weeks of graduated exercise. Their recurrent dislocation rate was 17.3%.

Rotator cuff tears in association with anterior dislocation

Rotator cuff tears are well documented in association with anterior dislocation of the shoulder and tend to occur with increasing frequency in the older patient. The incidence of rotator cuff tears in association with anterior dislocation is difficult to assess accurately because many authors' diagnoses were based on clinical impressions rather than proven arthrograms.

In 1969 Reeves reported the results of arthrograms performed on 47 patients with acute anterior dislocation of the shoulder and found ruptures of the rotator cuff in 26 of them (55%). He found it to be the predominant shoulder injury sustained at the time of dislocation in patients over 50 years of age. The arthrograms were repeated after 7–10 days, at which time 5 patients still showed rotator cuff defects. Two of these 5 patients had disability severe enough to warrant surgical exploration, at which time the diagnosis was confirmed. Only 1 patient in this group of 26 developed recurrent dislocation.

Simonet & Cofield (1984) found clinical evidence of rotator cuff tear in association with anterior dislocation in only 7 of 124 patients (6%). All resolved with time. However, in 1978 Pasila et al reported that this association occurred in 28 of 127 patients (22%), all aged over 50 years. This diagnosis was based on a clinical assessment at 3 weeks.

Craig (1984) quoted McLaughlin as suggesting that the incidence of rotator cuff tear may be as high as 70% in patients over 40 years of age after dislocation. Hawkins et al (1986) reported that 35 of 39 patients (90%) aged over 40 years had clinical findings indicative of an associated rotator cuff tear. These consisted of tenderness over the anterior rotator cuff, infraspinatus and supraspinatus muscle wasting, weakness of abduction and external rotation and a decrease in their active range of motion. After an average follow-up of 32 months, 9 patients reported a symptom-free shoulder, including 4 with a diagnosis of rotator cuff tear. The remaining 30 patients were still symptomatic with pain, weakness and decreased function. Fifteen of these patients had nocturnal pain and half the patients were significantly impaired when doing overhead work. Two-thirds had significant impairment of active motion with less than 120° of forward elevation and less than 30° of external rotation.

These figures suggest that 30 out of 39 patients aged over 40 years (77%) will have disability after 2½ years following a primary anterior dislocation, mainly due to a rotator cuff tear. Only 4 of 35 patients (11.5%) with an associated rotator cuff tear will be symptom-free.

Pasila et al (1980) found that 23 of their 26 patients with rotator cuff tears (88.5%) had permanent stiffness of the shoulder and in 14 of these the limitation was up to 40° in flexion. However, they stated that no patient had spontaneous pain or pain on movement of such severity as to indicate surgical treatment for rotator cuff rupture.

The results of the treatment of rotator cuff ruptures in association with anterior dislocation of the shoulder are disappointing. Hawkins et al (1986) reported on 14 patients referred as a result of pain, weakness and functional problems. Seven were treated with physiotherapy and none of these achieved adequate pain relief or improvement in function. Seven patients underwent decompressive acromioplasty and attempted cuff repair. Four had acceptable pain relief and 3 had an increase in strength and function.

Other complications

Nerve injury

The reported incidence of nerve injury following acute anterior dislocation is quite variable. In 1956 Rowe quoted an incidence of 5.4% nerve injury in 500 dislocations, whilst Hawkins et al (1986) reported an incidence of 18% axillary nerve injury in 39 patients aged over 40 years. Pasila et al (1978) had a 21% incidence of nerve injuries, of which 29 were brachial plexus injuries and 21 axillary nerve injuries. Kessel (1982) quoted a 10% incidence of axillary nerve injury, whilst Rockwood (1984a) claimed that the overall incidence of axillary nerve injury was in the order of 30%.

In Rowe's (1956) series 15% failed to recover. Pasila et al (1978) reported that 30% of the patients in their series had not recovered completely at 1 year. However all the patients aged under 51 years recovered, as compared with 58% of those aged over 51 years. They further stated that recovery occurred for up to 1 year after injury but quoted Assmus & Meirel, who stated that the prognosis was poor in those patients showing no recovery by 8–10 weeks after injury.

Rockwood (1984a) stated that regardless of whether the damage to the axillary nerve was transient or complete, the end result should yield a normal functioning shoulder.

Vascular damage

Damage to the axillary artery has been reported frequently enough in the literature to substantiate its place as an uncommon but grave complication of anterior dislocation. Although its overall incidence is difficult to ascertain, it is more common in the elderly patient with arteriosclerosis and it increases in incidence with the attempted closed reduction of chronic dislocations. The long-term prognosis depends on the result of arterial repair.

Summary

1. The younger patient with a treated primary anterior dislocation of the shoulder should have returned to full function by 3–4 months after injury.
2. Some 2–4% of patients aged under 30 had some residual stiffness after primary anterior dislocation.
3. A total of 77% of patients aged over 40 experienced some discomfort after anterior dislocation, and 25–66% had some permanent restriction of mobility.
4. Recovery time was increased by a factor of four when the dislocation persisted for over 12 hours.
5. Stiffness present after 1 year tended to be permanent.
6. From 8.5 to 88% (average 31%) of patients had a recurrence after primary anterior dislocation.
7. Some 69–70% of recurrences occurred within 2 years and a further 19–31% within 5 years.
8. Of patients under 20 years of age, 46–94% suffered a recurrence of their dislocation compared with 4.5–14.5% of patients aged over 40.
9. The length of immobilization of the shoulder in young patients with anterior dislocation does not appear to affect recurrence of dislocation, although 3 weeks' immobilization seems to be beneficial in the older age group.
10. There appears to be a decreasing incidence of recurrent dislocation with increasing severity of trauma, although this relationship in less certain in younger patients.
11. The sex of the patient with a primary anterior dislocation had an uncertain influence on the incidence of recurrence.
12. In all, 3–4.5% of patients with associated fractures of the greater tuberosity experienced recurrence of dislocation.
13. The presence of a humeral head defect was associated with an increased incidence of recurrent dislocation, although this association was less certain in younger patients.
14. Fractures of the glenoid rim had an uncertain association with recurrent dislocation.

15. An intensive period of rehabilitation decreased the incidence of recurrent dislocation in younger patients.
16. The incidence of rotator cuff tear in association with anterior dislocation was 6–55% but occurred in 22–90% of patients aged over 40 years.
17. Permanent disability persisted in 88.5% of patients sustaining a rotator cuff tear in association with their anterior dislocation.
18. Surgery for rotator cuff tear in association with anterior dislocation produced acceptable results in approximately 50% of patients.
19. The incidence of nerve damage in anterior dislocation of the shoulder was 5.4–30%.
20. Some 15–30% of nerve injuries failed to recover completely, although this incidence increased to 58% in patients aged over 50 years.
21. Recovery of axillary nerve injuries occurred up to 1 year after injury, although failure of any recovery after 8–10 weeks suggested a poor prognosis.
22. A normal functioning shoulder resulted whatever the eventual recovery of the axillary nerve.
23. Axillary artery damage was more common in the elderly and after attempted closed manipulation of chronic dislocation. The overall functional recovery depended upon the response of the artery to surgical repair.

RECURRENT ANTERIOR DISLOCATION AND SUBLUXATION

Recurrent anterior dislocation

The surgery of recurrent anterior dislocation of the shoulder is well documented. Many operations have been described, numerous modifications proposed and each operation has its proponents and critics. It is not the purpose of this section to select any particular operation as being ideal, but rather to tabulate the incidence of recurrence for those procedures as reported in the literature in order to assist in medicolegal reporting.

Rockwood (1984a) has already provided an extensive review of the literature and has shown that all of the reconstructions gave approximately 97% excellent results. His interpretation of excellent would appear to imply no redislocation and does not take into account residual pain and restricted movement. Table 3.18 records the incidence of recurrence following various reconstructions for anterior dislocation of the shoulder.

Failure to redislocate by no means implies an excellent result. Direct comparison between papers is impossible because of different criteria for assessing patients. In 1987 Ahmadain reported 66% excellent results with the Magnusson-Stack operation, with 31.5% of patients having more than

Table 3.18 Incidence of recurrence following various reconstructions for anterior dislocation of the shoulder

Procedure	Reference	Number of cases	Recurrence (%)
Magnusson-Stack	Ahmadain (1987)	38	2.6
	Day et al (1963)	24	0 at 5 years
	Day et al (1963)	14	14.3 at 16 years
	Rockwood (1984a)	571	4.1 average
Bristow	Halley & Olix (1975)	24	4
	Rockwood (1984a)	750	1.7 average
Bankart	Vidal et al (1984)	85	2.4
	Hovelius et al (1979)	46	4.3
	Morrey & Jones (1976)	16	0
	Day et al (1963)	17	0 at 5 years
	Day et al (1963)	9	33 at 16 years
	Werner & Reimers (1972)	77	6.5
	Rockwood (1984a)	513	3.3 average
Putti-platt	Hovelius et al (1979)	68	19
	Morrey & Jones (1976)	132	13.6%
	Werner & Reimer (1972)	28	0
	Rockwood (1984a)	432	3 average
Du-Toit stapling	Rao et al (1986)	65	1.5
	Sisk & Boyd (1974)	239	2.9
Boytchev	Ha'eri (1986)	26	0
Eden-Hybbinette	Werner & Reimers (1972)	15	20
	Solonen & Rokkanen (1972)	84	7
	Rockwood (1984a)	254	6 average

10° loss of external rotation. Hovelius et al (1983) had 90% (101 of 111 patients) excellent or good results with the Bristow procedure. Six patients in this series had redislocations and a further 8 had subluxations on one or two occasions. Some of these were presumably graded with his excellent results. The average loss of external rotation was 19° in abduction. Ahmadain rated any loss of external rotation of more than 10° as satisfactory only.

In 1984 Vidal et al reported 84% of their patients as excellent or good after the Bankart procedure. Some 21% had a 'significant loss of external rotation'. Loss of external rotation is also recorded in the majority of other procedures, but to varying degrees.

The length of follow-up is also important when comparing series. In their comparison of the Magnusson-Stack and the Bankart procedures, Day et al (1963) found no recurrences in the 41 procedures after a 5-year mean follow-up period, but found three recurrent dislocations and two subluxations in the 23 patients followed up for 16 years. In 1956 Rowe stated that 52% of recurrences following operative procedures occur in the first 2 years, 17% within 2–5 years, 28% within 5–10 years and 3% within 10–20 years.

Recurrent anterior subluxation

In recent years it has been recognized that there is a group of patients, usually athletes, who undergo episodes of recurrent anterior subluxation with or without true dislocation, the so-called dead arm syndrome (Rowe & Zarins 1981). Protzman (1980) classified these patients into two types: type I instability was present in the subluxating shoulder that had never been dislocated and type II instability was present in those shoulders with definite recurrent dislocation and episodes of chronic subluxation in the intervals between dislocations.

Patients may or may not experience a sensation of the shoulder slipping out of place, especially with external rotation and abduction. Pain may be felt in the overhead position and on throwing. In all, 55% of Rowe & Zarins' patients were unaware that the shoulder was dislocating. After the acute episode the patients were aware of numbness and tingling in the arm and hand, and the arm felt weak. They remained aware of weakness and a decreased range of motion for the next few hours.

Rowe & Zarins reported a 100% incidence of a positive apprehension test in external rotation–abduction, although Hastings & Coughlin (1981) found that this test was positive in only 50% of their patients. Evidence of bony changes on the anteroinferior glenoid rim were found in 68% of Hastings & Coughlin's patients, 43% of Blazina & Satzman's (1969) patients and 45% of those of Rowe & Zarins (1981). In addition, Rowe & Zarins found humeral head defects in 40%.

A period of intensive rehabilitation may be of benefit to these patients prior to consideration of surgical treatment, although Rowe & Zarins only achieved improvement by physiotherapy in 13% of their patients.

The results of the various surgical procedures for recurrent subluxation should be no different from those already reported for recurrent anterior dislocation.

Although athletic activities are a frequent precursor to this injury, forceful external rotation and a direct blow were a cause of 86% of Rowe & Zarins' cases and these injuries may therefore be the subject of litigation.

CHRONIC ANTERIOR DISLOCATION

Chronic anterior dislocation of the shoulder is less common today with the improved accident services, but may still be seen in the elderly patient or after unrecognized fractures of the glenoid (Kummel 1970). The major complaint in the elderly tends to be restriction of movement rather than pain. Younger patients tend to experience more in the way of pain due to the better condition of their muscles and ligaments. Not all patients necessarily require operation. Hejna et al (1969) treated 8 of their 15 cases non-operatively and these patients had an average total abduction of 82°. However, Rowe & Zarins (1982) used a points system to evaluate their results and found 3 poor and 1 fair result in 4 patients treated non-operatively.

Closed reduction may be successful but this becomes increasingly difficult and hazardous after 3–4 weeks due to the adherence by scar tissue of the brachial plexus and axillary artery to the capsule. In the elderly an arteriosclerotic axillary artery is especially at risk.

Open reduction may be achieved with or without preservation of the humeral head.

Hejna et al (1969) found that only one of their two patients improved the range of abduction after open reduction whilst Rowe & Zarins (1982) had one excellent, one good and one fair result in their chronic anterior dislocations. Neviaser (1963) reported on 16 patients who had operation for chronic dislocation (anterior and posterior). He did not indicate how many were anterior but the two reported cases of chronic anterior dislocation achieved abduction of 90 and 135°.

Summary

1. Recurrent dislocation after operative stabilization occurred in 1.7–6% of cases. Some 21–31% of these recurrences occurred after 5 years.
2. Excellent results occurred in 66–90% of patients after operative stabilization.
3. External rotation was reduced by most procedures, to varying degrees.
4. In all, 13% of recurrent subluxations may be 'cured' by intensive rehabilitation.
5. Elderly patients with chronic dislocation may be managed non-operatively and may achieve a reasonable range of active abduction.
6. Closed reduction should not be attempted after 3–4 weeks.
7. Open reduction produces variable return of function.

POSTERIOR DISLOCATION

Incidence and classification

Posterior dislocation of the shoulder is much less common than anterior dislocation yet the incidence of chronic dislocations from missed diagnosis is much greater.

Kessel (1982) quoted Rowe as reporting that 5% of shoulder dislocations are posterior, although Rowe (1956) quoted 2% as the true incidence. Rockwood (1984a) reviewed a number of series of posterior dislocations, and found the average incidence to be 2.17%.

Kessel (1982) classified posterior dislocation into:

1. Traumatic
   a. Acute
   b. Persistent (or chronic)
   c. Recurrent (dislocation and subluxation)
2. Habitual

Habitual dislocation need not be discussed further other than to emphasize the importance of distinguishing traumatic from habitual dislocation or subluxation. The habitual dislocators respond poorly to surgery due to commonly associated psychiatric problems.

Acute posterior dislocation

Little appears to have been written about prognostic indicators in acute posterior dislocation of the shoulder. Roberts & Wickstrom (1971) reviewed 14 cases of posterior dislocation treated conservatively. The delay in diagnosis in these patients was not mentioned and some may have been seen late. Nine (64%) achieved excellent or good results with slight limitation of movement. Their average age was 38 years. Five (36%) had fair or poor results. Their average age was 67 years. Thus functional results would appear to be good or excellent in patients under 40 years of age but diminished in quality in patients over this age. They also found that recurrence occurred in 9 of 24 patients (37.5%), with 5 of these 9 recurrences in patients immobilized for less than 3 weeks. Rowe (1956) reported a recurrence rate of 60% for his 10 cases of posterior dislocation.

Rockwood (1984a) stated that the incidence of associated fractures of the posterior glenoid and proximal humerus (including humeral head) was over 50% in posterior dislocation, and Roberts & Wickstrom (1971) found the incidence in their series to be 19 of 41 cases (46%). Of the 15 patients with adequate follow-up, 9 (60%) achieved a good or excellent result. They also reported 2 cases (5%) of neurological complication — a transient radial nerve palsy and an axillary nerve palsy with partial recovery — in 41 patients.

Chronic posterior dislocation

Considering the rarity of posterior dislocation of the shoulder, the incidence of late diagnosis is high. Rockwood (1984a) stated that 60% of posterior dislocations were not diagnosed at initial assessment.

Kessel (1982) reported 8 cases, and found the predominant complaint to be loss of movement. Some patients had been incorrectly labelled as 'frozen shoulder'. Pain was only significant in relatively recent dislocations. These patients were generally able to abduct to a right angle and one patient could abduct to 160°. Using a points system, Rowe & Zarins (1982) found that chronic posterior dislocation was less disabling than its anterior counterpart. Patients with minimal functional limitation could be managed non-operatively.

Hawkins et al (1987) found closed manipulation successful in 25% of 12 patients in whom it was attempted less than 6 weeks after injury. They also reported that transfer of the subscapularis muscle or lesser tuberosity into the humeral head defect was successful in maintaining reduction in all 8 cases performed at their units, with an average of 160–165° elevation, and internal rotation to the 12th thoracic vertebrae. However they had treated 5 failures of this procedure referred from other units.

Hemiarthroplasty was performed in 9 shoulders with good results in 66%. The 6 good results achieved ranges of motion similar to the group mentioned above. Failure occurred in those with degenerative changes of the glenoid.

Total arthroplasty was successful in 90% of 10 cases, with 1 failure dislocating and refusing further treatment. Of the 9 successful cases, 1 patient had moderate pain, but all were able to carry out the activities of daily living.

In their more complicated points system, Rowe & Zarins (1982) found excellent or good results in 40% of surgical reductions. Of 10 patients treated by surgery (open reduction, hemiarthroplasty or excision arthroplasty) the 6 fair results had moderate pain, 50% of elevation and only moderate limitation with overhead work.

Recurrent posterior dislocation and subluxation

Many operations are available for the treatment of recurrent posterior dislocation and subluxation but adequate information on each procedure to allow an adequate assessment of prognosis is lacking. Rockwood (1984a) reported that Tibone noted a 30% failure rate following posterior staple capsullorrhaphy. Hawkins et al (1984) reported on 50 cases of posterior instability of the shoulder, of which 80% had voluntary instability. Surgery was performed in 26 patients but recurrence occurred in 50%. It took 4 months for the patients to return to activities of daily living post-operatively and 6 months for those returning to sport. English & MacNab (1984) had 3 recurrences in 4 patients after posterior capsullorrhaphy but no recurrences in 4 patients after glenoid osteotomy. However, Pouget (1984) had 1 failure out of 5 patients after glenoid osteotomy, and Wilkinson & Thomas (1985) had 4 recurrences (19%) in 21 glenoid osteotomies.

Arthritis after dislocation

Samilson & Prieto (1983) reviewed 74 shoulders with glenohumeral arthropathy after single or multiple dislocations of the shoulder. As these patients were seen in a secondary referral centre they were unable to comment on the incidence of arthritis after dislocation, although they quoted Hindmarsh & Lindberg as noting a 7% incidence of moderate or severe arthritis after recurrent dislocations treated non-operatively. They found that posterior dislocation had a much higher incidence of moderate and severe arthritis than anterior dislocation, possibly related to a delay in the diagnosis of dislocation. The frequency of dislocation and the presence of a humeral head or glenoid rim defect was not related to the severity of arthritis.

Mild arthritis was noted to be asymptomatic. With increasing degrees of arthritis the degree of external rotation decreased.

Operations in which internal fixation devices intruded on the joint cartilage frequently resulted in moderate to severe arthritis.

Shoulder dislocation in children

Dislocation of the shoulder in children is exceedingly rare. Rowe (1956) noted 8 dislocations in children aged under 10 years of age out of 500 patients. Rockwood (1984b) reported 8 cases and Laskin & Sedlin (1971) reported a case of luxatioerecta in a child of 3 months with Erb–Duchenne brachial plexus palsy. Babbitt & Cassidy (1968) reported 2 cases of dislocation of the shoulder in infancy associated with obstetrical paralysis. Rockwood (1984b) had an incidence of recurrence of 50% in his cases but quoted Wagner & Lyne as noting a recurrence in 80% of 9 children with traumatic anterior dislocation. He also quoted Rowe as reporting 100% recurrence in children aged 1–10 years and 94% recurrence rate in children and young adults aged 11–20 years.

Summary

1. Some 2–5% of shoulder dislocations are posterior.
2. In all, 64% of acute posterior dislocations achieved excellent or good results. Increasing age mitigates against a good result.
3. Associated fractures occurred in about 50% of posterior dislocations but did not appear to affect the final result adversely unless a large humeral head defect was present.
4. Recurrent posterior dislocation occurred in 37.5–60% of cases.
5. Chronic posterior dislocation may cause minimal functional loss in the elderly.
6. Surgery for chronic posterior dislocation may produce 40–80% good results depending on the surgical operation and surgical expertise.
7. Surgery for recurrent posterior instability produced stable results in 20–50% of patients but voluntary subluxation would appear to mitigate against a good result.

8. It may take 4 months to return to the activities of daily living after surgical reconstruction for recurrent posterior instability.
9. The incidence of arthritis after anterior dislocation of the shoulder may be as high as 7%.
10. Arthritis after dislocation is more common in posterior dislocation.
11. Mild arthritis is asymptomatic.
12. Dislocation of the shoulder in children is rare and may be associated with obstetrical paralysis.
13. Recurrent shoulder dislocation occurred in 50–100% of children.

FRACTURES OF THE PROXIMAL HUMERUS

Incidence and classification

Fractures of the proximal humerus account for 3–5% of all injuries involving bone (Leyshon 1984). In 1970 Neer proposed a classification

DISPLACED FRACTURES OF PROXIMAL HUMERUS

(after NEER)

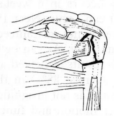

	Two-part	Three-part	Four-part
Anatomical Neck			
Surgical Neck			
Greater Tuberosity			
Lesser Tuberosity			
Fracture I Dislocation			

Fig. 3.1 Neer's four-segment classification (after Neer 1970a). Reprinted from Kessel (1982)

based on the four basic anatomical segments (Fig. 3.1) which took into account the presence or absence of *displacement* of one or more of these major segments (Neer 1970a). This classification will be used to assess prognosis in this section.

The six groups are:

1. Minimum displacement: no segment is displaced more than 1 cm or angulated more than 45°.
2. Anatomical neck fracture: a two-part fracture.
3. Surgical neck fracture: a two-part fracture with the fragment displaced more than 1 cm or angulated more than 45°.
4. Greater tuberosity displacement: a two-, three- or four-part fracture.
5. Lesser tuberosity displacement: a two-, three- or four-part fracture.
6. Fracture dislocations: a two-, three- or four-part injury with anterior or posterior dislocation.

Minimally displaced fractures

Minimally displaced proximal humeral fractures are usually managed conservatively. Union usually occurs in 6 weeks and the complication of avascular necrosis, although it can occur (Neer 1984), is very rare.

Functional recovery however is not guaranteed to return to normal and the recovery time may be quite slow. As can be seen from Table 3.19, the percentage of excellent/good results achieved (according to the various authors' criteria) is 85–95% (average 88%) in the five largest series. The disability time with these fractures is not insignificant. Neer (1984) observed that some patients did recover motion and function within 2 months but they were exceptional. Lingering stiffness, pain at the extreme of motion and 'weather ache' usually persist for at least 6 months. Strength and co-ordination return even more slowly. Poor mobility, rather than pain, seems to cause prolonged disability. In 1985 Young & Wallace reported that with their 34 patients with minimally displaced fractures, pain became

Table 3.19 Results following treatment of minimally displaced proximal humeral fractures

Reference	Number of patients	Number of excellent/ good results	%
Mills & Horne (1985)	57	54	95
Clifford (1981)	46	43	94
Ekström et al (1965)	100	90	90
Lundberg et al (1979)	42	36*	86
Stewart & Hundley (1955)	271†	231	85
Total (average)	516	454	(88)

*Result at 3 months.
†Patient group probably includes some displaced fractures.

insignificant with regard to interfering with sleep or activities of daily living by 6 months. They also found that it took 6 months to achieve maximum recovery of abduction as compared with 3 months to recover maximal internal rotation.

In 1965 Ekström et al reported the results of the treatment of 50 of their 100 patients with repeated procaine injections into the fracture and early mobilization. Overall 50% stabilized their movements by 3 months and 93% by 6 months, although 66% of the procaine-treated group had stabilized at 3 months. Similarly 63% were fit to return to work by the 3-month stage and 94% by 6 months, although 78% of the procaine-treated group returned to work at the 3-month stage.

Neer (1984) emphasized the importance of early functional exercises in the treatment of these patients. In 1981 Clifford reported a significant relationship between the time spent wearing a sling, the duration of physiotherapy and the final result in minimally displaced fractures. However Lundberg et al (1979) found no advantage in conventional physiotherapy over patients independently performing their own exercises, and Mills & Horne (1985) found no correlation between the duration of immobilization or duration of physiotherapy and the final result.

Two-part fractures

Anatomical neck fractures

Anatomical neck fractures are uncommon. Post (1980) stated that separation of the tuberosities in this group was rare whilst DePalma & Cantilli (1961) found that all of the 5 patients they reported had an associated fracture of the greater tuberosity or surgical neck. Three of their 5 cases achieved a good subjective result but only 2 were rated good objectively. They only reported avascular necrosis in 1 of these patients. However Post (1980) and Neer (1984) stated that the incidence of late avascular necrosis was high and was usually sufficiently disabling to require prosthetic replacement.

Surgical neck fractures

The results of the treatment of displaced surgical neck fractures are variable. Table 3.20 gives the results of conservative treatment. Overall 83% achieved a satisfactory result. Paavolainen et al (1983) reported excellent or satisfactory results from 14 of 15 patients (93%) treated by a plate and screws or screws alone. In 1980 Lentz & Meuser reported satisfactory results in 85 of 98 patients (87%) treated with a Rush pin, although the exact number of group III patients included in these figures is uncertain. These good results, however, were not achieved by Kristiansen & Christensen (1986) who found only 2 excellent results out of their 5 patients (40%) treated with plates.

Table 3.20   The results of the conservative treatment of displaced surgical neck fractures

Reference	Number of patients	Number of excellent/ good results	%
Mills & Horne (1985)	19	13	68.5
Young & Wallace (1985)	15	12	80*
Clifford (1981)	13	11	85
DePalma & Cantilli (1961)	28†	26	93
Total (average)	75	62	(83)

*Over 60° abduction was considered an acceptable (good) result.
†Includes 1 patient with operative fixation.

Greater tuberosity fractures

The unstable variety of fracture of the greater tuberosity should be considered as an avulsion of the attached rotator cuff muscles (Kessel 1982). The retracted tuberosity may impair motion by impinging under the acromion. Neer (1984) stated that a 1-cm displacement of this type in an active patient was best treated by open reduction and cuff repair. If the anatomy is restored the results should be good, as Young & Wallace (1985) found with a 100% acceptable/satisfactory result in 9 patients and DePalma & Cantilli (1961) with 86% good results in 14 cases. Delayed displacement of the greater tuberosity can occur and in 1983 Macpherson et al reported this occurrence in 10 of 89 cases (11%) in this type of fracture.

Lesser tuberosity fractures

This type of fracture is rare. Kessel (1982) stated that because complete avulsion of the lesser tuberosity carries with it the insertion of subscapularis it may lead to significant disability. Certainly Paavolainen et al (1983) noted an unsatisfactory result in the 1 case they reported which had been treated by internal fixation. However Neer (1984) stated that an avulsion of the lesser tuberosity has no clinical significance other than slight loss of internal rotation. This is borne out by the case reports of Andreasen (1948) and Labnola & Mohaghegh (1975). Post (1980) recommended internal fixation for large fragments.

Three-part fractures

There is disagreement in the literature as to whether three-part fractures of the proximal humerus are better treated by conservative or by operative means. Neer stated in 1984 that a prosthesis should be considered, with repair of the tuberosities and the rotator cuff, in the older patient with three-part greater tuberosity fractures. The results of those series in which conservative treatment was used are listed in Table 3.21. It can be seen

Table 3.21 The results of the conservative treatment of three-part fractures of the proximal humerus

Reference	Number of patients	Number of excellent/ satisfactory results	%
Neer (1970b)	20	0	0
Clifford (1981)	15	8–9*	56
Leyshon (1984)	34	24	70
Hawkins et al (1986)	13	10	77
DePalma & Cantilli (1961)	19	17†	89.5
Total (average)	101	59–60	(59)

*Figure obtained from results; including 1 four-part fracture.
†Two patients treated by internal fixation.

Table 3.22 The results of the surgical treatment of three-part fractures of the proximal humerus

References	Number of patients	Number of excellent/ satisfactory results	%
Kristiansen & Christensen (1986)	8	4	50
Neer (1970b)	22	13	59
Hawkins et al (1986)	15	13	86
Sturzenegger et al (1982)	8	7	87.5
Total (average)	53	37	(70)

that whilst Neer (1970b) had no successes with conservative management, DePalma & Cantilli (1961) found that they had reasonable results — although two of their patients were operated upon and their results were not removed from the overall figures.

The results of surgical treatment are shown in Table 3.22. Overall there appears to be a better final functional result after surgical treatment. Of those patients treated surgically, 70% obtained satisfactory or better results, as compared with 59% of the conservatively treated cases. These poor results of conservative treatment are heavily weighted by Neer's surprisingly poor results. If these are excluded, the results are similar to surgical treatment, with 72% satisfactory or better results. Kristiansen & Kofoed (1987) presented the results of 12 fractures — 2 two-part, 8 three-part and 2 four-part — treated by external fixation. In all, 82% achieved excellent or satisfactory results when reviewed 6–12 months after the operation.

Avascular necrosis was seen in 2 of 33 patients (6%) in Neer's (1970b) series and 2 of 8 patients (25%) in Kristiansen & Christensen's (1986) series. The overall incidence of avascular necrosis in the above papers is 11%.

Four-part fractures

In 1961 DePalma & Cantilli reported that all of the 7 cases of comminuted fracture of the proximal humerus in their series achieved good or fair results after conservative management, although they did not specifically state that these were four-part fractures. Neer (1984) however stated that he had found that avascular necrosis and reabsorption of the humeral head were so common after this type of fracture that he recommended primary replacement arthroplasty. In 1970 he reported a 100% failure rate in 12 cases of four-part fracture treated conservatively, as did Leyshon (1984) with 8 reported cases, of which 6 developed avascular necrosis.

Stableforth (1984) found that 11 of 17 patients (65%) with undisplaced four-part fractures treated conservatively recovered flexion to over 90°. Eleven (65%) were independent for activities of daily living by 6 months, 6 (35%) had no or only occasional pain whilst only 2 (12%) had constant pain. Of 16 patients with displaced four-part fractures only 1 (6%) had flexion beyond 90°, 7 (44%) were independent for daily activities by 6 months, 3 (19%) had no or occasional pain whilst 9 (56%) had constant pain. In a retrospective series 4 cases out of 32 (12.5%) had avascular necrosis.

A few reports of small series of these fractures treated by internal fixation suggest that surgery may produce better results. Sturzenegger et al (1982) reported 4 satisfactory results in 5 cases treated with a buttress plate with only 1 case of avascular necrosis, and Kristiansen & Christensen (1986) had 2 satisfactory cases in 3 surgically treated patients.

Fracture dislocation

Fracture dislocations may be two-, three- or four-part fractures in combination with anterior or posterior dislocations.

Two-part fracture dislocations, whether anterior or posterior, have a better prognosis than more comminuted fracture dislocations. DePalma & Cantilli (1961) reported 100% good results in 6 two-part fracture dislocations, whilst Einarsson (1958) had 14 acceptable results from 17 patients (82%). Knight & Mayne (1957) noted 56% acceptable results (9 of 16 patients) when large articular covered fragments remained intact. In the individual case reports of two-part posterior fracture dislocations (Prillaman et al 1969, Chattopadhyaya 1970), good results were obtained.

In 1970 Neer reported 45% (9 of 11 patients) acceptable results in three-part anterior dislocations and 66% (4 of 6 patients) in three-part posterior fracture dislocations. He noted a 100% failure rate in 9 cases of four-part anterior fracture dislocations and 3 four-part posterior fracture dislocations (Neer 1970b).

The results of the larger reported series of comminuted fracture dislocations are shown in Table 3.23. Results vary between 36 and 100%

Table 3.23 The results of the treatment of comminuted fracture dislocations of the proximal humerus

Reference	Number of patients	Number of satisfactory results	%
Knight & Mayne (1957)	9	5	55
Young & Wallace (1985)	5	5	100
Einarsson (1958)	13	5	38.5
DePalma & Cantilli (1961)	5	4	80
Mills (1974)	14	11	78.55
Sturzenegger et al (1982)	14	5	36

achieving a satisfactory outcome. These variable results presumably reflect the number of severely comminuted fracture dislocations in each group.

The results of replacement arthroplasty

The use of a replacement arthroplasty has been recommended for four-part fractures, fracture dislocations and some three-part injuries. The Neer prosthesis is widely reported in the literature. The results are however somewhat variable. Whilst pain relief is gratifying, occurring in all 16 of Tanner & Cofield's (1983) patients, 9 of 10 cases (90%) of Willems & Lim's (1985) series and 11 of 16 patients (69%) of Stableforth's (1984) series, and independence in daily activities is good — 9 of 10 cases (90%) of Willems & Lim (1985) and 14 of 16 cases (87.5%) of Stableforth (1984) — the ability to use the arm at shoulder level is less effective. In all, 75% (12 of 16 patients) achieved this ability in Tanner & Cofield's (1983) series. As a rule the range of movement is not especially restored by prosthetic replacement. Tanner & Cofield noted that the average active abduction in their series was 100°. The comparative results of the various series using the Neer (1970b) criteria are shown in Table 3.24. Only Neer has achieved such excellent results as he reported in 1970. However most of the poor results reported are due

Table 3.24 The results of the Neer hemiarthroplasty for fractures and fracture dislocations of the proximal humerus

Reference	Number of patients	Number of excellent/ satisfactory results	%
Neer (1970b)	42	39	93
Desmarchais et al (1984)	30	18	60
Willems & Lim (1985)	10	4	40
Paquet et al (1980)	18	7	39
Kraulis & Hunter (1976)	11	2	18
Total (average)	111	70	(63)

to a failure of restoration of a good range of movement, rather than being due to poor pain relief or failure to achieve independence in the activities of daily living.

The main complication appears to be pericapsular calcification which occurred in 36% of Kraulis & Hunter's (1976) series and 14% of Neer's (1970b) series. Neer (1963) pointed out that this especially tends to occur if surgery is delayed beyond 5 days after injury, and it causes a limitation in the range of movement.

Willems & Lim (1985) emphasized the importance of prolonged rehabilitation following prosthetic replacement and Stableforth (1984) stated that improvement occurs over a period of 18 months from surgery.

Non-union of proximal humeral fractures

Non-union of the proximal humerus is not often encountered, notwithstanding Neer's (1970b) reported incidence of 23% after certain types of fracture in this region. Not all require treatment; Bernstein's case (1963) was pain-free although active abduction was only to 60°. Treatment of non-union of fractures of the surgical neck has been recommended utilizing bone graft and blade plate (Crenshaw 1987) or Rush nails, screws or wires (Scheck 1982). More proximal non-unions can be treated by prosthetic replacement (Neer 1984). The reported results are too few to draw conclusions from, apart from saying that good function can result (Scheck 1982).

Epiphyseal fractures

Lesions of the proximal humeral epiphysis represent 3% of epiphyseal injuries (Neer & Horowitz 1965). The majority (91%) are Salter–Harris type II fractures, although type I fractures may occur in babies and infants (Dameron & Reibel 1969). Salter–Harris types III and IV injuries are very rare and type V injuries probably never occur. From a prognostic point of view the classification of Neer & Horowitz (1965) is more appropriate. These authors grade their fractures according to the displacement as follows:

Grade I: Less than 5 mm.
Grade II: To one-third the width of the shaft.
Grade III: To two-thirds the width of the shaft.
Grade IV: Greater than two-thirds of the shaft, including total displacement.

All reported series are unanimous in recording excellent functional results and open reduction is rarely required (see Table 3.25).

Even if anatomical reduction is poor, functional results appear good and

Table 3.25 The results of the treatment of proximal humeral epiphyseal fractures

Reference	Number of patients	Number of good results	%
Fraser et al (1967)*	10	9	90
Mcbride & Sisler (1965)	12	12	100
Neer & Horowitz (1965)	62	62	100
Nilsson & Svartholm (1965)	44	43	98
Smith (1956)	43	43	100
Baxter & Wiley (1986)	29	29	100

*All displaced fractures.

according to Sherk & Probst (1975) remodelling can occur over 6 years. Humeral shortening is not uncommon, occurring in 90% of Baxter & Wiley's (1986) cases. However, in only 30% of cases was this shortening more than 1 cm. In Dameron & Reibel's (1969) series, 14 of 46 patients (30.5%) had shortening, as did 23% (10 of 43 patients) in Smith's (1956) series. Neer & Horowitz (1965) found that shortening was rare under the age of 11 years, occurring in 11 of 67 cases (16.5%). Neer & Horowitz found shortening in 5 of 45 grade I and II injuries (11%); Baxter & Wiley (1968) found that in these grades the shortening averaged 3.5 mm. In grade III fractures the incidence of shortening was 25% (Neer & Horowitz 1965) and averaged 7.7 mm (Baxter & Wiley 1968). In grade IV injuries it occurred in 28% (Neer & Horowitz 1965) and averaged 12 mm, but could be as great as 7 cm.

Summary

1. Minimally displaced fractures usually unite in 6 weeks, and avascular necrosis is rare, although functional recovery can take up to 6 months.
2. Approximately 88% of minimally displaced fractures will achieve excellent/good results (minimal discomfort and abduction above 90°).
3. Some 50% of minimally displaced fractures stabilize their movements by 3 months and 93% do so by 6 months. In all, 63% return to work by 3 months and 94% by 6 months.
4. Anatomical neck fractures are rare but the incidence of avascular necrosis may be high.
5. A total of 83% of conservatively treated, displaced surgical neck fractures achieve satisfactory results. The results of surgical treatment are more variable.
6. Greater tuberosity fractures produce good results when not displaced under the acromion, thus blocking abduction. They result in 86–100% satisfactory results.

7. Approximately 11% of greater tuberosity fractures will displace with conservative treatment.
8. Lesser tuberosity fractures are rare. Large avulsed fragments may impair internal rotation.
9. Approximately 70% of patients with three-part proximal humeral fractures will achieve satisfactory or better results, although in conservatively treated patients this may be worse — 59%. External fixation may produce better results.
10. Avascular necrosis occurs in 11% of three-part fractures.
11. Conservatively treated, undisplaced four-part fractures have a 65% chance of achieving independent daily activity as compared with a 44% chance with displaced four-part fractures. Persistent stiffness, pain and functional disability are common.
12. Internal fixation of four-part fractures may yield better results, although only small series are reported.
13. The prognosis for fracture dislocations decreases as the degree of comminution increases.
14. A total of 82–100% of two-part fracture dislocations had satisfactory results.
15. Some 45% of three-part fracture dislocations had satisfactory results.
16. The results after four-part fracture dislocations were generally poor.
17. Of patients having prosthetic replacement, 69–100% achieved pain relief and 87.5–90% achieved independent daily living.
18. The overall results after prosthetic replacement according to Neer's criteria are disappointing, mainly due to an inability to restore full active movement. The active post-operative range of abduction averages 100°.
19. After prosthetic replacement for proximal humeral fractures 63% achieve excellent or satisfactory results and pericapsular calcification occurs in 14–36% of cases. Improvement in overall function occurs over 18 months after surgery.
20. A total of 90–100% of proximal humeral epiphyseal fractures had good functional results.
21. Anatomical malalignment rarely caused functional or cosmetic problems.
22. Shortening in grade I and II fractures occurred in 11% of patients and averaged 3.5 mm; in 25% of grade III fractures it averaged 7.7 mm, while in 28% of grade IV fractures it averaged 12 mm.

REFERENCES

Ahmadain A M 1987 The Magnusson-Stack operation for recurrent anterior dislocation of the shoulder. Journal of Bone and Joint Surgery 69B: 111–114
Alldredge R H 1965 Surgical treatment of acromioclavicular dislocations. Journal of Bone and Joint Surgery 47A: 1278

Allman F L 1967 Fractures and ligamentous injuries of the clavicle and its articulations. Journal of Bone and Joint Surgery 49A: 774–784

Andreasen A T 1948 Avulsion fracture of lesser tuberosity of humerus. Lancet i: 750–751

Anzel S H, Streitz W 1973 Closed management of acromioclavicular separations and dislocations. Journal of Bone and Joint Surgery 55A: 420

Arner O, Sandahl U, Orling H 1957 Dislocation of the acromio-clavicular joint. Acta Chirurgica Scandinavica 113: 140–152

Aronen J G, Regan K 1984 Decreasing the incidence of recurrence of first time anterior shoulder dislocations with rehabilitation. American Journal of Sports Medicine 12: 283–291

Aston J W, Gregory C F 1973 Dislocation of the shoulder with significant fracture of the glenoid. Journal of Bone and Joint Surgery 55A: 1531–1533

Babbitt D P, Cassidy R H 1968 Obstetrical paralysis and dislocation of the shoulder in infancy. Journal of Bone and Joint Surgery 50A: 1447–1452

Baker D M, Stryker W S 1965 Acute complete acromioclavicular separation. Journal of the American Medical Association 192: 105–108

Bargren J H, Erlanger S, Dick H M 1978 Biomechanics and comparison of two operative methods of treatment of complete acromioclavicular separation. Clinical Orthopaedics 130: 267–272

Bassett R W, Cofield R H 1983 Acute tears of the rotator cuff. Clinical Orthopaedics 175: 18–24

Bateman J E 1973 Cuff tears in athletes. Orthopaedic Clinics of North America 4: 721–745

Baxter M P, Wiley J J 1986 Fractures of the proximal humeral epiphysis. Journal of Bone and Joint Surgery 68B: 570–573

Beckman T 1923 Simultaneous luxation of both ends of clavicle. Acta Chirurgica Scandinavica 56: 156–163

Benchetit E, Friedman B 1979 Fracture of the coracoid process associated with subglenoid dislocation of the shoulder. Journal of Bone and Joint Surgery 61A: 295

Benton J, Nelson C 1971 Avulsion of the coracoid process in an athlete. Journal of Bone and Joint Surgery 53A: 356–358

Bernard T N, Brunet M E, Haddad R J 1983 Fractured coracoid process in acromioclavicular dislocations. Clinical Orthopaedics 175: 227–232

Bernstein S A (1963) Pseudarthrosis of the shoulder joint. Journal of Bone and Joint Surgery 45A: 216

Berson B L, Gilbert M S, Green S 1978 Acromioclavicular dislocations. Clinical Orthopaedics 135: 157–164

Bjerneld H, Hovelius L, Thorling J 1983 Acromioclavicular separations treated conservatively. Acta Orthopaedica Scandinavica 54: 743–745

Blazina M E, Satzman J S 1969 Recurrent anterior subluxation of the shoulder in athletics — a distinct entity. Journal of Bone and Joint Surgery 51A: 1037–1038

Bonnet J 1975 Fracture of the clavicle. Archivum Chirurgicum Neerlandicum 27: 143–151

Booth C M, Roper B A 1979 Chronic dislocation of the sternoclavicular joint. Clinical Orthopaedics 140: 17–20

Boucher P R, Morton K S 1968 Rupture of the distal biceps brachii tendon. Journal of Bone and Joint Surgery 50B: 436

Brooks A L, Hennings G D 1972 Injury to the proximal clavicular epiphysis. Journal of Bone and Joint Surgery 48A: 386

Brown J E 1961 Anterior sternoclavicular dislocation. A method of repair. American Journal of Orthopaedics 6: 184–189

Brown R 1927 Backward and inward dislocation of the clavicle. Surgical Clinics of North America 7: 1263

Buckerfield C T, Castle M E 1984 Acute traumatic retrosternal dislocation of the clavicle. Journal of Bone and Joint Surgery 66A: 379–385

Cahill B R 1982 Osteolysis of the distal part of the clavicle in male athletes. Journal of Bone and Joint Surgery 64A: 1053–1058

Cassels R E, Hamilton L R 1967 Rupture of the biceps brachii. Journal of Bone and Joint Surgery 49A: 1016

Cave A J E 1961 The nature and morphology of the costoclavicular ligament. Journal of Anatomy 95: 170–179

Chattopadhyaya P K 1970 Posterior fracture-dislocation of the shoulder. Journal of Bone and Joint Surgery 52B: 521–523

Clark R L, Milgram J W, Yawn D H 1974 Fatal aortic perforation and cardiac tamponade due to a Kirschner wire migrating from the right sternoclavicular joint. Southern Medical Journal 67: 316–318

Clifford P C 1981 Fractures of the neck of the humerus: a review of the late results. Injury 12: 91–95

Cofield R H 1985 Rotator cuff disease of the shoulder. Journal of Bone and Joint Surgery 67A: 974–979

Cofield R H, Lanzer W L 1985 Rotator cuff repair, results related to surgical pathology. Orthopaedic Transactions 9(3): 466

Craig E V 1984 The posterior mechanism of acute anterior shoulder dislocations. Clinical Orthopaedics 190: 212–216

Crenshaw A H 1987 Delayed union and non-union of fractures. In: Campbell's operative orthopaedics, 7th edn. CV Mosby, St Louis, Missouri, pp 2093–2094

Dameron T B, Reibel D B 1969 Fractures involving the proximal humeral epiphyseal plate. Journal of Bone and Joint Surgery 51A: 289–297

Dawe C J 1980 Acromioclavicular joint injuries. Journal of Bone and Joint Surgery 62B: 269

Day A J, MacDonnell J A, Pederson H E 1963 Recurrent anterior dislocation of the shoulder. Clinical Orthopaedics 45: 123–126

Denham R H, Dingley A F 1967 Epiphyseal separation of the medial end of the clavicle. Journal of Bone and Joint Surgery 49A: 1179–1183

De Orio J K, Cofield R H 1984 Results of a second attempt at surgical repair of a failed initial rotator-cuff repair. Journal of Bone and Joint Surgery 66A: 563–567

DePalma A F, Cantilli R A 1961 Fractures of the upper end of the humerus. Clinical Orthopaedics 20: 73–93

De Rosa G P, Kettelkamp D B 1977 Fracture of the coracoid process of the scapula. Journal of Bone and Joint Surgery 59A: 696–697

Desmarchais J E, Mauriad G, Benazet J P 1984 Treatment of complex fractures of the proximal humerus by Neer hemiarthroplasty. Journal of Bone and Joint Surgery 66B: 296

Deterbeck L C, Barnhart J M 1976 Complete dislocations of the acromioclavicular joint treated by mersilene tapping. Journal of Bone and Joint Surgery 58A: 280

Einarsson F 1958 Fractures of the upper end of the humerus. Acta Orthopaedica Scandinavica (suppl.) 32: 131–142

Ekström T, Lagergren C, von Schreeb T 1965 Procaine injections and early mobilisation for fractures of the neck of the humerus. Acta Chirurgica Scandinavica 130: 18–24

English E, MacNab I 1974 Recurrent posterior dislocation of the shoulder. Canadian Journal of Surgery 17: 147–151

Ferry A M, Rook F W, Masterson J H 1957 Retrosternal dislocation of the clavicle. Journal of Bone and Joint Surgery 39A: 905–910

Findlay R T 1981 Fractures of the scapula. Annals of Surgery 93: 1001–1008

Findlay R T 1987 Fractures of the scapula and ribs. American Journal of Surgery 38: 489–494

Fowler A W 1966 In: Report of ABC travelling fellows. Journal of Bone and Joint Surgery 48A: 386

Fraser R L, Haliburton R A, Barber J R 1967 Displaced epiphyseal fractures of the proximal humerus. Canadian Journal of Surgery 10: 427–430

Froimson A I 1978 Fracture of the coracoid process of the scapula. Journal of Bone and Joint Surgery 60A: 710–711

Froncioni J, Lenczner E 1985 Injuries to the distal biceps tendon. Journal of Bone and Joint Surgery 67B: 329

Galpin R D, Hawkins R J, Grainger R W 1985 A comparative analysis of operative versus nonoperative treatment of grade III acromioclavicular separations. Clinical Orthopaedics 193: 150–155

Garcia-Elias M, Salo J M 1985 Non-union of a fractured coracoid process after dislocation of the shoulder. Journal of Bone and Joint Surgery 67B: 722–723

Gearen P F, Petty W 1982 Panclavicular dislocation. Report of a case. Journal of Bone and Joint Surgery 64A: 454–455

Ghormley R K, Black J R, Cherry J H 1941 Ununited fractures of the clavicle. American Journal of Surgery 51: 343–349

Gilcreest E L 1934 The common syndrome of rupture, dislocation and elongation of the long head of the biceps brachii. Surgery, Gynaecology and Obstetrics 58: 322–340

Gillespie H S 1964 Excision of the outer end of the clavicle for dislocation of the acromioclavicular joint. Canadian Journal of Surgery 7: 18–20

Glick J M, Milburn L J, Haggerty J F, Nishimoto D 1977 Dislocated acromioclavicular joint: follow-up study of 35 unreduced acromioclavicular dislocations. American Journal of Sports Medicine 5: 264–270

Ha'eri G R 1986 Boytchev procedure for the treatment of anterior shoulder instability. Clinical Orthopaedics 206: 196–201

Halley D K, Olix M L 1975 A review of the Bristow operation for recurrent anterior subluxation and dislocation in athletes. Clinical Orthopaedics 106: 175–179

Halpern A A, Joseph R, Page J, Nagel D A 1979 Subclavian artery injury and fracture of the scapula. Journal of the American College of Emergency Physicians 8: 19–20

Hardegger F H, Simpsom L A, Weber B G 1984 The operative treatment of scapular fractures. Journal of Bone and Joint Surgery 66B: 725–731

Hastings D E, Coughlin L P 1981 Recurrent subluxation of the glenohumeral joint. American Journal of Sports Medicine 9: 352–355

Hastings D E, Horne J G 1977 Anterior dislocation of the acromioclavicular joint. Journal of Bone and Joint Surgery 59B: 507

Hawkins R J, Koppert G, Johnston G 1984 Recurrent posterior instability (subluxation) of the shoulder. Journal of Bone and Joint Surgery 66A: 169–174

Hawkins R J, Misamore G W, Hobeika P E 1985 Surgery for full thickness rotator cuff tears. Journal of Bone and Joint Surgery 67A: 1349–1355

Hawkins R J, Bell R H, Gurr K 1986 The three-part fracture of the proximal part of the humerus. Journal of Bone and Joint Surgery 68A: 1410–1414

Hawkins R J, Bell R H, Hawkins R H, Koppert G J 1986 Anterior dislocation of the shoulder in the older patient. Clinical Orthopaedics 206: 192–195

Hawkins R J, Neer C S, Pianta R M, Mendoza F X 1987 Locked posterior dislocation of the shoulder. Journal of Bone and Joint Surgery 69A: 9–18

Heckman J D, Levine M I 1978 Traumatic closed transection of the biceps brachii in the military parachutist. Journal of Bone and Joint Surgery 60A: 369–372

Heikel H V 1968 Rupture of the rotator cuff of the shoulder. Acta Orthopaedica Scandinavica 39: 477–492

Heinig C F 1968 Retrosternal dislocation of the clavicle. Journal of Bone and Joint Surgery 50A: 830

Hejna W F, Fossier C H, Goldstan T B, Ray R D 1969 Ancient anterior dislocation of the shoulder. Journal of Bone and Joint Surgery 51A: 1030–1031

Henry J H, Genung J A 1982 Natural history of glenohumeral dislocation — revisited. American Journal of Sports Medicine 10: 135–137

Hovelius L 1982 Incidence of shoulder dislocation in Sweden. Clinical Orthopaedics 166: 127–131

Hovelius L 1987 Anterior dislocation of the shoulder in teenagers and young adults. Journal of Bone and Joint Surgery 69A: 393–399

Hovelius L, Thorling J, Fredin H 1979 Recurrent anterior dislocation of the shoulder. Journal of Bone and Joint Surgery 61A: 566–569

Hovelius L, Lind B, Thorling J 1982 Primary dislocation of the shoulder. Clinical Orthopaedics 176: 181–185

Hovelius L, Akermark C, Albrektsson B 1983 Bristow–Latarjet procedure for recurrent anterior dislocation of the shoulder. Acta Orthopaedica Scandinavica 54: 284–290

Hovelius L, Eriksson K, Fredin H 1983 Recurrences after initial dislocation of the shoulder. Journal of Bone and Joint Surgery 65A: 343–349

Howard F M, Shafer S J 1965 Injuries to the clavicle with neurovascular complications. Journal of Bone and Joint Surgery 47A: 1335–1346

Imatani R J, Hanlon J J, Cady G W 1975 Acute, complete acromioclavicular separation. Journal of Bone and Joint Surgery 57A: 328–332

Ishizuki M, Yamaura I, Isobe Y, Furuya K, Tanabe K, Nagatsuka Y 1981 Avulsion fracture of the superior border of the scapula. Journal of Bone and Joint Surgery 63A: 820–822

Jacobs P 1984 Post-traumatic osteolysis of the outer end of the clavicle. Journal of Bone and Joint Surgery 46B: 705–707

Jacobs B, Wade P A 1966 Acromioclavicular joint injury. Journal of Bone and Joint Surgery 48A: 475–486

Jain A S 1984 Traumatic floating clavicle. A case report. Journal of Bone and Joint Surgery 66B: 560–561

Johnson E W, Collins H R 1963 Nonunion of the clavicle. Archives of Surgery 87: 963–966

Kappakas G S, McMaster J H 1978 Repair of acromioclavicular separation using a Dacron prosthesis graft. Clinical Orthopaedics 131: 247–251

Kavanagh T G, Sarkar S D, Phillips H 1985 Complications of displaced fractures (type II Neer) of the outer end of the clavicle. Journal of Bone and Joint Surgery 67B: 492–493

Kawabe N, Watanabe R, Sato M 1984 Treatment of complete acromioclavicular separation by coracoacromial ligament transfer. Clinical Orthopaedics 185: 222–227

Kazar B, Relovszky E 1969 Prognosis of primary dislocation of the shoulder. Acta Orthopaedica Scandinavica 40: 216–224

Kennedy J C 1949 Retrosternal dislocation of the clavicle. Journal of Bone and Joint Surgery 31B: 74–75

Kennedy J C, Cameron H 1954 Complete dislocation of the acromioclavicular joint. Journal of Bone and Joint Surgery 36B: 202–208

Kessel L 1982 In: Clinical disorders of the shoulder. Churchill Livingstone, Edinburgh

Khan A A, Lucas H K 1978 Plating of fractures of the middle third of the clavicle. Injury 9: 263–267

Kiviluoto O, Pasila M, Jaroma H, Sundholm A 1980 Immobilisation after primary dislocation of the shoulder. Acta Orthopaedica Scandinavica 51: 915–919

Knight R A, Mayne J A 1957 Comminuted fractures and fracture-dislocations involving the articular surface of the humeral head. Journal of Bone and Joint Surgery 39A: 1343–1355

Kraulis J, Hunter G 1976 The results of prosthetic replacement in fracture-dislocations of the upper end of the humerus. Injury 8: 129–131

Kristiansen B, Christensen S W 1986 Plate fixation of proximal humeral fractures. Acta Orthopaedica Scandinavica 57: 320–323

Kristiansen B, Kofoed H 1987 External fixation of displaced fractures of the proximal humerus. Journal of Bone and Joint Surgery 69B: 643–646

Kummel B M 1970 Fractures of the glenoid causing chronic dislocation of the shoulder. Clinical Orthopaedics 69: 189–191

Labnola J H, Mohaghegh H A 1975 Isolated avulsion fracture of the lesser tuberosity of the humerus. Journal of Bone and Joint Surgery 57A: 1011

Larsen E, Bjerg-Nielsen A, Christensen P 1986 Conservative or surgical treatment of acromioclavicular dislocation. Journal of Bone and Joint Surgery 68A: 552–555

Laskin R S, Sedhin E D 1971 Luxatio erecta in infancy. Clinical Orthopaedics 80: 126–129

Lazcano M A, Anzel S H, Kelly P J 1961 Complete dislocation and subluxation of the acromioclavicular joint. Journal of Bone and Joint Surgery 43A: 379–391

Lentz W, Meuser P 1980 The treatment of fractures of the proximal humerus. Archives of Orthopaedics and Traumatic Surgery 96: 283–285

Levine A H, Pais M J, Schwartz E E 1976 Post traumatic osteolysis of the distal clavicle with emphasis on early radiologic changes. American Journal of Roentgenology 127: 781–784

Leyshon R L 1984 Closed treatment of fractures of the proximal humerus. Acta Orthopaedica Scandinavica 55: 48–51

Lundberg B J, Svenungson-Hartwig E, Wikmark R 1979 Independent exercises versus physiotherapy in non displaced proximal humeral fractures. Scandinavian Journal of Rehabilitation Medicine 11: 133–136

Lunseth P A, Chapman K W, Frankel V H 1975 Surgical treatment of chronic dislocation of the sternoclavicular joint. Journal of Bone and Joint Surgery 57B: 193–196

Macpherson I, Crossan J F, Allister C A 1983 Unstable fractures of the greater tuberosity of the humerus. Journal of Bone and Joint Surgery 65B: 225

Malcapi C, Grassi G, Oretti D 1978 Posterior dislocation of the acromioclavicular joint: a rare or an easily overlooked lesion? Italian Journal of Orthopaedics and Traumatology 4: 79–88

Manske D J, Szabo R M 1985 The operative treatment of midshaft clavicular non unions. Journal of Bone and Joint Surgery 67A: 1367–1371

Marsh H O, Hazarion E 1970 Pseudarthrosis of the clavicle. Journal of Bone and Joint Surgery 52B: 793

McBride E D, Sisler J 1965 Fractures of the proximal humeral epiphysis and the juxta-epiphyseal humeral shaft. Clinical Orthopaedics 38: 143–153

McGahan J P, Rab G T 1980 Fracture of the acromion associated with an axillary nerve deficit. Clinical Orthopaedics 147: 216–218

McKenzie J M M 1963 Retrosternal dislocation of the clavicle. A report of two cases. Journal of Bone and Joint Surgery 45B: 138–141

McLennan J G, Ungersma J 1982 Pneumothorax complicating fracture of the scapula. Journal of Bone and Joint Surgery 64A: 598–599

Mehta J C, Sachder A, Collins J J 1973 Retrosternal dislocation of the clavicle. Injury 5: 79–83

Mills H J, Horne G 1985 Fractures of the proximal humerus in adults. Journal of Trauma 25: 801–805

Mills K L G 1974 Severe injuries of the upper end of the humerus. Injury 6: 13–21

Montgomery S P, Loyd R D 1977 Avulsion fracture of the coracoid epiphysis with acromioclavicular separation. Journal of Bone and Joint Surgery 59A: 963–965

Moore T O 1951 Internal pin fixation for fracture of the clavicle. American Surgeon 17: 580–583

Morrey B F, Jones J M 1976 Recurrent anterior dislocation of the shoulder. Journal of Bone and Joint Surgery 58A: 252–256

Moseley H F, Templeton J 1969 Dislocation of the acromio-clavicular joint. Journal of Bone and Joint Surgery 51B: 196

Neer C S 1960 Nonunion of the clavicle. Journal of the American Medical Association 172: 1006–1011

Neer C S 1963 Prosthetic replacement of the humeral head. Surgical Clinics of North America 43: 1581–1597

Neer C S 1968 Fractures of the distal third of the clavicle. Clinical Orthopaedics 58: 43–50

Neer C S 1970a Displaced proximal humeral fractures. Part 1. Classification and evaluation. Journal of Bone and Joint Surgery 52A: 1077–1089

Neer C S 1970b Displaced proximal humeral fractures. Part 2. Treatment of three-part and four-part displacement. Journal of Bone and Joint Surgery 52A: 1090–1103

Neer C S 1984 Fractures and dislocations of the shoulder. In: Rockwood C A, Green D P, (eds), Fractures in adults. J B Lippincott, Philadelphia, pp 675–721

Neer C S, Horowitz B S 1965 Fractures of the proximal humeral epiphysial plate. Clinical Orthopaedics 41: 24–31

Nettles J L, Linscheid R L 1968 Sternoclavicular dislocations. Journal of Trauma 8: 158–164

Neviaser J S 1952 Acromioclavicular dislocation treated by transference of the coracoacromial ligament. Archives of Surgery 64: 292–297

Neviaser J S 1963 The treatment of old unreduced dislocations of the shoulder. Surgical Clinics of North America 43: 1671–1678

Neviaser J S 1980 Injuries to the clavicle and its articulations. Orthopedic Clinics of North America 11: 233–237

Neviaser R J, Neviaser J S, Neviaser T J, Neviaser J S 1975 A simple technique for internal fixation of the clavicle. Clinical Orthopaedics 109: 103–107

Nilsson S, Svartholm F 1965 Fracture of the upper end of the humerus in children. Acta Chirurgica Scandinavica 130: 433–439

Nixon J E, DiStefano V 1975 Ruptures of the rotator cuff. Orthopedic Clinics of North America 6: 423–447

Norman W H 1985 Repair of avulsion of insertion of biceps brachii tendon. Clinical Orthopaedics 193: 189–194

Nogi J, Heckman J D, Hakala M, Sweet D E 1975 Non union of the clavicle in a child. Clinical Orthopaedics 110: 19–21

Ogden J A 1984 Distal clavicular physeal injury. Clinical Orthopaedics 188: 68–73

Omer G E 1967 Osteotomy of the clavicle in surgical reduction of anterior sternoclavicular dislocation. Journal of Trauma 7: 584–590

Oreck S L, Burgess A, Levine A M 1984 Traumatic lateral displacement of the scapula: a radiographic sign of neurovascular disruption. Journal of Bone and Joint Surgery 66A: 758–763

Paavolainen P, Bjorkenheim J M, Slätis P, Pauku P 1983 Operative treatment of severe proximal humeral fractures. Acta Orthopaedica Scandinavica 54: 374–379

Packer N P, Calvert P T, Bayley J I L, Kessel L 1983 Operative treatment of chronic ruptures of the rotator cuff of the shoulder. Journal of Bone and Joint Surgery 65B: 171–175

Paffen P J, Jansen E W L 1978 Surgical treatment of clavicular fractures with Kirschner wires: a comparative study. Archivum Chirurgicum Neerlandicum 30: 43–53

Paquet R, Desmarchais J E, Benazet J P 1980 Evaluation of the Neer prosthesis for humeral fracture. Journal of Bone and Joint Surgery 62B: 128

Pasila M, Jaroma H, Kiviluoto O, Sundholm A 1978 Early complications of primary shoulder dislocations. Acta Orthopaedica Scandinavica 49: 260–263

Pasila M, Kiviluoto O, Jaroma H, Sundholm A 1980 Recovery from primary shoulder dislocation and its complications. Acta Orthopaedica Scandinavica 51: 257–262

Pate J W, Wilhite J L 1969 Migration of a foreign body from the sternoclavicular joint to the heart. A case report. American Surgeon 35: 448–449

Paterson D C 1961 Retrosternal dislocation of the clavicle. Journal of Bone and Joint Surgery 43B: 90–94

Patterson W R 1967 Inferior dislocation of the distal end of the clavicle. Journal of Bone and Joint Surgery 49A: 1184–1186

Peacock H K, Brandon J R, Jones O L 1970 Retrosternal dislocation of the clavicle. Southern Medical Journal 63: 1324–1328

Penn I 1964 The vascular complications of fractures of the clavicle. Journal of Trauma 4: 819–831

Pierce R O 1979 Internal derangement of the sternoclavicular joint. Clinics in Orthopaedics 141: 247–250

Post M 1980 Fractures of the upper humerus. Orthopedic Clinics of North America 11: 239–252

Post M, Silver R, Singh M 1983 Rotator cuff tear. Clinical Orthopaedics 173: 78–91

Postacchini F, Ricciardi-Pollini P T 1977 Rupture of the short head tendon of the biceps brachii. Clinical Orthopaedics 124: 229–232

Pouget G 1984 Recurrent posterior dislocation of the shoulder treated by glenoid osteotomy. Journal of Bone and Joint Surgery 66B: 140

Powers J A, Bach P J 1974 Acromioclavicular separation. Clinical Orthopaedics 104: 213–223

Prillaman H A, Thompson R C 1969 Bilateral posterior fracture-dislocation of the shoulder. Journal of Bone and Joint Surgery 51A: 1627–1630

Protzman R R 1980 Anterior instability of the shoulder. Journal of Bone and Joint Surgery 62A: 909–918

Pyper J B 1978 Non union of fractures of the clavicle. Injury 9: 268–270

Rao J P, Francis A M, Hurley J, Daczkewycz R 1986 Treatment of recurrent anterior dislocation of the shoulder by du Toit Staple capsulorrhaphy. Clinical Orthopaedics 204: 169–176

Reeves B 1969 Acute anterior dislocation of the shoulder. Annals of the Royal College of Surgeons 44: 255–273

Roberts A, Wickstrom J 1971 Prognosis of posterior dislocation of the shoulder. Acta Orthopaedica Scandinavica 42: 328–337

Rockwood C A 1984a Fractures and dislocations of the shoulder. In: Rockwood C A, Green D P (eds), Fractures in adults. J B Lippincott, Philadelphia, pp 675–985

Rockwood C A 1984b Fractures and dislocations of the shoulder. In: Rockwood C A, Wilkins K E, King R E (eds), Fractures in children. J B Lippincott, Philadelphia, pp 577–682

Roscoe M A, Simmons E H 1984 The treatment of complete acromioclavicular dislocation. Journal of Bone and Joint Surgery 66B: 304

Rosenørm M, Pederson E B 1974 A comparison between conservative and operative treatment of acute acromioclavicular dislocation. Acta Orthopaedica Scandinavica 45: 50–59

Rowe C R 1956 Prognosis in dislocations of the shoulder. Journal of Bone and Joint Surgery 38A: 957–977

Rowe C R 1963 Fractures of the scapula. Surgical Clinics of North America 43: 1565–1571

Rowe C R 1968 An atlas of anatomy and treatment of midclavicular fractures. Clinical Orthopaedics 58: 29–42

Rowe C R 1980 Acute and recurrent anterior dislocations of the shoulder. Orthopedic Clinics of North America 11: 253–270

Rowe C R, Marble H C 1958 Sternoclavicular dislocations in fractures and other injuries. Chicago, Year Book Medical, p 258

Rowe C R, Zarins B 1981 Recurrent transient subluxation of the shoulder. Journal of Bone and Joint Surgery 63A: 863–872

Rowe C R, Zarins B 1982 Chronic unreduced dislocations of the shoulder. Journal of Bone and Joint Surgery 64A: 494–505

Rowe C R, Sakellarides H T 1961 Factors related to recurrences of anterior dislocations of the shoulder. Clinical Orthopaedics 20: 40–48

Sakellarides H 1961 Pseudarthrosis of the clavicle. Journal of Bone and Joint Surgery 43A: 130–138

Salvatore J E 1968 Sternoclavicular joint dislocation. Clinics in Orthopedics 58: 51–55

Samilson R L, Prieto V 1983 Dislocation arthropathy of the shoulder. Journal of Bone and Joint Surgery 65A: 456–460

Savastano A A, Stutz S J 1978 Traumatic sternoclavicular dislocation. International Surgery 63: 10–13

Scheck M 1982 Surgical treatment of non unions of the surgical neck of the humerus. Clinical Orthopaedics 167: 255–259

Selesnick F H, Jablon M, Frank C, Post M 1984 Retrosternal dislocation of the clavicle. Report of four cases. Journal of Bone and Joint Surgery 66A: 287–291

Sherk H H, Probst C 1975 Fractures of the proximal humeral epiphysis. Orthopedic Clinics of North America 6: 401–413

Simonet W T, Cofield R H 1984b Prognosis in anterior shoulder dislocation. American Journal of Sports Medicine 12: 19–24

Simonet W T, Melton L J, Cofield R H, Ilstrup D M 1984a Incidence of anterior shoulder dislocation of Olmsted County, Minnesota. Clinical Orthopaedics 186: 186–191

Simurda M A 1968 Retrosternal dislocation of the clavicle: a report of four cases and a method of repair. Canadian Journal of Surgery 11: 487–490

Sisk T D, Boyd H B 1974 Management of recurrent anterior dislocation of the shoulder. Du Toit type or staple capsulorrhaphy. Clinical Orthopaedics 103: 150–156

Smith D M 1975 Coracoid fracture associated with acromioclavicular dislocation. Clinical Orthopaedics 108: 165–167

Smith F M 1956 Fracture-separation of the proximal humeral epiphysis. American Journal of Surgery 91: 627–635

Smith R G 1963 Rupture of the distal tendon of the biceps brachii. Journal of Bone and Joint Surgery 45B: 628

Solonen K A, Rokkanen P 1972 The results of operative treatment for recurrent dislocation of the gleno-humeral joint. Acta Orthopaedica Scandinavica 43: 101–108

Soto-Hall R, Stroot J H 1960 Treatment of ruptures of the long head of biceps brachii. American Journal of Orthopedics 2: 192

Stableforth P G 1984 Four part fractures of the neck of the humerus. Journal of Bone and Joint Surgery 66B: 104–108

Stahl F 1954 Considerations on post-traumatic absorption of the outer end of the clavicle. Acta Orthopaedica Scandinavica 23: 9–13

Stein A H 1957 Retrosternal dislocation of the clavicle. Journal of Bone and Joint Surgery 39A: 656–660

Stewart M J, Hundley J M 1955 Fractures of the humerus. Journal of Bone and Joint Surgery 37A: 681–692

Sturzenegger M, Fornaro E, Jakob R P 1982 Results of surgical treatment of multifragmented fractures of the humeral head. Archives of Orthopaedics and Trauma Surgery 100: 249–259

Takagishi N 1978 Conservative treatment of the ruptures of the rotator cuff. Journal of the Japanese Orthopaedic Association 52: 781–787

Tanner M W, Cofield R H 1983 Prosthetic arthroplasty for fractures and fracture-dislocations of the proximal humerus. Clinical Orthopaedics 179: 116–128

Taylor A R 1967 Non union of fracture of the clavicle. Journal of Bone and Joint Surgery 49B: 383–384

Taylor A R 1969 Non union of fracture of the clavicle. Journal of Bone and Joint Surgery 51B: 568–569

Tibone J E, Elrod B, Jobe F W 1986 Surgical treatment of tears of the rotator cuff in athletes. Journal of Bone and Joint Surgery 68A: 887–891

Tossy J D, Mead N C, Sigmond H M 1963 Acromioclavicular separations: useful and practical classification for treatment. Clinical Orthopaedics 28: 111–119

Tregonning G, MacNab I 1976 Post-traumatic pseudarthrosis of the clavicle. Journal of Bone and Joint Surgery 58B: 264

Vidal J, Orst G, Denis P, Reboul C, Mamay T, Deguillaume P 1984 The Bankart procedure: its reliability among sportsmen. Journal of Bone and Joint Surgery 66B: 140

Wall J J 1970 Congenital pseudarthrosis of the clavicle. Journal of Bone and Joint Surgery 52A: 1003–1009

Wallace W A, Wiley A M 1986 The long-term results of conservative management of full thickness tears of the rotator cuff. Journal of Bone and Joint Surgery 68B: 162

Watson M 1985 Major ruptures of the rotator cuff. Journal of Bone and Joint Surgery 67B: 618–624

Waugh R L, Hathcock T A, Elliott J L 1949 Ruptures of muscles and tendons with particular reference to rupture or elongation of long tendon of biceps brachii. Surgery 25: 370–392

Weaver J K, Dunn H K 1972 Treatment of acromioclavicular injuries, especially complete acromioclavicular separations. Journal of Bone and Joint Surgery 54A: 1187–1194

Weiner D S, MacNab I 1970 Ruptures of the rotator cuff. Canadian Journal of Surgery 13: 219–227

Werner H H, Reimers J 1972 The operative treatment of recurrent anterior dislocation of the shoulder. Acta Orthopaedica Scandinavica 43: 375–383

Wheeler M E, Laaveg S J, Sprague B L 1979 Sternoclavicular joint disruption in an infant. Clinics in Orthopedics 139: 68–69

Wilber M C, Evans E B 1977 Fractures of the scapula. Journal of Bone and Joint Surgery 59A: 358–362

Wilkins R M, Johnston R M 1983 Ununited fractures of the clavicle. Journal of Bone and Joint Surgery 65A: 773–778

Wilkinson J A, Thomas W G 1985 Glenoid osteotomy for recurrent posterior dislocations of the shoulder. Journal of Bone and Joint Surgery 67B: 496

Willems W J, Lim T E A 1985 Neer arthroplasty for humeral fracture. Acta Orthopaedica Scandinavica 56: 394–395

Wolfgang G L 1978 Rupture of the musculotendinous cuff of the shoulder. Clinical Orthopaedics 134: 230–243

Worcester J N, Green D P Osteoarthritis of the acromioclavicular joint. Clinical Orthopaedics 58: 69–73

Yoneda B, Welsh R P, MacIntosh D L 1982 Conservative treatment of shoulder dislocation in young males. Journal of Bone and Joint Surgery 64B: 254–255

Young T B, Wallace W A 1985 Conservative treatment of fractures and fracture-dislocations of the upper end of the humerus. Journal of Bone and Joint Surgery 67B: 373–377

Zdravkovic D, Damholt V V 1974 Comminuted and severely displaced fractures of the scapula. Acta Orthopaedica Scandinavica 45: 60–65

Zenni E J, Kreig J K, Rosen M J 1981 Open reduction and internal fixation of clavicular fractures. Journal of Bone and Joint Surgery 63A: 147–151

Zilberman Z, Rejovitzky R 1981 Fracture of the coracoid process of the scapula. Injury 13: 203–206

Zlotsky N A, Ballard A 1966 Acromioclavicular injuries in athletes. Journal of Bone and Joint Surgery 48A: 1224–1225

4. The humerus

P. S. Fagg

INTRODUCTION

The shaft of the humerus is that part below the surgical neck and above the level of the epicondyles. The classification of these fractures is based on their anatomical location and the fracture pattern.

Fractures of the shaft of the humerus are uncommon. In 1958, Emmett & Breck stated that they had encountered only 166 fractures of the shaft of the humerus — approximately 1% of the 11 000 fractures seen in their practice.

Conservative management

In 1933 Caldwell introduced his concept of the hanging cast to produce dependent traction in the treatment of humeral shaft fractures. Prior to this, the humerus was the most common site of non-union. Many orthopaedic surgeons felt that the hanging cast was the treatment of choice for fractures of the humeral shaft at all anatomical levels. Some authors, however, considered that in certain circumstances the hanging cast was implicated as a contributory factor in the causation of non-union (Coventry & Laurnen 1970, Holm 1970).

Brachial U-splints (Klenerman 1966, Cartner 1973, Mast et al 1975), sugartong splints (Comfort 1973), or humeral braces (Sarmiento et al 1977, Balfour et al 1982) have been favoured by other surgeons because these methods stabilized the fractured bone without adding sufficient weight to cause distraction at the fracture site.

Lateral or overhead traction is not commonly used now, although it still has a place in the treatment of patients who have sustained other, often multiple injuries, or who have associated medical problems which mitigate against ambulatory treatment (Holm 1970, Vichare 1974, Mast et al 1975).

Thoracobrachial body casts are reserved, by those who use them, for special circumstances such as very comminuted, unstable fractures, although their use in the past was more widespread.

It can be seen that no single method of treatment is used for the conservative management of humeral shaft fractures, although these methods of treatment do seem to fall into the four main groups mentioned above — hanging cast, humeral splints or braces, traction and thoraco-brachial casts.

Hanging cast

The hanging cast gained widespread popularity in the USA after its introduction by Caldwell in 1933. In 1940 Caldwell reported 4 cases of delayed union and 1 of non-union in a series of 59 humeral fractures treated by this method. Its acceptance in the UK was less enthusiastic, no doubt due to the comments of Watson-Jones in *Fractures and Joint Injuries* (as quoted in Thompson et al 1965) in which he described it as a heavy plaster cast from the wrist to the axilla — sometimes even weighted with lumps of lead — slung and suspended from the neck. In *The Closed Treatment of Common Fractures* (1961), Charnley observed that the hanging cast method was open to serious mechanical criticism and that it readily produced over-distraction of the humerus.

However the published results of humeral shaft fractures treated by this method suggested that these pessimistic comments by the English authorities were misplaced. Table 4.1 records the incidence of delayed union and non-union after this method of treatment of humeral shaft fractures. It can be noted that Laferte & Rosenbaum (1937) reported no case of non-union in 58 fractures. In 1965 Mann & Neal reported the highest incidence of non-union — 6.5%. Thompson et al (1965) noted fragment distraction in some of these cases but found that these distracted fractures also healed solidly.

The average period of immobilization varied between 6 weeks (Laferte & Rosenbaum 1937, Stewart & Hundley 1955, Mann & Neal 1965) and 10 weeks (Scientific Research Committee, Pennsylvania Orthopaedic Society 1959). Mann & Neal reported that radiological union occurred in an average of 12.1 weeks.

Table 4.1 The incidence of delayed union and non-union after the hanging cast treatment of humeral shaft fractures

Reference	Number of patients	Number of delayed union	Number of non-union
Laferte & Rosenbaum (1937)	58		0
Caldwell (1940)	59	4 (6.8%)	1 (1.7%)
Stewart & Hundley (1955)	107		3 (2.8%)
Scientific Research Committee, Pennsylvania Orthopedic Society (1959)	69		3 (4.3%)
Mann & Neal (1965)	77		5 (6.5%)
Thompson et al (1965)	103*	1 (1%)	2 (1.9%)

*Includes 41 surgical neck fractures and 6 supracondylar fractures.

In 1955 Stewart & Hundley reported 81.3% excellent and 12.2% good results out of their 107 fractures. Excellent results had no pain or impairment of function and no radiological evidence of deformity. Good results had no pain or functional impairment for ordinary use, but 20% or less limitation of motion in the elbow or shoulder and angulation of not more than 10°. Laferte & Rosenbaum (1937) reported that 75% of their patients had an excellent functional result, and 82% had excellent radiological alignment.

Humeral splints or braces

The recent trend in the treatment of humeral shaft fractures has been away from hanging casts towards some form of humeral splinting by U-slab (Klenerman 1966), functional humeral brace (Sarmiento et al 1977), or by sugartong splints (Comfort 1973).

Table 4.2 records the incidence of delayed union and non-union by these methods of treatment. Klenerman's (1966) definition of delayed union — the absence of clinical union 8 weeks after fracture — has been used. The Scientific Research Committee, Pennsylvania Orthopedic Society (1959) reported 3 cases of non-union out of 26 cases (11.5%), but this figure is much higher than that of other published series.

The average healing time reported in these papers was similar to that reported for the hanging cast method. Bohler (1965) reported that union occurred in an average of 6–8 weeks, and Klenerman (1966) reported that 76% of fractures healed in this time. Sarmiento et al (1977) quoted 8.5 weeks as the healing time following the use of his functional brace and Cartner (1973) reported it as 9 weeks after using a U-slab and Gilchrist sling.

A comparison of the functional end-results recorded in these papers is difficult due to the different criteria adopted by the authors to assess their results. In 1966 Klenerman reported that 70% of his patients had an

Table 4.2 The incidence of delayed union and non-union with humeral splints and braces for humeral shaft fractures

Reference	Method	Number of patients	Number of delayed union	Number of non-union
Scientific Research Committee, Pennsylvania Orthopedic Society (1959)	Various	26		3 (11.5%)
Bohler (1965)	Desault cast	1019		4 (0.4%)
Klenerman (1966)	U-slab	87	8 (9.2%)	0
Cartner (1973)	U-slab	42		0
Mast et al (1975)	Sling and reverse sugartong splint	70	11 (15%)	4 (5%)

excellent result and 20% had a good result (90% in total). Balfour et al (1982) reported 81% excellent or good results, and Mast et al (1975) recorded 84% excellent and 8% satisfactory results using a modified Neer protocol, and slightly better results (80% excellent and 10% satisfactory) using an AEF (anatomy, economy, function) score. In 1982 Hunter reported 63% excellent and 27% good (90% total) in his 51 fractures assessed for function.

Traction

The use of either skin or skeletal traction in the management of the fractured humeral shaft is reserved for those patients with complex comminuted fractures or those who have alternative injuries which contraindicate ambulatory treatment.

In 1974 Vichare reported on 32 patients with multiple injuries including humeral shaft fracture. Describing his technique of skin traction as used on 5 patients, he stated that the fractures all united within 6 weeks with no deformity. In 1970 Holm reported 2 instances of non-union in his 12 patients with complex or compound humeral fractures treated by traction; the Scientific Research Committee, Pennsylvania Orthopedic Society (1959) had 1 non-union of 18 patients treated by either skin or skeletal traction.

Thoracobrachial cast

The use of a thoracobrachial cast is not now favoured in the routine treatment of humeral shaft fractures, but may still be used for complex injuries. The largest reported series appears to be that by Stewart & Hundley in 1955 who described the use of thoracobrachial cast in 53 cases. Of this number, 84.9% required a general anaesthetic during application, and the average period of immobilization was 10.4 weeks. Of the 9 cases reported by Vichare in 1974, 77.7% united in 10 weeks, and the Scientific Research Committee, Pennsylvania Orthopedic Group (1959) reported that the average healing time in 14 cases was 13 weeks. Stewart & Hundley (1955) and Vichare (1974) both reported 1 case of non-union whilst the Pennsylvania group had none. Stewart & Hundley (1955) found that 71.7% of their patients had an excellent or good result.

Results of conservative management related to compound injuries and anatomical site

Compound injuries. There is little in the literature on the results of the conservative management of compound fractures of the humeral shaft. Most series include compound fractures but fail to report the results seperately, or to suggest any major problems in their treatment.

The Scientific Research Committee, Pennsylvania Orthopedic Society (1959) included 10% compound injuries in their total of 159 cases. The healing time for these conservatively treated compound injuries averaged

13 weeks, as compared to an average of 12 weeks for the group as a whole. Of the 13 non-unions in the whole series, 3 (18.75%) occurred in compound fractures. Mann & Neal (1965) reported 1 non-union and 1 wound infection out of 20 compound fractures.

Anatomical site. In 1970 Holm reported that all non-unions in his series developed in transverse or short oblique mid-shaft fractures in young adults. In 1956 Laing reported the constancy of the arterial supply to the adult humerus at the junction of the middle and lower third and suggested that fractures at this level would probably destroy the main nutrient artery at the time of injury. This would result in the proximal end of the lower fragment depending for its arterial blood supply on vessels entering from the periosteum and ascending from the epicondyles. This might prejudice the results of internal fixation at this level but might not be so significant in conservatively treated fractures.

Klenerman (1966) reported 5 examples of delayed union out of 44 middle third fractures (11.3%); 2 of these had been treated by internal fixation. However, there were also 2 delayed unions out of 22 proximal third fractures (11%), and 1 out of 17 (5.9%) in the distal third. Mann & Neal (1965) reported non-union in 5 of 29 proximal fractures (17.2%), 4 of 52 (7.7%) middle third fractures and 1 of 15 (5.8%) distal third fractures.

Radiological alignment and functional end-result in humeral shaft fractures

Reporting on his extensive experience of the conservative management of humeral shaft fractures, Bohler in 1965 stated that: 'attaining adequate shortening of 1 to 10 mm is the most important task in fracture treatment. In transverse humeral shaft fractures, lateral displacement the full width of the shaft and shortening are functionally and cosmetically of no importance.'

In 1966 Klenerman reported that residual varus angulation occurred at the fracture site irrespective of its level, and that posterior bowing was found more often than anterior bowing. He found that anterior bowing of 20° or varus angulation of 30° could be present before deformity became clinically obvious and even then the function of the limb was good.

In 1982 Hunter confirmed this tendency to residual varus and posterior bowing and further found that the initial deformities of angulation and length were considerably reduced by treatment (with a U-slab), whether or not the fracture was manipulated. Thus it can be seen that accurate alignment is not essential for a good functional end-result. Rotation is probably the most important deformity to correct; Klenerman points out that this rotational deformity is prevented by supporting the hand on the lower part of the chest.

In a study of Royal Air Force personnel compiled in 1944, Doran reported that the power of the limb could be restored provided that the elbow permitted a total range of flexion and extension of about 70°. He stated that power did not recover with 'free use', even though the range of elbow movements was full. In the great majority of cases he found power to be restored to 75% of normal or better in an average of 4–6 weeks by resistance exercises. In 1975 Mast et al assessed 26 patients on a Cybex machine; only 2 of the 26 had an unsatisfactory functional result.

Summary

1. The incidence of non-union after hanging cast treatment of humeral shaft fractures was between 2.8 and 6.5%. Immobilization was required for 6–10 weeks and radiological union was seen at about 12 weeks.
2. Excellent or near normal function was found in 75–85% of humeral shaft fractures treated by the hanging cast method.
3. The average period of immobilization of humeral shaft fractures by humeral splints was 6–8 weeks, and the incidence of non-union was between 0.4 and 11.5%.
4. Excellent or near normal function was found in 80–90% of patients with humeral shaft fractures treated by humeral splints.
5. After the use of a thoracobrachial cast for humeral shaft fractures the average period of immobilization was 10–13 weeks. Excellent or good results occurred in 71.7%. The non-union rate varied from 1.8 to 11% with more complex injuries.
6. Compound humeral shaft fractures heal slightly slower than closed fractures and the incidence of non-union was higher, at 5–18.5%.
7. The delayed and non-union rate of proximal humeral fractures was 11–17%; of middle third fractures it was 7.5–11% and for lower third fractures it was about 6%.
8. Anterior bowing of 20°, varus angulation of 30° and complete lateral displacement did not alter the final outcome.

PRIMARY OPERATIVE MANAGEMENT

Primary operative management as the treatment of choice in humeral shaft fractures has not been championed by many. Early reports in the literature were almost unanimous in showing the inferior results of primary internal fixation compared with conservative treatment. In 1959 the Scientific Research Committee, of the Pennsylvania Orthopedic Society reported non-union rates of 9.4% after intramedullary fixation, 14.3% after screw fixation and 28.6% after the use of plates. The average healing time for this operative group as a whole was 17 weeks as compared with 12 weeks after closed treatment. In 1967 Christensen confirmed the longer disability time and the greater chance of non-union and secondary paresis of the radial nerve following surgery.

Even renowned exponents of internal fixation agree that the majority of closed humeral shaft fractures should be treated conservatively (Ruedi et al 1974). However, operative management does have its part to play in the treatment of humeral shaft fractures. The indications for open reduction and internal fixation of fractures of the humeral shaft include:

1. Multiple injured patients with humeral fracture.
2. Compound fractures.
3. Fractures with associated vascular or neural injury.
4. Injuries of the shoulder, elbow or forearm in the same limb.
5. Bilateral upper limb fractures.
6. Pathological fractures.
7. Failure of closed methods of treatment.

Operative fixation falls into three main groups:

1. Intramedullary fixation.
2. Plate fixation.
3. External fixation.

Intramedullary fixation

In 1986, Brumback et al reported that 55 out of 58 fractures (94%), treated by an intramedullary device, united in an average of 10.5 weeks (range 6–18 weeks). Three patients (6%) had delayed union requiring secondary plating and bone grafting — all resulted in union. The majority of these fractures were stabilized by a closed technique under image intensification. A total of 28 had proximal insertion of Rush nails, 7 epicondylar insertion of Rush nails and 23 distal insertion of Enders nails using a portal of entry just proximal to the olecranon fossa. Brumback et al found that 47 factures (81%) healed with less than 10° of angulation and only 3 (5.2%) with an angulation of more than 15°. Some 18 (64.3%) had excellent results from proximal insertion of the intramedullary device but too close an encroachment on the rotator cuff resulted in adhesive capsulitis being a problem in 28.6%. No patient with an epicondylar insertion had a good result, whereas 78.3% of those with a distal insertion proximal to the olecranon fossa had an excellent result.

In 1984 Stern et al reported on 60 patients treated mainly by Rush pins inserted either proximally or distally, by open, semi-open or closed techniques. In all, the fractures of 46 patients (76.6%) were united at 16 weeks. Nine of 60 patients (15%) had delayed union and united in an average of 22.7 weeks; 5 patients (8.3%) had non-union. Delayed union or non-union occurred in 4 of 17 proximal fractures (23.5%), 9 of 36 middle third fractures (25%) and 1 of 7 distal third fractures (14.5%). Thirty-one patients of the 51 (60.8%) who had an intramedullary device inserted from proximal to distal had adhesive capsulitis, which they defined as a painful, limited abduction of the shoulder, and forward flexion of less than 100°.

In Fenyo's series (1971), 33 of 55 patients underwent primary intramedullary fixation by Rush pin or Kuntschner nail. He reported 3 non-unions (11%) in the primary treatment group and 1 in the delayed treatment group. Of the 55 cases, 2 non-unions occurred in 14 proximal third fractures (14.5%) and 2 in 35 middle third fractures (5.7%). He found that the loss of working capacity averaged 8.8 months amongst the operated patients as compared with 5.5 months amongst conservatively treated patients. Fenyo reported 77.9% excellent or good results with his distally directed Rush nails and adhesive capsulitis did not appear to be a problem.

In 1983 Durbin et al described the results of Hackethal stacked nailing in 25 patients. The mean time for healing was 9.5 weeks, with 2 non-unions (8%). They found that 13 of their 21 patients (61.9%) regained a full range of movement. Seven patients (33.3%) lost less than 25° of elbow movement and 2 (9.5%) had loss of motion in the shoulder. These Hackethal nails were inserted from distal to proximal.

Transient radial nerve palsies occurred in 2 of Fenyo's cases and one of Stern et al, but recovery seemed to be the rule.

Plate fixation

Only three papers describe the use of compression plates in any large number of patients (Bell et al 1985, Foster et al 1985, Griend et al 1986). In all these series they were problem fractures and in Bell's series all patients had multiple injuries.

In Bell's series, 34 patients were followed up, with an average time to union of 19 weeks — defined as the time of the disappearance of the fracture line. Six fractures (17.6%) took 6 months or longer to unite and 1 case (2.9%) went on to a non-union. Bell et al reported 26 patients (76.5%) with a full range of shoulder movements and 33 (97%) with a fully functional shoulder. Thirty-one (91%) had full elbow movements, while the remaining 3 had severe elbow injuries.

In Griend's series of 34 patients, the fractures of 20 (58.8%) were united in 4 months and 28 (81.8%) within 6 months. Griend et al also reported 1 case (2.9%) of non-union. Their results in 31 patients with adequate records showed 100% return of shoulder movement, but there were 8 (25.8%) with up to a 20° loss of elbow extension and 6 (19.3%) with less than 50° movement at the elbow, although all of these had severe articular or soft tissue injury.

Both series had 1 transient radial nerve palsy which recovered, although Griend et al (1986) also had 1 complete iatrogenic nerve transection.

Bell et al (1985) had 1 infection (2.9%) and Griend et al had 2 (5.9%), both in compound fractures.

Foster et al (1985) reported 100% union in 34 cases.

There were two failure of implants in Bell's series, both of which subsequently healed with secondary procedures.

External fixation

Little has been published concerning the use of external fixators in humeral shaft fractures. In 1979 Sukhtian & Hughes reported on 1 case: solid union occurred in 3 months. In 1978 Kamhin et al presented 8 cases: union occurred between 8 and 14 weeks in the 4 cases reported as going on to union. In 2 cases the external fixation device was removed and AO compression plating instituted because of an increasing radial nerve paresis. The authors emphasized the risk of producing radial nerve lesions during manipulation for alignment.

Summary

1. After intramedullary fixation the fractures of 75–94% of patients were united by 16 weeks, whilst 5–11% of patients went on to a non-union.
2. Non-union was reported in up to 25% of proximal and middle third fractures.
3. Loss of shoulder movement occurred in up to 60% of proximally inserted devices and 33.3% lost up to 25° of elbow movement.
4. Transient radial nerve palsies were reported in 1.5–3.5% of cases treated by intramedullary devices.
5. Humeral shaft fractures treated by compression plating healed in an average of 19 weeks. In all, 82% were united (disappearance of fracture line) at 6 months, and there was a 3% non-union rate.
6. After plating humeral fractures there was a 95–100% return of a fully functioning shoulder, and a 75–90% chance of recovery of full elbow movement if there was no articular or severe soft tissue damage around the joint.
7. Infection occurred in 3–6% of plated humeral fractures.
8 There is insufficient literature on the use of external fixators in the treatment of humeral shaft fractures to draw any conclusions, but the radial nerve may be at risk from this technique.

RESULTS OF TREATMENT OF DELAYED OR NON-UNION

Delayed union or non-union of humeral shaft fractures are not common problems and the techniques of management have varied. At present the main methods of treatment are either intramedullary nailing techniques or compression plating with or without bone graft.

In 1949 D'Aubigne reported the results of 32 cases of non-union with a

10% failure rate. One out of 12 tibial onlay grafts failed to unite, but the others united in an average of 3.5 months. Two out of 4 Kuntschner nailings failed, but the other 2 united at an average of 3 months. The addition of bone grafts to the Kuntschner nailing resulted in 100% union, although at an average of 6 months.

In 1955 Horowitz reported 2 successful cases of non-union treated with 'intramedullary prostheses'. However Mnaymneh et al were less successful in 1963. In 47 cases their success rate was only 66%. They recommended excision of the pseudarthrosis, Kuntschner nailing and bone grafting in the upper two-thirds of the shaft, and onlay tibial graft and screws for the lower third.

In 1975 Christensen reported that 10 of his 13 Kuntschner nailings for non-union had united (77%). However, 3 required a second operation before union was achieved and only 2 cases had primary bone graft. A 70% success rate was reported by Stern et al (1984) using Rush pins in 9 cases and a Kuntschner nail in 1. The 2 cases without bone graft both went on to a non-union. In 1985 Pritchett reported a 10% non-union rate in the 10 cases treated by closed flexible intramedullary nailing, with union occurring in an average of 10.5 weeks. All these cases were treated for delayed union.

Murray et al (1964) reported 8 cases of union, at an average of 5 months, out of the 9 treated with double plating of the humerus.

In 1974 Titze reported 10 cases of non-union treated with compression plating. All united — 1 case after a second operation to replate a fracture after loosening had occurred. Time to union was not reported, but there were 2 transient radial nerve palsies. Also in 1974 Ruedi et al reported 5 cases of union in 5 patients who were followed up. One case, however, was for delayed union and the healing time was not reported. Chacha (1974) on the other hand had 1 non-union out of 17 cases treated with compression plates. The average time to union — defined as disappearance of a part or whole of the fracture line in the two standard radiographs as compared to the immediate post-operative radiographs — was 8.5 weeks, although 2 went on to delayed union (12%).

In Loomer & Kokan's paper (1976), the 9 cases of compression plating and bone graft which were adequately followed up all united by an average of 2.5 months.

In 1978 Kamhin et al reported the use of the AO external fixator with compression in 1 case of non-union of the humeral shaft. Union occurred in 8 weeks.

Summary

1. Open reduction and intramedullary nailing with bone graft of humeral shaft non-union had a success rate of 90%, whilst without bone graft there was a high failure rate.

2. Closed intramedullary nailing had a success rate of 90% with union occurring at an average of 10.5 weeks.
3. Compression plating of non-union had a union rate of 90–100% with delayed union occurring in 10–20% of cases.
4. The average healing time after compression plating of humeral shaft non-union was 8.5–10 weeks.
5. Transitory radial nerve palsies occurred in up to 20% of cases of compression plating of non-union, but full recovery usually occurred.

RADIAL NERVE PALSY

Radial nerve injury complicates closed fracture of the humerus in a significant number of cases, and strong arguments both for and against early exploration can be found in the literature. Many review articles were based on patients collected over a long period of time (in an article by Packer et al (1972) over a 40-year period) and the conclusions made by these authors were based on the accumulated results obtained over a period when changes in the management of these lesions occurred. Modern techniques, such as microscopic repair of nerve lacerations, are likely to affect the final outcome favourably.

The reported incidence of radial nerve palsy complicating humeral shaft fractures varies widely, from 1.8% (Holstein & Lewis 1963) to 17.6% (Branch 1955). Table 4.3 records the incidence of radial nerve palsy in those series which report 100 or more fractures of the humeral shaft. Taking these figures as a whole, there was an incidence of 10.5% of immediate radial nerve palsy following humeral shaft fracture. This wide variation in the incidence of radial nerve palsy is likely to be explained by population

Table 4.3 Incidence of radial nerve palsy in humeral shaft fractures

Reference	Number of fractures	Number of palsies	%
Holstein & Lewis (1963)	341	6	1.8
Thompson et al (1965)	103	3	2.9
Caldwell (1940)	108	4	3.7
Pollock et al (1981)	383*	23	6
Scientific Research Committee, Pennsylvania Orthopedic Society (1959)	159	19	11.3
Garcia & Maeck (1960)	226	27	11.9
Kettlekamp & Alexander (1967)	216	27	12.5
Mann & Neal (1965)	100	16	16
Mast et al (1975)	240	42	17.5
Branch (1955)	187	33*	17.6

*Indicates number estimated from available figures.

differences and the differing types of violence occurring in the catchment areas of the different reporting centres.

The true incidence of radial nerve palsy following open reduction and internal fixation is also difficult to ascertain. In 1960 Garcia & Maeck reviewed 31 years of radial nerve palsies occurring in New York and reported 24 cases of radial nerve palsy occurring after 102 cases of internal fixation — an incidence of 23.5%. The Pennsylvania group, reporting in 1959 on a 5-year study from 1952 to 1956, cited 3 cases of radial nerve palsy occurring after the internal fixation of 45 fractures (an incidence of 6.6%). However, Garcia & Maeck (1960) pointed out that over the last decade of their review there had been no cases of radial nerve palsy post-operatively, suggesting that the incidence was declining with modern surgical techniques.

It is therefore appropriate to quote only recent papers for a realistic figure. In 1984 Stern et al had 1 post-operative radial nerve palsy in 70 cases of intramedullary fixation (1.4%), and in 1971 Fenyo had 2 in 55 cases of Rush nail fixation (3.6%). An incidence of post-operative radial nerve palsy of 2.8% (Griend et al 1986) and 2.6% (Bell et al 1985) occurred after AO plating of humeral shaft fractures. These four series gave an overall incidence of post-operative radial nerve palsy of 2.5%.

The overall rate of radial nerve palsy after manipulation of fractures was about 2%. This figure is based on three papers which quote incidences of 1.25% (Mast et al 1975), 1.4% (Kettelkamp & Alexander 1967) and 3.5% (Scientific Research Committee, Pennsylvania Orthopedic Society 1959).

Table 4.4 shows the incidence of radial nerve palsy related to the site of the fracture. All of the reported series seem to agree that radial nerve palsy occurs less commonly in the proximal third of the humerus. Holstein & Lewis (1963) reported no radial nerve palsies in proximal shaft fractures out of 341 cases of humeral shaft fracture. However when those papers quoting incidences of radial nerve palsy with total numbers of fractures are compared there is an overall incidence of 7.3% of radial nerve palsy occurring with proximal humeral shaft fractures.

Table 4.4 Incidence of radial nerve palsy with fracture site

Reference	Proximal third	Middle third	Distal third
Mann & Neal (1965)	2/29 fractures	8/52 fractures	5/15 fractures
Klenerman (1966)	1/22 fractures	5/44 fractures	4/12 fractures
Mast et al (1975)	6/72 fractures	29/93 fractures	7/75 fractures
Garcia & Maeck (1960)	4	21	6
Holstein & Lewis (1963)	0	1	6
Kettelkamp & Alexander (1967)	5	23	5
Packer et al (1972)	2	14	10 (4 supracondylar)
Pollock et al (1981)	2	5	14

Table 4.4 further shows that all the quoted papers, except those of Holstein & Lewis (1963) and Pollock et al (1981), reported the highest percentage of radial nerve palsies as occurring after middle third fractures. However humeral shaft fractures are said to occur most commonly in the middle third. Therefore it may be that radial nerve palsies occur most readily after distal third fractures, as Klenerman (1966), Mann & Neal (1965) and Holstein & Lewis (1963) stated.

In 1954 Whitson reported that in 25 cadaveric dissections the radial nerve, as it left the front of the long head of triceps, was separated from the humerus in the region of the spiral groove by fibres of the medial head of triceps. As the lateral supracondylar ridge of the humerus was approached, he found that the radial nerve was in contact with the lower margin of the spiral groove for a variable distance; from 0 to 7 mm (average 3.3 mm). He felt that these observations offered an explanation for the fact that the radial nerve escapes injury in many fractures of the humerus in which nerve damage would be expected.

In 1963 Holstein & Lewis described a fracture syndrome occurring in the distal third of the humerus. A spiral fracture occurred in which the distal fragment was displaced proximally and the proximal fragment deviated radially. The radial nerve was caught in the fracture site, with the nerve fixed to the proximal fragment by the intermuscular septum. Nerve damage occurred from the distal end of the proximal fragment.

RECOVERY AFTER RADIAL NERVE PALSY

The place of operative or non-operative treatment in the management of humeral shaft fractures complicated by radial nerve palsy remains controversial.

Immediate radial nerve palsy

On reviewing those papers which recorded the results of over 10 cases of immediate radial nerve palsy, it can be seen that between 51.5 and 100% (average 79.9%) of cases achieved full recovery (see Table 4.5). It should be noted that the 1971 paper by Sim et al which gave a 51.5% recovery rate included cases of both immediate and late radial nerve palsies. There is disagreement as to whether early or delayed surgical exploration influences the final result. In 1955 Branch treated all of his 33 cases of radial nerve palsy by the hanging cast technique and achieved a 100% recovery rate without the need for surgical intervention. In 1981 Pollock et al reported that only 2 out of 24 of their cases required surgical intervention. They recommended that these patients should be observed for return of function over 3.5–4 months before considering surgery.

In 1967 Kettelkamp & Alexander explored 13 cases out of 33; 11 of these cases were explored within 2 weeks. They found interruption of the radial

Table 4.5 Overall recovery rate of immediate radial nerve palsies

Reference	Radial nerve palsies	Recovery	%
Sim et al (1971)	66*	34	51.5
Shaw & Sakellarides (1967)	31	20	64.5
Garcia & Maeck (1960)	31	21	67.7
Packer et al (1972)	31†	21	67.7
Klenerman (1966)	10	7	70
Mast et al (1975)	35	25	71.4
Kettlekamp & Alexander (1967)	27	25	92
Scientific Research Committee, Pennsylvania Orthopedic Society (1959)	19	18	94
Pollock et al (1981)	24	24	100
Mann & Neal (1965)	16	16	100
Branch (1955)	33‡	33	100

*Indicates some late-onset radial nerve palsies.
†Includes 5 occurring after manipulation of fracture.
‡Estimated figure from paper.

nerve in only 2 cases: one was caused by a gunshot wound, and the other was associated with an open fracture. They claimed that no surgically correctable nerve injury or mechanical impingement was found on exploration of their closed fractures. They recommended exploration of the radial nerve if there was no return of function after 8–12 weeks. Mast et al (1975) found it necessary to explore only 7 out of 35 cases and they reported that 24% of those radial nerves that recovered spontaneously did not start to show evidence of this recovery until 12 weeks after the injury. Packer et al (1972) explored 24 of their 31 cases; the 18 cases explored within 2 weeks had a far higher percentage of full recovery (16 cases), as compared with 1 out of 6 cases treated by late exploration. They stated that in several of their cases full nerve recovery was not evident for 8 months. They recommended exploration of the nerve after 6–8 weeks if there was no sign of recovery.

In 1960 Garcia & Maeck reported the results of exploration in 23 of 31 cases. Only 1 was severed, and it recovered completely after suture. Eighteen recovered completely after surgical exploration, compared with 3 of the 8 cases treated expectantly. They found that in patients with complete motor loss, the majority showed some visible sign of injury to the nerve at operation. They recommended that patients with complete nerve injuries should undergo surgery as soon after injury as possible, to inspect the nerve and repair it if necessary. On the other hand, they recommended that patients with incomplete palsies should be treated expectantly. They felt that surgery should be performed at the first sign of progression of the paralysis or if there was no sign of improvement after 4 months.

In 1967 Shaw & Sakellarides reported the results of exploration in 15 of their 25 patients with a complete paralysis of the radial nerve; they found the results of surgery discouraging. Only 1 of 8 cases having nerve suture or neurolysis recovered, although 5 procedures were undertaken in the 1930s, and three explorations were excessively delayed. They recommended that nerve exploration should be delayed for 7–8 weeks.

In open fractures that require debridement, or in those fractures that require an open reduction with a concomitant radial nerve palsy, the need to explore the nerve is obvious. The timing of surgery for closed humeral shaft fractures with radial nerve palsy has been recommended as being required immediately or with a delay of up to 4 months. The time at which radial nerve recovery commences may be as early as 24 hours. Pollock et al (1981) reported that in their slowest case, recovery did not commence until 7 months after injury, although from their series the commencement of the return of function occurred at an average of 7 weeks. Packer et al (1972) reported the start of recovery being delayed by up to 6 months, and Garcia & Maeck (1960) reported a delay of up to 4 months. Shaw & Sakellarides (1967) reported that the commencement of recovery occurred at an average of 5 weeks.

The time taken for full recovery to occur varied between 4 months (Mann & Neal 1965, Pollock et al 1981), 6 months (Scientific Research Committee, Pennsylvania Orthopaedic Society 1959), 6.6 months (Sim et al 1971) and 10 months (Shaw & Sakellarides 1967).

A delay of 8–16 weeks in the exploration of an immediate radial nerve palsy after closed humeral shaft fracture would appear acceptable.

Radial nerve palsy after fracture manipulation

There is little information available concerning radial nerve palsy developing after manipulation of the fracture. Fischer & Haine (1975) reported that 9 of their 13 cases had full recovery by 8 weeks after injury with a further 3 having partial recovery. Mast et al (1975) reported that 2 of their 3 cases recovered at 2 months; the third did not recover. The three in Kettelkamp and Alexander's (1967) series all recovered. Shaw & Sakellarides (1967) found 5 cases, 4 occurring in the so-called Holstein–Lewis fracture, for which early operation was performed. In all cases the nerve was found to be trapped within the fracture. These cases recovered at an average of 9 months. Packer et al (1972) had 3 cases related to humeral shaft fractures. All 3 were explored and recovered fully.

It would appear that radial nerve palsy occurring after a Holstein–Lewis fracture is manipulated should be explored, but expectant treatment is appropriate for those occurring after the other types of humeral shaft fractures.

Radial nerve palsy after internal fixation

As mentioned earlier in this section, with improvement in techniques the incidence of radial nerve palsy following internal fixation has lessened. It is reported to occur in 1.4–3.6% (average 2.5%) of cases. The majority of reported cases recovered within a few weeks. Shaw & Sakellarides (1967) reported on 9 cases of post-operative radial nerve palsy, 6 complete palsies and 3 partial palsies. All of these recovered; the average time for full recovery was 3 months for a partial palsy and 8 months for a complete palsy. Two cases required neurolysis for adherence within scar tissue.

Other neurovascular lesions

Injuries to the brachial artery, median nerve and ulnar nerve, singly or in any combination, have all been reported in the literature. The majority seem to occur with open fractures or gunshot wounds. In 1955 Branch reported a 3% incidence of ulnar nerve lesions in 187 humeral shaft fractures. No other figures can be gleaned from the literature.

Summary

1. The incidence of radial nerve palsy occurring immediately after humeral shaft fractures was 1.8–17.6% (average 10.5%).
2. The incidence of radial nerve palsy occurring after internal fixation was 1.4–3.6% (average 2.5%).
3. The incidence of radial nerve palsy occurring after manipulation of fractured humeral shafts was 1.25–3.5% (average 2%).
4. Radial nerve palsy occurred after proximal third fractures in approximately 5% of cases. These fractures were least likely to result in this palsy.
5. Radial nerve palsy occurred in an average of 14.6% of middle third fractures.
6. Distal third fractures were most likely to result in radial nerve palsy — it occurred in 19.4% of these fractures.
7. Full recovery of immediate radial nerve palsies occurred in 55.5–100% (average 79.9%) of cases.
8. A delay of 3–4 months between the time of injury and exploration of the radial nerve was acceptable.
9. Recovery of nerve function commenced at an average of 5–7 weeks after the initial injury but the first sign of nerve recovery could be delayed by up to 7 months.
10. Full nerve recovery usually occurred between 4 and 10 months.
11. Radial nerve palsy occurring after fracture manipulation recovered in 66–100% of cases at an average of 9 months.
12. Early exploration would appear to be indicated in radial nerve palsy occurring after manipulation of the Holstein–Lewis fracture.

13. Radial nerve palsy occurring after internal fixation tended to be transient, with a good prognosis.
14. Recovery was complete at 3 months for a partial radial nerve palsy and at 8 months for a complete palsy.

SPECIAL GROUPS

Humeral fractures in children

There is little written about the results of the treatment of humeral shaft fractures in children. In 1979 Sharrard pointed out that humeral shaft fractures can occur as a result of direct trauma in birth injury, the battered baby syndrome and as the result of a fall on the outstretched limb. Transverse or spiral fractures of the middle third of the shaft tend to occur in breech deliveries almost invariably during attempts to deliver the extended arm. They may also occur when trying to deliver impacted shoulders by axillary traction in vertex presentations. Union occurs rapidly, usually within 3 weeks.

Radial nerve palsy is common but less so than in adults (Dameron 1985). Nerve recovery usually occurs within 6–12 weeks (Catterall 1982, Dameron 1985).

Malunion is also reported to be common but lateral angulation will correct itself in the first 2–3 years of subsequent growth, even if it is up to 40–50°. If a humeral shaft fracture with complete separation is immobilized with the forearm across the trunk some internal rotation of the distal fragment can occur. If this rotational deformity measures less than 12° it should not be evident clinically (Dameron 1985).

Fractures in infancy and childhood can be treated with U-slabs, gutter slabs or spicas and union occurs in 4–6 weeks (Sharrard 1979). Thompson et al (1965) reported on two children whose fractures united in hanging casts.

In 1963 Devas reported on two cases of stress fracture of the humerus (both occurring in boys after they had thrown a cricket ball) which healed without complication.

Summary

1. Birth injury resulting in fracture of the humeral shaft heals rapidly in 3 weeks.
2. Fractures in infancy and childhood heal in 4–6 weeks.
3. Radial nerve palsy usually recovers in 6–12 weeks.

Fracture of the supracondyloid process

The supracondylar spur is said to occur in 1–3% of people (Kolb & Moore 1967). It is an occasional cause of median nerve and/or brachial artery compression.

The first English language description of a case of fracture of the supracondyloid process of the humerus was by Lund in 1930. In 1959 Genner described a case with complete recovery after periosteal excision of the spur. Kolb & Moore (1967) described two cases: one in a 4-year-old boy which was settled without treatment, and the second one was a 12-year-old boy in whom regeneration occurred after subperiosteal resection of the spur. They also drew attention to a case reported by Mardruzzato in 1938 of a 55-year-old woman with paraesthesia in the median nerve distribution of the hand with an established non-union near the apex of the supracondylar process. Excision of the process relieved her symptoms.

Summary

1. Supracondylar spurs were reported to occur in 1–3% of the population and fracture may occasionally occur.
2. Symptoms may resolve with conservative treatment.
3. If excision is required for local pain or median nerve or brachial artery compression, extraperiosteal excision is required, and full recovery is the rule.

REFERENCES

Balfour G W, Mooney V, Ashby M E 1982 Diaphyseal fractures of the humerus treated with a ready-made fracture brace. Journal of Bone and Joint Surgery 64A: 11–13
Bell M J, Beauchamp C G, Kellam J K, McMurty R Y 1985 The results of plating humeral shaft fractures in patients with multiple injuries. Journal of Bone and Joint Surgery 67B: 293–296
Bohler L 1965 Conservative treatment of fresh closed fractures of the shaft of the humerus. Journal of Trauma 5: 464–468
Branch H E 1955 Fractures of the humerus: ambulatory traction technique. Journal of Bone and Joint Surgery 37A: 1118
Brumback R J, Bosse M J, Poka A, Burgess A R 1986 Intramedullary stabilisation of humeral shaft fractures in patients with multiple trauma. Journal of Bone and Joint Surgery 68A: 960–970
Caldwell J A 1933 Treatment of fractures in the Cincinnati General Hospital. Annals of Surgery 97: 161–176
Caldwell J A 1940 Treatment of fractures of the shaft of the humerus by hanging-cast. Surgery, Gynaecology and Obstetrics 70: 421–425
Cartner M J 1973 Immobilisation of fractures of the shaft of the humerus. Injury 5: 175–179
Catterall A 1982 Fractures in children. In: Watson Jones' fractures and joint injuries, vol 1, 6th edn. Churchill Livingstone, Edinburgh, pp 484–512
Chacha P B 1974 Compression plating without bone grafts for delayed and non-union of humeral shaft fractures. Injury 5: 283–290
Charnley J 1961 The closed treatment of common fractures. Churchill Livingstone, Edinburgh
Christensen N O 1975 Kuntschner intramedullary reaming and nail fixation for non union of the humerus. Clinical Orthopaedics 116: 222–226
Christensen S 1967 Humeral shaft fractures, operative and conservative treatment. Acta Chirurgica Scandinavica 133: 455–460
Comfort T H 1973 The sugartong splint in humeral shaft fractures. Minnesota Medicine 56: 363–366

Coventry M B, Laurnen E L 1970 Ununited fractures of the middle and upper humerus. Special problems in treatment. Clinical Orthopaedics 69: 192–198

Dameron T B 1985 Fractures and dislocations of the shoulder. In: Rockwood C H, Wilkins K E, King R E (eds) Fractures in children. J B Lippincott, Philadelphia, pp 577–607

D'Aubigne R M 1949 Surgical treatment of non-union of long bones. Journal of Bone and Joint Surgery 31A: 256–266

Devas M B 1963 Stress fractures in children. Journal of Bone and Joint Surgery 45B: 534–536

Doran F S A 1944 The problems and principles of the restoration of limb function following injury as demonstrated by humeral shaft fractures. British Journal of Surgery 31: 351–368

Durbin R A, Gottesman M J, Saunders K C 1983 Hackethal stacked nailing of humeral shaft fractures. Experience with 30 patients. Clinical Orthopaedics 179: 168–174

Emmett J E, Breck L W 1958 A review and analysis of 11 000 fractures seen in private practice of orthopaedic surgery 1937–1956. Journal of Bone and Joint Surgery 40A: 1169–1175

Fenyo G 1971 On fractures of the shaft of the humerus. Acta Chirurgica Scandinavica 137: 221–226

Fischer D A, Haine J H 1975 Journal of Bone and Joint Surgery 55A: 1307

Foster R J, Dixon G L, Bach A W, Appleyard R W, Green T M 1985 Internal fixation of fractures and non-unions of the humeral shaft. Journal of Bone and Joint Surgery 67A: 857–864

Garcia A, Maeck B H 1960 Radial nerve injuries in fractures of the shaft of the humerus. American Journal of Surgery 99: 625–627

Genner B A 1959 Fracture of the supracondyloid process. Journal of Bone and Joint Surgery 41A: 1333–1335

Griend R V, Tomasin J, Ward E F 1986 Open reduction and internal fixation of humeral shaft fractures. Journal of Bone and Joint Surgery 68A: 430–433

Holm C L 1970 Management of humeral shaft fractures. Fundamental nonoperative techniques. Clinical Orthopaedics 71: 132–139

Holstein A, Lewis G P 1963 Fractures of the humerus with radial nerve paralysis. Journal of Bone and Joint Surgery 45A: 1382–1388

Horowitz J 1955 Resistant non union of the humerus. Journal of Bone and Joint Surgery 37A: 421

Hunter S G 1982 The closed treatment of fractures of the humeral shaft. Clinical Orthopaedics 164: 192–198

Kamhin M, Michaelson M, Waisbrod H 1978 The use of external skeletal fixation in the treatment of fractures of the humeral shaft. Injury 9: 245–248

Kettelkamp D B, Alexander H 1967 Clinical review of radial nerve injury. Journal of Trauma 7: 424–432

Klenerman L 1966 Fractures of the shaft of the humerus. Journal of Bone and Joint Surgery 48B: 105–111

Kolb L W, Moore R D 1967 Fractures of the supracondylar process of the humerus. Journal of Bone and Joint Surgery 49A: 532–534

Laferte M D, Rosenbaum M D 1937 The 'hanging cast' in the treatment of fractures of the humerus. Surgery, Gynaecology and Obstetrics 65: 231–237

Laing P G 1956 The arterial supply of the adult humerus. Journal of Bone and Joint Surgery 38A: 1105–1116

Loomer R, Kokan P 1976 Non union in fractures of the humeral shaft. Injury 7: 274–278

Lund H J 1930 Fracture of the supracondyloid process of the humerus — a case report. Journal of Bone and Joint Surgery 12: 925

Mann R J, Neal E G 1965 Fractures of the shaft of the humerus in adults. Southern Medical Journal 58: 264–268

Mast J W, Spiegel P G, Harvey J P, Harrison C 1975 Fractures of the humeral shaft. A retrospective study of 240 adult fractures. Clinical Orthopaedics 112: 254–262

Mnaymneh W A, Smith-Peterson M, Aufranc O E 1963 The treatment of non union of humeral shaft fractures. Journal of Bone and Joint Surgery 45A: 1548

Murray W R, Lucas D B, Inman V T 1964 Treatment of non-union of the fractures of the long bones by the two-plate method. Journal of Bone and Joint Surgery 46A: 1027–1048

Packer J W, Foster R R, Garcia A, Grantham S A 1972 The humeral fracture with radial nerve palsy: is exploration warranted? Clinical Orthopaedics 88: 34–38

Pollock F H, Drake D, Bovill E G, Day L, Trafton P G 1981 Treatment of radial neuropathy associated with fractures of the humerus. Journal of Bone and Joint Surgery 63A: 239–243

Pritchett J W 1985 Delayed union of humeral shaft fractures treated by closed flexible intramedullary nailing. Journal of Bone and Joint Surgery 67B: 715–718

Ruedi T, Moshfegh A, Pfeiffer K M, Allgower M 1974 Fresh factures of the shaft of the humerus. Conservative or operative treatment? Reconstruction Surgery and Traumatology 14: 65–74

Sarmiento A, Kinman P B, Galvin E G, Schmitt R H, Phillips J G 1977 Functional bracing of fractures of the shaft of the humerus. Journal of Bone and Joint Surgery 59A: 596–601

Scientific Research Committee, Pennsylvania Orthopedic Society 1959 Fresh midshaft fractures of the humerus in adults. Pennsylvania Medical Journal 62: 848–850

Sharrard W J W 1979 Paediatric orthopaedics and fractures, 2nd edn. Blackwell Scientific, Oxford, pp 1506–1508

Shaw J L, Sakellarides H 1967 Radial nerve paralysis associated with fractures of the humerus. A review of 45 cases. Journal of Bone and Joint Surgery 49A: 899–902

Sim F H, Kelly P J, Henderson E D 1971 Journal of Bone and Joint Surgery 53A: 1023

Stern J, Mattingly D A, Pomeroy D L, Zenni E J, Kreig J K 1984 Intramedullary fixation of humeral shaft fractures. Journal of Bone and Joint Surgery 66A: 639–646

Stewart M J, Hundley J M 1955 Fractures of the humerus. A comparative study in methods of treatment. Journal of Bone and Joint Surgery 37A: 681–692

Sukhtian W, Hughes S 1979 An external fixation device. Journal of the Royal Society of Medicine 72: 831–834

Thompson R G, Compere E L, Schnute W J, Compere C L, Kernaham W T, Keagy R D 1965 The treatment of humeral shaft fractures by the hanging cast method. Journal of the International College of Surgeons 43: 52–60

Titze A 1974 The operative treatment of fractures of the shaft of the humerus. Reconstruction Surgery and Traumatology 14: 75–83

Vichare N A 1974 Fractures of the humeral shaft associated with multiple injuries. Injury 5: 279–282

Whitson R O 1954 Relation of the radial nerve to the shaft of the humerus. Journal of Bone and Joint Surgery 36A: 85

5. The elbow

T. G. Wadsworth

INTRODUCTION

Development

There are six secondary centres of ossification at the elbow in the developing child; rarely, extra ossicles may also be present. The normal secondary centres can be useful in determining the skeletal age of a child. They appear in the following order: capitulum, radial head, internal epicondyle, trochlea, olecranon and external epicondyle (Fig. 5.1).

Unusual accessory bones at the elbow are antecubital, paratrochlear, accessory coronoid and the patella cubiti.

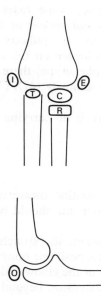

Fig. 5.1 Secondary centres of ossification. I = internal epicondyle; T = trochlea; C = capitulum; R = radial head; E = external epicondyle; O = olecranon

Confusion about radiographic appearances in the child may occur and it is frequently useful to take X-ray films of the opposite elbow. This is particularly so when determining whether the medial epicondyle has become trapped within the elbow joint.

Anatomy

There is normally a lower humeral angle seen in the lateral projection on X-ray; the articular surface lies at about 45° forward on the vertical axis of the humeral shaft (Fig. 5.2).

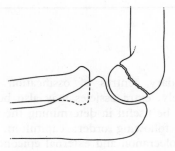

Fig. 5.2 The lower humeral angle

The 'carrying angle' is in the coronal plane and is variable. The elbows are typically equal, except for some cases of unilateral elbow trauma. Usually, the angle is valgus and greater in the female than the male; this difference becomes obvious at puberty. Certain sex chromosome anomalies have a distinct influence on the carrying angle; for instance in Turner's syndrome (45XO phenotype) there is gross valgus deformity and in another sex chromosome anomaly (47XYY phenotype) there is a varus angle.

In some individuals, there is no carrying angle and there is said to be cubitus rectus.

Measurement

It is important to employ routine measurement (Fig. 5.3). Following a unilateral injury the measurements should be compared with the opposite arm.

In the case of elbow motion, the straight position is 0° and range of flexion is measured from this position: however, in some individuals there is normal hyperextensibility of the elbow and a + sign is then employed for the number of degrees of extension beyond the 0° position.

In measuring forearm rotation, the elbow should be held at 90° of flexion at the side of the body: measurement should be started in the 0 position

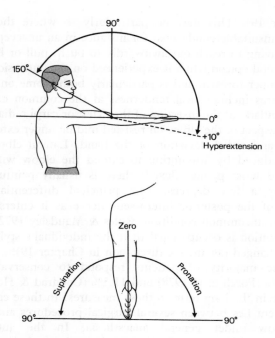

90°

150°

0°

+10°
Hyperextension

Zero

Supination   Pronation

90°   90°

Fig. 5.3 Measurement of elbow and forearm rotation motion

with the thumb up. Supination and pronation are measured from this 0 position and should be compared with the opposite arm.

A goniometer should be used to measure elbow motion accurately.

Vascular and neurological status should always be checked.

ADULT INJURIES

Insertion tendonopathy (see discussion in Chapter 19)

The commonest example is lateral epicondylitis, so-called tennis elbow, and the least common is distal biceps tendonitis at the front of the elbow. Medial epicondylitis, golfer's elbow, is much less common than tennis elbow. These conditions are typically due to repetitive strain causing pathological changes at the specialized junction of tendon and periosteum: each may be called an enthesopathy (Wadsworth 1987).

Although lateral and medial epicondylitis have been described in tennis players and golfers respectively, in actual fact the considerable majority of cases in average clinical experience occur in people who do not have any sports interest.

The importance of these conditions in medicolegal reporting is that they may be associated with frequently repetitive awkward tasks at work (see Chapter 19). This may be particularly so where the individual is working in unsuitable conditions, for instance in an unacceptably confined space and having to reach out awkwardly to push, pull or lift objects.

Pain in lateral epicondylitis is experienced on the outer side of the elbow and in the upper forearm and is particularly bothersome on gripping. The clinical features include local tenderness at the common extensor muscle origin, particularly at the insertion of the extensor carpi radialis brevis, pain in the outer aspect of the elbow on resisted middle finger extension, resisted dorsiflexion and radial deviation of the hand. Lateral elbow pain is also typically produced by attempting to extend the elbow with the forearm pronated and wrist palmar flexed; there is usually painful limitation of extension by a few degrees. The principal differential diagnosis is entrapment of the posterior interosseus nerve as it enters the supinator muscle — an uncommon condition (Roles & Maudsley 1972).

If the condition is occupational then the individual's style of work may have to be changed (again, see discussion in Chapter 19).

Whilst the majority of patients respond to conservative measures, between 3.3% (Posch et al 1978) and 11.5% (Coonrad & Hooper 1973) are unresponsive in the long term to these measures. In these cases, the choice of management lies between several surgical procedures and manipulation of the elbow under general anaesthesia. In the author's opinion manipulation achieves a satisfactory result in the majority of patients. It is simple to perform and relatively inexpensive.

Limbers (1980) claimed that 28% of patients with tennis elbow were not improved whatever operative procedure was chosen.

Table 5.1 The results of modifications of the extensor release for tennis elbow

Reference	Number of patients	Number of excellent/ satisfactory results	%
Verhaar & Walenkamp (1986)	165	119	72
Posch et al (1978)	43	37	86
Nirschl & Pettrone (1979)	88	75	85
Total (average)	296	231	(78)

Table 5.1 records the results of modifications of the extensor release on tennis elbow. Overall, 78% achieved a satisfactory result. Coonrad & Hooper (1973) felt that recovery could occur up to 1 year after surgery. Verhaar & Walenkamp (1986) reported that 57% of their 165 patients had some loss of muscular strength after surgery.

Neurological trauma

While laceration of nerves can occur in open trauma at the elbow, it is much more common to see closed neurological trauma. Mention has already been made of neurological damage associated with ischaemic changes following supracondylar fracture of the elbow in the child. This may involve the medial and ulnar nerves, with appropriate loss of sensation and muscle-wasting and weakness in the hand. This is typically associated with clawing of the digits, palmar flexion deformity of the wrist and serious impairment of function. Volkmann's ischaemic contracture can also occur due to tight upper limb casts.

Compression neuropathy of the radial nerve at the elbow and lower humerus is most often associated with external compression, e.g. in 'Saturday night palsy' where an inebriated individual falls asleep awkwardly in a chair. Such external compression can also be delivered to the unconscious patient on the operating table and in bed in hospital: steps should be taken to guard against such external compression. Radial palsy may also be associated with humeral shaft fractures. The majority of cases of external compression neuropathy of the radial nerve fully recover extension power in the wrist and digits. There is sometimes a small residual area of sensory deficit in the distal cutaneous distribution of the radial nerve on the back of the hand. While recovery is awaited, the wrist should be maintained in modest dorsiflexion with a short cock-up splint; muscle bulk may be maintained by daily electrical stimulation to the extensor muscles of the forearm.

From the medicolegal point of view there are two conditions of particular importance: tardy ulnar palsy and external compression neuropathy.

Tardy ulnar palsy

This usually follows a fracture of the lateral condyle of the humerus in the child. It is explained in the section on childhood injuries, below, how injuries to the capitular epiphysis can result in cubitus valgus due to deficiency or absence of the lateral lip of the trochlea, resulting from damage to the trochlear–capitular ossific link. This may be due to malunion, premature epiphyseal fusion or non-union. Damage to the outer lip of the trochlea allows the ulna to slide laterally, with resultant cubitus valgus deformity. When the ulna migrates laterally, the roof of the cubital tunnel, the arcuate ligament, approaches the floor of the tunnel and so the stage is set for compression of the ulnar nerve (Fig. 5.4).

The association between childhood trauma and tardy ulnar palsy in adult life was discussed by Panas (1878) and Mouchet (1898). The interesting fact is that, on average, the palsy manifests itself 22 years after injury to the elbow. The reason for this typical interval is unknown. It may be that mild neuropathy occurred at the time of the initial injury and an external compression stimulus in adult life triggers off clinical ulnar nerve palsy. On the other hand, it may be that developing osteophytic formation

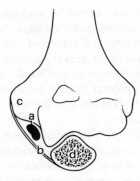

Fig. 5.4   Schematic representation of the cubital tunnel. a = ulnar nerve; b = arcuate ligament; c = medial epicondyle; d = olecranon. Note that the tunnel will narrow if the ulna moves laterally

of the medial lip of the trochlea can result in late compression of the already compromised ulnar nerve.

Clearly, a child with injury to the capitular epiphysis, the lateral condyle of the humerus, may develop ulnar compression neuropathy in adult life with impairment of sensory and motor function of the hand. If the unstable types I, II and III injury are not properly treated by internal fixation, then the risk of such important long-term ill effects is much increased (see p. 125). Premature epiphyseal fusion (particularly the second type) may occur even after expert treatment and, therefore, the risk is still a distinct although less common possibility in the well treated case. The clinical features are of cubitus valgus and neurological deficit ranging from sensory loss alone to severe wasting and weakness of the muscles supplied by the ulnar nerve in the hand and the medial half of the flexor digitorum profundus and flexor carpi ulnaris muscles. The dorsal cutaneous branch of the ulnar nerve is included in the neurological deficit. Additionally, swelling of the ulnar nerve may be palpable proximal to the arcuate ligament and pressure over the damaged ulnar nerve produces discomfort as well as paraesthesiae in the inner part of the hand. The elbow flexion test (Wadsworth 1982) can be useful in diagnosis.

External compression neuropathy

This may be acute where a single blow is delivered to the ulnar nerve. However, those cases where subacute external compression is delivered to the cubital tunnel over a period of minutes or hours are more common. This is a particular hazard of hospitalization and is potentially litigious. When a patient is unconscious on the operating table or in the intensive care unit, or when depression of consciousness is present when in bed in the ward, there is risk to the ulnar nerve within the cubital tunnel if pressure is delivered to this part of the elbow.

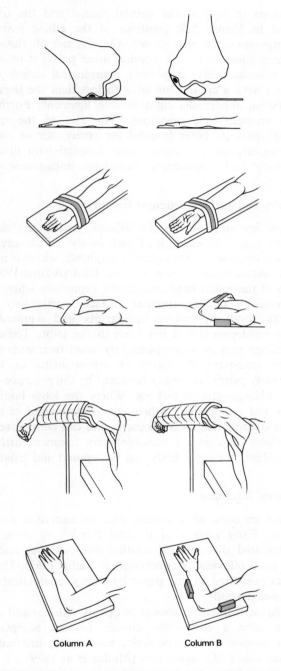

Column A   Column B

Fig. 5.5 The cubital tunnel external compression syndrome: positions of risk are shown in column A and safe positions in column B

The positions of risk to the cubital tunnel and the ulnar nerve are demonstrated in Figure 5.5; positions of the elbow with avoidance of external compression are also shown. Clearly, not all those at risk from external compression do in fact develop ulnar palsy; it may be that those individuals who do suffer important neurological deficit as a result of hospitalization have a cubital tunnel with less than the normal volume or there may be an abnormally tight arcuate ligament. Further research is required to answer these questions. The fact of the matter is that, unfortunately, patients enter hospital for emergency or elective reasons, some non-surgical, and sometimes leave hospital with ulnar nerve palsy and occasionally with considerable functional impairment of the hand.

Chondropathy and surface articular fractures

These injuries are most often sports-related, particularly in patients aged from 15 to 30 years. An example of such injury has already been given in the fourth type of injury to the capitular epiphysis, which is most commonly seen in little league baseball players in the USA (Adams 1965). Here there is impaction of the radial head against the capitulum when the baseball is thrown. Contusion of the articular surface, particularly of the lower humerus, can result in surface incongruity and segments of articular cartilage can be detached and left loose in the joint. These fragments of articular cartilage may be accompanied by small fragments of bone. Apart from remote long-term ill effects of osteoarthritis in some of these individuals, early painful disability is caused by the presence of loose bodies in the joint and episodes of locking. Where the loose bodies are entirely cartilaginous and radiopaque, arthroscopic examination of the elbow may be helpful in eliciting diagnosis. Loose bodies can be removed and in some instances, where there is a reasonable bony fragment included with the detached cartilage, the loose body can be reposed and fixed into position.

Lower humeral fractures

These injuries are quite often severe, with comminution and displacement (Evans 1953). Early reports of internal fixation of these intra-articular fractures suggested that internal fixation was not easy and offered little chance of a good outcome (Riseborough & Radin 1969). However, all the surgical cases presented in this paper had a non-anatomical reduction and a poor functional result.

Ideally, displaced fractures should be openly reduced and internally fixed in order to give a reasonable chance for an acceptable range of humeroulnar motion with early active movement. Internal fixation may be carried out using AO techniques (Muller et al 1979).

Pure supracondylar fractures without an intra-articular extension appear to give a satisfactory functional recovery whether closed or operative treatment is utilized (Soltanpur 1978, Aitken & Rorabeck 1986, Browne et al 1986). Intra-articular fractures of the distal humerus present more difficult problems and surgical treatment produces better functional results.

In some, it is only possible to get the medial and lateral condyles together, ideally with two screws for bicortical fixation, and to treat the injury as a simple supracondylar fracture where there is gross comminution of bone proximal to the condyles. In others, comminution is so great that 'bag of bones' treatment is the only available choice, with the elbow being immobilized in a collar and cuff for several weeks and then an active exercise programme instituted.

In 1986 Zagorski et al reported the superior results of internal fixation of these intra-articular fractures as compared with those achieved after conservative measures. In all, 76% of 29 fractures achieved a satisfactory result after internal fixation compared with 8% of 13 patients after conservative treatment. This paper used the functional assessment of Bickel & Perry (1963) which accepted a total range of flexion–extension of 60° in the good grading.

A number of papers report the long-term follow-up of intra-articular fractures after internal fixation (Table 5.2). Overall, 78% of patients achieved a satisfactory result after internal fixation, although the criteria for assessment did vary between these series.

With stable fixation of awkward intra-articular lower humeral fractures, there is the opportunity for an early active exercise programme. An alternative to this, and one gaining some popularity, is for continuous passive motion with an appropriate motorized hinged brace (Salter 1982). The importance of early mobilization was stressed by Aitken & Rorabeck (1986).

Ulnar compression neuropathy at the cubital tunnel is a possibility. A

Table 5.2 The results of the internal fixation of intercondylar fractures of the distal humerus

Reference	Number of patients	Number of excellent/ good results	%	Number of fair/poor results	%
Henley (1987)*	25	23	92	2	8
Zagorski et al (1986)[†]	29	22	76	7	24
Aitken & Rorabeck (1986)[‡]	16	12	75	4	25
Tregonning & Mackie (1986)*	21	11	52	10	48
Browne et al (1986)[†]	25	21	84	4	16
Jupiter et al (1985)*	34	27	79	7	21
Shetty (1982)*	19	15	79	4	21
Total (average)	169	131	(78)	38	(22)

*Excellent/good result: 30° extension to 120° flexion.
[†]Excellent/good result: at least 60° of extension–flexion.
[‡]Excellent/good result: up to 75° arc of flexion.

further important complication is post-traumatic osteoarthritic change which, in the course of time, can result in further painful limitation of movement. In 1985 Jupiter et al reported, after an average of 5.8 years follow-up, a normal articular width on follow-up radiographs in 11 patients (32%), slight to moderate narrowing in 19 patients (56%) and extensive post-traumatic arthritis in four patients (12%). They felt that the clinical evaluation did not correlate with the follow-up radiograph. Deterioration in the state of these elbows is presumed to occur but has not been adequately documented. Such individuals are often unable to hold down their usual job and a frequent problem is limitation of various activities of daily living and sports activities.

Surgery for non-union of the distal humerus utilizing AO plates with or without bone graft resulted in union in 17 of 18 cases (94%) (Ackerman & Jupiter 1988). However, function after an average of a 3.6 year follow-up was poor, with only 35% of patients achieving a satisfactory result with extension–flexion from 30° to 120°.

Olecranon fractures

Undisplaced olecranon fractures are easily treated by immobilization of the limb in a collar and cuff. However, most fractures of the adult olecranon are displaced and are, in effect, ruptures of the extensor mechanism of the elbow with important disability and loss of active extension.

Such injuries may be classified into four types (Fig. 5.6). In the first type there is a small fragment avulsed and it is best in this circumstance to

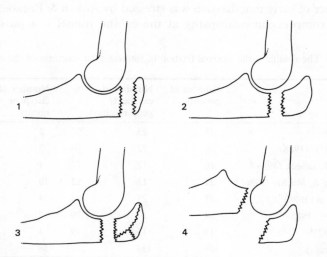

Fig. 5.6 Classification of displaced fractures of the olecranon. 1 = avulsion of a small fragment; 2 = simple fracture with a large proximal fragment; 3 = comminuted fracture; 4 = distal fracture with instability of the radius and ulna

remove the fragment and to suture the damaged triceps tendon into the body of the olecranon through drill holes.

In the second type the fracture is situated about the centre of the articular surface of the olecranon and in the third type the fracture is similarly placed but not comminuted. Open reduction and internal fixation are required in these two types: a popular method is that of the AO technique with encircling wire and two Kirschner wires placed longitudinally across the fracture site and the encircling wires incorporated around the ends of these at the proximal part of the olecranon (Muller et al 1979). Sometimes this method also has to be accompanied by screw fixation. If expertly performed, results are good, but on occasions failure of bony union occurs with disruption of the articular surface and fibrous union.

The author's preferred method is bicortical screw fixation, the screw being placed from the point of the olecranon obliquely across the fracture site into the anterior ulna (Wadsworth 1976). Early active movement sets the stage for useful motion and an excellent result is usual.

The fourth type of olecranon fracture is more distally placed and the ulnar shaft and the radius have a potential for displacing forwards, sometimes severely; this is in effect an anterior-type Monteggia injury. It is mandatory for these cases to be reduced and fixed just as in types II and III cases.

The majority of these injuries, properly treated, should result in virtually full elbow movement. In 1987 Helm et al reported no difference in the final functional result whether a tension band technique or screw fixation was used. They found that very few patients complained of pain after their olecranon fracture was treated. Holdsworth & Mossad (1984) found that 73% of their 52 patients treated by a tension band technique were asymptomatic whilst 17% only complained of pain when the elbow was knocked. The remainder had occasional spontaneous pain. Kiviluoto & Santavirta (1978) found a slightly lower number of patients were symptom-free — 61% of 33 patients, with the rest experiencing occasional pain.

Flexion is rarely lost after the treatment of these fractures, although extension may be lost to some degree in from 50% (Ericksson et al 1957) to 75% (Holdsworth & Mossad 1984). Between 81% (Kiviluoto & Santavirta 1978) and 94% (Holdsworth & Mossad 1984) lost less than 30° of extension. Eriksson et al (1957) noted that only 3% of patients are consciously aware of any limitation of movement. Most patients recover final movement by 3 months (Gartsman et al 1981).

Holdsworth & Mossad (1984) measured extensor peak strength and reported that 38% of their patients had 75% or more strength than that of the contralateral side, whilst 78% of patients recovered more than 50% of the extensor peak strength of the contralateral limb. Worse functional results were seen in older patients in this series.

Complications due to the backing out of tension band wires were common. In 1986 Jensen & Olsen reported 55% complications after tension band techniques in 53 patients and, in 1985, Macko & Szabo had 80% complications in 20 patients.

However, there is the potential risk of progressive osteoarthritic change in future years, particularly if accurate reduction has not been accomplished. In 1987 Helm et al reported only 1 patient out of 48 (2%) showing evidence of degenerative changes after internal fixation of these fractures. However both Kiviluoto & Santavirta (1978) and Gartsman et al (1981) reported a 20% incidence of degenerative changes after these fractures. The more severe the injury, the more likely it is to result in long-term degenerative changes. Morris et al (1978) reported on 9 'combined force' injuries of the elbow with fractured olecranon and radial head. Seven of these 9 patients developed degenerative changes. Such osteoarthritis will cause painful limitation of elbow movement which can compromise activities of daily living and work and also leisure pursuits. Of the 20 patients in Macko & Szabo's series (1985), 70% were united at 3 months after tension band techniques and 90% were united by 5 months. Non-union can occur and it was reported in 3% of Eriksson et al's series (1957). Simple excision of the olecranon fragment and triceps advancement seems to produce good results (Waldram & Porter 1987).

Radial head and neck fractures

These injuries can conveniently be classified into five types (Bakalim 1970; Fig. 5.7):

1. Undisplaced segmental fracture of the radial head.
2. Displaced fracture segment with a step in the articular surface at the radiohumeral joint.
3. Gross comminution of the whole radial head.
4. Undisplaced radial neck fracture.

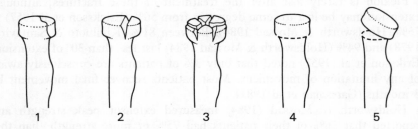

Fig. 5.7 Classification of adult radial head and neck fractures, adapted from Bakalim (1970). 1 = undisplaced segmental fracture of the radial head; 2 = fracture segment displaced with a step in the articular surface at the radiohumeral joint; 3 = gross comminution of the whole radial head; 4 = undisplaced radial neck fracture; 5 = angular displacement of the radial head with a fracture through the radial neck

5. Angular displacement of the radial head with a fracture through the radial neck.

The majority of radial head and neck fractures should be treated conservatively, most often with excellent results. Radin & Riseborough (1966) classified their results into one of three groups:

1. Good, if there was less than 10° of loss of motion in any direction and no symptoms.
2. Fair, if there was up to 30° of loss of motion in any direction or minor complaints or both.
3. Poor, if there were major complaints or more than 30° of loss of motion in any direction, or both.

They found that 15 of 30 type I fractures had a good result and 11 a fair result (87% satisfactory result).

In 1981 Miller et al looked at the long-term follow-up of the conservative treatment of type II fractures. Using the above criteria they reported that 29 of their 34 patients (81%) treated conservatively achieved satisfactory results. They further reported that there was only rarely a deterioration in the short-term result.

Even better results were reported by Mathur & Sharma in 1984. They used a plaster cast to immobilize the elbow, yet allowing free rotation of the forearm. Forty-three of their 50 patients returned to a full range of motion and a further 6 only lost less than 10° of motion (96% good result).

It is useful to aspirate the elbow, using a lateral approach into the radiohumeral articulation, some 24 hours after the injury. Removal of blood at this time is quite effective in significantly reducing pain and if performed at this stage there is not much risk of significant build-up of further haemoarthrosis. Pinder (1969) and Fleetcroft (1984) suggested that the long-term functional result was permanently improved after aspiration of the haematoma. Fleetcroft (1984) reported that full flexion and extension were achieved in 83% of those patients aspirated and rotation was full in all. On the other hand, in his non-aspirated group only 58% had full flexion and extension and 86% had full rotation.

However, Holdsworth et al (1987), whilst confirming that pain relief was immediate and lasting, were unable to show any long-term difference in the final outcome after aspiration of the haematoma. They found that the older the patient, the worse the functional results and noted that loss of extension of the elbow was the main disability after fracture of the radial head and correlated well with the residual symptoms.

In displaced segmental radial head fractures, causing significant limitation of forearm rotation, the fragment may be reduced and screwed into position or in some instances it may simply be excised. Gerard et al (1984) reported good results after screw fixation in 21 patients. In 1985

Bunker & Newman reported good results in 10 patients whose radial head fractures were treated with the Herbert bone screw (Herbert & Fisher 1984).

It is often best to leave the comminuted type III injury alone and opt for an early active exercise programme for the elbow and forearm.

Type IV cases are best treated conservatively; the injured limb should be immobilized in a collar and cuff for 4 weeks with early active movement at 2 weeks.

The unusual type V injury carries a poor prognosis, as the blood supply of the separated radial head is lost, and there is grave risk of avascular necrosis even if the fracture can be adequately reduced and maintained in good position.

Radial head and neck fractures are sometimes associated with elbow dislocation and surgery is best avoided in these circumstances, in order to minimize the risk of myositis ossificans with resultant gross limitation of elbow movement. Total separation of the radial head through a radial neck fracture in the adult is best treated by removal of the radial head: consideration can be given to its replacement with a prosthesis.

If there is significant restriction of forearm rotation in the type III injury 3 months after the injury, then consideration should be given to removal of the radial head and its possible replacement with a prosthesis. In 1983 Mikic & Vukadinovic reported that only 50% of their 60 patients had a satisfactory result after the radial head was excised. On the other hand, Goldberg et al (1986) reported that 31 of their 36 patients (86%) were satisfied with the results of radial head excision and 92% had satisfactory function. Broberg & Morrey (1986) reported the results of delayed excision of the radial head in 21 patients. In all, 90% of their patients were functionally satisfied and 77% were rated objectively as having an excellent or good result. Grip strength was reduced by 7% after radial head excision (Coleman et al 1987).

Subluxation of the distal radioulnar joint as a complication of excision of the radial head was reported to occur in 37 of 58 wrists (64%) by Taylor & O'Conner in 1964. Some 50% of these 58 patients had symptoms of weakness or pain at the wrist. McDougal & White (1957) reported that 12 of 44 patients (27%) with radial head excision had wrist symptoms, as did 30% of the 60 patients of Mikic & Vukadinovic (1983).

However, Radin & Riseborough (1966) reported that although subluxation occurred in 14 of 36 wrists (39%), only 3 patients had mild symptoms. These authors could find no correlation between the degree of subluxation at the distal radioulnar joint and symptoms.

A similar lack of correlation between proximal migration of the radius and wrist symptoms was reported by Morrey et al (1979), Stephen (1981) and Waddell & Campbell (1980).

The results of the use of a silastic prosthesis after radial head excision have been variable. In 1979 Mackay et al reported that 17 of their 18 cases

(94%) had satisfactory results. Harrington & Tountas (1981) reported on the use of a radial head prosthesis in 17 patients with radial head fracture and gross instability of the elbow. Fourteen (82%) of patients had a satisfactory result.

In 1986 Carn et al found that only 70% of their 10 patients had a satisfactory result. Their patients had an average 8% loss of grip strength. In 1981 Morrey et al reported 5 failures out of 17 cases of silastic replacement (70% satisfactory results). They concluded that the indications for the use of the silastic radial head prosthesis after fracture are extremely limited.

Fracture of the prosthesis is not uncommon (Mackay et al 1979) and it may be the cause of symptoms (Mayhall et al 1981).

The long-term complications of types II, III and IV injuries of the radial head are osteoarthritis with resultant painful limitation of elbow motion and forearm rotation. The risk is greater the worse the damage to the articular surface of the radial head. The reported incidence of degeneration at the elbow after radial head fracture varies between 52% of 60 patients (Mikic & Vukadinovic 1983) and 100% of 36 patients (Goldberg et al 1986). Although Mikic & Vukadinovic (1983) reported that 43% of their 60 patients had symptoms from the elbow, most authors report no correlation between the presence of radiographic degeneration and elbow symptoms (Morrey et al 1979, Carn et al 1986, Goldberg et al 1986).

In some cases, particularly where the radial head has been removed and not replaced by a prosthesis, there is a risk of cubitus valgus developing. This gives rise to the long-term possibility of compression ulnar neuropathy within the cubital tunnel, because the ulna displaces outwards with approximation of the roof of the cubital tunnel to the floor. Mikic & Vukadinovic (1983) reported that 15 of their 55 adult patients (27%) developed increase of their cubitus valgus after radial head resection. This increase averaged 5° (Goldberg et al 1986) to 20° (Coleman et al 1987).

Ulnar nerve symptoms occurred in 5 (8%) of Mikic & Vukadinovic's (1983) patients and in 1 (8%) of Stephen's (1981) 12 patients.

Monteggia injuries (see also Chapter 6)

This is a combination of fracture of the ulnar shaft, usually in the upper third, with displacement of the radial head (Monteggia 1813). If a fracture of the ulna is present with over-riding or angular deformity or even a curved deformity, where there is no radial shaft fracture, then there must be a high degree of suspicion of displacement of the radial head. Curved deformity of the ulna is more often seen in the child. Otherwise, the extent of this injury may not be fully recognized and it may be improperly treated, with resulting persistent deformity and limitation of function of the elbow and forearm. Open reduction and internal fixation of the ulna is the usual treatment. Sometimes the radial head has to be stabilized by appropriate soft tissue surgery.

In the child this important injury can be treated conservatively after appropriate reduction of the ulna and repositioning of the radial head: the limb is then immobilized in an above-elbow plaster of Paris cast for 4–6 weeks. The final result is excellent in the properly treated case.

Dislocation

In the adult, unlike the child, avulsion fractures medially and laterally are frequently seen, occurring in from 12 to 62% of elbow dislocations (De Lee et al 1984). These do not appear to prejudice the final functional result (Protzman 1978). Usually the dislocation occurs with the olecranon and radial head lying posteriorly and it is most unusual to see an anterior dislocation.

Reduction is easily accomplished, usually under general anaesthesia. It is necessary to immobilize the elbow at 90° with the forearm in neutral rotation with a well padded posterior plaster of Paris splint and a collar and cuff for at least 2 weeks, and to opt for an active elbow exercise programme thereafter. In 1987 Josefsson et al reported the results of a prospective randomized study comparing surgical and non-surgical treatment in 30 patients with simple dislocation of the elbow. They found no evidence that the results were improved by surgical repair.

Following elbow dislocations the main movement to suffer some permanent loss is extension. In 1978 Protzman found the average loss of extension in 47 patients to be 7°. He noted a direct correlation between the duration of immobilization, the loss of extension and the period of disability. The 27 patients immobilized for less than 5 days had an average 3° loss of extension and an average disability period of 6 weeks. Those 7 patients immobilized for longer than 3 weeks lost an average 21° extension and had a disability period averaging 24 weeks. This association of an unsatisfactory result after prolonged immobilization was also reported by Mehlhoff et al (1988). These authors reported an average of 12° loss of extension in 52 patients, which was the same as the extension loss reported in 52 patients by Josefsson et al (1984).

Improvement in the range of movement normally occurs within 6 months (Wadsworth 1982) but improvement has continued to occur up to 1 year after treatment (Mehlhoff et al 1988).

Periarticular calcification occurred in 60% (Protzman 1978) to 95% (Josefsson et al 1984) of patients but did not affect the final functional result. Mehlhoff et al (1988) noted that 45% of their 52 patients had some residual pain at follow-up at an average of 34 months.

Signs of early degenerative joint disease were reported in 38% of 50 patients in Josefsson et al's 1984 study after an average of 24 years' follow-up.

Recurrent or habitual dislocation of the elbow is much less common than recurrent dislocation of the glenohumeral joint of the shoulder and is in fact rarely seen. Usually the condition appears to commence with childhood or adolescent dislocation. The capitulum and trochlear notch may be mis-shaped and loose bodies may be present.

Several operative procedures are available to restore stability to the elbow joint (Wadsworth 1982).

Summary

1. Conservative treatment fails to cure tennis elbow in 3–11.5% of cases.
2. In all, 78% of patients with tennis elbow achieved a satisfactory result with surgery: 57% had some loss of muscle strength after surgery.
3. The majority of cases of external compression neuropathy of the radial nerve recovered full muscle power.
4. Tardy ulnar palsy occurs 22 years after injury to the elbow.
5. A total of 78% of intra-articular distal humeral fractures achieved a satisfactory result after internal fixation.
6. Degenerative changes were reported in 68% of intra-articular distal humeral fractures at 6-year follow-up.
7. A total of 35% of patients achieved a satisfactory functional result after surgery for non-union of the distal humerus.
8. The functional results after internal fixation of olecranon fractures are generally good. Degenerative changes were reported to occur in 2–20% of patients after olecranon fractures.
9. Types I and II radial head fractures had up to a 96% satisfactory result.
10. From 50 to 90% of patients had a satisfactory result after radial head excision. Subluxation of the distal radioulnar joint may be a problem.
11. Some 52–100% of radial head fractures had degenerative changes.
12. Loss of extension after simple dislocation of the elbow in the adult averaged 7–12°. Degenerative changes were reported in 38% of patients at 24-year follow-up.

POST-TRAUMATIC OSTEOARTHRITIS

This is the second commonest type of arthritis of the elbow, the most common being rheumatoid disease. Other causes are rare.

After childhood injury, osteoarthritis can result from incongruity of the articular surface of the lower humerus after trauma to the capitular epiphysis. This is most likely to happen after non-union of the lateral condyle and when the fracture through the metaphysis of the lower humerus passes through the ossification centre rather than its more usual situation at the inner side of the ossification centre. More commonly, adult intra-articular lower humeral fractures are the cause.

Less commonly, osteoarthritic change can occur after a fracture of the olecranon and certain radial head fractures. Usually the pain is not so severe when compared with osteoarthritis of the hip and knee. This is probably because the elbow is a non-weight-bearing joint and osteoarthritic disability of the elbow can to some extent be compensated for by mobility of the shoulder, wrist and digital joints.

However, individuals with advanced osteoarthritic change in the elbow may face serious painful disability to such an extent that work activity and certain activities of daily living are seriously compromised. Leisure pursuits may also be severely affected.

Apart from painful limitation of range of motion of the elbow, loose bodies may form in the osteoarthritic joint and these may lead to painful locking of the elbow. Loose bodies may require removal arthroscopically or at arthrotomy.

Special X-ray views of the elbow may be required in order to determine the presence of loose bodies. Arthrography, computerized tomography and arthroscopy can be useful.

Typically, in the established case of osteoarthritis of the elbow joint, there may be deformity of the radial head, the distal humeral and olecranon articular surfaces and the coronoid process. There may be obvious loose body formation. In some, the most seriously involved part of the joint is the humeroradial articulation, often accompanied by enlargement and deformity of the radial head.

Osteoarthritic changes in the humeroulnar articulation at the inner side may cause ulnar compression neuropathy in the cubital tunnel.

It is usual for limitation of extension of the elbow to be present and in more advanced cases there may be considerable restriction of flexion and, in some, limitation of forearm rotation.

There may be major restriction of the elbow motion in the presence of mild osteoarthritic change: in these individuals, surgical release of the elbow may be considered, followed by an intensive active exercise programme. Consideration can be given to the use of a continuous passive motion machine. Sometimes a satisfactory result can be obtained, but increase in range of movement tends to be unpredictable in most individuals and surgery is not without risk to the neurovascular structures.

Apart from removal of loose bodies and surgical release of the stiff elbow, other operative procedures to consider are various forms of arthroplasty. Resection arthroplasty can be useful in certain cases, but results are unpredictable.

Replacement prosthetic arthroplasty of the elbow joint can be performed and a number of prostheses are available, although this is a difficult area of replacement surgery and results are unpredictable.

Furthermore, it is unwise to replace the arthritic elbow with a prosthesis in an individual who is likely to have to perform hard manual work.

CHILDHOOD INJURIES

Epiphyseal separations

Injuries of the medial and lateral epicondyles are usually of little practical importance. It is unusual to have to reposition an injury of the lateral epicondyle. However, separation of the medial epicondylar epiphysis may be of importance for the following reasons:

1. Considerable separation of the epiphysis can lead to non-union and deformity of the cubital tunnel: this may result in ulnar compression neuropathy and neurological deficit in the hand in later life.
   Therefore, severe displacement needs to be corrected.
2. The medial epicondylar epiphysis may be displaced in association with dislocation of the elbow.

Josefsson and Danielsson (1986) reviewed 56 unreduced conservatively treated medial humeral epicondylar fractures at an average of 35 years after the injury. They found a 55% incidence of non-union and a 10% incidence of ulnar nerve symptoms in those patients with non-unions. Function and range of elbow movement were good in all cases.

Separation of the olecranon epiphysis is rare. Occasionally a fragment may be avulsed with the triceps tendon; this represents a severe injury to the extensor apparatus of the elbow and, in these circumstances, open reduction and Kirschner wire fixation of the fragment are required. Complications are uncommon.

Total separation of the lower humeral epiphyses is very rare and can be confused with injuries of the lateral humeral condyle and dislocation of the elbow joint (Marmor & Bechtol 1960). These injuries may be distinguished by X-raying the opposite elbow and drawing a line up through the radial shaft. The line should pass through the capitulum on the anteroposterior X-ray unless there is dislocation.

The capitular epiphysis accounts for ossification of the outer lip of the trochlea. This trochlear–capitular ossific link is of considerable importance. The carrying angle is dependent upon the varying depth of the lateral lip of the trochlea. The configuration of this lip is such that a valgus angle is eliminated when the elbow is flexed. Injuries of the capitular epiphysis, the lateral condyle, are common and are an important cause of loss of elbow function. Post-traumatic osteoarthritis and tardy ulnar nerve palsy may also follow these injuries.

The author has divided such injuries to the capitular epiphysis into four types (Wadsworth 1972; Fig. 5.8a). In the first three types, the fracture usually lies to the inner side of the ossification centre and, less commonly,

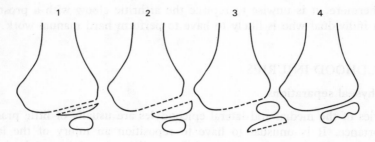

Fig. 5.8a Classification of injuries to the capitular epiphysis. 1 = undisplaced; 2 = moderate displacement; 3 = severe displacement with rotary deformity; 4 = direct trauma to the articular surface of the capitular epiphysis by impingement of the radial head

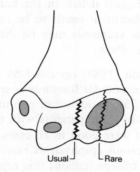

Fig. 5.8b In the first three types of injuries to the capitular epiphysis, the fracture usually extends to the joint surface, medial to the ossification centre. The type 1 injury is occasionally unstable

through it (Fig. 5.8b). In the first type the injury is usually stable, but there is the potential in some of these cases for displacement. This is more likely if the lateral fracture gap is 3 mm or more. Under these circumstances, the fracture is completely through the articular cartilage. These patients should be reviewed carefully with repeat X-rays to check the position at weekly intervals until a month after the injury.

In the second type where there is moderate displacement and in the third type where there is gross displacement with rotatory deformity, open reduction and internal fixation either by two Kirschner wires or a cancellous screw are mandatory. In the fourth type there is impingement of the radial head against the capitulum — as occurs in little league baseball players (Adams 1965) and the articular surface is damaged. In some cases, there may simply be chondropathy. This is seen more often in the USA than the UK.

Injuries to the lateral condyle of the humerus in the child have the potential for serious complications (Flynn et al 1975, Jakob et al 1975):

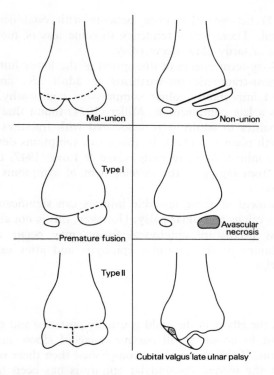

Mal-union

Non-union

Type I

Premature fusion

Avascular
necrosis

Type II

Cubital valgus 'late ulnar palsy'

Fig. 5.9 Complications of injuries to the capitular epiphysis

malunion, particularly in types II and III, non-union in types I, II and III and premature epiphyseal fusion in all (Wadsworth 1964; Fig. 5.9).

Lateral condylar overgrowth with spur formation is a common sequel to these injuries. Maylahn & Fahey (1958) found that it occurred in 28% of children with this injury. However, it is of no significant functional or cosmetic importance (Cotton 1902, Wadsworth 1972).

In the first three types, premature fusion may occur in two ways. Firstly, fusion may affect the capitular epiphysis and the metaphysis of the humerus only, with consequent fish-tail deformity. Secondly, the normal pattern of fusion is followed by the capitular and trochlear epiphysis fusing with each other and then to the lower humerus. However, fusion is often accelerated on the capitular side in the latter situation and even here valgus deformity may occur. Valgus deformity always follows the first type of epiphyseal fusion because loss of the lateral lip of the trochlea allows the olecranon to displace laterally. Accelerated fusion may even occur in the fourth type of injury to the capitular epiphysis and again there is potential for valgus deformity.

Non-union is a serious hazard of the unstable types I, II and III injuries, with loss of the lateral lip of the trochlea and consequent valgus deformity.

Wilkins (1984) believed that even patients with established non-union functioned well. There was a tendency to some loss of movement and a high incidence of tardy ulnar nerve palsy.

Important long-term effects of disruption of the lower humeral articular surface are post-traumatic osteoarthritis in adult life, and even more frequently and importantly, ulnar compression neuropathy. Tardy ulnar nerve palsy is a late complication. Miller (1924) found that 47% of tardy ulnar nerve palsies in adults were associated with fractures of the lateral condylar growth plate as a child. In this series symptoms developed 30–40 years after the injury. More recently, Gaye & Love (1947) found that the average time from injury to the development of symptoms was 22 years in 100 patients.

Proper treatment of these unstable injuries can significantly lessen the risk of cubitus valgus and ulnar palsy. However, this is not always the case, particularly as premature epiphyseal fusion may occur even with an undisplaced injury to the capitular epiphysis and after expertly treated unstable injuries.

Dislocation

Dislocation of the elbow in the child is usually posterior and easily reduced. It is important to obtain a full passive range of elbow movement after elbow reduction. If this cannot be accomplished then there must be strong suspicion that the medial epicondylar epiphysis has been trapped in the humeroulnar articulation. Check X-rays should demonstrate this, particularly if compared with the opposite elbow. A major problem occurs when the dislocation occurs before ossification of the medial epicondylar epiphysis and then one has to rely on the sign of incomplete elbow motion after reduction.

Wilkins (1984) described four major complications which may follow elbow dislocation in the child:

1. *Nerve injuries*: In reviewing three large series of 285 patients she found that the incidence of nerve injury was 11%. The ulnar nerve was most commonly injured. The prognosis for these injuries was good and only 1 patient failed to make a full recovery.
2. *Arterial injuries*: These are rare. Eliason & Brown (1937) found 20 cases reported in the literature and added a further case. Three-quarters of the arterial injuries occurred in open dislocations. Four of the children required amputation and 6 had a severe Volkmann's contracture.
3. *Myositis ossificans*: Wilkins pointed out that true myositis ossificans — ossification within the muscle sheath leading to significant stiffness — was rare; heterotopic ossification in the ligaments and capsule of the elbow joint was more common. However, this latter condition rarely

caused impaired elbow function. Thompson & Garcia (1967) found a 3% incidence of myositis ossificans in elbow dislocations without fracture. Where dislocation was associated with a fracture the incidence increased to 18%.
4. *Recurrent dislocation*: In the combined series of 285 cases described by Wilkins (1984) the incidence was 0.7%.

Supracondylar fracture

This is a common and potentially grave injury. Unfortunately, a considerable proportion of these fractures are severely displaced with the lower humeral fragment lying 'in space' posteriorly. Only 1% of supracondylar fractures in the child are in flexion, or anterior.

The major problem is with the severely displaced extension-type supracondylar fracture where all contact is lost between the lower humeral fragment and the metaphysis of the humerus.

The distal humeral fragment is usually internally rotated in the displaced extension-type injuries. This deformity tends to persist and accentuate the varus which may develop.

After careful reduction, the elbow should be flexed fully: a posterior well padded plaster of Paris splint should be applied together with a collar and cuff. Unfortunately, the fully reduced position quite often cannot be held and treatment may be difficult in these children.

Other methods of treatment for the difficult fracture include:

1. Overhead olecranon skeletal traction (Edmon & Lohr 1963, Worlock & Colton 1987).
2. Percutaneous wiring of the lower humeral fragment. The procedure is performed under general anaesthesia and fluoroscopy. This method can only be used where the lower humeral fragment can be completely reduced. Otherwise overhead skeletal traction should be used initially.
3. Internal fixation. Where reduction cannot be completely achieved, consideration can be given to open reduction and internal fixation through a posterior approach. This is probably best performed by Kirschner wires engaging the cortices of the humerus in the young child. This method of reduction and fixation *must* be employed where vascular surgery is required.

Residual tilting of the lower fragment may be determined by constructing Baumann's angle on an anteroposterior radiograph of the injured elbow and the opposite elbow: a line is drawn along the epiphyseal surface of the lateral part of lower humeral metaphysis (Baumann 1929). The second line is drawn along the axis of the humerus and the angle formed by the two lines joining is compared at the two elbows (Fig. 5.10).

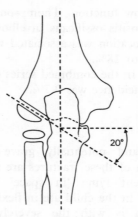

Fig. 5.10 Baumann's angle, compared with the opposite elbow, is useful to measure tilting of the lower humeral fragment

Range of elbow motion after severe supracondylar fracture tends to be best where full reduction has been achieved. The principal aim of treatment in dispaced supracondylar fractures of the elbow in the child is *prevention of vascular impairment*, well known in its severe form as Volkmann's ischaemic contracture.

Careful observation is required for at least 48 hours, in particular of the colour and mobility of the digits and quality of the radial pulse.

If vascular impairment goes untreated then there is potential for very serious functional deficit in the limb. Muscle infarction principally involves the deep finger flexors and the long flexor to the thumb. This results in the digits being clawed and sensation is impaired, particularly in the median nerve distribution. There is intrinsic muscle weakness in the hand. The end-result is a virtually non-functioning hand and upper limb. This sad situation is preventable by proper management of the injury.

Another complication of supracondylar fracture of the humerus in the child is varus, or gunstock, deformity. This is not only cosmetically unacceptable but in many cases causes an important functional disability. If the varus deformity is 20° or more then corrective supracondylar osteotomy should be considered at or near skeletal maturity. There are several methods available, and probably the best are the French (1959) and the Lloyd-Roberts (personal communication) techniques.

The largest series of supracondylar fractures in children reported in the English literature was Henrickson's (1966) follow-up of 545 cases. This is a thorough appraisal of the long-term results after these injuries and may be worth consulting in the difficult case. The patients in these series were treated by immobilization (224 cases), reduction followed by immobilization (232 cases), open reduction and internal fixation (73 cases) and skeletal or skin traction (6 cases). Wilkins (1984) pointed out the difficulties of comparing results of differing treatment methods in this condition because of the varied experience of the authors and the poor definition of the fracture types involved.

The important conclusions in Henrickson's (1966) series were:

1. The end-results were excellent in 73%, good in 21% and poor in 6% of patients. The criteria used in the evaluation of the end-results are shown in Table 5.3. In the report the results are broken down according to the degree of primary displacement and the adequacy of reduction. It is interesting to note that there was a 3% incidence of poor results in the undisplaced fractures.

   The majority of excellent results were found in those patients in whom a perfect reduction had been achieved, irrespective of the degree of primary displacement.

2. The incidence of permanent ischaemic contracture was 0.4%. This figure is similar to the 0.5% incidence described by Wilkins (1984) in 4520 cases.

3. Nerve injuries occurred in 3% of patients. The most commonly injured nerve was the median, followed by the ulnar and the radial. Wilkins (1984) described a 7% incidence of nerve injury and reported that the radial nerve was most frequently affected. Severe impairment of neurological function persisted in only 1 of the 18 patients in Henrickson's (1966) series. Wilkins described near complete recovery in these cases.

4. Osteoarthritis occurred in 2% of the patients (11 cases) in Henrickson's series.

5. The highest frequency of poor results occurred in boys with severe displacement.

Table 5.3 Criteria used in the evaluation of the end-results of supracondylar fractures (from Henrickson 1966 with permission)

	Excellent	Good	Poor
Difference in carrying angle	±10°	±15–20°	±25° or more
Limited flexion, extension, pronation and/or supination	0–10°	15–20°	25° or more
Pain	none	on exertion or with change of weather	on exertion and with change of weather
Symptoms during work	none	mild	severe
Muscle contracture	none	none	yes
Persistent nerve injury	no	no	yes

6. Loss of flexion or extension of 5° or more occurred in less than 5% of patients.
7. Henrikson found a 20% incidence of cubitus varus of over 10° following extension supracondylar fractures. The incidence was much higher in those patients with an inadequate final reduction. The incidence of cubitus valgus in excess of 10° was 0.8%. These measurements represent the difference between the carrying angles of the injured and uninjured arms.

After the much less common flexion-type of supracondylar fracture the incidences of cubitus varus and valgus were 5.5% and 3% respectively.

Proximal radial epiphysis

Injuries of the upper radial epiphysis are common in the child. In many, the injuries are either undisplaced or minimally displaced and in these cases treatment is simply with collar and cuff. Complications are rare.

The older the child the less acceptable is deformity (Fig. 5.11): in some, closed reduction can be obtained to an acceptable position and in others open reduction is required.

There is a rare variant of this injury in which the upper radial epiphysis is totally displaced. It may be that the elbow is first dislocated by a fall on to the outstretched hand and then the child falls on to the point of the elbow: at this moment, the radial head is impacted against the capitulum and knocked off, and the elbow is spontaneously reduced. The epiphysis can only be repositioned by open reduction, but there is a grave risk of

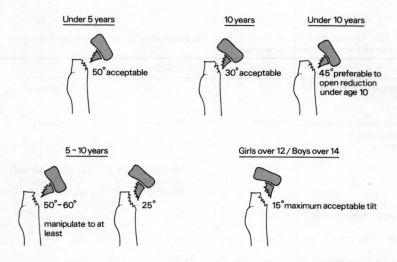

Fig. 5.11 The older the child, the less acceptable is deformity of the radial head

avascular necrosis of the upper radial epiphysis, however well the injury is treated.

Premature epiphyseal fusion can sometimes occur in these injuries. When avascular necrosis occurs then cubitus valgus is a particular problem, with the risk in adult life of ulnar compression neuropathy in the cubital tunnel (Jeffrey 1972).

Wilkins (1984) reviewed the literature and found an overall incidence of poor results in 15–23% of cases despite apparently adequate treatment. The most common cause of a poor result was loss of movement.

Summary

1. Lateral condylar overgrowth is quite common after injuries to this structure. It does not usually cause any significant functional or cosmetic problems.
2. Tardy ulnar nerve palsy is a late complication of injuries to the lateral humeral condyle. It may take 20 years or more for symptoms to develop.
3. The end-results of supracondylar fractures are excellent or good in over 90% of patients (see Henrickson's criteria, Table 5.3). Better results were found after accurate fracture reduction.
4. Henrickson (1966) found a 2% incidence of osteoarthritis after supracondylar fractures of the humerus.

REFERENCES

Ackerman G, Jupiter J B 1988 Nonunion of fracture of the distal end of the humerus. Journal of Bone and Joint Surgery 70A: 75–83
Adams J E 1965 Injury to the throwing arm (a study of traumatic changes in the elbow joints of boy baseball players). California Medicine 102: 127
Aitken G K, Rorabeck C H 1986 Distal humeral fractures in the adult. Clinical Orthopaedics 207: 191–197
Bakalim G 1970 Fractures of radial head and their treatment. Acta Orthopaedica Scandinavica 41: 320
Baumann E 1929 Beitrage zur Kenntnis der Frakturen am Ellbogengelenk. Unter besonderer Beruscksichtigung der Spatfolgen. I. Allgemeiner und Fractura supracondylica. Brun's Beitrage zur Klinischen Chirurgie 146: 1
Bickel W E, Perry R E 1963 Comminuted fractures of the distal humerus. Journal of the American Medical Association 184: 553–557
Broberg M A, Morrey B F 1986 Results of delayed excision of the radial head after fracture. Journal of Bone and Joint Surgery 68A: 669–674
Browne A O, O'Riordan M, Quinland W 1986 Supracondylar fractures of the humerus in adults. Injury 17: 184–186
Bunker T D, Newman J H 1985 The Herbert differential pitch bone screw in displaced radial head fractures. Injury 16: 621–623
Carn R M, Medige J, Curtain D, Koenig A 1986 Silicone rubber replacement of the severely fractured radial head. Clinical Orthopaedics 209: 259–269
Coleman D A, Blair W F, Shurr D 1987 Resection of the radial head for fracture of the radial head. Journal of Bone and Joint Surgery 69A: 385–392
Coonrad R W, Hooper W R 1973 Tennis elbow; its course, natural history, conservative and surgical management. Journal of Bone and Joint Surgery 55A: 1177–1182

Cotton F J 1902 Elbow fractures in children. Annals of Surgery 35: 75–104
De Lee J C, Green D P, Wilkins K E 1984 Fractures and dislocations of the elbow. In: Rockwood C A, Green D P (eds) Fractures in adults, vol 1. J. B. Lippincott, Philadelphia
Edmon P, Lohr G 1963 Supracondylar fractures of the humerus treated with olecranon traction. Acta Orthopaedica Scandinavica 125: 505
Eliason E L, Brown R B 1937 Posterior dislocation of the elbow with rupture of the radial and ulnar arteries. Annals of Surgery 106: 1111–1115
Eriksson E, Sahlen O, Sandahl U 1957 Late results of conservative and surgical treatment of fracture of the olecranon. Acta Chirurgica Scandinavica 113: 153–156
Evans E M 1953 Supracondylar-Y fractures of the humerus. Journal of Bone and Joint Surgery 35B: 381
Fleetcroft J P 1984 Fractures of the radial head: early aspiration and mobilisation. Journal of Bone and Joint Surgery 66B: 141–142
Flynn J C, Richards J R, Salzman R I 1975 Prevention and treatment of non-union of slightly displaced fractures of the lateral humeral condyle in children. Journal of Bone and Joint Surgery 57A: 1087
French P R 1959 Varus deformity of the elbow following supracondylar fractures of the humerus in children. Lancet ii: 439
Gartsman G M, Sculco T P, Otis J C 1981 Operative treatment of olecranon fractures. Journal of Bone and Joint Surgery 63A: 718–721
Gaye J R, Love J G 1947 Diagnosis and treatment of tardy palsy of the ulnar nerve. Journal of Bone and Joint Surgery 29: 1087–1097
Gerard Y, Schernburg F, Nerot C 1984 Anatomical, pathological and therapeutic investigation of fractures of the radial head in adults. Journal of Bone and Joint Surgery 66B: 141
Goldberg I, Peylon J, Yosipovitch Z 1986 Late results of excision of the radial head for an isolated closed fracture. Journal of Bone and Joint Surgery 68A: 675–679
Harrington I J, Tountas A A 1981 Replacement of the radial head in the treatment of unstable elbow fractures. Injury 12: 405–312
Helm R H, Hornby R, Miller S W M 1987 The complications of surgical treatment of displaced fractures of the olecranon. Injury 18: 48–50
Henley M B 1987 Intra-articular distal humeral fractures in adults. Orthopedic Clinics of North America 18: 11–23
Henrickson B 1966 Supracondylar fracture of the humerus in children. Acta Chirurgica Scandinavica (Suppl): 369
Herbert T J, Fisher W E 1984 Management of the fractured scaphoid using a new bone screw. Journal of Bone and Joint Surgery 66B: 114
Holdsworth B J, Mossad M M 1984 Elbow function following tension band fixation of displaced fractures of the olecranon. Injury 16: 182–187
Holdsworth B J, Clement D A, Rothwell P N R 1987 Fractures of the radial head — the benefit of aspiration. Injury 18: 44–47
Jakob R, Fowles J V, Rang M, Kassab M T 1975 Observations concerning fractures of the lateral humeral condyle in children. Journal of Bone and Joint Surgery 57B: 430
Jeffrey C C 1972 Fractures of the neck of the radius in children. Journal of Bone and Joint Surgery 54B: 717
Jensen C M, Olsen B B 1986 Drawbacks of traction-absorbing wiring (TAW) in displaced fractures of the olecranon. Injury 17: 174–175
Josefsson P O, Danielsson L G 1986 Epicondylar elbow fracture in children: 35 year follow up of 56 cases. Acta Orthopaedica Scandinavica 57: 313–315
Josefsson P O, Johnell O, Gentz C-F 1984 Long-term sequelae of simple dislocation of the elbow. Journal of Bone and Joint Surgery 66A: 927–930
Josefsson P O, Gentz C-F, Johnell O, Wendeberg A B 1987 Surgical versus non-surgical treatment of ligamentous injuries following dislocation of the elbow. Journal of Bone and Joint Surgery 69A: 605–608
Jupiter J B, Neff U, Holzach P, Allgauer M 1985 Intercondylar fracture of the humerus. Journal of Bone and Joint Surgery 67A: 226–239
Kiviluoto O, Santavirta S 1978 Fractures of the olecranon. Acta Orthopaedica Scandinavica 49: 28–31
Limbers P A 1980 Tennis elbow. Journal of Bone and Joint Surgery 62B: 262

Mackay I, Fitzgerald B, Miller J H 1979 Silastic replacement of the head of the radius in trauma. Journal of Bone and Joint Surgery 61B: 494–497

Macko D, Szabo R M 1985 Complications of tension-band wiring of olecranon fractures. Journal of Bone and Joint Surgery 67A: 1396–1401

Marmor L, Bechtol C O 1960 Fracture separation of the lower humeral epiphysis. Journal of Bone and Joint Surgery 42A: 333

Mathur N, Sharma C S 1984 Fracture of the head of the radius treated by elbow cast. Acta Orthopaedica Scandinavica 55: 567–568

Mayhall W S T, Tiley F T, Paluska D J 1981 Fracture of silastic radial-head prosthesis. Journal of Bone and Joint Surgery 63A: 459–460

Maylahn D J, Fahy J J 1958 Fractures of the elbow in children. Journal of the American Medical Association 166: 220–228

McDougall A, White J 1957 Subluxation of the inferior radio-ulnar joint complicating fracture of the radial head. Journal of Bone and Joint Surgery 39B: 278–287

Mehlhoff T L, Noble P C, Bennett J B, Tullos H S 1988 Simple dislocation of the elbow in the adult. Journal of Bone and Joint Surgery 70A: 244–249

Mikic Z D, Vukadinovic S M 1983 Late results in fractures of the radial head treated by excision. Clinical Orthopaedics 181: 220–228

Miller E M 1924 Later ulnar nerve palsy. Surgery, Gynaecology and Obstetrics 38: 37–46

Miller G K, Drennan D B, Maylahn D J 1981 Treatment of displaced segmental radial-head fractures. Journal of Bone and Joint Surgery 63A: 712–717

Monteggia G B 1813 Instituzione chirurgiche, 2nd edn. G Maspero, Milan

Morrey B F, Chao E Y, Hui F C 1979 Biomechanical study of the elbow following excision of the radial head. Journal of Bone and Joint Surgery 61A: 63–68

Morrey B F, Askew L, Chao E Y 1981 Silastic prosthetic replacement for the radial head. Journal of Bone and Joint Surgery 63A: 454–458

Morris E W, Miller J H, McLatchie G R, Amis A 1978 Combined force injuries of the elbow joint. Journal of Bone and Joint Surgery 60B: 444

Mouchet A 1898 Thèse de docteur, Paris

Muller M E, Allgower M, Schneider R, Willenegger H 1979 Manual of internal fixation; techniques recommended by the AO group, 2nd edn. Springer-Verlag, Berlin

Nirschl R P, Pettrone F A 1979 Tennis elbow: the surgical treatment of lateral epicondylitis. Journal of Bone and Joint Surgery 61A: 832–839

Panas J (1878) Sur une cause peu connue de paralysie du nerf cubital. Archives Générals de Medecine (Paris) 2: 5

Pinder I M 1969 Fracture of the head of the radius in adults. Journal of Bone and Joint Surgery 51B: 386

Posch J N, Goldberg V M, Larrey R 1978 Extensor fasciotomy for tennis elbow; a long term follow-up study. Clinical Orthopaedics 135: 179–182

Protzman R R 1978 Dislocation of the elbow joint. Journal of Bone and Joint Surgery 60A: 539–541

Radin E L, Riseborough E J 1966 Fractures of the radial head. Journal of Bone and Joint Surgery 48A: 1055–1064

Riseborough E J, Radin E L 1969 Intercondylar T fracture of the humerus in the adult. Journal of Bone and Joint Surgery 51A: 130–141

Roles N C, Maudsley R H 1972 Radial tunnel syndrome. Resistant tennis elbow as a nerve entrapment. Journal of Bone and Joint Surgery 54B: 499–508

Salter R B 1982 Motion versus rest: why immobilize joints? Journal of Bone and Joint Surgery 64B: 251

Shetty S 1982 Surgical treatment of T and Y fractures of the distal humerus. Injury 14: 345–348

Soltanpur A 1978 Anterior supracondylar fracture of the humerus (flexion type). Journal of Bone and Joint Surgery 60B: 383–386

Stephen I B M 1981 Excision of the radial head for closed fracture. Acta Orthopaedica Scandinavica 52: 409–412

Taylor T K F, O'Conner B T 1964 The effect upon the inferior radio-ulnar joint of excision of the head of the radius in adults. Journal of Bone and Joint Surgery 46B: 83–88

Thompson H C, Garcia A 1967 Mysotis ossificans. Aftermath of elbow injuries. Clinical Orthopaedics 50: 129–134

Tregonning G D, Mackie C E J 1986 Displaced Y-shaped intercondylar fractures of the humerus. Journal of Bone and Joint Surgery 68B: 677

Verhaar J A N, Walenkamp G H I M 1986 Operative therapy of radial humeral epicondylitis. Acta Orthopaedica Scandinavica 57: 451

Waddell J P, Campbell V 1980 Surgical treatment of radial head fracture. Journal of Bone and Joint Surgery 62B: 130

Wadsworth T G 1964 Premature epiphyseal fusion after injury of the capitulum. Journal of Bone and Joint Surgery 46B: 46

Wadsworth T G 1972 Injuries of the capitular (lateral humeral condylar) epiphysis. Clinical Orthopaedics and Related Research 85: 127–142

Wadsworth T G 1976 Screw fixation of the olecranon. Lancet ii: 118

Wadsworth T G (ed) 1982 The elbow. Churchill Livingstone, Edinburgh

Wadsworth T G 1987 Tennis elbow; conservative, surgical and manipulative treatment. British Medical Journal 294: 251

Waldram M A, Porter K M 1987 Late treatment of non-union of fracture of the olecranon. Injury 18: 419–420

Wilkins K E 1984 Fractures and dislocations in the elbow region. In: Rockwood C A Jnr, Wilkins K E, King R E (eds) Fractures in children, vol 3. J B Lippincott, Philadelphia

Worlock P H, Colton C L 1987 Severely displaced supracondylar fractures of the humerus in children. A simple method of treatment. Journal of Paediatric Orthopaedics 7: 49–53

Zagorski J B, Jennings J J, Burkhalter W E, Uribe J W 1986 Comminuted intraarticular fractures of the distal humeral condyles. Clinical Orthopaedics 202: 197–204

FURTHER READING

Blount W P 1963 The enigma of elbow fractures in children. Bulletin of the Hospital for Joint Diseases 24: 22

Kashiwagi D 1985 Osteoarthritis of the elbow joint. Proceedings of International Seminar on the Elbow Joint, Kobe, Japan. Elsevier Science Publishers, Amsterdam

Morrey B F 1985 The elbow and its disorders. W B Saunders, Philadelphia

Wadsworth T G 1986 The elbow. Churchill Livingstone, Edinburgh (Spanish edn)

6. The forearm

P. S. Fagg

FRACTURES OF BOTH BONES IN THE ADULT

Conservative treatment

Undisplaced fractures of the forearm in adults are adequately treated in an above-elbow plaster of Paris cast, and union should occur in 6–8 weeks (Creuss 1973).

The results of the conservative treatment of displaced fractures appear to be far from satisfactory. In 1949 Knight & Purvis reviewed 100 cases of fresh fracture of the shafts of both bones of the forearm in adults, 41 of which were treated conservatively. Only 12 of these 41 cases (29%) achieved a satisfactory result. There were 5 cases (12%) of non-union and in 60% of the cases a residual deformity of rotation of from 25 to 60° was present. The authors found that the average time to solid union was 18–20 weeks. Mervyn Evans (1951) drew attention to the importance of correcting the rotational deformity of these fractures. Of 50 cases he described, 21 were in adults of which there was 1 malunion requiring an osteotomy and bone graft. Unfortunately he did not separate the results of these adult fractures from those of the children in his series when reporting his overall results.

In 1952 Bolton & Quinlan reported that the mean healing time in 90 cases of adult forearm fractures treated conservatively was 13 weeks. There were 4 cases of non-union (4.5%) and 2 cases of malunion (2%). Fifty-six (62%) healed in good anatomical alignment, 53 cases (59%) had good function and 61 cases (55%) had full or only minimal restriction of rotation. Acceptable rotation was achieved in 90% of lower third fractures, 57.5% of middle third fractures and 60% of proximal third fractures. In all, 59% returned to their former employment.

In 1953 Bradford et al reported the results of manipulation in 19 displaced fractures, of which 12 cases (63%) achieved a satisfactory position. However in 7 of these 12 fractures (58%) the position was lost over the course of the next 3 weeks, leaving only 5 of the original 19 cases (26%) in an acceptable reduced position.

Matthews & Saunders (1979) reported on 22 cases of fracture of the forearm in adults treated by closed methods. A total of 36% had

137

complications; there were 2 cases of non-union (9%), 4 cases of delayed union beyond 6 months (18%) and 2 cases of malunion (9%). In contrast, when reporting the results of 45 fractures treated with a forearm functional brace, Sarmiento et al (1975) found only 1 non-union (2%) and 2 cases of malunion (4.5%). The healing time averaged 9.9 weeks for isolated ulna fractures, 11 weeks for isolated radial fractures and 15.1 weeks for fractures of both bones. The average loss of pronation and supination in these fractures was less than 10° — only 2 cases lost more than 10° of rotation in pronation or supination.

Intramedullary fixation

Many varieties of intramedullary fixation have been used in the treatment of forearm fractures. In 1957 Smith & Sage reviewed 555 forearm fractures in 338 patients treated by Rush pins, Kirschner wires, Steinman pins, Kuntschner nails or Lottes nails. They found an overall non-union rate of 20%. When the 38% of non-unions from the use of Kirschner wires were excluded this overall non-union rate fell to 14%. Table 6.1 records the rate of non-union in the larger reported series of intramedullary fixation for forearm fractures. The overall non-union rate from these five series was

Table 6.1   The non-union rate after intramedullary forearm fixation

Reference	Number of fractures	Number of non-union	%	Nail
Caden (1961)	157	26	16.6	Rush pin
Street (1986)	137	10	7	Square
Cotler et al (1971)	125	8	6.4	Schneider
Sage (1959)	82	5	6.2	Sage
Marek (1961)	52	0	0	Square
Total (average)	553	49	(8.9)	

Table 6.2   The functional results after intramedullary forearm fixation

Reference	Number of patients	Number of satisfactory results	%	Nail
Street (1986)	103	86*	83.5	Square
Cotler et al (1971)	87	82	94	Schneider
Michels & Weissman (1976)	80	67	84	Rush pin
Sage (1959)	39	27†	69	Sage
Marek (1961)	32	27‡	84	Square
Total (average)	341	289	(84.7)	

*Less than 50% loss of pronation–supination.
†Pronation and supination each lacking less than 45°.
‡70–90% normal rotation.

8.9%. The average time to union, in these series, varied between 15 and 20 weeks.

The functional results obtained by the use of the various fixation devices reviewed in Smith & Sage's (1957) paper showed that 82% achieved a satisfactory result, by which was implied less than a 20° reduction in elbow flexion–extension and less than a 60° reduction in pronation–supination. Table 6.2 records the functional results reported by the authors of five of the larger series.

Thus, overall, 84.7% achieved a satisfactory functional result following intramedullary fixation although, as can be seen, these authors did vary in their interpretation of what constituted a reasonable result.

Plate fixation

In the series reported by Knight & Purvis in 1949, there was a 20% non-union rate in the 20 cases of forearm fracture treated by plate fixation and only 35% of these 20 patients had a satisfactory end-result. Using a rigid plate Hicks (1961) was able to reduce the non-union rate to 6% in 66 fractures. Although earlier papers had shown a significant complication rate with plate fixation, Burwell & Charnley (1964), using Burns and Shermans plates on 218 forearm fractures, showed that failure was due to poor anatomical reduction and the use of inappropriately short plates. Their overall non-union rate was 9.6% in 218 fractures. However in those cases where fixation was intact this fell to 2.2%; where fixation was inadequate this non-union rate rose to 44.7%.

Table 6.3 records the results of the treatment of forearm fractures with rigid plates in some of the larger series. The overall union rate was 96.8%. In view of the fact that primary bone union occurs after rigid plate fixation it can be difficult to be sure at what point radiological union has occurred. That this depends on author interpretation probably explains why Anderson et al (1975) found the average time to union to be 7.4 weeks in their 330 fractures whilst Dodge & Cady (1972) reported it to be 12 weeks for a radius plated when both bones were fractured, but 18 weeks when isolated fractures of the forearm bones were plated.

Table 6.3 The results of compression plating of forearm fractures

Reference	Number of fractures	Number united	% united
Anderson et al (1975)	330	321	97.3
Hadden et al (1983)	177	172	97.2
Dodge & Cady (1972)	106	103	97.2
Grace & Eversmann (1980)	92	90	97.8
Stern & Drury (1983)	87	81	94.2
Total (average)	792	767	(96.8)

Table 6.4   The functional results after compression plating of forearm fractures

Reference	Number of forearms	Number with satisfactory results	%
Anderson et al (1975)	223	200*	89.7
Hadden et al (1983)	111	89†	80.2
Dodge & Cady (1972)	71	61‡	85.9
Grace & Eversmann (1980)	64	58§	90.6
Lui et al (1985)	42	36	85.7
Total (average)	511	444	(86.9)

*Less than 50% loss of pronation–supination.
†Less than 30% loss of pronation–supination.
‡Less than 20% loss of forearm rotation.
§Less than 40% loss of forearm rotation.

Table 6.4 records the functional results achieved after forearm plating in the larger series. Overall, 86.9% achieved a satisfactory result. The infection rate after plating of forearm fractures varied between 2.4% (Anderson & Bacastow 1984) and 5.5% (Hadden et al 1983). In 1986, Moed et al reported the results of immediate internal fixation of open fractures of the diaphysis of the forearm in 50 patients. A total of 72 of 79 fractures united (91%). As would be expected, the grade I compound injuries had a better union rate (96.7%) than the grade II (89.6%) or grade III injuries (84.2%). The average time to union was 13.2 weeks (12.8 weeks for grade I injuries and 13.8 weeks for grade III injuries). Excellent or satisfactory results were achieved in 85% of patients. In all, 90% of patients with grade I injuries achieved satisfactory results as compared with 88% of grade II and 70% of grade III injuries.

Summary

1. Undisplaced forearm fractures in adults unite in 6–8 weeks, and displaced fractures heal in 13–20 weeks. Some 29–62% of patients with displaced fractures treated in above-elbow plaster of Paris had a satisfactory result.
2. Conservatively treated adult forearm fractures had a non-union rate of 4.5–12%, a malunion rate of 2–9% and a delayed union rate of 4.5–18%. Rotation was significantly restricted in 45–60% of patients treated in an above-elbow plaster. Rotation was most restricted in middle third fractures.
3. The functional bracing of adult forearm fractures has been reported as achieving excellent results, with a 2% non-union rate, a 4.5% malunion rate and significant limitation in rotation in 4.5% of patients.
4. Union occurred in 91% of adult forearm fractures treated by intramedullary fixation within 15–20 weeks.

5. A satisfactory functional end-result was achieved in 85% of adult patients after intramedullary fixation of their forearm fractures.
6. A union rate of 96.8% occurred following the adequate plating of forearm fractures. The average time to union was variably reported at 7.4–18 weeks. A satisfactory functional result was obtained in 86.9% of patients.
7. A 2.4–5.5% infection rate occurred after the plating of forearm fractures.
8. There was a 96.7% union rate and a 90% satisfactory functional level achieved after the plating of grade I compound fractures.
9. A 89.6% union rate and an 88% satisfactory functional level were reported after the plating of grade II compound fractures.
10. There was an 84.2% union rate and a 70% satisfactory functional level after the plating of grade III compound forearm fractures.
11. The average time to union after the plating of compound forearm fractures was 13.2 weeks.

FRACTURE OF BOTH BONES IN CHILDREN

Fractures of the forearm bones in children respond more readily to conservative treatment than their equivalent fracture in adults. In 1917 Whipple & St John reported on the conservative treatment of 95 forearm fractures in children: 97.9% had a good anatomical result and 96.8% had a good functional result after an average 18-month follow-up.

Thomas et al (1975) found that 65 patients out of 285 (23%) had an unsatisfactory result at 3 months after fracture but at their 4-year review this number of unsatisfactory results had fallen to 8 (2.9%). All 8 patients had incomplete recovery of rotation; none was aware of any functional limitation.

Proximal third fractures

Proximal third fractures account for 6.9% (Blount et al 1942) to 10% (Cooper 1964) of forearm fractures in children. In the study of Thomas et al (1975), 50% of 8 patients with proximal forearm fractures had unsatisfactory results at 3 months and 37.5% (3 patients) still had a residual loss of rotation at 4 years, although none of them was aware of any functional disability. Holdsworth & Sloan (1983) reviewed 51 proximal forearm fractures. Ten patients (19.6%) had lost more than 15° of pronation or supination but only 3 were felt to have significant restriction of rotation. Fifteen (29%) had mild symptoms of minor discomfort or aching in cold weather.

Middle third fractures

Middle third fractures constitute 15–17.7% of forearm fractures in children.

Greenstick fractures of the middle third require 4–6 weeks in plaster. In 1976 Van Herpe stated that since the diaphysis was the most slowly growing area of bone, virtually no angulation was acceptable at this level. He further stated that there was a great tendency to reangulation after manipulation unless the intact dorsal bony bridge was broken at the time of reduction. However Kaya Alpar et al in 1981 stated that in their 56 greenstick fractures with angular deformity alone, no subsequent deformity occurred despite leaving the concave cortex intact. Thomas et al (1975) reported that 11 of their 28 middle third fractures (39%) had unsatisfactory results at 3 months but only 2 (7%) had a significant restriction of rotation at 4 years. Kaya Alpar et al (1981) found that 10% of their 80 midshaft forearm fractures were angulated by 15° or more and all of these had decreased rotation. In those fractures with only one bone displaced in the initial radiograph, conservative treatment was used but there was a tendency for the fracture to slip, requiring remanipulation. When both bones were displaced the results of conservative treatment were always unsatisfactory, with more than 15° of residual angulation being usual.

Distal third fractures

Distal third forearm fractures account for 75% of forearm fractures in children. Buckle fractures require only 2–3 weeks in a below-elbow plaster. In 1964 Cooper stated that 20° of angulation of the distal third of the forearm could be accepted without requiring reduction and Van Herpe (1976) felt that 30° angulation could be accepted in children under the age of 7. These angulated greenstick fractures and those undisplaced fractures with both cortices broken required an above-elbow plaster for 6 weeks. Davis & Green (1976) found that 10% of their fractures reangulated.

Table 6.5 Signs suggesting impending problems after forearm fractures in children (after Creasman et al 1984)

Factor	Number of patients with sign	Number (%) unsatisfactory
Angulation 10–30° in any plane	16	5 (31)
Anteroposterior bow straightened or reversed	10	6 (60)
Abnormal bow in lateral plane	8	3 (37.5)
Displacement >50%	8	2 (25)
Shortening at distal radioulnar joint	9	3 (33)
Up to 45° malrotation	9	2 (22)
Single bone injuries	19	2 (10.5)
Proximal fractures	6	2 (33)
Midshaft fractures	31	3 (9.7)
Distal fractures	20	3 (15)

Displaced distal third fractures required 6 weeks in plaster after reduction but 25% of these redisplaced (Davis & Green 1976).

In 1975 Thomas et al reported that 45 of 249 patients (18%) with distal third fractures had unsatisfactory results at 3 months but only 3 of 40 patients (7.5%) had an unsatisfactory result at 4 years.

In 1984 Creasman et al analysed those factors which might mitigate against a good result (Table 6.5).

Internal fixation

In 1984 Nielsen & Simonsen reported the results of 29 children with displaced forearm fractures treated with AO plates. All united; there was 1 case of deep infection. Of 27 patients reviewed, 22 (81.5%) had no loss of rotation and none had lost more than 20° of rotation. Nielsen & Simonsen noted a mean total increase in the linear growth of the plated bones of 2.4 mm (range 15 mm lengthening to 6.5 mm shortening), and an average of 4.5 mm discrepancy in the lengths of the radius and ulna. This alteration in growth had no obvious effect on function.

Malunion

The remodelling ability of fractures in children is well known but there is debate over the degree of residual angulation that it is acceptable to leave, in the knowledge that remodelling will occur.

Midshaft fractures

Angular deformity resulting from fracture of the midshaft of the forearm will correct poorly with a resultant reduction in the range of pronation and supination (Gandhi et al 1962). In 1976 Högström et al reviewed 25 patients with mainly midshaft fractures, with a minimal angulation at union of 10° (average angulation 20° for the whole group). At final follow-up an average of 10° correction (50% of the original deformity) had occurred. The authors found that only children under the age of 10 years were able to produce large corrections of growth. They felt that all deformities exceeding 10° in the midshaft should be corrected. Daruwalla (1979) agreed that 10° was the upper limit of angulation acceptable in midshaft fractures. Matthews et al (1982) and Tarr et al (1984) confirmed in cadaver studies that a 10° angulation in the midshaft of forearm bones produced less than 20° loss of rotation. In 1982 Fuller & McCullough stated that in children aged over 11 years with midshaft fractures spontaneous correction of the malunion could not be anticipated. Roberts (1986) felt that radial deviation of over 15° at the fracture site rather than dorsal angulation was significant in reducing rotation after midshaft fractures.

Distal third fractures

There seems to be a better chance of achieving a correction of the malunion of distal third fractures if there are enough years left for remodelling to occur before the distal radial epiphysis fuses. This occurs between 15 and 25 years of age (Gandhi et al 1962). These authors found that after 5 years of remodelling there was a 98% correction of the distal third malalignment. Daruwalla (1979) felt that 15° of angulation of the distal third could be expected to remodel and Friberg (1979) reported that only 2 of his 4 patients with 20° of angulation achieved full correction. In 1982 Fuller et al reported that a 20° residual angulation produced a 30° loss of rotation; they felt that limitation of rotation of the forearm was directly related to the angular deformity.

However, in 1977 Nilsson & Obrant reported an approximate 20° loss of rotation in 18 fractures that had healed with no angular deformity, implying that factors other than residual deformity were responsible for this dysfunction.

Blackburn et al (1984) reported the results of a drill osteoclasis in 15 children with significant malunion of the forearm. Eleven of these children regained full pronation and supination.

Plastic deformation

Plastic deformation was first described by Barton in 1821 (King 1984). In 1974 Borden described 8 cases but found manipulative reduction of little benefit in 6 of these patients. Sanders & Heckman (1984) however achieved an average correction of 85% of the angulation but stressed that many minutes of sustained manipulation may be required to reduce the deformity. They described 1 case in an adult, as did Greene (1982). Residual deformity will be related to residual angulation, as discussed above.

Summary

1. In all, 97–98% of children had a satisfactory functional result after the conservative treatment of forearm fractures in children.
2. Some 20–37.5% of proximal third fractures had more than 15° loss of rotation, although there could still be normal function.
3. A total of 7–10% of middle third forearm fractures in children lost more than 15° of rotation.
4. In all, 10% of angulated distal third fractures and 25% of displaced distal third fractures will reangulate in plaster. Significant rotation is lost in 7.5%.
5. Narrowing of the interosseous distance is the significant factor causing a poor result in children.

6. Children's forearm fractures treated with AO plates achieved full rotation in 81.5% of cases.
7. Only 10° of angulation of midshaft forearm fractures in children aged under 10 was acceptable. In children over the age of 10 less angulation was acceptable, depending on age.
8. Angulation of 15° was acceptable in distal third fractures unless the patient was close to cessation of bone growth.
9. Loss of rotation may be related to factors other than residual angulation.
10. Osteotomy for malunion may result in an excellent result in over 70% of patients.
11. An 85% improvement of angulation can be expected in plastic deformation after manipulation.

ISOLATED FRACTURE OF THE ULNA

Isolated fractures of the shaft of the ulna, without dislocation of the radial head, have a reputation for being slow to heal and having a high incidence of non-union. This has led some authors to recommend internal fixation as the routine treatment for these fractures (Creuss 1973).

In 1957 Smith & Sage noted a non-union rate of 20% in 79 isolated ulnar fractures treated by various intramedullary fixation devices. However Richey et al (1958) achieved 100% union in 13 fractures treated by an intramedullary nail.

In 1974 Hooper reported union in all the 16 patients whose isolated ulnar fractures were plated. However Anderson et al (1975) had a 4.3% non-union rate in 45 plated ulnar fractures whilst Corea et al (1981) had a non-union rate of 10% after 47 plated fractures.

After internal fixation the time to union is variably recorded as between 8 (Richey et al 1958) and 16.7 weeks (Burwell & Charnley 1964). Corea and co-workers (1981) reported that the mean time to union in their 254 cases was 12.7 weeks, with little difference being noticed between conservative treatment or internal fixation.

An above-elbow plaster of Paris cast has been the traditional conservative method of treatment. Altner & Hartman (1972) treated 151 fractures in this way and found only 1 case of non-union (0.6%). A satisfactory functional result was achieved in 93% of the patients and the healing time was 7 weeks in the distal third, increasing to 10 weeks in the proximal third. Du Toit and Gräbe (1979) treated 63 patients in this manner, all uniting in an average of 7.6 weeks, although the proximal fractures united faster than the distal ones.

In 1976 Sarmiento et al reported no non-unions after using a forearm brace in 72 isolated ulnar fractures. The fractures healed in 9.9 weeks and the average loss of motion was 7° of rotation in middle third fractures and

12° loss of rotation in the distal third fractures. Pollock et al (1983) had similar good results after treating 59 isolated ulnar fractures without immobilization. The average healing time for this group was 6.7 weeks and the average loss of forearm rotation was 5°.

Brakenbury et al (1981) reported 21 non-unions out of 254 isolated ulnar fractures, the incidence being higher in midshaft fractures. A 20% non-union rate was seen in fractures with more than 50% shaft displacement and open reduction had three times the non-union rate of conservatively treated fractures (4.9% compared with 17.4%).

Summary

1. Conservatively treated isolated ulnar shaft fractures had a low non-union rate (4.9%) and healed in 7–10 weeks. Satisfactory function can be expected in over 90% of patients.
2. Rigid plating of isolated ulnar shaft fractures produced a slower rate to radiological union, excellent functional results, but a higher non-union rate (17.4%).

COMPLICATIONS OF FOREARM FRACTURES

Non-union

The incidence of non-union in forearm fractures is discussed under the various sections. Good reports of union following surgery for non-union of forearm fractures have been reported by various authors. In 1962 De Buren reported 34 successes in 36 non-unions (94%) treated with a plate and cancellous bone graft, with 27 uniting in 4 months. Rosen (1979) reported a 95% success rate in 21 non-unions treated with compression plates applied with and without cancellous bone graft. Union occurred in an average of about 6 months with hypertrophic non-unions healing in approximately 4 months and atrophic non-unions in 5–8 months.

In 1965 Scaglietti et al reported a 92% union rate in 102 non-unions treated with onlay cortical grafts. Christensen (1976) had less success with intramedullary Kuntschner nails without grafting. Only 75% of 20 fractures healed primarily; in 4 of these the X-rays were not consolidated at 1 year.

Heppenstall et al (1983) had an 80% union rate in 40 non-unions treated with DC electrical stimulation but cautioned against its use when large fracture gaps or infections were present. Encouraging results have been reported by Dell et al (1984) in the use of vascularized fibular grafts in 4 infected non-unions, converting them to 1-bone forearms.

Nerve and tendon lesions

In 1957 Smith & Sage reported 53 nerve lesions (31 radial, 10 ulnar, 4 median, 8 mixed) in 338 fractures (15.7%) treated by intramedullary nailing, but one-third of these patients had compound injuries. The true incidence in close forearm fractures is much lower than this, and lies somewhere between 0.9% (Davis & Green 1976) and 5% (Hadden et al 1983). These lesions are usually transient and all the main nerve trunks have been involved. In 1972 Altner & Hartman reported the case of a patient whose flexor tendons to the index and middle finger were adherent to the callus of an isolated ulnar fracture, causing impaired function; Mackay & Simpson (1980) reported the closed rupture of the extensor digitorum communis tendon following a fracture of the lower end of the radius with anterior displacement.

Synostosis

In 1987 Vince & Miller reported the results of the treatment of 28 adult patients and 10 children with cross-union as a complication of forearm fractures (Vince & Miller 1987a, 1987b). They found that the overall incidence in adults was 2%. In children the incidence was 5.7% for proximal fractures whilst it was very rare in middle and distal third injuries. They divided cross-union into three types. Type 1 occurred in the distal intra-articular part of the radius and ulna, type 2 in the middle, or the non-articular part of the distal third of the radius and ulna, and type 3 cross-union occurred in the proximal third. The type 1 injuries in adults were uncommon (4 cases) and none occurred in children. This type occurred after Colles' fractures in each case; all 4 underwent surgery but only 1 had a satisfactory result.

Type 2 injuries were commonest in adults (14 cases), with only 3 cases occurring in children. These cases tended to occur after severe trauma and an associated head injury was common. This association with head injury had been noted by Hadden et al (1983) and Stern & Drury (1983). Ten type 2 cross-unions in adults were excised. In all, 70% had satisfactory functional results and there were no recurrences. Three were excised in children, with 1 satisfactory result and 1 recurrence.

Ten type 3 cross-unions occurred in adults, again associated with severe trauma. Six occurred in children, only 2 after high-energy injuries, and 3 of these 6 children had undergone open reduction. Surgery was performed in 3 of the adult cases and two synostoses recurred. In 3 children the radial head was excised in an attempt to improve movement, but a satisfactory result was only achieved in the patient who had a prosthesis inserted to replace the excised radial head. In 1973 Creuss reported 50% satisfactory results after the excision of 6 cross-unions; however, he did not specify their location.

Refracture after plate removal

There seems to be a significant incidence of refracture after plate removal, especially if the plate is removed less than 1 year from its application.

Andersen et al (1975) removed the plates routinely from less than 10% of their 244 patients; they had 8 refractures when the plates were removed before 1 year. They now leave the plate for 12–18 months and apply a protective splint for 4–6 weeks after plate removal. They do not, however, recommend the routine removal of plates, a view endorsed by Teipner & Mast (1980) who had an incidence of refracture of 10% after plate removal from 69 forearm bones. However, the majority of these had had double plates applied. Hidaka & Gustilo (1984) noted 7 refractures in 32 forearm bones (21.8%) after plate removal. A total of 40% of forearm bones in which the plate was removed before 1 year refractured, as opposed to 13.6% when the plates were removed after 1–5 years. Nielsen & Simonsen (1984) reported a 3.4% refracture rate after plate removal in 29 children.

Summary

1. Non-union of forearm fractures treated with compression plates with and without bone graft healed in 94–95% of cases. Hypertrophic non-unions healed in 4 months and atrophic non-unions in 5–8 months.
2. Nerve injuries were associated with 0.9–5% of closed forearm fractures, although these injuries were invariably transient.
3. Rarely, flexor or extensor tendons may be compromised by forearm fractures.
4. Synostosis occurred in 2% of adults and 5.7% of proximal third fractures in children.
5. Of cross-unions in adults, 50–52% had satisfactory function after surgery. Most success occurred in the type 2 injuries (70% success rate).
6. Of cross-unions in children, 33% had satisfactory function after surgery.
7. Refracture after plate removal occurred in up to 21.8% of forearms. Plates should not be removed before 18 months if possible.

MONTEGGIA FRACTURE DISLOCATION

Incidence and classification

Although uncommon, Monteggia fracture dislocations of the forearm are by no means rare, occurring in 0.7% of elbow injuries (Bruce et al 1974) and from 5% (Altner 1981) to 9.9% (May & Mauck 1961) of fractures of the radius and ulna. However, judging from the reported series, on presentation a large number are not diagnosed. In 1940 Speed & Boyd reported that 52% of Monteggia fractures were diagnosed 4 weeks or longer after the accident, although the number from the same centre had dropped to 23% by 1969 (Boyd & Boals 1969). Other articles however quoted the incidence at between 16% (Smith 1947) and 21% (Edwards 1952). More recent papers tend not to quote figures for delayed diagnosis, suggesting continued improvement in making the initial diagnosis.

Bado's classification (1967) is most widely used for these fractures. He classified Monteggia fractures or lesions into the following groups:

Type I: Anterior dislocation of the radial head with a fracture of the ulnar diaphysis at any level with anterior angulation.

Type II: Posterior or posterolateral dislocation of the radial head with a fracture of the ulnar diaphysis with posterior angulation.

Type III: Lateral or anterolateral dislocation of the radial head with a fracture of the ulnar metaphysis.

Type IV: Anterior dislocation of the radial head with a fracture of the proximal third of the radius and a fracture of the ulna at the same level.

He also described some Monteggia equivalent lesions which will not be considered further in this section. Bado pointed out that in the type II Monteggia lesion there frequently coexisted a lesion at the wrist.

Monteggia fracture dislocations in adults

The incidence of the different types of Monteggia fracture dislocations in adults is shown in Table 6.6. Overall 76% are type I, 22% type II and 2% are type IV. In 1951 Penrose reported a 70% incidence of the posterior (type II) fracture dislocation, although this figure is exceptionally high compared with other reported series.

Table 6.6   The incidence of the different types of Monteggia fracture dislocation in adults

Reference	Type I	Type II	Type IV
Reckling (1982)	19 of 24 (79%)	5 of 24 (21%)	
Jessing (1975)	5 of 6 (83%)	1 of 6 (17%)	
Bruce et al (1974)	11 of 15 (73%)	3 of 15 (20%)	1 of 15 (7%)
Reckling & Cordell (1968)	10 of 14 (71%)	4 of 14 (29%)	
Total	45 of 59 (76%)	13 of 59 (22%)	1 of 59 (2%)

No type III lesions in adults were found in the literature, although Anderson (1984) states that he remembers seeing a case.

It is difficult to compare these series because of the differing criteria for functional assessment. Reckling & Cordell (1968) based their final result on the active range of motion of the wrist, forearm and elbow. A good result was one with less than a 10° loss of motion, a fair result had more than 10 but less than 30° loss of motion and a poor result had more than 30° loss of motion in either plane. This system was used by Reckling (1982) and has been applied by the present author to Jessing's (1975) results. Boyd & Boals' (1969) criteria were:

Excellent: A full range of flexion–extension and pronation–supination.
Good: At least 75° motion in flexion–extension and pronation–supination 50% of normal or better.
Fair: At least 50° motion in flexion–extension and 50% of pronation–supination.
Poor: Less than 50° motion in flexion–extension, and less than 50% pronation–supination.

Bruce et al (1974) used a points system (readers should refer to the original paper for more details).

Table 6.7   Overall results of the treatment of Monteggia fracture dislocations in adults

Reference	Excellent/good	Fair	Poor
Reckling & Cordell (1968)	4 of 14 (29%)	8 of 14 (57%)	2 of 14 (14%)
Boyd & Boals (1969)	57 of 74 (77%)	9 of 74 (12%)	8 of 74 (11%)
Bruce et al (1974)	5 of 21 (24%)	5 of 21 (24%)	11 of 21 (52%)
Jessing (1975)	1 of 11 (9%)	4 of 11 (36%)	6 of 11 (55%)
Reckling (1982)	6 of 30 (20%)	18 of 30 (60%)	6 of 30 (20%)
Total (average)	73 of 150 (49%)	44 of 150 (29%)	33 of 150 (22%)

Table 6.7 is thus constructed using the individual authors' grading for comparison. It can be seen that 49% of patients achieved an excellent or good result as compared with 51% who achieved a fair or poor result.

Although the number of patients reported on is small, no patient achieved a good result by closed methods of treatment of the ulnar fracture. Some form of internal fixation of the ulna gave superior results to closed treatment. Most series used a variety of non-rigid internal fixation, such as intramedullary rods. Barquet & Caresani (1981) stated that the best way to provide rigid fixation of type IV fractures in adults was by means of compression plates. This preference for compression plates was also expressed by Boyd & Boals (1969) and by Anderson (1984). A closed reduction of the radial head was considered acceptable. If it was not reduced after fixation of the ulna, an open reduction was required to remove portions of torn annular ligament or radial head fragments which were blocking reduction.

There is insufficient data in the literature from which to draw any strong conclusions as to the results to be expected from the various types of Monteggia fracture dislocation. Penrose (1951) looked exclusively at the posterior (type II) Monteggia fracture and found that all had an associated fracture of the radial head. He reported excellent functional results in all his cases but with some permanent restriction of movement. These would all however be rated poor using the above functional assessments.

Barquet & Caresani (1981) reported 14 cases of fracture of the shaft of ulna and radius with associated dislocation of the radial head (type IV). Five of these 14 patients (36%) achieved an excellent/good result by various methods of internal fixation.

Monteggia fracture dislocation in children

The incidence of the different types of Monteggia fracture dislocation in children is shown in Table 6.8. Comparison with Table 6.7 shows that the lateral displacement (type III) injury was more common in children whilst the posterior displacement (type II) injury was more common in adults.

A comparison of those series reporting the treatment of these fractures in children is given in Table 6.9. Whilst excellent/good results are the rule, poor results do occur, although none were recorded in the larger series that have been shown in Table 6.9. In 1974 Bruce et al reported 2 poor results in 12 children, 1 being due to the development of a synostosis.

Results appeared to be good no matter which type of fracture dislocation was being reported or which method of treatment was used. Closed reduction of the dislocated radial head and closed manipulation of the fracture with plaster immobilization seem to be the treatment of choice.

Table 6.8 The incidence of the different types of Monteggia fracture dislocation in children

Reference	Type I	Type II	Type III	Type IV
Wiley & Galey (1985)	22 of 46 (48%)	5 of 46 (11%)	18 of 46 (39%)	1 of 46 (2%)
Letts et al (1985)	28 of 33 (85%)	1 of 33 (3%)	4 of 33 (12%)	
Peiró et al (1977)	18 of 25 (72%)	1 of 25 (4%)	6 of 25 (24%)	
Fowles et al (1983)	14 of 15 (93%)		1 of 15 (7%)	
Ramsey & Pederson (1962)	11 of 15 (73%)		4 of 15 (27%)	
Total (average)	93 of 134 (69%)	7 of 134 (5%)	33 of 134 (25%)	1 of 134 (0.75%)

Table 6.9 The results of treatment of Monteggia fracture dislocation in children

Reference	Number of patients	Excellent/good	Fair
Wiley & Galey (1985)	31	31 (100%)	0
Peiró et al (1977)	25	25 (100%)	0
Letts et al (1985)	23	22 (96%)	1 (4%)
Smith (1947)	21	20 (95%)	1 (5%)
Bado (1967)	18	18 (100%)	0
Total (average)	118	116 (98%)	2 (2%)

There were no poor results in any of these series.

Open reduction of a radial head which remains dislocated despite attempts at closed reduction is occasionally required, as is intramedullary fixation or compression plating for unstable fractures.

Normal function was usually restored 2–3 months after injury.

Wiley & Galey (1985) found increased hyperextension of the elbow by 5–10° in 12 out of their series of 31 patients (39%). Similarly, Letts et al (1985) noted that 10 of their 22 patients (45%) were noted to have a mild hyperextension of the elbow of 5° more than the uninjured side.

Complications of Monteggia fracture dislocations

Malunion

Although patients with persistent subluxation and dislocation of the radial head could obtain almost perfect function in the elbow, the majority had limited movements of flexion–extension and pronation–supination, muscle atrophy, weakness of the extremity, pain on heavy lifting, arthritic changes about the head of the radius and, in children, usually an increase in the carrying angle (Speed & Boyd 1940).

McGuire & Myers (1986) reported the restoration of normal elbow function in 7 cases of missed Monteggia fracture treated by simple ulnar osteotomy without a direct operation on the radial head.

Kalamchi (1986) reported 2 children in whom he performed a drill osteotomy of the ulna and repair of the annular ligament. This resulted in an improved range of movement.

Bell Tawse (1965) utilized a strip of fascia from the triceps tendon to refashion the annular ligament. No osteotomy of the ulna was performed. Almost full movements were restored apart from slight limitation of pronation in some patients.

Tardy palsy of the posterior interosseous nerve has been described following untreated Monteggia lesions. Lichter & Jacobsen (1975) described a case developing 39 years after injury which was treated by radial head excision and decompression with almost full return of function. Austin's case (1976) occurred 65 years after initial injury. Holst-Nielson & Jensen (1984) treated their 2 cases by splitting the ligament of Frohse with full return of function. Their cases occurred 30 and 39 years after the initial injury.

Nerve lesions

Although the incidence of nerve lesions in Monteggia fracture dislocations varied from series to series, in those series reviewed in this chapter the overall incidence was 16%, which correlated well with the 17% occurrence reported by Altner (1981). Although the radial nerve or posterior interosseous nerve are usually involved, Wiley & Galey (1985) reported involvement of the anterior interosseous nerve and Stein et al (1971) reported ulnar nerve involvement. The posterior interosseous nerve is also vulnerable at the time of open reduction of the radial head. In the case reported by Spar (1977) it was actually wrapped round the radial head and was acting as a block to reduction.

Spontaneous recovery of function seems to be the rule following neuropraxia at the time of injury or peroperatively. This had usually occurred by 2–3 months. Although Stein et al (1971) explored 6 of their 7 nerve lesions and recommend surgical decompression of involved nerves, the majority of reported cases have resolved without recourse to decompression.

Summary

1. Monteggia fracture dislocations occurred in 0.7% of elbow injuries and 5–9.9% of fractures of the radius and ulna.
2. Wrist lesions have been seen in association with type II injuries.
3. In all, 76% of Monteggia fracture dislocations in adults were of type I, 22% were of type II, type III was very rare, and 2% were of type IV.
4. Overall, 49% of adult Monteggia fracture dislocations achieved an excellent or good result.
5. Stable internal fixation with closed or open reduction of the radial head gave the best functional result.
6. A total of 70% of Monteggia fracture dislocations in children were of type I, 5% were of type II, 25% type III and type IV lesions rarely occurred.
7. An excellent/good result occurred in 98% of children whatever the type of fracture or the method of treatment. The disability time was from 6 to 12 weeks.
8. A mild hyperextension deformity was seen in 39–45% of children after Monteggia fracture dislocation.
9. Persistent dislocation of the radial head limited elbow movement and caused an increase in the carrying angle in some children.
10. Satisfactory improvement in function has been reported following various surgical treatments for persistent malunion.
11. Tardy palsy of the posterior interosseous nerve has been reported up to 65 years after initial injury.
12. Nerve lesions (usually posterior interosseous) occurred in 16% of Monteggia fracture dislocations. Spontaneous recovery was the rule.

GALEAZZI FRACTURE DISLOCATION

The term *Galeazzi fracture* was originally applied to radial fractures occurring at the junction of the middle and distal thirds of the shaft associated with disruption of the inferior radio-ulnar joint. It is now more generally used to describe radial fractures at any level associated with this disruption.

In 1975 Mikic reported that 57% of the fractures in his series of mainly adult patients occurred at the junction of the middle and distal thirds of the radius and 31% in the middle third of the radial shaft. Only 4% occurred in the distal third of the radius.

Moore et al (1985) reported a 6.8% incidence of Galeazzi fracture (84 cases) out of a series of 1236 forearm fractures in adults. Wong (1967) found the incidence in adults to be slightly higher in Singapore where 38 cases out of a series of 364 forearm fractures (10.4%) were of the Galeazzi type.

Galeazzi fracture dislocation in adults

The conservative treatment of this type of fracture in adults has produced poor results. In 1957 Hughston reported only 3 good results out of 38 patients (8%) treated by closed reduction and immobilization. A similar poor result following conservative treatment was reported from Singapore where Wong (1967) had 3 satisfactory results out of 34 patients (9%). Mikic (1975) found that the healing time for these fractures in adults was 2–3 months.

Intramedullary fixation devices and compression plates have been utilized in the operative treatment of this type of fracture. Although Mikic reported 68% excellent results from 19 Rush intramedullary pins, compared with 50% excellent results from 12 cases plated, more recently published papers suggested that rigid fixation for this fracture gave better results. In 1982 Reckling reported good results in all 17 of his patients treated by immediate open reduction. Krause & Horne (1984) reported 22 satisfactory results in 23 patients (95.5%) treated by plate fixation. In 1985 Moore et al reported 2 non-unions in 36 fractures (5.5%) treated with compression plates, although both united after second plates and bone graft were applied. Final healing was rated as excellent in 35 of 36 fractures (97%). A total of 80% of these patients had an excellent range of movement — less than 10° loss of wrist flexion–extension and less than 25° loss of pronation–supination. Similarly, function was rated as excellent in 78% of patients whilst only 1 patient (3%) had a poor functional result. Grip strength however was normal in only 7 patients (20%). The average loss of grip strength was 33% in males and 20% in females.

Ulnar and anterior interosseous nerve lesions are occasionally reported in association with Galeazzi fracture dislocation. Mikic (1975) found only 1 ulnar nerve injury in his 125 patients with this fracture.

Galeazzi fracture dislocation in children

The reported results of the treatment of Galeazzi fracture dislocations in children tend to be better than those for adults, although Wong (1967) reported that all 6 children in his series had unsatisfactory results after conservative management.

Better results were reported by Walsh et al in 1987. In 17 of the 41 patients (41%) in this series the injury to the distal radioulnar joint was not recognized initially. Of 39 fractures treated conservatively, 24 (61.5%) had excellent results and 12 (30.5%) had fair results. Excellent results were more readily achieved when the fracture was at the junction of the middle and distal third (75%) than with fractures of the distal third (47.5%). Below-elbow plasters gave excellent results in 7 of 16 cases (43.5%) whilst above-elbow plasters gave excellent results in 17 of 23 cases (74%). Walsh et al found that the healing time for children with these fractures was 4–6 weeks.

In 1984 King stated that 10° of angulation in these radial shaft fractures in children was acceptable and no loss of pronation or supination would result.

Summary

1. Only 8–9% of adult patients achieved a satisfactory result after the conservative treatment of Galeazzi fracture dislocations. Satisfactory results were reported in 68% of patients following intramedullary fixation, and in 80–100% of patients after compression plates.
2. Grip strength was impaired by 33% in males and 20% in females after the compression plating of these fractures.
3. Nerve palsies were infrequent following this fracture.
4. An excellent result was achieved in 61.5% of conservatively treated Galeazzi fractures in children whilst 30.5% achieved a fair result.
5. Distal third fractures and treatment in below-elbow plasters resulted in a worse result than fractures at the junction of the middle and distal third and above-elbow immobilization.
6. Healing time in children was from 4 to 6 weeks.
7. Ten degrees of angulation can be accepted with no anticipated loss of function.

REFERENCES

Altner P C 1981 Monteggia fractures. Orthopaedic Review 10: 115–120
Altner P C, Hartman J T 1972 Isolated fractures of the ulnar shaft in the adult. Surgical Clinics of North America 52: 155–170
Anderson L D 1984 Fractures of the shafts of the radius and ulna. In: Rockwood C A, Green D P (eds) Fractures in adults, Vol 1. J B Lippincott, Philadelphia, pp 511–558
Anderson L D, Bacastow D W 1984 Treatment of forearm shaft fractures with compression plates. Contemporary Orthopaedics 8: 17–25
Anderson L D, Sisk T D, Tooms R E, Park W I 1975 Compression plate fixation in acute diaphyseal fractures of the radius and ulna. Journal of Bone and Joint Surgery 57A: 287–297
Austin R 1976 Tardy palsy of the radial nerve from a Monteggia fracture. Injury 7: 202–204
Bado J L 1967 The Monteggia lesion. Clinical Orthopaedics 50: 71–86
Barquet A, Caresani J 1981 Fracture of the shaft of the ulna and radius with associated dislocation of the radial head. Injury 12: 471–476

Bell Tawse A J S 1965 The treatment of malunited anterior Monteggia fractures in children. Journal of Bone and Joint Surgery 47B: 718–723

Blackburn N, Ziv I, Rang M 1984 Correction of the malunited forearm fracture. Clinical Orthopaedics 188: 54–57

Blount W P, Schaefer A A, Johnson J H 1942 Fractures of the forearm in children. Journal of the American Medical Association 120: 111–117

Bolton H, Quinlan A G 1952 The conservative treatment of fractures of the shaft of the radius and ulna in adults. Lancet ii: 700–705

Borden S 1974 Traumatic bowing of the forearm in children. Journal of Bone and Joint Surgery 56A: 611–616

Boyd H B, Boals J C 1969 The Monteggia lesion. Clinical Orthopaedics 66: 94–100

Bradford E H, Adams R W, Kilfoyle R M 1953 Fractures of both bones of the forearm in adults. Surgery, Gynaecology and Obstetrics 96: 240–244

Brakenbury P H, Corea J R, Blakemore M E 1981 Non union of the isolated fracture of the ulnar shaft in adults. Injury 12: 371–375

Bruce H E, Harvey J P, Wilson J C 1974 Monteggia fractures. Journal of Bone and Joint Surgery 56A: 1563–1576

Burwell H N, Charnley A D 1964 Treatment of forearm fractures in adults with particular reference to plate fixation. Journal of Bone and Joint Surgery 46B: 404–425

Caden J G 1961 Internal fixation of fractures of the forearm. Journal of Bone and Joint Surgery 43A: 1115–1121

Cotler J M, Ingemi B J, Prabhaker M P 1971 Experience with Schneider nailing in forearm fractures. Journal of Bone and Joint Surgery 53A: 1228–1229

Christensen N O 1976 Küntschner intramedullary reaming and nail fixation for non union of the forearm. Clinical Orthopaedics 116: 215–221

Cooper R R 1964 Management of common forearm fractures in children. Journal of the Iowa Medical Society 54: 589–598

Corea J R, Brakenbury P H, Blakemore M E 1981 The treatment of isolated fractures of the ulnar shaft in adults. Injury 12: 365–370

Creasman C, Zaleske D J, Ehrlich M G 1984 Analyzing forearm fractures in children. Clinical Orthopaedics 188: 40–53

Creuss R L 1973 The management of forearm injuries. Orthopedic Clinics of North America 4: 969–982

Daruwalla, J S 1979 A study of radioulnar movements following fractures of the forearm in children. Clinical Orthopaedics 139: 114–120

Davis D R, Green D P 1976 Forearm fractures in children. Clinical Orthopaedics 120: 172–184

De Buren N 1962 Causes and treatment of non union in fractures of the radius and ulna. Journal of Bone and Joint Surgery 44B: 614–625

Dell P C, Sheppard J E 1984 Vascularized bone grafts in the treatment of infected forearm non unions. Journal of Hand Surgery 9A: 653–658

Dodge H S, Cady G W 1972 Treatment of fractures of the radius and ulna with compression plates. Journal of Bone and Joint Surgery 54A: 1167–1176

Du Toit F P, Gräbe R P 1979 Isolated fractures of the shaft of the ulna. South African Medical Journal 56: 21–25

Edwards E G 1952 The posterior Monteggia fracture. American Surgeon 18: 323–327

Evans E M 1951 Fractures of the radius and ulna. Journal of Bone and Joint Surgery 33B: 548–561

Fowles J V, Sliman N, Kassab M T 1983 The Monteggia lesion in children. Journal of Bone and Joint Surgery 65A: 1276–1283

Friberg K S I 1979 Remodelling after distal forearm fractures in children. Acta Orthopaedica Scandinavica 50: 731–739

Fuller D S, McCullough C J 1982 Malunited fractures of the forearm in children. Journal of Bone and Joint Surgery 64B: 341–367

Gandhi R K, Wilson P, Mason Brown J J, Macleod W 1962 Spontaneous correction of deformity following fractures of the forearm in children. British Journal of Surgery 50: 5–10

Grace T G, Eversmann W W 1980 Forearm fractures. Journal of Bone and Joint Surgery 62A: 433–438

Greene W B 1982 Traumatic bowing of the forearm in an adult. Clinical Orthopaedics 168: 31–34

Hadden W A, Reschauer R, Segl W 1983 Results of AO plate fixation of forearm shaft fractures in adults. Injury 15: 44–52

Heppenstall R B, Brighton C T, Esterhai J L, Becker C T 1983 Clinical and roentgenographic evaluation of non union of the forearm in relation to treatment with DC electrical stimulation. Journal of Trauma 23: 740–744

Hicks J H 1961 Fractures of the forearm treated by rigid fixation. Journal of Bone and Joint Surgery 43B: 680–687

Hidaka S, Gustilo R B 1984 Refracture of bones of the forearm after plate removal. Journal of Bone and Joint Surgery 66A: 1241–1243

Högström H, Nilsson B E, Willner S 1976 Correction with growth following diaphyseal forearm fracture. Acta Orthopaedica Scandinavica 47: 299–303

Holdsworth B J, Sloan J P 1983 Proximal forearm fractures in children: residual disability. Injury 14: 174–179

Holst-Nielson F, Jensen V 1984 Tardy posterior interosseous nerve palsy as a result of an unreduced radial head dislocation in Monteggia fractures: a report of two cases. Journal of Hand Surgery 9A: 572–575

Hooper G 1988 Isolated fractures of the shaft of the ulna. Injury 6: 180–184

Hughston J C 1957 Fractures of the distal radial shaft. Journal of Bone and Joint Surgery 39A: 249–264

Jessing P 1975 Monteggia lesions and their complicating nerve damage. Acta Orthopaedica Scandinavica 46: 601–609

Kalamchi A 1986 Monteggia fracture-dislocation in children. Journal of Bone and Joint Surgery 68A: 615–619

Kaya Alpar E, Thompson K, Owen R, Taylor J F 1981 Midshaft fractures of the forearm bones in children. Injury 13: 153–158

King R E 1984 Fractures of the shafts of the radius and ulna. In: Rockwood C A, Wilkins K E, King R E (eds) Fractures in children. J B Lippincott, Philadelphia, pp 301–362

Knight R A, Purvis G D 1949 Fractures of both bones of the forearm in adults. Journal of Bone and Joint Surgery 31A: 755–764

Krause B C, Horne J G 1984 Galeazzi fracture dislocation revisited. Journal of Bone and Joint Surgery 66B: 613

Letts M, Locht R, Wiens J 1985 Monteggia fracture-dislocations in children. Journal of Bone and Joint Surgery 67B: 724–727

Lichter R L, Jacobsen T 1975 Tardy palsy of the posterior interosseous nerve with a Monteggia fracture. Journal of Bone and Joint Surgery 57A: 124–125

Lui S, Barrington T W, Evans D C, Harrington I J, Malcolm B W, Simmons E H 1985 Fractures of the forearm treated by compression plating: a retrospective review. Journal of Bone and Joint Surgery 67B: 326

Mackay I, Simpson R G 1980 Closed rupture of extensor digitorum communis tendon following fracture of the radius. The Hand 12: 214–216

Marek F M 1961 Axial fixation of forearm fractures. Journal of Bone and Joint Surgery 43A: 1099–1114

Matthews L S, Kaufer H, Garver D F, Sonstegard D A 1982 The effect on supination–pronation of angular malalignment of fractures of both bones of the forearm. Journal of Bone and Joint Surgery 64A: 14–17

Matthews W E, Saunders E A 1979 Fractures of the radius and ulna: part II. American Surgeon 45: 321–324

May V R, Mauck W 1961 Dislocation of the radial head with associated fracture of the ulna. Southern Medical Journal 54: 1255–1261

McGuire T P, Myers P 1986 Ulna osteotomy for missed Monteggia fracture. Journal of Bone and Joint Surgery 68B: 336

Michels C, Weissman S L 1976 Intramedullary nailing in fractures of the forearm. Journal of Bone and Joint Surgery 58B: 380

Mikic Z 1975 Galeazzi fracture-dislocation. Journal of Bone and Joint Surgery 57A: 1071–1080

Moed, B R, Kellam J F, Foster R J, Tile M, Hansen S T 1986 Immediate internal fixation of open fractures of the diaphysis of the forearm. Journal of Bone and Joint Surgery 68A: 1008–1017

Moore T M, Klein J P, Patzakis M J, Harvey J P 1985 Results of compression-plating of closed Galeazzi fractures. Journal of Bone and Joint Surgery 67A: 1015–1021

Nielsen A B, Simonsen O 1984 Displaced forearm fractures in children treated with AO plates. Injury 15: 393–396

Nilsson B E, Obrant K 1977 The range of motion following fracture of the shaft of the forearm in children. Acta Orthopaedica Scandinavica 48: 600–602

Peiró A, Andres F, Fernandez-Esteve F 1977 Acute Monteggia lesions in children. Journal of Bone and Joint Surgery 59A: 92–97

Penrose J H 1951 The Monteggia fracture with posterior dislocation of the radial head. Journal of Bone and Joint Surgery 33B: 65–73

Pollock F H, Pankovich A M, Prieto J J, Lorenz M 1983 The isolated fracture of the ulnar shaft. Journal of Bone and Joint Surgery 65A: 339–342

Ramsey R H, Pederson H E 1962 The Monteggia fracture-dislocation in children. Journal of the American Medical Association 182: 1091–1093

Reckling F W, Cordell L D 1968 Unstable fracture-dislocations of the forearm. Archives of Surgery 96: 999–1007

Richey S J, Richardson J P, Thompson M S 1958 Rigid medullary fixation of forearm fractures. Southern Medical Journal 7: 852–856

Reckling F W 1982 Unstable fracture-dislocations of the forearm (Monteggia and Galeazzi lesions). Journal of Bone and Joint Surgery 64A: 857–863

Roberts J A 1986 Angulation of the radius in children's fractures. Journal of Bone and Joint Surgery 68B: 751–754

Rosen H 1979 Compression treatment of long bone pseudarthroses. Clinical Orthopaedics 138: 154–166

Sage F P 1959 Medullary fixation of fractures of the forearm. Journal of Bone and Joint Surgery 41A: 1489–1516

Sanders W E, Heckman J D 1984 Traumatic plastic deformation of the radius and ulna. Clinical Orthopaedics 188: 58–67

Sarmiento A, Cooper J S, Sinclair W F 1975 Forearm fractures: early functional bracing. Journal of Bone and Joint Surgery 57A: 297–304

Sarmiento A, Kinman P B, Murphy R B, Phillips J G 1976 Treatment of ulnar fractures by functional bracing. Journal of Bone and Joint Surgery 58A: 1104–1107

Scaglietti O, Stringa G, Mizzau M 1965 Bone grafting in non union of the forearm. Clinical Orthopaedics 43: 65–76

Smith F M 1947 Monteggia fractures. Surgery, Gynaecology and Obstetrics 85: 630–640

Smith H, Sage F P 1957 Medullary fixation of forearm fractures. Journal of Bone and Joint Surgery 39A: 91–98

Spar I 1977 A neurologic complication following Monteggia fracture. Clinical Orthopaedics 122: 207–209

Speed J S, Boyd H B 1940 Treatment of fractures of ulna with dislocation of head of radius. Journal of the American Medical Association 115: 1699–1705

Stein F, Grabias S L, Deffer P A 1971 Nerve injuries complicating Monteggia lesions. Journal of Bone and Joint Surgery 53A: 1432–1436

Stern P J, Drury W J 1983 Complications of plate fixation of forearm fractures. Clinical Orthopaedics 175: 25–29

Street D M 1986 Intramedullary forearm nailing. Clinical Orthopaedics 212: 219–230

Tarr R R, Garfinkel R I, Sarmiento A 1984 The effects of angular and rotational deformities of both bones of the forearm. Journal of Bone and Joint Surgery 66A: 65–70

Teipner W A, Mast J W 1980 Internal fixation of forearm diaphyseal fractures: double plating versus single compression (tension band plating) —a comparative study. Orthopaedic Clinics of North America 11: 381–391

Thomas E M, Tuson K W R, Browne P S H 1975 Fractures of the radius and ulna in children. Injury 7: 120–124

Van Herpe L B 1976 Fractures of the forearm and wrist. Orthopaedic Clinics of North America 7: 543–556

Vince K G, Miller J E 1987a Cross-union complicating fracture of the forearm. Part I: adults. Journal of Bone and Joint Surgery 69A: 640–653

Vince K G, Miller J E 1987b Cross-union complicating fracture of the forearm. Part II: children. Journal of Bone and Joint Surgery 69A: 654–661

Walsh H P J, McLaren C A N, Owen R 1987 Galeazzi fractures in children. Journal of Bone and Joint Surgery 69B: 730–733

Whipple A O, St John F B 1917 A study of 100 consecutive fractures of the shafts of both bones of the forearm with the end results in 95. Surgery, Gynaecology and Obstetrics 25: 77–91

Wiley J J, Galey J P 1985 Monteggia injuries in children. Journal of Bone and Joint Surgery 67B: 728–731

Wong P C N 1967 Galeazzi fracture-dislocations in Singapore 1960–1964. Incidence and results of treatment. Singapore Medical Journal 8: 186–193

7. The wrist

P. S. Fagg

FRACTURES OF THE DISTAL RADIUS

Fractures of the distal radius may be divided into:

1. Undisplaced fractures.
2. Fractures of the distal radius with dorsal displacement (Colles' fracture).
3. Fractures of the distal radius with palmar displacement (Smith's fracture).
4. Marginal articular (Barton's) fractures.

The first two groups will be considered together for convenience.

Fractures of the distal radius — undisplaced and with dorsal displacement

In 1814 Colles gave his description of the fracture of the distal radius with dorsal displacement which bears his name. He stated: 'that the limb will at some remote period again enjoy perfect freedom in all its motions, and be completely exempt from pain: the deformity, however, will remain undiminished through life' (Dobyns & Linscheid 1984). Since this statement many articles have appeared on the subject, reporting good and bad overall results, enthusing over a variety of conservative and operative methods of treatment, and reporting factors both radiological and clinical pertaining to good or bad overall results. A full spectrum of opinions can be found with diligent research of the literature. Reports of the overall results are further hampered by the wide variety of classifications of these fractures.

It is proposed not to comment on the benefits of each variety of plaster type or functional brace but to look at the overall results of conservative treatment, and then to look more closely at the results as they relate to those factors more widely regarded as important by various authors. The results of operative treatment will be reported later.

161

162 MEDICOLEGAL REPORTING IN ORTHOPAEDIC TRAUMA

The overall functional results of conservative treatment

In this section it is proposed to look at the overall results of the conservative treatment of Colles' fractures. Table 7.1 shows the results of the five larger series. These series had either used the points system of Gartland & Werley (1951) or Lidström's (1959) grading to evaluate their functional results. These results show that 76% of patients with Colles' fractures achieved a satisfactory result. Lidström (1959), Smaill (1965) and Frykman (1967) all reported that there was no significant deterioration in the overall functional result with time once recovery had occurred after the injury. Recovery time was variably reported as occurring from 3 to 6 months after the initial fracture.

Table 7.1 The functional results of conservative treatment

Reference	Total fractures	Excellent total,	%	Good total,	%	Fair total,	%	Poor total,	%
Lidström (1959)*	515	214	41.5	195	37.9	61	11.9	45	8.7
Frykman (1967)*	430	105	24.4	218	50.7	81	18.8	26	6.1
Altissimi et al (1986)†	297	113	38.0	145	48.8	35	11.8	4	1.4
Dias et al (1987)†	187	25	13.4	76	40.6	74	39.6	12	6.4
Gartland & Werley (1951)†	60	13	21.7	28	46.7	17	28.3	2	3.3
Overall	1489	470	31.6	662	44.4	268	18.0	89	6.0
		76% satisfactory					24% unsatisfactory		

*Lidström categories.
†Gartland & Werley categories.

Subjective symptoms

A high percentage of patients appear to suffer from subjective symptoms following Colles' fractures despite achieving a reasonable functional result. Bacorn & Kurtzke (1953) retrospectively reviewed 2132 cases from the files of the Workmen's Compensation Board of New York state and found that only 62 cases (2.9%) had no subjective symptoms. Eelma & McElfresh (1983) reported that 82% of 56 patients with Colles' fractures had subjective symptoms whilst Frykman (1967) reported that 52.3% of 430 patients had symptoms, although just over 28% of the total study group had very mild symptoms. Similarly Lidström (1959) found 45.8% of 515 patients with subjective symptoms although 25.8% had very mild symptoms.

Thus subjective symptoms have been reported as occurring in between 46 and 97% of patients with Colles' fractures. Bacorn & Kurtzke (1953) felt that there was an average disability of 24% loss of function of the hand after such a fracture, whereas Green & Gay (1956) estimated the average disability to be 17.7% in 75 fractures.

Table 7.2   The incidence and type of painful subjective symptoms following Colles' fractures

Reference	Total sample	Number with symptoms	%
Pain on strenuous use			
Lidström (1959)	515	59	11.5
Smaill (1965)	41	3	7.3
Frykman (1967)	430	58	13.5
Pain on loading the wrist			
Lidström (1959)	515	54	10.5
Frykman (1967)	430	61	14.2
Pain with weather change			
Smaill (1965)	41	9	22.0
Frykman (1967)	430	23	5.4
Eelma & McElfresh (1983)	58	23	39.7
Pain from the radioulnar joint			
Frykman (1967)	430	59	13.7
Eelma & McElfresh (1983)	58	13	22.4
Altissimi et al (1986)	297	108	36.4
Pain on forced dorsiflexion			
Eelma & McElfresh (1983)	58	19	32.8

Pain. Pain, from a variety of causes, is a common subjective complaint and the various types and incidences are shown in Table 7.2. Of the 56 patients in Eelma & McElfresh's (1983) study, 75% had subjective symptoms of pain compared to only 34% in Smaill's (1965) series.

Fatiguability. A sensation of weakness of the wrist and hand with strenuous activity was noted in 2.3% of Frykman's (1967) 430 cases and 6.6% of the 515 patients in Lidström's (1959) series.

Loss of grip strength. Table 7.3 records those larger series which specifically reported loss of grip strength in their functional assessment. Between 18 and 35% of patients were aware of a feeling of subjective

Table 7.3   The incidence of weakness of grip in Colles' fractures

Reference	Total sample	Number with symptoms	%
Bacorn & Kurtzke (1953)	2130	737	34.6
Lidström (1959)			
subjective	515	141	27.4
objective	481	84	17.5
Frykman (1967)	430	154	35.8
Altissimi et al (1986)	297	53	17.9
Eelma & McElfresh (1983)			
subjective	56	36	64.2
objective	56	5	8.9

Only 3% of Bacon & Kurtzke's (1953) sample had severe weakness.

weakness, although objectively the incidence was lower. In 1983 Eelma & McElfresh reported a higher subjective incidence of weakness (64.2%) but this was in a younger patient population who tend to be more demanding than older patients. However only 8.9% of these patients had any evidence of objective weakness.

Finger stiffness. Residual finger stiffness after Colles' fracture was noted in 47.5% of the 2130 patients in Bacorn & Kurtzke's (1953) series. This figure is surprisingly high. Gartland & Werley (1951) reported an incidence of 18% which was also high when compared to more recent studies. Thus Older et al (1965) found a 6% incidence in 100 fractures, Altissimi et al (1986) a 4.4% incidence in 297 fractures whilst in Frykman's (1967) series his incidence was as low as 0.7% after 430 fractures.

Table 7.4   Loss of motion after Colles' fractures

Reference	Patient sample	Palmar flexion		Dorsiflexion	
		Number decreased	%	Number decreased	%
Bacorn & Kurtzke (1953)	2130		94.5		80
Lidström (1959)	515	210	40.8	73	14.2
more than 20°		92	17.9	43	8.4
Frykman (1967)	430	223	51.9	122	28.4
more than 20°		132	30.7	97	22.6
Eelma & McElfresh (1983)	58	8	13.8	25	43
more than 20°		3	5.2	11	19

Reference	Patient sample	Ulnar deviation		Radial deviation	
		Number decreased	%	Number decreased	%
Lidström (1959)	515	78	15.2	36	7
more than 20°		64	12.4	36	7
Frykman (1967)	430	173	40.2	90	20.9
more than 20°		127	29.5	76	17.7
Eelma & McElfresh (1983)	58	11	19	6	10.4
more than 20°		2	3.5	1	1.7

Reference	Patient sample	Pronation		Supination	
		Number decreased	%	Number decreased	%
Bacorn & Kurtzke (1953)	2130		28.2		36.9
Lidström (1959)	515	38	7.4	47	9.1
more than 20°		26	5.1	26	5.1
Frykman (1967)	430	19	4.4	66	15.4
more than 20°		13	3	49	11.4
Eelma & McElfresh (1983)	58	3	5.2	18	31
more than 20°		2	3.5	6	10.4

Loss of motion. In 1965 Smaill reported very little difference in the range of motion of the injured wrist when it was compared with the uninjured one in his 41 patients. Table 7.4 records the percentage loss of wrist movement after these fractures. It can be seen that no clear pattern emerges. Generally palmar flexion, ulnar deviation and supination were more restricted than dorsiflexion, radial deviation and pronation. The degree of the loss of motion varied widely.

Cosmetic appearance. The final cosmetic appearance was found to appear normal in 39% (Smaill 1965) to 60% (Lidström 1959) of patients. The incidence of residual cosmetic deformity varied widely with a prominent ulna being reported in 7.9% (Frykman 1967) to 46.3% (Smaill 1965) of fractures; radial deviation was noted in 18.3% (Frykman 1967) to 37.9% (Lidström 1959) while dinner fork deformity was cited in from 5.6% (Lidström 1959) to 10.9% (Frykman 1967) of cases.

McAuliffe et al (1987) and Stewart et al (1985a) have drawn attention to the importance to the elderly female patient of a good cosmetic result.

Factors affecting functional results

The age of the patient. There appears to be general agreement in the literature that there is a lower incidence of impaired function in the younger age group than the older groups. Bacorn & Kutzke (1953) further stated that the percentage disability in Colles' fractures increased directly with age at a rate of approximately 4% loss of function per decade. Frykman (1967) and Lidström (1959) agreed that the younger age group had better functional results but they felt that the importance of the age factor on this end-result was slight. Stewart et al (1985a) showed that improvement of function between 3 and 6 months after fracture was statistically more significant in patients aged under 64. As stated previously, Eelma & McElfresh (1983) found a high incidence of subjective symptoms (82%) in their 56 patients aged under 45 years as compared with the larger series of Frykman (1967) and Lidström (1959) where the incidence was 52% and 45% respectively. In these young patients they found that 86% of those aged 18 to 25 years had a good or excellent result as compared with 62% in those aged 36 to 45 years.

The fracture pattern. Many different classifications have been applied to Colles' fractures (Gartland & Werley 1951, Lidström 1959, Older et al 1965, Frykman 1967). Of these, Frykman's is now most widely used but is too complicated to form the basis for discussion in this section.

For simplicity, we will look at the results following fissure fractures, extra-articular fractures, intra-articular fractures involving the radiocarpal joint, intra-articular fractures involving the radioulnar joint and comminuted fractures.

The original amount of dorsal tilt has been shown to have no appreciable effect on the ultimate end-result (Gartland & Werley 1951, Lidström 1959,

Villar et al 1987). Stewart et al (1984) however felt that the functional result was related to the severity of initial displacement but that the type of fracture did not influence the final anatomical result.

Table 7.5 shows how the different published classifications fall into the categories that will be assessed in this section. It is obviously difficult to combine classifications and some overlap must occur.

Table 7.5 Correlation of previous fracture classifications to the categories used in this section

Fissure fracture	
Frykman (1967)	Fissure fracture
Older et al (1965)	Type I
Lidström (1959)	Type I
Extra-articular	
Frykman (1967)	Types I and II
Older et al (1965)	Type II
Lidström (1959)	Types IIA and IIC
Gartland & Werley (1951)	Type I
Involving radiocarpal joint	
Frykman (1967)	Types III and IV
Lidström (1959)	Types IIB and IID
Gartland & Werley (1951)	Type II
Involving radioulnar joint	
Frykman (1967)	Types V and VI
Comminuted	
Frykman (1967)	Types VII and VIII
Older er al (1965)	Type IV
Lidström (1959)	Type IIE
Gartland & Werley (1951)	Type III

Table 7.6 shows the functional results related to fracture type. These figures show no great correlation between fracture pattern and final functional outcome. This view was also held by Stewart et al (1984) and Altissimi et al (1986). Certainly undisplaced fissure fractures gave the best functional results (see Table 7.6) with 89–100% satisfactory results. Comminuted fractures tended to have the worst functional scores with 25–80.7% satisfactory results. Green & Gay (1956) agreed that the end-results in non-comminuted fractures were generally better, and Cooney et al (1980) found that comminuted fractures had a higher incidence of complications. The other aspects of the fracture pattern do not appear greatly to affect the final functional outcome, although Frykman (1967) felt that involvement of the radioulnar joint was an important contribution to poor functional results. In his series this group had the lowest percentage of satisfactory results (62.7%), even lower than that for comminuted fractures (69%). The contribution of the involvement

Table 7.6 Functional result related to fracture pattern

Reference	Total	Excellent		Good		Fair		Poor	
		n	%	n	%	n	%	n	%
Fissure fracture									
Lidström (1959)	40	40	100						
Older et al (1965)	13	13	100						
Frykman (1967)	19	11	57.9	6	31.5	1	5.3	1	5.3
Extra-articular fractures									
Gartland & Werley (1951)	7	6 satisfactory results (85.7%)				1 unsatisfactory result (14.3%)			
Lidström (1959)	339	159	46.9	117	34.5	36	10.6	27	8.0
Older et al (1965)	25	18	72	6	24			1	4
Frykman (1967)	156	56	35.9	80	51.2	17	10.9	3	2
Eelma & McElfresh (1983)	23	8	34.8	14	60.9	1	4.3		
Altissimi et al (1986)	90	79 satisfactory results (88%)				11 unsatisfactory results (12%)			
Involving radiocarpal joint									
Gartland & Werley (1951)	27	20 satisfactory results (74%)				7 unsatisfactory results (16%)			
Lidström (1959)	107	39	36.5	51	47.7	12	11.2	5	4.6
Frykman (1967)	98	19	19.4	53	54.1	19	19.4	7	7.1
Eelma & McElfresh (1983)	18	2	11.1	13	72.2	3	16.7		
Altissimi et al (1986)	73	66 satisfactory results (90.4%)				7 unsatisfactory results (9.6%)			
Involving radioulnar joint									
Frykman (1967)	102	19	18.6	45	44.1	26	25.5	12	11.8
Eelma & McElfresh (1983)	9	2	22.2	5	55.6	2	22.2		
Altissimi et al (1986)	41	38 satisfactory results (92.7%)				3 unsatisfactory results (7.3%)			
Comminuted fractures									
Gartland & Werley (1951)	26	15 satisfactory results (58%)				11 unsatisfactory results (42%)			
Lidström (1959)	32	2	6.3	12	37.5	8	25	10	31.2
Older et al (1965)	14	6	42.9	5	35.7			3	21.4
Frykman (1967)	74	11	14.9	40	54.1	19	25.7	4	5.3
Eelma & McElfresh (1983)	8			2	25	4	50	2	25
Altissimi et al (1986)	93	75 satisfactory results (80.7%)				18 unsatisfactory results (19.3%)			

of the radioulnar joint to an inferior functional result has also been commented on by Gartland & Werley (1951), who found that 39% had unsatisfactory results, Mason (1953) and Older et al (1965), with 70% poor results from involvement of the radioulnar joint, and Hollingsworth & Morris (1976). In 1979 Mohati & Kar reported that 60 of their 200 patients (30%) had pain and tenderness over the radioulnar joint after fracture healing. Arthrograms of the inferior radioulnar joint were performed and tears of the triangular fibrocartilage complex were found in 27 (45%). This abnormality was found even in well reduced Colles' fractures. Villar et al (1987) reported that involvement of the radioulnar joint resulted in an increased loss of grip strength when compared with fractures involving the radiocarpal joint.

Malunion. In 1953 Mason stated that a united, fully reduced Colles' fracture was always accompanied by an excellent functional and cosmetic end-result. However, both Cassebaum (1950) and Frykman (1967) reported 2–5% poor functional results in association with excellent anatomical results. Many authors, however, have reported excellent functional results with poor anatomical healing. In 1959 Lidström reported that 52% of his patients with a poor anatomical result had good function, whilst Frykman (1967) reported a 64% incidence, Stewart et al (1985a) an 81% incidence at 6-month review, and Cassebaum (1950) over 85% satisfactory results. However, there is no doubt that the functional end-result deteriorates with increasing deformity. What is disputed in the literature is the radiological parameters which are important with regards to ultimate function.

Dorsal angulation. Villar et al (1987) felt that residual dorsal angulation was not significant in producing unsatisfactory results and Frykman (1967) felt that residual dorsal angulation only slightly increased the incidence of unsatisfactory end-results. Lidström (1959) felt that a dorsal angulation of less than 10° was of no consequence but that any larger angulation caused a rapid decline in the functional results. Hollingsworth & Morris (1976) found that 6% of patients with 0° dorsal angulation had unsatisfactory results, whilst with 1–10° dorsal angulation there were 19% unsatisfactory results and with over 10° dorsal angulation this rose to 42%. Altissimi et al (1986) reported 50% unsatisfactory results when dorsal angulation measured more that 15°. Green & Gay (1956) estimated that with up to 10° dorsal angulation there was an average 14% permanent loss of function and with over 10° angulation this rose to an average of 34% permanent disability. Rubinovich & Rennie (1983) found that a loss of volar tilt adversely affected the functional result by decreasing grip and pinch strength, whilst Porter & Stockley (1986) found that this occurred only if the dorsal angulation exceeded 20°.

Radial deviation. Villar et al (1987) and Gartland & Werley (1951) felt that abnormal radial deviation did not affect the functional end-result. Rubinovich & Rennie (1983) felt that a radial deviation of less than 10° affected the outcome by weakening grip whilst Altissimi et al (1986) reported 100% unsatisfactory results when the radial deviation was less than 5°.

Radial shortening. Lidström (1959), Frykman (1967) and Green (1975) felt that increasing radial shortening caused increasing unsatisfactory results, although Frykman (1967) found that this was more so when radial shortening was combined with a degree of dorsal angulation. Villar et al (1987) found that increasing radial shortening caused decreasing grip strength.

The value of remanipulation. In 1973 Pool reported that there was no progression of the deformity after 6 weeks from the initial reduction although Dias et al (1987a,b) found that it progressed over a 3-month period even after plaster casts had been removed. Lidström (1959) reported that 28% of reduced fractures redisplaced whilst Porter & Stockley (1986) reported a 59% incidence. Redisplacement after remanipulation was reported to occur in 40% (Lidström 1959), 52% (McQueen et al 1986) and 57.5% (Collert & Isacson 1978) of cases.

The results of operative treatment

The operative treatment of Colles' fractures falls into four basic groups:

1. Bipolar fixation with pins and casts.
2. External fixation.
3. Internal fixation with pins or nails.
4. Internal fixation with plates.

Bipolar fixation with pin and casts. Many papers describe this technique of fixation, in which pins are placed proximal and distal to the fracture, reduction is obtained and then held by incorporating the pins in the plaster. Subtle differences in the technique are described but for simplicity they will be considered together. Table 7.7 shows the functional results obtained by using this technique. Satisfactory functional results were obtained in 92.9% of patients. The anatomy was generally better maintained than with pure plaster immobilization. Between 75% (Scheck 1962) and 88% (Rauis et al 1979) had satisfactory anatomical results. Green (1975) and Weber & Scabo (1986) pointed out that volar angulation was rarely corrected by this technique.

This technique is not without its complication rate. Chapman et al (1982) reported a 21% incidence of loose pins in 80 cases, a 20% incidence of pin tract infections, a 9% incidence of osteomyelitis requiring curettage and a 9% incidence of iatrogenic fracture of the metacarpal or ulna. The figures from Weber & Szabo's (1986) paper for these complications in 76 cases

Table 7.7 The functional results of bipolar fixation

Reference	Number of patients	Excellent		Good		Fair		Poor	
		n	%	n	%	n	%	n	%
Scheck (1962)	24	10	41.7	13	54.2			1	4.1
Cole & Obletz (1966)	33	17	51.5	14	42.4	2	6.1	0	
Green (1975) objective	45	10	22.2	29	64.4	2	4.4	4	9
Rauis et al (1979)	102	98	96.1	3	2.9			1	1
Suman (1983)	37	8	21.6	22	59.5			7	18.9
Overall	241	143	59.3	81	33.6	4	1.7	13	5.4
		92.9% satisfactory				7.1% unsatisfactory			

were 21% loose pins, 8% pin tract infections, 4% osteomyelitis and 7% iatrogenic fracture.

External fixation. The functional results of the larger reported series of patients treated by various external fixation devices are shown in Table 7.8. Overall 87% of patients achieved a satisfactory result. These figures appear slightly inferior to those for bipolar fixation. However the fractures treated by this method tended to be those with greater disturbance of anatomy. Thus in Cooney et al's (1979) paper 48% of the fractures were comminuted (Frykman types VII and VIII), whilst 40% of Vaughan et al's (1985) series were Frykman type VIII. Final grip strength varied between 54% (Cooney 1983) and 72% (Nakata et al 1985) that of the uninjured side. Again there are risks of pin loosening, pin tract infection, osteomyelitis and iatrogenic fracture. Cooney et al (1979) reported complications in 27% of their patients.

Table 7.8 The functional results of external fixation

Reference	Number of patients	Excellent		Good		Fair		Poor	
		n	%	n	%	n	%	n	%
Cooney et al (1979)	60	28	46.7	26	43.3	5	8.3	1	1.7
Jonsson (1983)	57	18	31.6	25	43.9	11	19.3	3	5.2
Cooney (1983)	100	22	22	64	64	10	10	4	4
D'Anca et al (1984)	81	55	68	21	26	3	4	2	2
Vaughan et al (1985)	52	15	28.9	31	59.6	6	11.5		
Overall	350	138	39.4	167	47.7	35	10	10	2.9
		87.1% satisfactory				12.9% unsatisfactory			

Internal fixation with pins and rods. A number of reports record the results of percutaneous pinning of Colles' fractures. Satisfactory results were recorded in 82% (De Palma 1952), 84% (Dowling & Sawyer 1961), and 96% (Clancey 1984) of cases. Similarly, Munson & Gainor (1981) recorded 95% satisfactory anatomical results by this method. Other recorded techniques include Rush pins (Rush 1954), when 84% of patients had full function immediately after surgery, an intramedullary screw (Myles 1978), and tension band wiring (Katznelson et al 1980).

Internal fixation with plates and screws. Internal fixation is not commonly used for Colles' fractures. Kristianson & Gjersøe (1968) described a specially designed plate for fractures of the distal radius with 57% satisfactory anatomical results and 91% satisfactory functional results.

Melone (1984) classified intra-articular fractures of the radius into four types. In 1986 he reported the results of internal fixation of 15 patients with his type 4 injury — the severest grade with wide separation or rotation of the intra-articular fragments. In all 80% achieved satisfactory functional results and 93% had satisfactory anatomical results. All lost some mobility, as they were intra-articular fractures. Grip strength averaged 84% of that of the uninjured hand.

Complications of Colles' fractures

Nerve injuries. The median and ulnar nerves are at risk from compression within their respective tunnels at the wrist as a consequence of Colles' fractures. Table 7.9 records the incidence of median nerve compression in the larger reported series. This incidence varies from 0.2% (Bacorn & Kurtzke 1953) to 17.4% (Stewart et al 1985b). According to the authors, this high figure was a reflection of the fact that the patients in their series were reviewed by a hand surgeon. The overall incidence from these largest series was 2.6%.

Although the majority of compressions of the median nerve were noted early on after the fracture, symptoms of compression can be delayed. In nearly 25% of the cases noted by Stewart et al (1985b) and 10.5% of those reported by Lynch & Lipscomb (1963) the symptoms developed after 3 months, and 2 cases developed 19 and 24 years after the injury, although it is not certain whether the original fracture can be implicated in these 2 cases. Stewart et al (1985b) noted that their cases of median nerve irritability occurred in the older patient and in those who had a greater residual dorsal angulation (average 12.6° in patients with symptoms compared with 7° in those without). Frykman (1967) found that all 10 cases of median nerve compression in his series were associated with intra-articular fractures. Melone (1984) divided the intra-articular fractures of the distal radius into four types. The type I fracture was stable with minimal comminution and the type II fracture was comminuted and unstable. Of 70 type II fractures, 10 (14%) had median nerve compression. His rare type III fracture was comminuted with a ventral spike from the proximal radius which compressed the median nerve in all three cases of

Table 7.9 Incidence of median and ulnar nerve compression with Colles' fracture

Reference	Number of patients	Median nerve		Ulnar nerve	
		n	%	n	%
Bacorn & Kurtzke (1953)	2130	4	0.2	1	0.05
Lynch & Lipscomb (1963)	600	19	3.2	not recorded	
Lidström (1959)	515	1	0.5	5	1
Frykman (1967)	430	10	2.3	4	0.9
Altissimi et al (1986)	297	31	10.4	9	3
Pool (1973)	239	13	5.4	not recorded	
Stewart et al (1985)	213	37	17.4	2	0.9
Overall median	4424	115	2.6		
ulnar	3585			21	0.6

this type until the spike was excised. In the type IV injury, with wide separation of the fragments, 13 of 15 patients (87%) had median nerve compression (Melone 1986).

The majority of median nerve compressions settled down with conservative treatment. A few cases came to carpal tunnel decompression, and the results were usually good although Lewis (1978) pointed out that the nerve could be compressed by fibrosis as a consequence of haematoma beneath the deep fascia, at the level of the fracture site, well away from the carpal tunnel.

Ulnar nerve compression was less frequent, with an overall incidence of 0.6%.

Tendon injuries. The incidence of rupture of the extensor pollicis longus tendon after Colles' fracture is low, varying between 0.5% (Stewart et al 1985b), 0.7% (Frykman 1967) and 1% (Mason 1953). Engkvist & Lundberg (1979) noted that 39 of the 54 cases they presented (72%) occurred in undisplaced fractures. However, Trevor (1950) noted only 4 undisplaced fractures in his 9 cases (44%) of extensor pollicis longus rupture. Thirty-four of 52 cases from Engkvist & Lundberg's (1979) series (65%) ruptured within 8 weeks as did 8 of 9 (89%) of Trevor's (1950) series. Rarely, the tendons of extensor communis may rupture as a late consequence of Colles' fracture (Sadr 1984).

Flexor tendons are rarely affected by Colles' fractures. Stuart & Beckenbaugh (1987) have reported entrapment of the flexor digitorum profundus tendons to the long and ring fingers in a displaced comminuted Colles' fracture. Melone (1984, 1986) has reported rupture of flexor pollicis longus and the long flexor to the index finger. Broder (1954) reported rupture of the long flexors to the long, ring and little fingers. Diamond & Newman (1987) reported sequential rupture of all flexor tendons, except the flexor digitorum profundus tendons to the little finger, occurring over the course of 20 weeks.

Post-traumatic osteoarthritis. The incidence of post-traumatic arthritis following Colles' fractures is shown in Table 7.10. As can be seen, there is wide variation between an incidence of 3% (Cooney 1983) and 21.6%

Table 7.10　The incidence of post-traumatic osteoarthritis following Colles' fractures

Reference	Number of patients	Incidence of arthritis	
		n	%
Lidström (1959)	515	65	12.6
Altissimi et al (1986)	297	53	17.8
Mason (1953)	100	4	4
Cooney (1983)	100	3	3
Gartland & Werley (1951)	60	13	21.6
Overall	1072	138	12.9

(Gartland & Werley 1951). Certainly 35 of Lidström's (1959) 65 cases included patients with only minute osteophytic change. Frykman (1964) described involvement of the radioulnar joint in 18.3% of cases. The cases of Altissimi et al (1986) all involved the radiocarpal joint but there was a longer follow-up of up to 6 years. After a 5–6-year follow-up Smaill (1965) found a 24% incidence of arthritis in 41 patients. There was, however, insufficient data available to suggest an increasing incidence of degenerative changes with increasing length of follow-up. Only 30% of Smaill's 10 patients with radiological signs of osteoarthrosis were symptomatic, and only 32% of those patients in Altissimi et al's (1986) paper had functional results in the fair or poor group.

The comminuted intra-articular fractures had a greater incidence of degenerative change following fracture. In all, 14 of 15 patients with type 4 (Melone 1986) intra-articular fractures had changes. In Gartland & Werley's (1951) series these changes were seen in none of the 7 patients with their type 1 (simple Colles' fracture) and 10 of the 26 patients with type 3 (displaced and comminuted) fractures. Similarly, only 1 of 339 patients in Lidström's extra-articular groups (IIA, IIC) had changes as compared with 14 of 32 patients with the comminuted (IIE) fracture.

Dupuytren's contracture. Bacorn & Kurtzke (1953) found 4 cases of Dupuytren's contracture (0.2%) in association with 2130 cases of Colles' fracture. Stewart et al (1985b) found that 9 patients (4.2%) of 213 had palmar fascia nodules or bands at 3-month follow-up, increasing to 23 patients (11%) of 209 patients at 6-month follow-up. In all cases the Dupuytren's contracture was mild, and occurred in old patients.

Carpal instability. Carpal instability will be discussed more fully in a later section of this chapter. Taleisnik (1985) described three types of proximal carpal instability occurring after trauma. These were dorsal carpal and palmar carpal translocation occurring at the radiocarpal joint and mid-carpal instability. Cooney et al (1980) described corrective osteotomy in 14 patients with symptomatic malunion causing pain, deformity and a decreased range of motion. Thirteen of these patients had improved grip strength and motion after surgery. Fernandez (1982) reported satisfactory results in 15 of 20 corrective osteotomies.

Taleisnik & Watson (1984) described surgery for 10 patients with a mid-carpal instability secondary to malunited fracture of the distal radius. Following corrective osteotomy 9 patients had complete relief of pain and dynamic subluxation, but the 1 patient having a ligament reconstruction developed a recurrence of symptoms.

Cooney et al (1980) and Jones (1987) both described scapholunate dissociation in combination with Colles' fractures. In Rosenthal et al's (1983) series of 190 consecutive fractures of the distal radius 14 cases (7.4%) of scapholunate dissociation were found although some of these fractures had palmar displacement.

Summary

1. A total of 76% of patients with Colles' fractures had a satisfactory end-result.
2. Subjective symptoms occurred in 46–97% of patients after a Colles' fracture.
3. It has been estimated that the average disability following a Colles' fracture is 17.7–24%.
4. Up to 75% of patients had reported experiencing some subjective symptoms of pain with various activities after Colles' fracture.
5. Fatiguability occurred in 2.3–6.6% of wrists after Colles' fracture.
6. Some 18–35% of patients experienced feelings of subjective weakness after Colles' fracture, although objective weakness occurred in 9–17.5%.
7. Residual finger stiffness had been reported as occurring in 0.7–47.5% of patients after Colles' fractures.
8. Palmar flexion, ulnar deviation and supination were most restricted following Colles' fractures.
9. In all, 39–60% of patients had a normal appearance to their wrist.
10. The younger the patient, the better the overall functional result after Colles' fracture.
11. Undisplaced fissure fractures had 89–100% satisfactory results.
12. Comminuted fractures had 25–80% satisfactory results.
13. Involvement of the radioulnar joint resulted in 30–70% unsatisfactory results.
14. Tears of the triangular fibrocartilage complex in the distal radioulnar joint may cause poor results in well reduced Colles' fractures.
15. Some 2–5% of patients with an excellent anatomical result had a poor functional result.
16. A total of 52–85% of patients with poor anatomical results had satisfactory functional results.
17. A dorsal tilt of over 10° adversely affected the functional end-result.
18. A radial deviation of less than 10° and increased radial shortening probably affected the functional end-result.
19. From 28% to 59% of manipulated fractures redisplaced, and this displacement occurred up to 3 months after initial reduction.
20. From 40% to 57.5% of remanipulated fractures redisplaced.
21. Bipolar fixation resulted in 93% satisfactory functional result and 75–88% satisfactory anatomical results.
22. After external fixation 87% of patients achieved a satisfactory result although these fractures were often more severe.
23. Median nerve compression has been reported in 0.2–17.4% (average 2.6%) of Colles' fractures: in 10–25% of these cases the symptoms developed after 3 months.

24. Intra-articular fractures, older patients and residual dorsal angulation are associated with a higher incidence of median nerve compression.
25. Ulnar nerve compression occurred in 0.6% of distal radial fractures.
26. Rupture of extensor pollicis longus occurred in 0.5–1% of distal radial fractures.
27. From 44% to 72% of ruptures of extensor pollicis longus occurred in undisplaced fractures and 65–89% occurred within 8 weeks of fracture.
28. Some 3–18% of fractures of the distal radius resulted in post-traumatic arthritis.
29. Of patients with radiological signs of post-traumatic arthritis, 30% were symptomatic.
30. The incidence of post-traumatic arthritis was higher in comminuted intra-articular fractures.
31. There may be an increased incidence of Dupuytren's disease after Colles' fractures.
32. Proximal carpal instability may follow malunited fracture of the distal radius. Corrective osteotomy was successful in over 75% of cases.
33. Of distal radial fractures, 5–7.4% may have associated scapholunate dissociation.

Fracture of the distal radius with palmar displacement

The description of a fracture of the distal radius with palmar displacement was made by R. W. Smith in 1847. J. R. Barton in 1838 described dorsal marginal fracture of the distal radius and drew attention to the occurrence of the less frequent palmar marginal fracture (Thompson & Grant 1977). Controversy exists as to whether dorsal marginal fracture alone or dorsal and palmar marginal fractures constitute the true Barton's fracture.

In all, 5% of distal radial fractures were of the palmar displacement (Smith's) type (Lidström 1959) and 1.3–2.2% were marginal articular fractures (King 1975, Thompson & Grant 1977).

Fractures with palmar displacement are unstable and redisplacement during the course of plaster treatment is common. Thomas (1957) emphasized the importance of maintaining the forearm in supination. Only 3 of 8 cases (37.5%) maintained anatomical reduction with plaster treatment in Flandreau et al's (1962) series, and 2 of 7 cases (28.6%) in Thompson & Grant's (1977) series.

Table 7.11 shows the results of conservative treatment in three series. Overall 68.4% had satisfactory functional results. In 1975 King reported that all 17 of the marginal articular fractures in his series had some pain, weather sensitivity or discomfort with heavy labour, mild weakness and some minor loss of movement. On the other hand Thomas (1957) who

Table 7.11   The conservative treatment of distal radial fractures with palmar displacement

Reference	Number of patients	Excellent		Good		Fair		Poor	
		n	%	n	%	n	%	n	%
Lidström (1959)	13	1	7.7	6	46.2	4	30.8	2	15.3
Flandreau et al (1962)	8	4	50	3	37.5			1	12.5
Frykman (1967)*	17	4	23.5	8	47	4	23.5	1	6
Overall	38	9	23.7	17	44.7	8	21	4	10.6
		68.4% satisfactory				31.6% unsatisfactory			

*Involves four operated cases.

treated his patients with the forearm in full supination, only had 1 of 11 patients who did not achieve full pronation. The healing time was 6 weeks (Benjamin 1982).

In 1965 Ellis described a technique of internal fixation of these fractures with a buttress plate. In 1973 De Oliveira reported 20 satisfactory results in 24 patients (83%) after the use of internal fixation and Fuller (1973) had satisfactory results in 28 of 31 fractures (90%). The average period of incapacity after internal fixation was 4 months (De Oliveira 1973).

Subsequent radiocarpal arthritis was noted in 2 of 13 cases (15.4%) of Lidström's (1959) series and 3 of 24 patients (12.5%) of De Oliveira's cases.

Occasionally the tendon of extensor pollicis longus has been reported as being trapped within these fractures (Morrissey & Nalebuff 1977, Murakami & Todani 1981).

Summary

1. Anatomical reduction was lost in 28–37% of conservatively treated fractures of the distal radius with palmar displacement.
2. A satisfactory result was achieved in 68.4% of distal radial fractures with palmar displacement after conservative treatment. The healing time was 6 weeks.
3. In all, 83–90% of these fractures had satisfactory results after internal fixation. The average period of incapacity was 4 months.
4. Post-traumatic arthritis occurred in 12–15% of these fractures.

Epiphyseal fractures of the distal radius and ulna

Epiphyseal fractures of the distal radius and ulna are common injuries in childhood. The incidence is variably reported as having occurred in 8.5% (Harbison et al 1978) to 17.9% (Thomas et al 1975) of forearm fractures in children and in 54.8% of 911 wrist injuries reported by Lee et al (1984).

The majority are Salter type II injuries. In the series of 499 epiphyseal injuries presented by Lee et al (1984), 110 (22%) were Salter type I injuries, 288 (57.7%) type II, 13 (2.6%) type III, 10 (2%) type IV, 2 (0.4%) type V and 76 (15.3%) were unclassified.

Accurate reduction of the fracture was not necessary for a good functional result. Both Blount et al (1942) and Bragdon (1965) stated that only 50% apposition was required to give a good functional result and O'Brien (1984) quoted Aitken as having found no residual deformity in 58 patients reviewed. Plaster immobilization was required for up to 3–6 weeks. Redisplacement can occur and this happened in 4 of 53 cases (7.5%) reported by Davis & Green (1976). Blount et al (1942), Bragdon (1965) and O'Brien (1984) warned of the danger of premature fusion of the epiphyseal plate after repeated manipulation of these fractures. Lee et al (1984) found that 6 patients out of 22 (27.3%) who underwent two or more attempts at closed reduction had premature fusion.

Open reduction was rarely required but irreducible fractures have been reported, with the block to reduction being the flexor digitorum profundus tendon to the ring and little fingers (Manoli 1982) or the median nerve and flexor pollicis longus tendon (Sumner & Khun 1984).

Although 5 of 67 patients (7.5%) in Thomas et al's (1975) series were felt to have unsatisfactory results on discharge from review, most patients eventually achieved full function following these injuries (Harbison et al 1978).

Table 7.12 Incidence of premature epiphyseal fusion in fractures of the distal radial epiphysis

Reference	Number of patients	Number of premature fusions	%
Thomas et al (1975)	42	3	7.1
Davis & Green (1976)	53	1	1.9
Harbison et al (1978)	88	2	2.3
Lee et al (1984)	100	7	7
Overall	283	13	4.6

Premature epiphyseal arrest was the main complication. Table 7.12 records the incidence of this complication in reported series (4.6% overall). Although this problem usually arose as the result of the compression type V injury, this injury was often not diagnosed at initial presentation (Benjamin 1982, O'Brien 1984). It also occurred in types IV and II injuries (Lee et al 1984). The present author could find no record of premature fusion occurring in the rare type III injury. Premature fusion may be partial or complete and produces deformity, weakness of grip and occasional loss of motion. The results of various surgical procedures for this complication were generally good (Lee et al 1984).

Summary

1. Accurate reduction of distal radial epiphyseal fractures was not necessary for a good functional result.
2. Redisplacement occurred in 7.5% of cases.
3. Repeated manipulation resulted in premature fusion of the epiphysis in 27.3% of cases.
4. Premature epiphyseal arrest occurred in 4.6% of cases, and occurred in Salter types II, IV and V injuries.

Isolated injury of the distal radioulnar joint

Pure dislocation of the distal radioulnar joint and tears of the triangular fibrocartilage complex do occur in isolation but are not common injuries.

Dislocation of the distal radioulnar joint

Isolated dorsal or palmar dislocation of the distal ulna can occur. However this isolated lesion was missed at initial assessment in up to 50% of cases (Alexander 1977). Dorsal dislocation results in a prominent ulna with painful and limited supination. The dislocation is easily reduced when seen in the acute stage and plaster immobilization is required for 4–6 weeks. Manipulative reduction of a dorsal dislocation has been performed successfully 60 days after initial injury (Dameron 1972), although Dobyns & Linscheid (1984) felt that if reduction was delayed beyond 2 weeks then laxity of the distal radioulnar joint could occur. This would result in recurrent subluxation in pronation, which might require ligamentous reconstruction or distal excision of the ulna in some cases. Late presentation may require open reduction or excision of the distal ulna.

Palmar dislocation causes the wrist to appear narrow on the anteroposterior X-ray, and pronation is painful or impossible. This type of dislocation tends to be stable when reduced early, although habitual volar subluxation has been reported (Birch-Jensen 1951, Rose-Innes 1960). Late diagnosis may necessitate open reduction or excision of the distal ulna.

Tears of the triangular fibrocartilage complex (TFC)

Tears of the TFC can occur in isolation or in combination with fractures of the distal radius and ulna. Degeneration and perforation of the TFC can also occur with ageing and 30.6–53% of TFCs in cadavers show perforation (Coleman 1960, Fisk 1984).

Strickner et al (1980) found 53 confirmed lesions of the triangular disc on arthrography in 153 patients (34.6%) with post-traumatic ulnar pain. Moharti & Kar (1979) found arthrographically proven tears of the TFC in 27 of 60 patients after a Colles' fracture (45%).

In 1984 Dobyns & Linscheid suggested that if an acute tear of the TFC was suspected then the wrist should be immobilized for 4–6 weeks. They reported that these injuries often improved with time.

Coleman (1960) reported that removal of the disc relieved symptoms and did not prejudice function. In 1984 Merion et al found that 11 of 16 patients (69%) were relieved of their symptoms by the partial excision of the disc, although the results were poor in those patients aged over 40 years. In 1986 Van der Linden reported even better results after excision of the disc with 30 satisfied patients out of 33 (91%).

Fisk (1984) however suggested that the results of disc excision were disappointing and he felt that instability of the distal radioulnar joint was almost inevitable.

Summary

1. Isolated dislocations of the radioulnar joint were frequently missed at initial presentation.
2. Early reduction of dorsal dislocation resulted in good functional recovery but late presentation may require distal ulnar excision.
3. Prompt reduction of volar dislocation tended to be stable although recurrent subluxation can occur.
4. Perforations in the triangular fibrocartilage complex were seen in 30.6–53% of cadavers.
5. Of patients with post-traumatic ulnar pain, 35% had lesions of the triangular disc.
6. Of patients with Colles' fractures, 45% had tears of the triangular fibrocartilage.
7. Acute tears of the triangular disc may settle with 4–6 weeks in plaster.
8. From 69% to 91% of patients may have successful results following triangular disc excision, although results were poor in those aged over 40 years.

Scaphoid fractures

Fractures of the carpal scaphoid are relatively common. Their classification into anatomical thirds (distal, middle and proximal) is adequate to enable consideration of their prognosis. These fractures can be further divided into undisplaced or displaced fractures.

The incidence of scaphoid fractures at these three anatomical sites in some of the larger series is shown in Table 7.13. Overall, 22.4% of these fractures occurred in the distal third, 71% in the middle third and 6.6% in the proximal third.

The majority of scaphoid fractures are treated by conservative methods, although there is no agreement as to which position of immobilization is correct. The overall results of conservative treatment will be presented

Table 7.13 The incidence of scaphoid fractures according to anatomical location

Reference	Number of patients	Distal third		Middle third		Proximal third	
		n	%	n	%	n	%
London (1961)	300	73	24.3	218	72.7	9	3
Stewart (1954)	258	44	17.1	207	80.2	7	2.7
Leslie & Dickson (1981)	222	63	28.4	146	65.8	13	5.8
Eddeland et al (1975)	134	22	16.5	85	63.4	27	20.1
Borgeskov et al (1966)	102	26	25.5	66	64.7	10	9.8
Overall	1016	228	22.4	722	71	66	6.6

with no consideration to the position of immobilization. A later section will deal with the results of surgical treatment.

The results of conservative treatment

The overall rate of non-union in conservatively treated scaphoid fractures from 6 of the larger reported series is shown in Table 7.14. This gives an overall non-union rate of 3.4%. Herbert & Fisher (1984), writing in support of their compression screw, claimed a non-union rate in the order of 50% after conservative treatment.

The rate at which union occurs at the various anatomical locations will be discussed later in this section. It is perhaps appropriate at this point to stress how unreliable interobserver agreement is when attempting to assess radiographic criteria for scaphoid union (Dias et al 1988).

Although the functional results are generally good, Borgeskov et al (1966) reported 3 patients (4%) with complaints severe enough to reduce their working capacity. Some 30% had slight impairment of function and Eddeland et al (1975) found that 28% of their patients had a slight decrease in grip strength. In 1954 Stewart reported that function recovered very quickly after removal of plaster following scaphoid fractures, and had generally recovered in $3\frac{1}{2}$ weeks.

Table 7.14 The non-union rate in conservatively treated scaphoid fractures

Reference	Number of patients	Number of non-unions	%
Stewart (1954)*	306	3	1
London (1961)	227	11	5
Leslie & Dickson (1981)	222	11	5
Russe (1960)	220	6	2.7
Eddeland et al (1975)	92	4	4.3
Borgeskov et al (1966)	71	4	5.6
Overall	1138	39	3.4

*The end-result of some of his reported fractures was uncertain.

There is an increased frequency of non-union with increased delay in treatment after injury (Eddeland et al 1975). However in 1961 Mazet & Hohl reported that union could occur when treatment was delayed by over 8 months, although the period of plaster immobilization was over 1 year in 2 of his cases.

Undisplaced fractures of the scaphoid have a significantly higher union rate than displaced fractures. Table 7.15 shows the reported incidences in those series distinguishing the rates of union between these two groups of fractures. Although these are not large series it can be seen that the non-union rate in displaced scaphoid fractures varied between 45% and 83%.

Mazet & Hohl (1963) described conservative treatment in 7 displaced fractures with only 1 non-union (14%); however, all 6 that healed did so with deformity.

Table 7.15 The comparative rates of union between undisplaced and displaced scaphoid fractures

Reference	Undisplaced fractures			Displaced fractures		
	Patients (n)	Non-unions	%	Patients (n)	Non-unions	%
Dickison & Shannon (1944)				8	6	75
Eddeland et al (1975)	82	11	13.4	30	36	83
Cooney et al (1980)	32	2	6	13	6	46
Weber (1980)	19	0	0	11	6	54.5

Leslie & Dickson (1981) felt that non-union was not related to the initial displacement of the fracture but more to those fractures which displaced during treatment.

However, Mclaughlin & Parkes (1969), Fisk (1984b) and Taleisnik (1985) regarded internal fixation of the fractured scaphoid as mandatory when there was displacement of the fracture.

Avascular necrosis was variably reported as occurring in from less than 1% of scaphoid fractures (Borgeskov et al 1966) to up to 39% of proximal scaphoid fractures (Taleisnik 1985). It seems to cause delay in union; in Stewart's paper (1954) fractures with avascular necrosis healed in an average of 21 weeks as compared with 10–16 weeks for other fractures. Avascular necrosis is not a sign of impending non-union.

Results in distal third fractures. The overall incidence of distal third fractures is 22.4%. These fractures may be further subdivided into fractures of the scaphoid tubercle, the intra-articular distal pole fractures and true distal third fractures.

Fractures of the tubercle are stable, extra-articular and tend to heal rapidly in 3–6 weeks. Occasionally non-union occurs, as in 3 of 23 cases (13%) reported by Dickison & Shannon (1944).

Ripperger et al (1980) described the intra-articular distal pole fracture. Eight radiodistal cases were diagnosed early and healed in 6–7 weeks with good results. Four ulnodistal cases were diagnosed late and all went on to symptomatic non-union.

Other distal third fractures tend to unite in 4–8 weeks. Borgeskov et al (1966) reported excellent functional results in 11 of 17 patients (64.7%), good results in 5 patients (29.4%) and fair results in 1 patient (5.9%).

Results in middle third fractures. Union occurred in 95–100% of wrist fractures (Taleisnik 1985) although London (1961) reported the incidence of union to be lower — 92.5%.

The union time was reported at between 6 and 16 weeks. Borgeskov et al (1966) found excellent functional results in 32 of 44 patients (72.7%), satisfactory results in 11 patients (25%) and fair results in 1 (2.3%).

Results in proximal third fractures. The incidence of non-union in proximal fractures was twice that at the more distal sites (Eddeland et al 1975). Avascular necrosis occurred in 14–39% of cases (Taleisnik 1985). Union was reported as occurring at 10–24 weeks. The functional results in these fractures (Borgeskov et al 1966) were 30% excellent, 60% good and 10% fair in 10 patients.

The results of the operative treatment of fresh scaphoid fractures

Internal fixation of the fractured scaphoid is recommended in displaced fractures, fractures associated with carpal instability and where the fracture is part of a complicated fracture dislocation.

In 1969 Mclaughlin & Parkes reported 100% union in a series of 16 fresh scaphoid fractures treated by screw fixation. In 22 fresh fractures treated with a screw Maudsley & Chen (1972) had 19 unions (86.4%) with all the patients achieving bony union having excellent function, and 2 of the non-unions nonetheless having good function post-operatively. In 1979 Huere reported a 92.3% union rate in 13 fractures.

Herbert (1986) reported excellent results with his compression screw, with 97.5% union in 40 cases; patients returned to work in an average of 3.7 weeks. Bunker et al (1987) achieved union in 10 of 11 fresh fracture dislocations (90.9%) using the Herbert screw. They experienced technical difficulties with this device, however, as did Pring et al (1987) and Ford at al (1987).

Non-union of the scaphoid

Not every case of scaphoid non-union is necessarily a cause of symptoms. In some cases symptoms are provoked by a second injury and may rapidly resolve with conservative measures. This has led some authors (London 1961, McDonald & Petrie 1975) to recommend no surgical treatment for established non-union in the absence of significant clinical symptoms. However a number of more recent publications have suggested that there is progressive degeneration with an increased period of non-union.

Mack et al (1984) looked at 47 symptomatic scaphoid non-unions. They divided the stages of degeneration into three groups. Group I, with scaphoid changes only, was seen in 23 patients with an average duration of their non-union of 8.2 years. Fourteen patients in group II with radioscaphoid degeneration had had their non-union for 17 years. The third group with generalized arthritis (10 patients) had had their non-unions for an average of 31.6 years. The authors commented that after 5–10 years of non-union almost all scaphoids showed cyst formation and resorptive changes within the scaphoid.

Ruby et al (1985) also found an increased incidence and severity of degenerative changes with increasing duration of non-union. Only 1 (4%) of 23 non-unions of 1–4 years' duration had arthritis, whilst 92% of 13 patients with non-union of 5–9 years and all 19 patients with non-union of 10 or more years had degenerative changes.

Vender et al (1987) reported progressive arthritis in 64 patients with scaphoid non-union: 100% had scaphoid cysts when the non-union was over 18 months old. A total of 75% had radioscaphoid arthritis at 4 years whilst only 38% had mid-carpal arthritis after this period of non-union. These and similar findings have led these authors and others (Cooney et al 1980, Melone 1981, Kleinart & Zenni 1984, Stark et al 1986) to the conclusion that at least symptomatic and probably asymptomatic scaphoid non-unions should be treated surgically.

Fisk (1970) noted the adverse effects that carpal instability had on scaphoid union. Black et al (1986) reported that 10 of their 64 non-unions had a scapholunate gap and the instability was progressive and associated with the earlier onset of arthritis. The presence of displacement at the fracture site and the scapholunate gap did not change in frequency with time but the incidence of increased scapholunate angle and the dorsal intercalated segmental instability pattern increased significantly with a longer duration of non-union.

Monsivais et al (1986) performed wrist arthrograms or plain X-rays in 20 consecutive scaphoid non-unions. They found that an intercalated segmental instability was consistently found in wrists with non-union of scaphoid fractures and probably predicted those patients with a greater chance of non-union. Failure to correct this instability and subsequent malunion increased the chances of developing arthritis (Vender et al 1987). Fernandez (1984) and Nakamura et al (1987) described good correction of malalignment, and union with anterior wedge-shaped bone grafts and internal fixation.

Many techniques have been described for the surgical treatment of scaphoid non-union. A few of the more commonly used techniques will be briefly described.

Bone graft. Cancellous or corticocancellous bone grafts are inserted using a variety of techniques via dorsal or volar approaches. Table 7.16

Table 7.16   The results of bone grafts for scaphoid non-union

Reference	Number of patients	Number united	%
Mulder (1968)	100	97	97
Cooney et al (1980)	66	58	87.9
Verdan & Narakas (1968)	45	44	97.7
Green (1985)	45	33	73.3
Fisk (1984a)	41	30*	73.1
Herness & Posner (1977)	40	40	100
Overall	337	302	89.6

* A further 7 were described as incomplete union.

documents the results from the larger reported series. These reported series are describing slightly differing techniques. Overall the union rate was about 90%. Union occurred in 15.8–18 weeks.

Green (1985) described 92% union in his cases which had good vascularity of the proximal pole of the scaphoid, as compared with no cases of union when the proximal pole was totally avascular

Screw fixation. Maudsley & Chen (1972) performed screw fixation in 19 cases of non-union. Although 17 patients were satisfied with the results of treatment, only 2 actually achieved radiological union. The use of compression screws had produced improved rates of union. In 16 cases of non-union Gasser (1965) had 9 cases uniting (56.2%). Kvarnes & Reikeras (1983) reported that 42 of their 44 patients united (95.5%) with a compression screw, and Leyshon et al (1984) had 28 of 32 patients (87.5%) united. From these three papers an overall union rate of 85.9% was achieved with compression screws.

More recently the Herbert screw has been introduced; this can be combined with cancellous bone graft (Herbert & Fisher 1984). In this paper, of 103 non-unions, 84 (81.5%) were probably united. In a later paper Herbert (1986) described failure of surgery in 12 of 200 reconstructions — a union rate of 94%. In 1987 Bunker et al reported that 28 of their 33 cases (84.8%) united. Ford et al (1987) had less success — 8 of 11 patients united (72.7%) — as did Pring et al (1987) with 8 of 14 patients (57.1%) uniting. Both these authors stressed the technical difficulties of this technique.

Electrical stimulation. Electrical stimulation has been used to good effect in the treatment of scaphoid non-unions. Two basic concepts of electrical treatment exist. One concept has a constant current delivered via electrodes implanted directly into the fracture site via invasive or semi-invasive techniques. The second technique employs a totally non-invasive system, using electromagnetic coils placed outside the cast.

Taylor et al (1985) reported 6 cases of union out of 11 (54.5%) treated by direct current stimulation, and union occurred in an average of 4.3 months. Bora et al (1981) achieved 12 unions in 17 cases (70.6%) using a semi-invasive direct current technique; these fractures healed in an average of 12 weeks. Frykman et al (1986) reported a 79.6% union rate (35 of 44 fractures) using a pulsed electromagnetic field and cast, and union occurred in an average of 4.3 months.

Proximal row carpectomy. Neviaser (1983) reported the results of 24 patients who underwent a proximal row carpectomy for various carpal disorders. The results were surprisingly good, with 23 patients achieving relief of pain. Grip strength equalled that of the normal wrist and 50–70% of normal dorsiflexion or palmar flexion was achieved. Ulnar deviation was 85% of normal and radial deviation 17%. Most patients, however, felt a lack of confidence in the wrist, with a sense of weakness on gripping.

Soft tissue interposition arthroplasty. Soft tissue interposition arthroplasty was reported by Boeckstyns & Busch (1984) as producing no or minimal symptoms in 11 of 13 patients (84.6%) as compared with 27 of 28 patients (96.4%) with a Matti–Russe type of bone graft. The soft tissue arthroplasty group returned to work after an average of 6.2 weeks as compared with 15.5 weeks for the bone graft group. In 1985 Boeckstyns et al reported that 25 of 26 patients were satisfied following this procedure. Mobility was decreased by 20–25% and grip strength was reduced by 8%. Carpal collapse occurred in 15 patients and degenerative changes were seen in 7 of 25 cases (28%).

Vascularized bone graft. Kuhlmann et al (1987) reported the successful treatment of 3 patients with scaphoid non-union treated by a vascularized bone graft pedicled on the volar carpal artery.

Tendon rupture

Mahring et al (1985) and Thomsen & Falstei-Jensen (1988) have reported attritional rupture of flexor pollicis longus and in 1 case, the flexor profundus to the index finger after long-standing non-union of the scaphoid.

Scaphoid fracture in children

Scaphoid fractures in children are not common. On occasions they have been reported in children under 6 years of age (Larson et al 1987). These occur most commonly in the distal third of the scaphoid. Müssbichler (1961) reported 100 scaphoid fractures in children: 85% occurred in the distal third and 52% were avulsions from the dorsoradial surface of the scaphoid. Of Vahvanen & Westerland's (1980) 108 cases, 94 (87%) were distal third and 41 (38%) were avulsion fractures. In Christodoulou & Colton's (1986) series of 64 patients, 38 (59.4%) were distal third fractures and a further 24 (37.5%) were waist fractures. Proximal third fractures in children are uncommon.

Scaphoid fractures in children generally heal well with conservative measures in 4–7 weeks.

Non-union occasionally occurs and was seen in 2% of Müssbichler's (1961) series, 1.6% of Christodoulou & Colton's (1986) series and in no patients in Vahvanen & Westerland's (1980) series.

Southcott & Rosman (1977) described 8 cases of scaphoid non-union in children: all united after cancellous bone grafts.

Summary

1. The incidence of fresh scaphoid fractures was 22.4% in the distal third, 71% in the middle third and 6.6% in the proximal third.
2. The overall reported incidence of non-union after conservative treatment was 3.4%, although some authorities quoted rates of up to 50%.
3. In all, 30% of scaphoid fractures had slight functional impairment and 4% had to reduce their working capacity. Some 28% had some decrease in grip strength. Function recovered about 3.5 weeks after plaster removal.
4. There was an increased incidence of non-union with delay in treatment, although union has occurred with delayed conservative treatment.
5. Displaced fractures had an increased rate of non-union of 45–83%.
6. Avascular necrosis causes delayed union rather than non-union.
7. Fractures of the scaphoid tubercle healed rapidly in 3–6 weeks and non-union was uncommon. Radial distal intra-articular fractures healed well, whereas ulnar distal articular fractures tended to go on to non-union.
8. Distal third fractures tended to unite in 4–8 weeks with 94.1% excellent or good results.
9. Some 92–95% of middle third fractures united in an average of 6–16 weeks. Satisfactory functional results were seen in 97.7%.
10. Proximal third fractures had an increased incidence of non-union and avascular necrosis. Union in proximal third fractures occurred in 10–24 weeks, with 90% satisfactory results.
11. Union rates of 86.4–100% were achieved with screw fixation of fresh fractures. The Herbert screw has achieved union rates of 91–95% in fresh fractures.
12. Although scaphoid non-unions may be asymptomatic, degenerative changes slowly develop.
13. After 5–10 years of non-union almost all patients show degenerative changes within the scaphoid; radioscaphoid degeneration is generally seen after 17 years and generalized arthritis after 31.6 years.
14. Carpal instability increases the incidence of non-union and the rate of development of degenerative changes.
15. There was an overall union rate of 90% after various bone grafting

techniques for non-union of the scaphoid. Union occurred in 15.8–18 weeks. Avascularity of the proximal pole increased the chances of failure to achieve union.
16. Compression screws produced union rates of 85.9%.
17. In scaphoid non-union Herbert screw fixation has produced union rates of 57.1–94%.
18. Flexor tendon rupture after scaphoid non-union has been reported.
19. Scaphoid fractures in children are uncommon, and the majority are distal third fractures.
20. Scaphoid fractures in children unite in 4–7 weeks.
21. Scaphoid non-union in children occurred in up to 2% but united well with cancellous bone grafts.

Lunate fractures and Kienböck's disease

Aetiology

The cause of Kienböck's disease and its relation to trauma remains controversial. In 1910 Kienböck maintained that at the moment of injury a transient perilunar dislocation with ligamentous tear occurred, interfering with the vascular supply to the lunate bone. Subsequent reports have suggested the infrequent occurrence of osteonecrosis following perilunar dislocations and fracture dislocation.

White & Omer (1984) reviewed 24 fracture dislocations and found 3 cases (12.5%) of transient vascular compromise of the lunate, suggested by a relative increase in the radiodensity of this bone. They found that natural resolution of the avascular necrosis was the rule and none of these cases progressed to the classic avascular necrosis of Kienböck's disease.

Whether osteonecrosis occurs prior to fracture or whether a single fracture or multiple stress fractures cause the osteonecrosis and secondary avascular changes is disputed.

In 1987 Amadio et al described a patient in whom they showed that suspected osteonecrosis preceded a fracture of the lunate. Histological evidence of this osteonecrosis, however, was not obtained.

Therkelsen & Andersen (1949) were of the opinion that repetitive trauma played the predominant role in the causation of osteonecrosis. Of 109 cases of Kienböck's disease a history of fairly definite trauma was found in only 42 cases (38%). Almquist & Burns (1982) also felt that Kienböck's disease was probably caused by microfractures or stress fractures developing within the lunate. That the avascular process is due to repetitive trauma and ischaemia is a view also held by Fisk (1984). According to Lee (1963), over 30% of lunates are vulnerable to an avascular process due to the pattern of vascularity of the lunate.

Taleisnik (1985) quoted Hulten who in 1928 described the ulnar-minus variant as occurring in 23% of 400 normal wrists and 18 of 23 patients (78%) with Kienböck's disease. Gelberman et al (1975) also showed a statistically significant association between negative ulnar variance and Kienböck's disease. They showed negative ulnar variance in 21% of normal blacks, 29% of normal whites and 13 of 15 (87%) of affected wrists of patients with Kienböck's disease. The disease is less likely to occur in blacks. This racial difference had previously been noted by Chan & Huang (1971) who commented upon its absence in Chinese patients despite the same distribution of negative ulnar variance as in Hulten's series.

Negative ulnar variance is believed to subject the lunate to a 'nutcracker' effect between the ulnar border of the radius and the head of the capitate. Fisk (1984) pointed out that there was no 'step' between the ulna and radius since the triangular fibrocartilage is thicker with a short ulna and thinner with a long one. However, there may be altered resistance between the cartilaginous end of the radius and this fibrocartilage complex.

In 1986 Kristensen et al suggested that in 8 of 47 cases of Kienböck's disease they could demonstrate subchondral bone formation in the distal radius opposite the lunate bone (Kristensen et al 1986a). If these 8 wrists were excluded, no statistical difference could be found in the incidence of the ulnar-minus variant in the diseased wrists when compared with normal wrists.

Beckenbaugh et al (1980) and Dobyns & Linscheid (1984) suggested that a primary fracture and subsequent non-union and avascular necrosis were the main cause of Kienböck's disease. In the paper by Beckenbaugh et al, 72% of 46 patients had a history of wrist injury and 67% had evidence of fracture or fragmentation of the lunate.

Fresh lunate fractures however are rarely reported. Cetti et al (1982) reported 3 cases of fresh lunate fracture and they could find only 3 well documented cases on reviewing the literature. None of their 3 cases (1 died) went on to develop Kienböck's disease.

However, Beckenbaugh et al (1980) with 2 cases, Brolin (1964) with 4 cases, and Stahl (1947) with 4 cases have all reported that fresh lunate fractures have gone on to produce the full-blown radiological picture of Kienböck's disease.

The treatment of Kienböck's disease

The treatment of Kienböck's disease remains controversial. Proponents may be found for both conservative and surgical treatment.

The results of conservative treatment. Some authors (Lichtman et al 1977, Almquist 1986) have reported the failure of conservative treatment to produce significant improvement or to prevent collapse of the lunate. In fact Lichtman et al (1977) reported that 19 of their 22 patients (86.4%) had unsatisfactory results after non-operative treatment.

In 1986 Kristensen et al reported the 20-year follow-up of 49 patients treated by either plaster immobilization alone or receiving no treatment (Kristensen et al 1986b). Just under 80% (39 of 49 patients) were pain-free or had pain only on heavy work. Most patients reported that the pain gradually subsided after some years. All had deformed lunates and 67% developed osteoarthritic changes. These authors found however that there was little correlation between the symptomatic and radiographic status of the patient. This poor correlation between symptoms and radiographic findings has been confirmed by Mirabello et al (1987).

Evans et al (1986) reported on 16 conservatively treated wrists with a 20-year follow-up. Ten patients (62.5%) had a satisfactory result. Two-thirds of these patients showed no progression of their radiological changes.

In 1949 Therkelsen & Andersen reported that 36 of 48 patients (75%) had satisfactory results. Tajima (1966) found no appreciable difference in the end-results of non-operative versus surgical treatment in 80 wrists seen during a 42-year period.

The results of surgical treatment. Many surgical techniques have been proposed for Kienböck's disease. Only the more commonly used lunate excision and prosthetic replacement, joint levelling operations and arthrodesis will be considered.

Lunate excision and prosthetic replacement. Because simple lunate excision is followed by progressive carpal collapse, various lunate implants have been proposed to replace the excised bone. Silicone implants were most commonly used, although recently they have fallen into disfavour because of the reported incidence of silastic synovitis (Palmer 1987).

Stark et al (1981) used a hand-carved silicone rubber spacer in 36 patients and achieved satisfactory relief of pain in 29 of 32 (90.6%) who were followed up for over 2 years. Progressive loss of carpal height was seen in 77% of these patients.

In 1977 Lichtman et al reported 14 satisfactory results out of 20 patients (70%) using the initial Swanson silastic prosthesis. These results improved to 93.8% satisfactory (15 of 16 patients) using the newer version (Lichtman et al 1982).

Similar good results have been reported by Beckenbaugh et al (1980) with 100% satisfactory results in 9 patients, by Bertini et al (1982) with 94.5% good results in 21 patients and by Pardini (1984) with 95% satisfactory results in 20 patients.

However Kato et al (1986) reported that whilst silicone replacement arthroplasty gave excellent results in those wrists with only mild preoperative carpal collapse, two-thirds of patients with advanced preoperative carpal collapse had poor results, due to the progression of osteoarthritic changes or subluxation of the prosthesis.

In 1986 Evans et al had 43% good, 33% fair and 24% poor results in 21 patients treated by silicone relacement arthroplasty. More than half of these cases had radiological abnormalities, including carpal collapse, scapholunate diastasis and generalized degenerative changes in the carpus. Two patients had changes resembling silicone synovitis.

Joint levelling procedures. Joint levelling procedures are aimed at neutralizing the ulnar-minus variant at the wrist by either ulnar-lengthening or radial-shortening operations.

In 1986 Almquist quoted the results of radial shortening from 7 separate papers and found that 69 of 79 reported cases (87%) had a satisfactory clinical result. Similarly, Ovesen in 1981 reported 86% satisfactory results in 7 cases of radial shortening.

Good results have also been reported following ulnar-lengthening procedures. This operation is technically easier but the rate of non-union of the osteotomy is higher.

In 1982 Armistead et al reported 90% satisfactory pain relief in 20 patients, with some increase in the range of movement and a 17% improvement in grip strength. Although 13 patients showed no change in the degree of sclerosis of their lunates, 6 showed decreased sclerosis but only 1 showed increased sclerosis.

Sundberg & Linscheid (1984) had 18 of 19 patients (95%) with satisfactory pain relief and a 20% improvement in grip strength. Eight showed less sclerosis of the lunate at follow-up whilst 3 showed increased sclerosis.

Arthrodesis. Radiocarpal arthrodesis for severe disease and various intercarpal arthrodeses have been suggested as means of treating Kienböck's disease. There is little information in the literature concerning long-term results but Taleisnik (1985) and Almquist (1986) provide some discussion on the various techniques.

Summary

1. Kienböck's disease is unlikely to be the result of a transient perilunar dislocation. Transient vascular compromise without progression to osteonecrosis occurred in only 12.5% of cases.

2. Repetitive trauma may be a cause of Kienböck's disease. An ulnar-minus variant may predispose to this repetitive trauma, which occurred in 78–87% of patients with Kienböck's disease. However, it may be an apparent abnormality secondary to degeneration rather than a primary abnormality.

3. It is suggested by some authors that a primary fracture causes Kienböck's disease.

4. The failure rate after the conservative treatment of Kienböck's disease has been reported to be as high as 86.4%, although other authors have reported 62.5–80% satisfactory symptomatic results after the long-term follow-up of such treatment.

5. Silicone replacement arthroplasty has produced satisfactory results in 90–100% of patients. However progressive radiological abnormalities and silicone synovitis are causing silicone replacement arthroplasty to fall into disfavour.

6. Joint levelling procedures have produced satisfactory results in 86–95% of patients.

Isolated injury to other carpal bones

Although uncommon when compared with the frequency with which the scaphoid is fractured, every carpal bone is capable of being fractured or dislocated in isolation.

Triquetrum

Fractures of the triquetrum are said to be the next most common carpal fracture after the scaphoid. The reported incidence varies between 3.5% (Bonnin & Greening 1943) and 20.2% (Borgeskov et al 1966).

The importance of triquetral fractures is not so much the problems that occur when the fracture is in isolation, but the fact that dorsal chip fractures or fractures through the body of the triquetrum may be the only sign of a spontaneously reduced complex carpal dislocation (Green & O'Brien 1979, O'Brien 1984, Taleisnik 1985).

Triquetral fractures fall into two main types — dorsal chip and body fractures. Dorsal chip fractures are common. In Bonnin & Greening's (1943) series of 60 triquetral fractures, 49 (82%) were of this kind, as were 28 of the 29 triquetral fractures (97%) in Borgeskov et al's (1966) series. In 1956 Bartone & Grieco reported on 46 triquetral fractures: 70% were isolated chip fractures, 2% were isolated body fractures and the other 28% were combined body and dorsal chip fractures.

Dorsal chip fractures require immobilization for 2–4 weeks. There is a relatively high incidence of non-union of these chip fractures but complete functional recovery is the rule despite this non-union. However, Bartone & Grieco (1956) suggested that if these fractures are misdiagnosed and not immobilized then chronic residual pain may persist for several months, although this does not interfere with ordinary use of the wrist.

Fractures of the body tend to be undisplaced and unite after 4–6 weeks' immobilization in a plaster cast. Herbert (1986) has reported the use of his compression screw in the treatment of these fractures. Complete functional recovery is the rule.

Avascular necrosis has not been reported. Non-union is rare after fractures of the body but has been reported (Durbin 1950) although in this patient it caused only a slight decrease in the range of motion and no pain.

Isolated dislocation of the triquetrum is rare but can occur volarly (Frykman 1980, Soucacos & Hartefilakidis-Garofalidis 1981) or dorsally (Bieber & Weiland 1984, Goldberg & Heller 1987). Excision of the triquetrum has been used to treat these dislocations with no obvious functional impairment, although reduction, either closed or open, is to be preferred (Taleisnik 1985).

Summary

1. Triquetral injuries comprise 3.5–20.2% of carpal fractures, and they may be the only radiological sign of a complex carpal dislocation.
2. Dorsal chip fractures are common, heal in 2–4 weeks and rarely cause any functional disturbances even though non-union is common.
3. Triquetral body fractures are common but heal in 6 weeks and cause little functional disturbance.
4. Non-union in body fractures is rare but causes little disability.
5. Dislocation, either dorsal or volar, is rare and causes little long-term disability.

Pisiform

Injuries to the pisiform are rare, and occurred in 0.7% (Borgeskov et al 1966) to 3% (Dobyns & Linscheid 1984) of reported series. Fracture patterns include avulsions of the distal portion, vertical fractures or osteochondral fractures of the articular surface (Dobyns & Linscheid 1984). Immobilization for 3–4 weeks is all that is required for the fracture to become asymptomatic. Post-traumatic degenerative changes in the pisotriquetral joint have been reported following intra-articular fracture (Jenkins 1951). Should pain persist, or degeneration develop following a pisiform fracture, excision of the whole bone produces excellent results (Palmieri 1982).

Occasionally a dislocation of the pisiform bone occurs. Minami et al (1984) reported a case which, despite open reduction and Kirschner wire fixation, went on to redislocate, requiring excision of the bone. They reviewed the 6 previous reported cases, 3 of which were excised. These authors recommended that the pisiform should be removed in cases of isolated dislocation.

Ulnar nerve palsy has been reported to occur in association with a fracture of the pisiform (Howard 1964).

Summary

1. Pisiform fractures and dislocations occurred in 0.7–3% of carpal injuries.
2. Immobilization for 3–4 weeks is generally sufficient.
3. Symptomatic fractures, degeneration of the pisotriquetral joint and isolated dislocation of the pisiform were treated by excision of the pisiform with excellent results.

Trapezium

The incidence of fractures of the trapezium has been reported as occurring in 1% (Dobyns & Linscheid 1984) to 5% (Cordrey & Ferrer-Torrels 1960) of carpal fractures. Two main fracture patterns are seen; vertical fractures running through the articular surface of the first carpometacarpal joint often accompanied by subluxation of the first metacarpal, and trapezial ridge fractures.

Cordrey & Ferrer-Torrels (1960) reviewed the world literature and found 75 reported cases. Of these, 60% had persistent pain and swelling with diminished movement of the wrist and thumb at the end of treatment. In none of these reported cases was open reduction and internal fixation advocated. More recently, Jones & Ghorbal (1985) reported 3 vertical fractures: 2 were treated with plaster cast immobilization and 1 had percutaneous Kirschner wire fixation without accurate reduction of the fracture. All 3 had residual symptoms, with approximately 50% loss of movement and strength of power, pinch and key grip. They all experienced aching with prolonged writing and repetitive work.

In contrast to these poor results after conservative treatment, the results of open reduction and internal fixation have been good. Cordrey & Ferrer-Torrels (1960) reported excellent results in 5 vertical fractures treated with open reduction and Kirschner wire fixation. They reported that the fractures healed in 8 weeks. In 1984 Freeland & Finley reported full function after fixation of a vertical fracture with an AO 4.0 mm cancellous screw. Holdsworth & Shackleford (1987) reported only minimal loss of movement after the use of a Herbert screw in a fracture dislocation of the trapezium.

Trapezial ridge fractures were described as the 'missed fracture' by McClain & Boyes (1966), as all 4 of their cases (plus 2 of the 3 reported by Palmer in 1981) were diagnosed late. In 1981 Palmer described two types. The type I trapezial ridge fracture occurs at the base of the ridge of the trapezium and Palmer's 1 case healed with immobilization. The commoner type II (an avulsion fracture from the tip of the volar ridge) tends to progress to non-union. In the 4 cases reported by McClain & Boyes (1966) and in 1 of the 2 cases of non-union reported by Palmer (1981), excision of the avulsed fragment was performed. However late surgical treatment did not result in immediate relief of symptoms and a relatively long delay in returning to normal work was the rule (McClain & Boyes 1966). In over one-half of the cases reported in these two papers there were signs and symptoms of irritability of the median nerve within the carpal tunnel.

Dislocation of the trapezium may occur in an ulnar volar or dorsal radial direction and seems to occur with equal frequency in both directions. In 1969 Siegel & Hertzberg reviewed the literature and found only 2 cases of true dislocation, previously reported by Peterson; these had been treated by excision of the trapezium. Goldberg et al (1981) excised the trapezium in their case of an ulnar–volar dislocation but found some shortening of the thumb with reasonable preservation of pinch grip but poor opposition. Closed reduction if possible is the ideal treatment but this is rarely achieved, and when achieved is often unstable. Open reduction and Kirschner wire fixation have produced good results (Boe 1979, Brewood 1985, Sherlock 1987) but two cases of ulnar–volar dislocation treated in this way resulted in fusion of the first carpometacarpal joint with some loss of movement and poor opposition (Siegel & Hertzberg 1969, Seiman 1972).

Summary

1. The incidence of fractures of the trapezium was 1–5%.
2. Conservative treatment of displaced vertical fractures produced over 60% residual symptoms.
3. The results of the operative fixation of vertical fractures were good.
4. Trapezial ridge fractures were often overlooked, often went on to non-union, and recovery, even after surgical excision of the non-union, was slow.
5. Over 50% of trapezial ridge fractures were associated with median nerve irritability.
6. Dislocations of the trapezium generally did well with open reduction and Kirschner wire fixation, although premature fusion of the first carpometacarpal joint has occurred.

Trapezoid

Less than 0.7% of carpal fractures occurred at the trapezoid (Borgeskov et al 1966). Fractures of the trapezoid are rarely reported. Isolated fractures may be treated in a plaster cast for 3–6 weeks but secondary degenerative changes may occur between the trapezoid and second metacarpal, necessitating a later arthrodesis (Bryan & Dobyns 1980).

Dislocation of the trapezoid, whilst uncommon, seems to be more frequent than fracture. Dislocation may occur in a dorsal or volar direction. Treatment consists of closed manipulation and plaster immobilization (Meyn & Roth 1980), open reduction and Kirschner wire fixation (Stein 1971), or open reduction and primary limited arthrodesis (Goodman & Shankman 1984). Kopp (1985) stated that the shape of the trapezoid prevented closed reduction in palmar dislocations.

Avascular necrosis of the trapezoid may occur after open reduction (Meyn & Roth 1980).

If further surgery is required due to secondary degenerative changes, limited arthrodesis is to be preferred to simple excision of the trapezoid because the second metacarpal and trapezium will migrate into the defect, producing symptomatic disability (Meyn & Roth 1980, Kopp 1985, Taleisnik 1985).

Summary

1. Trapezoid fractures occurred in less than 0.7% of carpal fractures.

2. Trapezoid fractures heal with plaster immobilization in 3–6 weeks, although secondary arthritis may occur.
3. Dislocation may occur in a dorsal or volar direction. Avascular necrosis may occur following open reduction.
4. If secondary symptoms require surgery, limited arthrodesis is to be preferred to excision of the trapezoid.

Capitate

The incidence of capitate fractures was 0.4–1.4% of all carpal fractures (Borgeskov et al 1966, Dobyns & Linscheid 1984). Fractures of the capitate may occur as isolated injuries, as part of the scaphocapitate (naviculocapitate) syndrome, or in association with other carpal or metacarpal fractures.

Although Adler & Shafton (1962) found 79 reported cases in the world's literature, of which 48 were isolated capitate fractures, there have been few reports of the isolated fracture since then. The authors added 5 of their own cases, 3 of which had been followed up. These 5 healed after plaster immobilization for 3–6 weeks, the 2 without previous arthritis had full function. In 1982 Rand et al reported 3 isolated capitate fractures with non-union occurring in 2 of them. In a previous article from the same centre, Bryan & Dobyns (1982) had reported that non-union of the capitate was common. Non-union of the capitate healed well with bone grafting (Freeman & Hay 1985).

In 1982 Rand et al found that 5 of their 7 patients without a perilunar dislocation had a mean range of motion of 73% and a grip strength of 78% of the contralateral normal hand. Four of 6 patients with follow-up radiographs revealed post-traumatic arthritis. The 2 patients without arthritis had a shorter follow-up period (less than 3 years) as compared with a mean follow-up of 10 years 5 months for the 4 patients with arthritis.

The scaphocapitate syndrome has previously been well described (Stein & Siegel 1969). It involves a fracture of the scaphoid, with a fracture of the proximal pole of the capitate rotated 90 or 180° to its long axis, with or without an associated perilunar dislocation.

Plaster immobilization in the rotated position has resulted in union with no pain and 25% loss of full motion (Jones 1955). However, non-union and avascular necrosis of the proximal pole are more likely to occur (Marsh & Lampros 1959). In 1956 Fenton recommended excision of the proximal pole with reasonable preservation of function but some loss of movement. In 1971 Meyers et al performed an open reduction with wire fixation and reported the return of full function.

Vance et al (1980) resorted to open reduction and pin fixation in 4 cases after the failure of attempts at closed reduction in each case. In 1982 Rand et al reported that 4 of 5 patients with trans-scaphoid, transcapitate perilunar fracture dislocations had a mean range of 65% and grip strength of 68% of the contralateral hand. Three of the 4 patients with adequate follow-up had degenerative arthritis (mean follow-up 3 years 9 months) and only 1 followed up for 1 year was free of this.

A case of volar dislocation of the capitate in a complex wrist injury has been reported (Lowrey et al 1984).

A rare injury involving disruption of the carpal arch through the capitate–hamate articulation distally and pisotriquetral joint proximally has been reported after severe crush injuries. Reduction of the diastasis is required to avoid rotational abnormalities of the fourth and fifth metacarpals. The prognosis however is related to the severity of initiating trauma (Adler & Shafton 1962, Primiano & Reef 1974, Garcia-Elias et al 1985, Norbeck et al 1987).

Summary

1. Capitate fractures occurred in 0.4–1.4% of carpal injuries.
2. Fractures of the body of the capitate resulted in a range of motion of 73% of the contralateral wrist whilst grip strength was 78% of the opposite wrist.
3. Non-union is not uncommon and degenerative change was the rule after a 10-year follow up.
4. Open reduction of the scaphocapitate syndrome was the treatment of choice.
5. Perilunar scaphocapitate fracture dislocations resulted in 65% motion and 68% grip strength of the contralateral wrist at follow-up. Degenerative changes were common after a 4-year follow-up.

Hamate

Fractures of the hamate occurred in from 0.5% (Dobyns & Linscheid 1984) to 4.6% (Taleisnik 1985) of carpal fractures.

These fractures occur either through the body or the hook of the hamate. Fractures of the body are uncommon, although in 1973 Bowen reviewed the literature and found 44 recorded cases — 29 of the body, 5 of the hook and 10 whose site was unrecorded. Although only 5 fractures of the hook of the hamate were recorded, these types now appear to occur more frequently than body fractures. This is probably due to increased recognition of this type of fracture as well as their increasing frequency from racquet and club sports.

Fractures of the body may be dorsal oblique in association with subluxation of the base of the ulnar metacarpals. This may be treated with Kirschner wire fixation (Bowen 1973, Thomas & Birch 1983) or a cortical mini-lag screw (Freeland & Finley 1986) with good functional results.

True body fractures may pass to the ulnar side or, more commonly, radial to the hook of the hamate. These fractures are usually stable and require

4–6 weeks in plaster cast to become asymptomatic even if fibrous union alone is achieved (Taleisnik 1985). Open reduction and internal fixation are required if the fracture is displaced (Ogunro 1983, Taleisnik 1985, Ali 1986). Proximal pole osteochondral fractures may occur (Dobyns & Linscheid 1984). In 1964 Howard described 2 patients with fractures of the body of the hamate who had associated ulnar nerve palsies.

Fractures of the hook of the hamate are more common and there is an almost 100% progression to non-union. This is not only due to the fact that these fractures are often diagnosed late, as even after immediate treatment non-union is not uncommon (Nisenfield & Neviaser 1974, Blair et al 1982). The present author could find no record of primary bone union of hook of hamate fractures until the recent report of Bishop & Beckenbaugh (1988) in which they recorded 2 cases.

Non-union of the hook of the hamate tends to result in local tenderness and pain on gripping. However, cast immobilization can sometimes resolve these symptoms, presumably due to fibrous union (Egawa & Asai 1983). In 90% of the 20 patients in Stark et al's (1977) series surgery was required. Occasionally bone graft and screw fixation have been performed (Fisk 1984, Bishop & Beckenbaugh 1988) although 1 of the 3 cases in the 1988 series went on to non-union. Excision of the ununited fragment gives universally good results (Carter et al 1977, Stark et al 1977, Egawa & Asai 1983, Foucher et al 1985, Bishop & Beckenbaugh 1988). In the 1988 series all 18 employed patients returned to work and sport. Eight (42%) had no symptoms, 6 (32%) had mild symptoms and 5 (26%) had moderate or multiple symptoms.

Flexor tendon tendinitis or rupture has been reported in association with ununited hook of hamate fractures (Clayton 1969, Crosby & Linscheid 1974, Okuhara et al 1982, Takami et al 1983, Foucher et al 1985). In 1985 Foucher et al reported that 5 of their 6 patients with non-union had fraying or rupture of flexor tendons, whereas Stark et al (1977) reported only 1 case of flexor tendon involvement in 20 patients. Bishop & Beckenbaugh (1988) have estimated that 15–20% of hook of hamate non-unions are associated with flexor tendon involvement. In my review I have found 19 reported cases of flexor tendon injury in 86 reported cases of fracture of the hook of the hamate — an incidence of 22%.

Involvement of the ulnar nerve with hook of hamate fractures was reported by Howard (1964). Egawa & Asai (1983) reported that 4 of their 6 cases of hook of hamate fracture had hypoaesthesia in an ulnar nerve distribution. Bishop & Beckenbaugh (1988) reported ulnar nerve involvement in 5 of 21 cases (23.8%). Occasionally median nerve irritability has been noted (Manske 1978, Bishop & Beckenbaugh 1988). Tardy ulnar nerve palsy has been reported due to perineural fibrosis (Baird & Friedenberg 1968). No case of avascular necrosis has been reported.

Dislocation of the hamate can occur in a volar or dorsal direction. It can sometimes be reduced closed (Duke 1963) but usually open reduction is required (Gunn 1985, Ohshio et al 1986). The functional result after reduction is usually good.

Summary

1. The incidence of hamate fractures was 0.5–4.6%.
2. Dorsal oblique fractures heal with good functional results if reduced well.
3. True body fractures tend to be stable and heal in 4–6 weeks in a plaster cast.
4. Fractures of the hook of the hamate have an almost 100% non-union rate. Excision of the ununited fragment is the procedure of choice. Some 42% will be asymptomatic and 32% will have mild symptoms.
5. Ulnar nerve neuropathy may occur with body and hook fractures. Tardy ulnar palsy can occur, as can median nerve neuropathy.
6. Flexor tendinitis or rupture was reported in 15–22% of hook of hamate non-unions.
7. Dislocation of the hamate occasionally occurs.

Dislocations and fracture dislocations of the carpus

Dislocations and fracture dislocations of the carpus comprised 1–2% of all fractures (Morawa et al 1976) and 4.8–13.8% of all carpal injuries (Dobyns & Linscheid 1984). Many varieties and combinations of dislocations or fracture dislocations can occur.

Most carpal dislocations and fractures are confined to an area contained within a lesser arc that closely hugs the lunate and a greater arc that crosses the middle third of the scaphoid and runs distal to the mid-carpal joint in an ulnar direction to cross the triquetrum (Taleisnik 1985). Based on these two arcs, carpal dislocations and fracture dislocations can be classified into four main groups (Fig. 7.1):

Group I: Perilunate and lunate dislocations.
Group II: Trans-scaphoid perilunate fracture dislocation (with or without other carpal bones in the greater arc).
Group III: Variants of the above pattern, including scaphocapitate syndrome and isolated dislocation of other carpal bones.
Group IV: Radiocarpal dislocations.

Lunate and perilunate dislocations

Mayfield et al (1980) investigated the pathomechanics of carpal instability in perilunate and lunate dislocations in 32 cadaver wrists. The authors described four stages in a progressive perilunar instability, ranging from

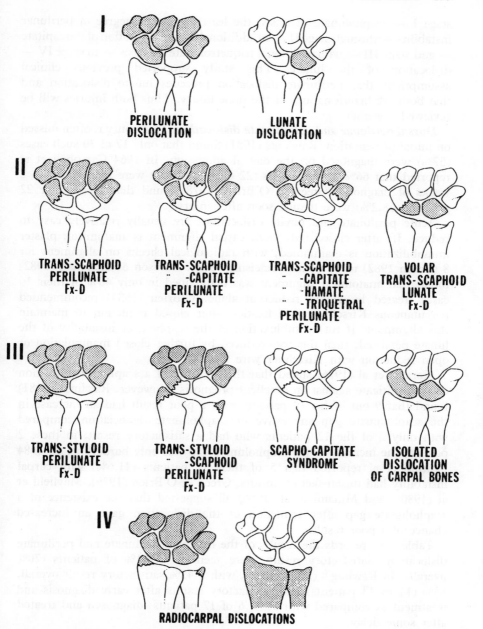

Fig. 7.1 Classification of common carpal dislocations and fracture dislocations (from Taleisnik (1985)).

Group I: Perilunate and lunate dislocations.
Group II: Dislocations and fracture dislocations of the greater arc.
Group III: Variants.
Group IV: Radiocarpal dislocations.

stage I — scapholunate diastasis, the least significant degree of perilunar instability — through stage II — an additional dorsal dislocation of the capitate — and stage III — with additional triquetrolunate diastasis — to stage IV — dislocation of the lunate. This study supported previous clinical assumptions that perilunate dislocation precedes lunate dislocation and that both are manifestations of the same injury. Thus both injuries will be reviewed together.

Dorsal perilunar and volar lunate dislocation. This injury is often missed on initial presentation. Rawlings (1981) found that only 17 of 30 such cases (57%) were diagnosed on the day of admission. In 1964 Campbell et al reported that 66% of their cases (22 of 33 patients) were treated within 2 weeks of diagnosis; Green & O'Brien (1978) found that 15 of their 22 patients (68.2%) were treated soon after injury.

Acute perilunate and lunate dislocations are usually relatively easy to reduce. If, after closed reduction, carpal alignment is anatomical, plaster immobilization is maintained, with radiological checks on alignment for 8 (Green 1982) to 10 weeks (Taleisnik 1985). Adkison & Chapman (1982) found that anatomical alignment was maintained in only 40% of their 10 cases treated by closed reduction alone. O'Brien (1984) recommended percutaneous Kirschner wire fixation after closed reduction to maintain this alignment. If rotary subluxation of the scaphoid or instability of the lunate persisted, then this was reduced by further closed manipulation or open reduction with Kirschner wire fixation.

Morawa et al (1976) stated that the presence of a scaphoid subluxation did not mitigate against an excellent prognosis. However, Rawlings (1981) found that 9 out of his 12 patients with a poor result had an increase in the scapholunate gap suggestive of scapholunate dissociation compared with only 2 of the 12 patients who had a satisfactory result; in these 2 patients the increase in the scapholunate gap was only borderline. In 1984 Panting et al reported that 5 of their 12 patients (41.6%) with carpal instability had unsatisfactory results. Green & O'Brien (1979), Mayfield et al (1980), and Minami et al (1986) all suggested that the existence of a scapholunate gap after reduction of the dislocation gave an increased chance of a poor result.

Table 7.17 records the results of the treatment of lunate and perilunate dislocation. Satisfactory results were seen in 43–91% of patients (70% overall). In Rawling's (1981) series, with a 43% satisfactory result overall, 85% (11 of 13 patients) had satisfactory results after early diagnosis and treatment as compared with 35% (6 of 17 patients) diagnosed and treated after some delay.

Green & O'Brien (1978) stressed the fact that virtually all of these patients had some permanent limitation of motion, and it took several months before the maximum benefit of rehabilitation was obtained. They found that only rarely were their patients able to return to an occupation requiring the heavy use of the hands before 6 months.

Table 7.17 Results of the treatment of lunate and perilunate dislocations

Reference	Number of patients	Satisfactory		Unsatisfactory	
		n	%	n	%
Campbell et al (1964)	15	12	80	3	20
Morawa et al (1976)	24	22	91	2	9
Green & O'Brien (1978)	16	9	56	7	44
Rawlings (1981)	30	13	43	17	57
Panting et al (1984)	29	24	83	5	17
Overall	114	80	70	34	30

Campbell et al (1964, 1965) reported good results following proximal row carpectomy for some cases of chronic dislocation. Excision of the lunate was seldom felt to be indicated and reduction of the chronically displaced lunate, if possible, was also felt to give a satisfactory wrist. In 1988 Siegert et al reported on 16 cases of chronic dislocation and felt that open reduction should be the treatment of choice. All 6 of their patients so treated had a satisfactory result. In these chronic cases, proximal row carpectomy and wrist fusion were preferred to isolated lunate excision.

Avascular necrosis of the lunate with collapse is extremely uncommon. White & Omer (1984) recorded only 3 cases of transient ischaemia in 24 fracture dislocations (12.5%). The clinical course of these cases was for resolution to occur and none progressed to collapse.

The incidence of symptoms related to median nerve compression within the carpal tunnel is reported as occurring in from 16% (Adkison & Chapman 1982) to 56.6% (Rawlings 1981) of all perilunate dislocations and fracture dislocations. These symptoms are usually transient but the longer the symptoms persist the worse the final outcome.

Stern (1981) reported the rupture of the flexor pollicis longus and flexor digitorum superficialis and profundus tendons to the index and long fingers in a case of chronic volar dislocation of the lunate.

Volar perilunar and dorsal lunate dislocation. Dorsal dislocation of the lunate is extremely rare and isolated case reports are recorded (Seidenstein 1956, Bilos & Hui 1981). Volar perilunar dislocation is only slightly more common (Pournaras & Kappas 1979, Taleisnik 1985). Treatment of these injuries is along the lines of the more common dorsal perilunar and volar lunar dislocations. Closed reduction of the volar perilunar dislocation is said to be more difficult and it is more unstable once reduced (Taleisnik 1985).

Dislocations and fracture dislocations of the greater arc

Trans-scaphoid perilunar fracture dislocation of the carpus is the common injury in this group. In many ways, with regards to treatment, it may be looked upon as a variety of perilunate dislocation but the displacement occurs through the body of the scaphoid rather than the scapholunate ligament.

Closed treatment may be considered if anatomical reduction of the scaphoid can be achieved and maintained. Healing of the scaphoid fracture may be delayed and avascular necrosis of the proximal scaphoid fragment is common. However avascular necrosis does not imply non-union. In Adkison & Chapman's (1982) series, 13 of 19 cases (68%) lost the anatomical position with conservative treatment.

If an anatomical position of the scaphoid cannot be maintained, then the incidence of non-union of the scaphoid is increased. In Adkison & Chapman's (1982) series the incidence of non-union with non-anatomical reduction of the scaphoid was 75%.

In 1956 Wagner recommended primary wrist arthrodesis for the displaced trans-scaphoid perilunate fracture dislocation. However, most authors recommend open reduction with the scaphoid being held reduced with wires or screws with or without bone graft (Worland & Dick 1975, Morawa et al 1976, Green & O'Brien 1978, Herbert 1986, Cooney et al 1987).

Occasionally these fracture dislocations have proved to be irreducible by closed means, either due to the proximal pole of the scaphoid dislocating volar to the lunate (Weiss et al 1970) or to interposition of the dorsal capsule (Jasmine et al 1988).

The incidence of median nerve irritation after trans-scaphoid perilunate fracture dislocations varied between 30% (Cooney et al 1987) and 43.75% (Moneim et al 1984). These injuries were usually transient.

Table 7.18 records the results of the treatment of trans-scaphoid perilunate fracture dislocations. Overall, 76% of these patients achieved a satisfactory result. This table includes patients treated both surgically and conservatively. Morawa et al (1976), Adkison & Chapman (1982) and Cooney et al (1987) all emphasized the improved results obtained by the operative treatment of these injuries as compared to the results of

Table 7.18 The results of the treatment of trans-scaphoid perilunate fracture dislocations

Reference	Number of patients	Satisfactory		Unsatisfactory	
		n	%	n	%
Morawa et al (1976)	21	18	86	3	14
Green & O'Brien (1978)	18	12	67	6	33
Moneim et al (1984)*	12	10	83	2	17
Panting et al (1984)	19	13	68	6	32
Cooney et al (1987)†	26	20	77	6	23
Overall	96	73	76	23	24

*Includes some group III variants.
†This series includes patients treated by open reduction only.

conservative treatment. Moneim et al (1984) found that after internal fixation the scaphoid united in an average of 13 weeks.

In 1975 Worland & Dick reported that only one of their cases had more than 50% of normal wrist motion, and Cooney et al (1987) found the average wrist flexion to be 40° and the average extension 36° in 22 patients treated operatively. Only 9 of the 22 patients (41%) had no pain, 9 (41%) had mild but tolerable pain and 4 (18%) had severe pain. Thirteen (59%) of patients in this same group had no weakness, 6 (27%) had mild to moderate weakness and 3 (14%) had severe weakness. Of cases seen at an average of 4.3 years following treatment, 56% had radiographic evidence of intercarpal arthritis and 54% evidence of radiocarpal arthritis. Green (1982) pointed out that return to heavy work occurred 6 months to 1 year after these injuries.

In 1984 Lowdon et al described a case of recurrent dorsal trans-scaphoid perilunate dislocation through a scaphoid non-union.

Occasionally a palmar trans-scaphoid lunate fracture dislocation occurs. Green & O'Brien (1978) and Viegas et al (1987) reported poor results in a total of 4 cases treated by surgery. However, Stern (1984) reported good results following surgery in 2 cases.

Palmar trans-scaphoid perilunate fracture dislocation is also occasionally reported. Saunier & Chamay (1980), Green & O'Brien (1978) and Fernandes et al (1983) had a good result with their cases treated by screw fixation, whilst Aitken & Nalebuff (1960) had a good functional result despite a scaphoid non-union after closed treatment in their case. Cooney et al (1987) had a poor result with their case.

Variants

Many of these have been discussed in the sections on fracture and dislocation of the individual carpal bone. Isolated dislocation of the scaphoid or scaphoid and lunate will be discussed in this section.

Isolated dislocations of the scaphoid are rare injuries. The dislocation may be radial or dorsoradial (Connell & Dyson 1955, Taylor 1969, Maki et al 1982, Amamilo et al 1985) or anterior or anterolateral (Taylor 1969, Murakami 1977, Thomas 1977). Reduction was generally achieved closed — in 16 of 20 reported cases (Amamilo et al 1985) — and the functional end-result was usually good with only occasional discomfort. Avascular necrosis of the scaphoid was not reported.

In the case reported by Murakami (1977), a capsular flap prevented closed reduction, therefore open reduction with no fixation was performed but subluxation of the scaphoid occurred. It seems that if open reduction is required Kirschner wire fixation should be utilized (Green 1982, Amamilo et al 1985).

Dislocation of the scaphoid and lunate may occur as a unit (Küpfer 1986, Coll 1987) or with both bones in isolation from each other (Gordon

1972, Brown & Muddu 1981). In all reported cases open reduction was required, avascular necrosis of the lunate was common and the functional results were poor.

Radiocarpal dislocation

Isolated radiocarpal dislocations are rare. In 1985 Varodompun et al reported the fourth case of isolated dorsal dislocation. Closed reduction was usually easy and full function was restored (Freund & Ovesen 1977).

Isolated volar dislocation is also rare. In 1988 Moore & McMahon reported the fifth case. Closed reduction was usually easy and function was invariably fully restored (Rosardo 1966, Fehring & Milek 1984), although Moore & McMahon's case described a feeling of occasional weakness, and early degenerative changes were noted.

With increasing severity of injury there is an increasingly complex fracture dislocation. Moneim et al (1983) described 4 patients with isolated radiocarpal dislocation with marginal fractures of the radius and ulna. Closed reduction was successful in 3 cases and the functional end-results were generally good. Three cases had associated intercarpal injuries, open reduction was required and the results were inferior, with 2 unsatisfactory results.

In 1977 Bilos et al described 5 patients with severe radiocarpal dislocations. Although reasonable function was achieved, all cases showed some irregularity of the radiocarpal or intercarpal joints. Similarly, Schoenecker et al (1984) and Nyquist & Stern (1984) have remarked on a guarded prognosis for the severe compound or comminuted fracture dislocations of the radiocarpal joint.

Summary

1. Lunate and perilunate dislocation were missed on initial presentation in 32–43% of cases.
2. Anatomical alignment was only maintained in 40% of cases of lunate and perilunate dislocation treated by closed reduction and plaster immobilization.
3. An increased scapholunate gap or scapholunate angle gave a poor result in 42–75% of cases of lunate and perilunate dislocation.
4. A satisfactory result was seen in 70% of cases of lunate and perilunate dislocation, and delay in treatment increased the risk of a poor result. It took many months of rehabilitation to achieve return of function after these injuries and some restriction of motion was the rule.
5. Median nerve symptoms were seen in 16–57% of cases of lunate and perilunate dislocation but were usually transient.
6. Flexor tendon rupture has been reported in an old unreduced case of volar dislocation.

7. Of conservatively treated trans-scaphoid perilunate fracture dislocations, 68% lost their anatomical position. The incidence of non-union of the scaphoid with non-anatomical reduction was at least 75%.
8. Median nerve irritation occurred in 30–44% of cases of trans-scaphoid perilunate fracture dislocation, although these symptoms were usually transient.
9. Of trans-scaphoid perilunate fracture dislocations, 76% achieved a satisfactory result. Better results were achieved by surgical treatment. These patients tended to lose approximately 50% of wrist movement; pain was absent in 41% and grip strength was normal in 59% after treatment. Return to heavy work occurred in 6 months to 1 year.
10. Degenerative changes were seen in over 50% of wrists after trans-scaphoid perilunate fracture dislocation at an average of 4.3 years after the injury.
11 Isolated scaphoid dislocations were usually easily reduced by closed manipulation and the functional results were generally good.
12. Isolated scaphoid lunate dislocation usually required open reduction and the functional results were generally poor.
13. Isolated radiocarpal dislocations had a good prognosis, whereas comminuted or compound fracture dislocations had a guarded prognosis.

Traumatic carpal instability

Classification

Post-traumatic carpal instability was first referred to by Gilford and associates in 1943 (Linscheid et al 1972). Fisk (1970) used the term carpal instability when referring to the concertina deformity seen in some wrists after scaphoid fractures. In 1972 Linscheid et al classified carpal instabilities into dorsiflexed intercalated segment instability (DISI) and volar palmar flexed intercalated segment instability (VISI). Since this paper, much has been written about the classification of these carpal instabilities. Taleisnik (1985) has written in detail about these classifications and interested readers should refer to this book. He divides them into lateral, medial and proximal carpal instabilities. These may be subdivided into static forms of carpal instability, where the collapse patterns may be recognized on routine radiographs, and dynamic forms which are only apparent on routine radiographs when the patient has actively assumed the pattern of carpal collapse. They are classified as follows:

1. Lateral carpal instability
   a. Scapholunate dissociation (rotary subluxation of the scaphoid)
   b. Scaphocapitate diastasis
   c. Scaphotrapezium — trapezoid instability

2. Medial carpal instability
   a. Triquetrolunate dissociation
   b. Triquetrohamate dissociation
3. Proximal carpal instability

These proximal carpal instabilities occur without primary intracarpal pathology and are secondary to disruption of the radiocarpal ligaments or malunions of the distal radius:

1. Radiocarpal
   Ulnar translocation
   Dorsal radiocarpal subluxation
   Volar radiocarpal subluxation
2. A dynamic mid-carpal dorsal instability pattern

Lateral carpal instability

Scapholunate dissociation is the commonest form of carpal instability. It may be primary, secondary to more extensive injury or disease, or associated with extracarpal injuries. It usually occurs following trauma but is also seen in association with rheumatoid arthritis, infection, spastic paralysis and congenital ligament laxity (Vance et al 1979, Hergenröeder & Penix 1981).

Persistence of intercarpal collapse seems to result in significant degenerative changes although the rate of progression of this degeneration is not recorded (Crittenden et al 1970, Linscheid et al 1972, Howard et al 1974, Hudson et al 1976). Hudson et al (1976) found evidence of articular cartilage narrowing and osteophyte formation in 11 of 19 cases (58%).

Treatment of scapholunate dissociation is more successful if initiated early. The aim of treatment is to re-establish the anatomical alignment of the carpus. This can be achieved by closed reduction alone, although this should probably be supplemented by percutaneous Kirschner wires (Rask 1979, O'Brien 1984). Open reduction may be required and again percutaneous Kirschner wires may be used to provide stability (Howard et al 1974, Nielsen & Hedeboe 1984). In 1978 Palmer et al reported on 17 patients treated within 1 month of injury by closed reduction, open reduction alone or combined with direct suture of torn ligaments or ligament reconstruction. Of these 17 patients, 9 (53%) had no pain whilst 6 (35%) had only slight pain. Grip strength was 53–80% of normal and the average range of movement was decreased from normal by almost 50%. Patient satisfaction was good in 9 cases (53%), fair in 5 (29%) and poor in 3 (18%).

Chronic scapholunate dissociation without radiocarpal arthritis may be treated either by ligament reconstruction or intercarpal arthrodesis if surgical treatment is required.

The results of ligament reconstruction were reported by Palmar et al in 1978. Of the 30 patients with chronic scapholunate dissociation without arthritis, 20 (66%) had no pain, 9 (30%) had slight pain and only 1 had moderate pain. The range of wrist movement was decreased to approximately 45° of palmar flexion and dorsiflexion. Grip strength was improved in 19 patients (63%) and averaged 76% of normal. The scapholunate gap and scapholunate angle were restored to normal in 24% of the patients.

In 1982 Glickel & Millender reported the results of ligament reconstruction in 21 patients. Only 2 were pain-free although 18 patients (86%) noticed a decrease in their pain. They found that grip strength was generally only slightly increased and the range of motion was reduced to an average of 41° palmar flexion and 53° of dorsiflexion. They also found that whilst the scapholunate angle was initially improved, as follow-up continued the scapholunate gap and scapholunate angle increased, suggesting that the repairs 'stretch out' with time and use.

Jackson & Protas (1981) described ligament reconstruction in 3 cases of snapping scapholunate subluxation but they suggested that limited intercarpal fusion was a better choice of procedure, particularly for labourers.

Limited intercarpal fusion produced satisfactory results in 66% of patients (Uematsu 1978, Kleinman et al 1982). Union of the arthrodesis was sometimes difficult to achieve and in Hastings & Silver's (1984) series of 6 patients, 3 had a non-union. Range of motion was decreased but averaged approximately 80% of the preoperative range (Kleinman et al 1982, Hastings & Silver 1984). Grip strength was also improved as compared with the preoperative strength and Eckenrode et al (1986) reported that grip strength was 74% of normal whilst pinch grip was 86% of normal.

Scaphotrapezium–trapezoid instability is rare and only isolated cases have been reported (Taleisnik 1980, Kuur & Boe 1986). Taleisnik (1985) believes that many cases of osteoarthritis of the scaphotrapezium–trapezoid joint may be the result of an unstable articulation.

Medial carpal instability

Medial carpal instabilities take place between the triquetrum (medial column) and the hamate and lunate (central column). Two types of medial instability are recognized:

1. Triquetrohamate, which occurs across the mid-carpal joint with loss of stability of the central column, present only during ulnar or radial deviation (dynamic DISI and VISI).
2. Triquetrolunate, producing a static type of VISI collapse (Taleisnik 1984). Lichtman et al (1984) and Reagan et al (1984) have described dynamic types of triquetrolunate instability.

In triquetrohamate instability tenodesis and ligament reconstruction or limited carpal arthrodesis should be considered (Lichtman et al 1981,

Taleisnik 1985) if conservative measures fail to control the symptoms.

Triquetrolunate instability often exhibits minimal disability after acute injury and the need for surgical correction is infrequent (Taleisnik 1985). If surgery is required then ligament reconstruction or intercarpal fusion produced good results in the majority of patients (Reagan et al 1984).

In 1988 Trumble et al described 7 patients with static or dynamic VISI. They felt that the instability occurred between the proximal lunate and triquetrum, and distal hamate and capitate. Arthrodesis of the proximal and distal rows of the ulnar carpus provided relief of wrist pain in 5 of 6 patients. Flexion–extension was 63% of normal, radial and ulnar deviation 57% of normal and grip strength 74% of normal.

Proximal carpal instability

Proximal carpal instability follows major disruption of the radiocarpal ligament support or changes in the alignment of the distal articular surface of the radius. There are two main types. Radiocarpal instabilities follow a disturbance of the relationship of the proximal carpal row to the radius and ulna. Mid-carpal instabilities include patients with a dynamic type of DISI without scapholunate dissociation secondary to malunion of fractures of the distal radius.

Radiocarpal instabilities
Ulnar translocation. Ulnar translocation usually follows inflammatory arthritis but may occur as a post-traumatic event. According to Taleisnik (1985) there are two types. Type I involves an ulnar shift of the whole carpus and in type II the scaphoid remains in its normal relationship to the radius. This produces a scapholunate gap which must not be confused with the gap seen in scapholunate dissociation.

Taleisnik (1985) describes the acute injury as being associated with marked swelling and an extreme loss of the range of movement and grip strength. There is often a cosmetic deformity. He feels that surgical correction is invariably required and should involve either radiolunate or radioscapholunate fusion.

In 1987 Rayhack et al described traumatic ulnar translocation in 8 cases. The initial diagnosis was delayed by an average of 7.3 months. Seven patients underwent ligament repair with or without tendon augmentation. Three achieved a good result, 2 a fair result and 2 required conversion to a wrist arthrodesis at an average follow-up of 32 months.

Dorsal carpal translocation. This occurs secondary to intra-articular or extra-articular malunited fractures of the distal radius. Extra-articular malunions are treated by a dorsal open wedge osteotomy to correct the dorsal angulation of the distal articular surface. Intra-articular fractures without degenerative changes require an osteotomy along the plane of the fracture. In the presence of degeneration a radioscapholunate fusion may be required.

Palmar carpal translocation. Palmar carpal translocation also occurs in association with intra-articular malunited fractures of the distal radius. Smith's fractures do not appear to result in this type of instability. Bellinghausen et al (1983) have described 2 patients with a pure post-traumatic palmar carpal subluxation. In both these patients there was an associated ulnar translocation. Both cases were treated by plaster immobilization. In both patients recurrent subluxation occurred but there was discomfort in the wrist only after heavy work. If surgical treatment is required, osteotomy through the plane of the fracture or arthrodesis should be considered.

Mid-carpal instability. In 1972 Linscheid et al described a static form of DISI occurring without scapholunate dissociation after fractures of the distal radius. A dynamic form of DISI can occur in association with a painful synovitis localized to the mid-carpal area (Taleisnik & Watson 1984). They performed a corrective osteotomy of the distal radius in 9 cases resulting in relief of symptoms and correction of the deformity.

Johnson & Carrera (1986) described a chronic capitolunate instability in 12 patients, all with a remote dorsiflexion injury to the symptomatic wrist. They described a dorsal displacement stress test to show dorsal subluxation of the capitate out of the cup of the lunate. Eleven patients had surgery which involved shortening of the radial capitate ligament, with satisfactory results in 9 of the 11 patients. However the significance of the stress test is uncertain as some of the asymptomatic contralateral wrists tested had more displacement than did the symptomatic wrists.

Summary

1. Scapholunate dissociation resulted in significant degenerative changes in up to 58% of cases.
2. Early treatment of scapholunate dissociation involves closed or open reduction with or without percutaneous wire fixation. Early treatment resulted in minimal or no pain in 88% of patients, almost a 50% reduction in wrist movement and a 53–80% reduction in grip strength.
3. Ligament reconstruction for chronic scapholunate dissociation produced early relief of symptoms with no or little pain in 86–96% of patients, almost a 50% loss of motion and 76% of normal grip strength. These ligament repairs may stretch out.
4. Intercarpal arthrodesis for chronic scapholunate dissociation produced satisfactory results in 66–75% of cases. Non-union occurred in up to 50% of cases. Range of motion averaged 80% of normal. Grip strength improved to 74% of normal and pinch grip improved to 86% of normal.

5. Scaphotrapezium–trapezoid instability is rare.
6. Triquetrohamate instability produces a dynamic DISI or VISI deformity. Tenodesis, ligament reconstruction or limited carpal arthrodesis are required if conservative treatment fails.
7. Triquetrolunate instability produces a dynamic or static VISI deformity. Triquetrolunate instability often produces few symptoms. If surgery is required, ligament reconstruction or limited arthrodesis produces satisfactory results.
8. Ulnar translocation is a rare injury which resulted in reasonable early results after ligament repair and tendon augmentation. Arthrodesis may be used primarily or to treat failed ligament repairs.
9. Dorsal carpal translocation and palmar carpal translocation require distal radial osteotomy or fusion.
10. Static or dynamic mid-carpal instabilities respond well to distal radial osteotomy.
11. Chronic capitolunate instability may be a post-traumatic instability and appeared to produce a reasonable result from shortening of the radial capitate ligament.

REFERENCES

Adkison J W, Chapman M W 1982 Treatment of acute lunate and perilunate dislocations. Clinical Orthopaedics 164: 199–207
Adler J B, Shafton G W 1962 Fractures of the capitate. Journal of Bone and Joint Surgery 44A: 1537–1547
Aitken A P, Nalebuff E A 1960 Volar transnavicular perilunar dislocation of the carpus. Journal of Bone and Joint Surgery 42A: 1051–1057
Alexander A H 1977 Bilateral traumatic dislocation of the distal radioulnar joint, ulna dorsal. Clinical Orthopaedics 129: 238–244
Ali M A 1986 Fracture of the body of the hamate bone associated with compartment syndrome and dorsal decompression of the carpal tunnel. Journal of Hand Surgery 11B: 207–210
Almquist E E 1986 Kienböck's disease. Clinical Orthopaedics 202: 68–78
Almquist E E, Burns J F 1982 Radial shortening for the treatment of Kienböck's disease — a 5 to 10 year follow-up. Journal of Hand Surgery 7: 348–352
Altissimi M, Anterucci R, Fiacca C, Mancini G B 1986 Long-term results of conservative treatment of fractures of the distal radius. Clinics in Orthopaedics 206: 202–210
Amadio P C, Hanssen A D, Berquist T H 1987 The genesis of Kienböck's disease: evaluation of a case by magnetic resonance imaging. Journal of Hand Surgery 12A:1044–1049
Amamilo S C, Uppal R, Samuel A W 1985 Isolated dislocation of carpal scaphoid. Journal of Hand Surgery 10B: 385–388
Armistead R B, Linscheid R L, Dobyns J H, Beckenbaugh R D 1982 Ulnar lengthening in the treatment of Kienböck's disease. Journal of Bone and Joint Surgery 64A: 170–178
Bacorn R W, Kurtzke J F 1953 Colles' fracture. Journal of Bone and Joint Surgery 35A: 643–658
Baird D B, Friedenberg Z B 1968 Delayed ulnar-nerve palsy following a fracture of the hamate. Journal of Bone and Joint Surgery 50A: 570–572
Bartone N F, Grieco R V 1956 Fractures of the triquetrum. Journal of Bone and Joint Surgery 38A: 353–356
Beckenbaugh R D, Shives T C, Dobyns J H, Linscheid R L 1980 Kienböck's disease: the natural history of Kienböck's disease and consideration of lunate fractures. Clinical Orthopaedics 149: 98–106

Bellinghausen H W, Gilula L A, Young L V, Weeks P M 1983 Post-traumatic palmar carpal subluxation. Journal of Bone and Joint Surgery 65A: 998–1006

Benjamin A 1982 Injuries of the forearm. In Watson Jones' Fractures and joint injuries Wilson J N (ed) Churchill Livingstone, Edinburgh, pp 650–709

Bertini S, Capanna R, Vitale C 1982 Use of the Swanson prosthesis in Kienböck's disease. Italian Journal of Orthopaedics and Traumatology 8: 33–41

Bieber E J, Weiland A J 1984 Traumatic dorsal dislocation of the triquetrum: a case report. Journal of Hand Surgery 9A: 840–842

Bilos Z J, Hui P W T 1981 Dorsal dislocation of the lunate with carpal collapse. Journal of Bone and Joint Surgery 63A: 1484–1486

Bilos Z J, Pankovich A M, Yelda S 1977 Fracture–dislocation of the radiocarpal joint. Journal of Bone and Joint Surgery 59A: 192–203

Birch-Jensen A 1951 Luxation of the distal radio-ulnar joint. Acta Chirurgica Scandinavica 101: 312–317

Bishop A T, Beckenbaugh R D 1988 Fracture of the hamate hook. Journal of Hand Surgery 13A: 135–139

Black D M, Watson H K, Vender M I 1986 Scapholunate gap with scaphoid non union. Clinical Orthopaedics 224: 205–209

Blair W F, Kilpatrick W C, Omer G E 1982 Open fracture of the hook of the hamate. Clinical Orthopaedics 163: 180–184

Blount W P, Schaefer A A, Johnson J H 1942 Fracture of the forearm in children. Journal of the American Medical Association 120: 111–116

Boe S 1979 Dislocation of the trapezium. Acta Orthopaedica Scandinavica 50: 85–86

Boeckstyns M E H, Busch P 1984 Surgical treatment of scaphoid pseudarthrosis; evaluation of the results after soft tissue arthroplasty and inlay bone grafting. Journal of Hand Surgery 9A: 378–382

Boeckstyns M E H, Kjäer L, Busch P, Holst-Nielsen F 1985 Soft tissue interposition arthroplasty for scaphoid non union. Journal of Hand Surgery 10A: 109–114

Bonnin J G, Greening W P 1943 Fractures of the triquetrum. British Journal of Surgery 31: 278–283

Bora F W, Osterman A L, Brighton C T 1981 The electrical treatment of scaphoid non union. Clinical Orthopaedics 161: 33–38

Borgeskov S, Christiansen B, Kjäer A, Balslev I 1966 Fractures of the carpal bones. Acta Orthopaedica Scandinavica 37: 276–287

Bowen T L 1973 Injuries of the hamate bone. The Hand 5: 235–237

Bragdon R A 1965 Fractures of the distal radial epiphysis. Clinical Orthopaedics 41: 59–63

Brewood A F M 1985 Complete dislocation of the trapezium; a case report. Injury 16: 303–304

Broder H 1954 Rupture of flexor tendons, associated with a mal-united Colles' fracture. Journal of Bone and Joint Surgery 36A: 404–405

Brolin I 1964 Post-traumatic lesions of the lunate bone. Acta Orthopaedica Scandinavica 34: 167–182

Brown R H L, Muddu B N 1981 Scaphoid and lunate dislocation. The Hand 13: 303–307

Bryan R S, Dobyns J H 1981 Fractures of the carpal bones other than lunate and navicular. Clinical Orthopaedics 149: 107–111

Bunker T D, McNamee P B, Scott T D 1987 The Herbert screw for scaphoid fractures. Journal of Bone and Joint Surgery 69B: 631–634

Campbell R D, Lance E M, Yeoh C B 1964 Lunate and perilunar dislocations. Journal of Bone and Joint Surgery 46B: 55–72

Campbell R D, Thompson T C, Lance E M, Adler J B 1965 Indications for open reduction of lunate and perilunate dislocations of the carpal bones. Journal of Bone and Joint Surgery 47A: 915–937

Carter P R, Eaton R G, Littler J W 1977 Ununited fracture of the hook of the hamate. Journal of Bone and Joint Surgery 59A: 583–588

Cassebaum W H 1950 Colles' fracture. Journal of the American Medical Association 143: 963–965

Cetti R, Christensen S-E, Reuther K 1982 Fracture of the lunate bone. The Hand 14: 80–84

Chan K P, Huang P 1971 Anatomic variations in radial and ulnar lengths in the wrists of Chinese. Clinical Orthopaedics 80: 17–20

Chapman D R, Bennett J B, Bryan W J, Tullos H S 1982 Complications of distal radial fractures: pins and plaster treatment. Journal of Hand Surgery 7: 509–512

Christodoulou A G, Colton C L 1986 Scaphoid fractures in children. Journal of Pediatric Orthopaedics 6: 37–39

Clancey G J 1984 Percutaneous Kirschner-wire fixation of Colles' fractures. Journal of Bone and Joint Surgery 66A: 1008–1014

Clayton M L 1969 Rupture of the flexor tendons in carpal tunnel (non rheumatoid with specific reference to fractures of the hook of the hamate). Journal of Bone and Joint Surgery 51A: 798–799

Cole J M, Obletz B E 1966 Comminuted fractures of the distal end of the radius treated by skeletal transfixion in plaster cast. Journal of Bone and Joint Surgery 48A: 931–945

Coleman H M 1960 Injuries of the articular disc at the wrist. Journal of Bone and Joint Surgery 42B: 522–529

Coll G A 1987 Palmar dislocation of the scaphoid and lunate. Journal of Hand Surgery 12A: 476–480

Collert S, Isacson J 1978 Management of redislocated Colles' fractures. Clinical Orthopaedics 135: 183–186

Connell M C, Dyson R P 1955 Dislocations of the carpal scaphoid. Journal of Bone and Joint Surgery 37B: 252–253

Cooney W P 1983 External fixation of distal radial fractures. Clinical Orthopaedics 180: 44–49

Cooney W P, Linscheid R L, Dobyns J H 1979 External pin fixation for unstable Colles' fractures. Journal of Bone and Joint Surgery 61A: 840–845

Cooney W P, Dobyns J H, Linscheid R L 1980 Complications of Colles' fractures. Journal of Bone and Joint Surgery 62A: 613–619

Cooney W P, Dobyns J H, Linscheid R L 1980 Fractures of the scaphoid: a rational approach to management. Clinical Orthopaedics 149: 90–97

Cooney W P, Bussey R, Dobyns J H, Linscheid R L 1987 Difficult wrist fractures. Perilunate fracture–dislocations of the wrist. Clinical Orthopaedics 214: 136–147

Cordrey L J, Ferrer-Torrels M 1960 Management of fractures of the greater multangular. Journal of Bone and Joint Surgery 42A: 1111–1118

Crittenden J J, Jones D M, Santarelli A G 1970 Bilateral rotational dislocation of the carpal navicular. Radiology 94: 629–630

Crosby E B, Linscheid R L 1974 Rupture of the flexor profundus tendon of the ring finger secondary to ancient fracture of the hook of the hamate. Journal of Bone and Joint Surgery 56A: 1076–1078

Dameron T B 1972 Traumatic dislocation of the distal radio-ulnar joint. Clinical Orthopaedics 83: 55–63

D'Anca A F, Sternlieb S B, Byron T W, Feinstein P A 1984 External fixator management of unstable Colles' fractures. Orthopaedics 7: 853–859

Davis D R, Green D P 1976 Forearm fractures in children. Clinical Orthopaedics 120: 172–184

De Oliveira J C 1973 Barton's fractures. Journal of Bone and Joint Surgery 55A: 586–594

De Palma A F 1952 Comminuted fractures of the distal end of the radius treated by ulnar pinning. Journal of Bone and Joint Surgery 34A: 651–662

Diamond J P, Newman J H 1987 Multiple flexor tendon ruptures following Colles' fracture: a case report. Journal of Hand Surgery 12B: 112–114

Dias J J, Wray C C, Jones J M, Gregg P J 1987a The value of early mobilisation in the treatment of Colles' fractures. Journal of Bone and Joint Surgery 69B: 463–467

Dias J J, Wray C C, Jones J M 1987b The radiological deformity of Colles' fractures. Injury 18: 304–308

Dias J J, Taylor M, Thompson J, Brenkel I J, Gregg P J 1988 Radiographic signs of union of scaphoid fractures. Journal of Bone and Joint Surgery 70B: 299–301

Dickson J C, Shannon J G 1944 Fractures of the carpal scaphoid in the Canadian army. Surgery, Gynecology and Obstetrics 79: 225–239

Dobyns J H, Linscheid R L 1984 Fractures and dislocations of the wrist. In: Rockwood C A, Green D P (eds) Fractures in adults. J B Lippincott, Philadelphia, pp 411–510

Dowling J J, Sawyer B 1961 Comminuted Colles' fractures. Journal of Bone and Joint Surgery 43A: 657–668

Duke R 1963 Dislocation of the hamate bone. Journal of Bone and Joint Surgery 45B: 744

Durbin F C 1950 Non-union of the triquetrum. Journal of Bone and Joint Surgery 32B: 388

Eckenrode J F, Louis D S, Greene T L 1986 Scaphoid-trapezium-trapezoid fusion in the treatment of chronic scapholunate instability. Journal of Hand Surgery 11A: 497–502

Eddeland A, Eiken O, Hellgren E, Ohlsson N-M 1975 Fractures of the scaphoid. Scandinavian Journal of Reconstructive Surgery 9: 234–239

Eelma J, McElfresh E C 1983 Colles' fractures in young adults. Minnesota Medicine 66: 487–490

Egawa M, Asai T 1983 Fracture of the hook of the hamate. Journal of Hand Surgery 8: 393–398

Ellis J 1965 Smith's and Barton's fractures. Journal of Bone and Joint Surgery 47B: 724–727

Engkvist O, Lundberg G 1979 Rupture of the extensor pollicis longus tendon after fracture of the lower end of the radius — a clinical and microangiographic study. The Hand 11: 76–85

Evans G, Burke F D, Barton N J 1986 A comparison of conservative treatment and silicone replacement arthroplasty in Kienböck's disease. Journal of Hand Surgery 11B: 92–102

Fehring T K, Milek M A 1984 Isolated volar dislocation of the radiocarpal joint. Journal of Bone and Joint Surgery 66A: 464–466

Fenton R L 1956 The naviculo-capitate fracture syndrome. Journal of Bone and Joint Surgery 38A: 681–684

Fernandes H J A, Köberle G, Ferreira G H S, Camargo J N 1983 Volar transscaphoid perilunar dislocation. The Hand 15: 276–280

Fernandez D L 1982 Correction of post-traumatic wrist deformity in adults by osteotomy, bone grafting, and internal fixation. Journal of Bone and Joint Surgery 64A: 1164–1178

Fernandez D J 1984 A technique for anterior wedge-shaped grafts for scaphoid non unions with carpal instability. Journal of Hand Surgery 9A: 733–737

Fisk G R 1970 Carpal instability and the fractured scaphoid. Annals of the Royal College of Surgeons 46: 63–76

Fisk G R 1984a Non union of the carpal scaphoid treated by wedge grafting. Journal of Bone and Joint Surgery 66B: 277

Fisk G R 1984b The wrist. Journal of Bone and Joint Surgery 66B: 396–407

Flandreau R H, Sweeney R M, O'Sullivan W D 1962 Clinical experience with a series of Smith's fractures. Archives of Surgery 84: 36–39

Ford D J, Khoury G, El-Hadidi S, Lunn P G, Burke F D 1987 The Herbert screw for fractures of the scaphoid. Journal of Bone and Joint Surgery 69B: 124–127

Foucher G, Schuind F, Merle M, Brunelli F 1985 Fractures of the hook of the hamate. Journal of Hand Surgery 10B: 205–210

Freeland A E, Finley J S 1984 Displaced vertical fracture of the trapezium treated with a small cancellous lag screw. Journal of Hand Surgery 9A: 843–844

Freeland A E, Finley J S 1986 Displaced dorsal oblique fracture of the hamate treated with a cortical mini lag screw. Journal of Hand Surgery 11A: 656–658

Freeland B H, Hay H L 1985 Non union of the capitate. Journal of Hand Surgery 10A: 187–190

Freund L G, Ovesen J 1977 Isolated dorsal dislocation of the radiocarpal joint. Journal of Bone and Joint Surgery 59A: 277

Frykman E 1980 Dislocation of the triquetrum. Scandinavian Journal of Plastic Reconstructive Surgery 14: 205

Frykman G 1964 Arthritis of the distal radio-ulnar joint after injury. Journal of Bone and Joint Surgery 46B: 359

Frykman G 1967 Fracture of the distal radius including sequelae. Acta Orthopaedica Scandinavica (suppl) 108

Frykman G K, Taleisnik J, Peters G et al 1986 Treatment of nonunited scaphoid fractures by pulsed electromagnetic field and cast. Journal of Hand Surgery 11A: 344–349

Fuller D J 1973 The Ellis plate operation for Smith's fracture. Journal of Bone and Joint Surgery 55B: 173–178

Garcia-Elias M, Abanco J, Salvador E, Sanchez R 1985 Crush injury of the carpus. Journal of Bone and Joint Surgery 67B: 286–289

Gartland J J, Werley C W 1951 Evaluation of healed Colles' fractures. Journal of Bone and Joint Surgery 33A: 895–907

Gasser H 1965 Delayed union and pseudarthrosis of the carpal navicular: treatment by

compression-screw osteosynthesis. Journal of Bone and Joint Surgery 47A: 249–266
Gelberman R H, Salaman P B, Jurist J M, Posch J L 1975 Ulnar variance in Kienböck's disease. Journal of Bone and Joint Surgery 37A: 674–676
Glickel S Z, Millender L H 1982 Ligamentous reconstruction for chronic intercarpal instability. Orthopaedic Transactions 6: 167
Goldberg B, Heller A P 1987 Dorsal dislocation of the triquetrum with rotary subluxation of the scaphoid. Journal of Hand Surgery 12A: 119–122
Goldberg I, Amit S, Bahar A, Seelenfreund M 1981 Complete dislocation of the trapezium. Journal of Hand Surgery 6: 193–195
Goodman M L, Shankman G B 1984 Palmar dislocation of the trapezoid. Journal of Hand Surgery 9A: 127–131
Gordon S L 1972 Scaphoid and lunate dislocation. Journal of Bone and Joint Surgery 54A: 1769–1772
Green D P 1975 Pins and plaster treatment of comminuted fractures of the distal end of the radius. Journal of Bone and Joint Surgery 57A: 304–310
Green D P 1982 Operative hand surgery, vol 1. Churchill Livingstone, Edinburgh
Green D P 1985 The effect of avascular necrosis on Russe bone grafting for scaphoid non union. Journal of Hand Surgery 10A: 597–605
Green D P, O'Brien E T 1978 Open reduction of carpal dislocations: indications and operative techniques. Journal of Hand Surgery 3: 250–265
Green D P, O'Brien E T 1979 Classification and management of carpal dislocations. Clinical Orthopaedics 149: 55–72
Green J T, Gay F H 1956 Colles' fracture — residual disability. American Journal of Surgery 91: 636–642
Gunn R S 1985 Dislocation of the hamate bone. Journal of Hand Surgery 10B: 107–108
Harbison J S, Stevenson T M, Lipert J R 1978 Forearm fractures in children. Australia and New Zealand Journal of Surgery 48: 84–88
Hastings D E, Silber R L 1984 Intercarpal arthrodesis in the management of chronic carpal instability after trauma. Journal of Hand Surgery 9A: 834–840
Herbert T J 1986 Use of the Herbert bone screw in surgery of the wrist. Clinical Orthopaedics 202: 79–92
Herbert T J, Fisher W E 1984 Management of the fractured scaphoid using a new bone screw. Journal of Bone and Joint Surgery 66B: 114–123
Hergenröeder P T, Penix A R 1981 Bilateral scapholunate dissociation with degenerative arthritis. Journal of Hand Surgery 6: 620–622
Herness D, Posner M A 1977 Some aspects of bone grafting for non union of the carpal navicular. Acta Orthopaedica Scandinavica 48: 373–378
Holdsworth B J, Shackleford I 1987 Fracture dislocation of the trapezio-scaphoid joint — the missing link? Journal of Hand Surgery 12B: 40–42
Hollingsworth R, Morris J 1976 The importance of the ulnar side of the wrist in fractures of the distal end of the radius. Injury 7: 263–266
Howard F M 1964 Ulnar-nerve palsy in wrist fractures. Journal of Bone and Joint Surgery 43A: 1197–1201
Howard F M, Fahey T, Wojcik E 1974 Rotary subluxation of the navicular. Clinical Orthopaedics 104: 134–139
Hudson T M, Caragol W J, Kaye J J 1976 Isolated rotatory subluxation of the carpal navicular. American Journal of Roentgenology 126: 601–611
Huere D R 1979 Primary internal fixation of carpal navicular fractures in the athlete. American Journal of Sports Medicine 7: 175–177
Jackson W T, Protas J M 1981 Snapping scapholunate subluxation. Journal of Hand Surgery 6: 590–594
Jasmine M S, Packer J W, Edwards G S 1988 Irreducible trans-scaphoid perilunate dislocation. Journal of Hand Surgery 13A: 212–215
Jenkins S A 1951 Osteoarthritis of the pisiform-triquetral joint. Journal of Bone and Joint Surgery 33B: 532
Johnson R P, Carrera G F 1986 Chronic capitolunate instability. Journal of Bone and Joint Surgery 68A: 1164–1176
Jones G B 1955 An unusual fracture–dislocation of the carpus. Journal of Bone and Joint Surgery 37B: 146–147
Jones W A 1987 Beware the sprained wrist. Journal of Bone and Joint Surgery 70B: 293–297

Jones W A, Ghorbal M S 1985 Fractures of the trapezium. A report of three cases. Journal of Hand Surgery 10B: 227–230

Jonsson U 1983 External fixation for redislocated Colles' fractures. Acta Orthopaedica Scandinavica 54: 878–883

Kato H, Usui M, Minami A 1986 Long-term results of Kienböck's disease treated by excisional arthroplasty with a silicone implant or coiled palmaris longus tendon. Journal of Hand Surgery 11A: 645–653

Katznelson A, Volpin G, Lin E 1980 Tension band wiring for fixation of comminuted fractures of the distal radius. Injury 12: 239–242

Kienböck R 1910 Concerning traumatic malacia of the lunate and its consequences: degeneration and compression fractures. The classic. Clinical Orthopaedics 149: 4–8

King R E 1975 Barton's fracture–dislocation of the wrist. Current Practice in Orthopaedic Surgery 6: 133–144

Kleinart J M, Zenni E J 1984 Non union of the scaphoid. Orthopaedic Review 13: 125–141

Kleinman W B, Steichen J B, Strickland J W 1982 Management of chronic rotary subluxation of the scaphoid by scapho-trapezio-trapezoid arthrodesis. Journal of Hand Surgery 7: 125–136

Kopp J R 1985 Isolated palmar dislocation of the trapezoid. Journal of Hand Surgery 10A: 91–93

Kristensen S S, Thomassen E, Christensen F 1986a Ulnar variance in Kienböck's disease. Journal of Hand Surgery 11B: 258–260

Kristensen S S, Thomassen E, Christensen F 1986b Kienböck's disease — late results by non-surgical treatment. Journal of Hand Surgery 11B: 422–425

Kristianson A, Gjersøe E 1968 Colles' fracture operative treatment, indications and results. Acta Orthopaedica Scandinavica 39: 33–46

Kuhlmann J N, Mimour M, Buabighi A, Baux S 1987 Vascularised bone graft pedicled on the volar carpal artery for non union of the scaphoid. Journal of Hand Surgery 12B: 203–210

Küpfer K 1986 Palmar dislocation of scaphoid and lunate as a unit: case report with special reference to carpal instability and treatment. Journal of Hand Surgery 11A: 130–134

Kuur E, Boe A M 1986 Scaphoid-trapezium-trapezoid subluxation. Journal of Hand Surgery 11B: 434–435

Kvarnes L, Reikeras O 1983 Non union of the carpal navicular. The Hand 15: 252–257

Larson B, Light T R, Ogden J A 1987 Fracture and ischemic necrosis of the immature scaphoid. Journal of Hand Surgery 12A: 122–127

Lee B S, Esterhai J L, Das M 1984 Fracture of the distal radial epiphysis. Clinical Orthopaedics 185: 90–96

Lee M L H 1963 The intraosseous arterial pattern of the carpal lunate bone and its relationship to avascular necrosis. Acta Orthopaedica Scandinavica 33: 43–55

Leslie I J, Dickson R A 1981 The fractured carpal scaphoid. Journal of Bone and Joint Surgery 63B: 225–230

Lewis M H 1978 Median nerve decompression after Colles' fracture. Journal of Bone and Joint Surgery 60B: 195–196

Leyshon A, Ireland J, Trickey E L 1984 The treatment of delayed union and non union of the carpal scaphoid by screw fixation. Journal of Bone and Joint Surgery 66B: 124–127

Lichtman D M, Mack G R, Macdonald R I, Gunther S F, Wilson J N 1977 Kienböck's disease: the role of silicone replacement arthroplasty. Journal of Bone and Joint Surgery 59A: 899–908

Lichtman D M, Schneider J R, Swafford A R, Mack G K 1981 Ulnar midcarpal instability — clinical and laboratory analysis. Journal of Hand Surgery 6: 515–523

Lichtman D M, Alexander H, Mack G R, Gunther S F 1982 Kienböck's disease — update on silicone replacement arthroplasty. Journal of Hand Surgery 7: 343–347

Lichtman D M, Noble W H, Alexander C E 1984 Dynamic triquetrolunate instability; case report. Journal of Hand Surgery 9A: 185–187

Lidström A 1959 Fractures of the distal end of the radius. Acta Orthopaedica Scandinavica (suppl) 41

Linscheid R L, Dobyns J H, Beabout J W, Bryan R S 1972 Traumatic instability of the wrist. Journal of Bone and Joint Surgery 54A: 1612–1632

London P S 1961 The broken scaphoid bone. Journal of Bone and Joint Surgery 43B: 237–244

Lowdon I M R, Simpson A H R W, Burge P 1984 Recurrent dorsal trans-scaphoid perilunate dislocation. Journal of Hand Surgery 9B: 307–310

Lowrey D G, Moss S H, Wolff T W 1984 Volar dislocation of the capitate. Journal of Bone and Joint Surgery 66A: 611–613

Lynch A C, Lipscomb P R 1963 The carpal tunnel syndrome and Colles' fracture. Journal of the American Medical Association 185: 363–366

Mack G R, Bosse M J, Gelberman R H, Yu E 1984 The natural history of scaphoid non union. Journal of Bone and Joint Surgery 66A: 504–509

Mahring M, Semple C, Gray I C M 1985 Attritional flexor tendon rupture due to a scaphoid non union imitating an anterior interosseous nerve syndrome. A case report. Journal of Hand Surgery 10B: 62–64

Maki N J, Chuinard R G, D'Ambrosia R 1982 Isolated, complete radial dislocation of the scaphoid. Journal of Bone and Joint Surgery 64A: 615–616

Manoli A 1982 Irreducible fracture-separation of the distal radial epiphysis. Journal of Bone and Joint Surgery 64A: 1095–1096

Manske P R 1978 Fracture of the hook of the hamate presenting as carpal tunnel syndrome. The Hand 10: 181–183

Marsh A P, Lampros P J 1959 The naviculo-capitate fracture syndrome. American Journal of Roentgenology 82: 255–256

Mason M L 1953 Colles' fracture. British Journal of Surgery 40: 340–346

Maudsley R H, Chen S C 1972 Screw fixation in the management of the fractured carpal scaphoid. Journal of Bone and Joint Surgery 54B: 432–441

Mayfield J K, Johnson R P, Kilcoyne R K 1980 Carpal dislocations: pathomechanics and progressive perilunar instability. Journal of Hand Surgery 5: 226–241

Mazet R, Hohl M 1961 Conservative treatment of old factures of the carpal scaphoid. Journal of Trauma 1: 115–127

Mazet R, Hohl M 1963 Fractures of the carpal navicular. Journal of Bone and Joint Surgery 45A: 82–112

McAuliffe T B, Hilliar K M, Coates C J, Grange W J 1987 Early mobilisation of Colles' fractures. Journal of Bone and Joint Surgery 69B: 727–729

McClain E J, Boyes J H 1966 Missed fractures of the greater multangular. Journal of Bone and Joint Surgery 48A: 1525–1528

McDonald G, Petrie D 1975 Un-united fracture of the scaphoid. Clinical Orthopaedics 108: 110–114

Mclaughlin H L, Parkes J C 1969 Fracture of the carpal navicular bone: gradations in therapy based upon pathology. Journal of Trauma 9: 311–319

McQueen M M, Maclaren A, Chalmers J 1986 The value of remanipulating Colles' fractures. Journal of Bone and Joint Surgery 68B: 232–233

Melone C P 1981 Scaphoid fractures: concepts in management. Clinics in Plastic Surgery 8: 83–94

Melone C P 1984 Articular fractures of the distal radius. Orthopedic Clinics of North America 15 (2): 217–236

Melone C P 1986 Open treatment for displaced articular fractures of the distal radius. Clinical Orthopaedics 202: 103–111

Merion J, Wood V E, Schoene H R, Frykman G K, Hohl J C, Bestard E A 1984 Isolated tears of the triangular fibrocartilage of the wrist; results of partial excision. Journal of Hand Surgery 9A: 527–530

Meyers M H, Wells R, Harvey J P 1971 Naviculo-capitate fracture syndrome. Journal of Bone and Joint Surgery 53A: 1383–1386

Meyn M A, Roth A M 1980 Isolated dislocation of the trapezoid bone. Journal of Hand Surgery 5: 602–604

Minami A, Ogino T, Ohshio I, Minami M 1986 Correlation between clinical results and carpal instabilities in patients after reduction of lunate and perilunar dislocation. Journal of Hand Surgery 11B: 213–220

Minami M, Yamazaki J, Ishii S 1984 Isolated dislocation of the pisiform. Journal of Hand Surgery 9A: 125–127

Mirabello S C, Rosenthal D I, Smith R J 1987 Correlation of clinical and radiographic findings in Kienböck's disease. Journal of Hand Surgery 12A: 1049–1054

Moharti R C, Kar N 1979 Study of the triangular fibrocartilage of the wrist joint in Colles' fracture. Injury 11: 321–324

Moneim M S, Boger J T, Omer G E 1983 Radiocarpal dislocation — classification and rationale for management. Clinical Orthopaedics 192: 199–209

Moneim M S, Hofammann K E, Omer G E 1984 Transscaphoid perilunate fracture–dislocation. Clinical Orthopaedics 190: 227–235

Monsivais J J, Nitz P A, Scully T J 1986 The role of carpal instability in scaphoid non union: casual or causal? Journal of Hand Surgery 11B: 201–206

Moore D P, McMahon B A 1988 Anterior radio-carpal dislocation: an isolated injury. Journal of Hand Surgery 13B: 215–217

Morawal L G, Ross P M, Schock C C 1976 Fractures and dislocations involving the navicular–lunate axis. Clinical Orthopaedics 118: 48–53

Morrissey R T, Nalebuff E A 1977 Distal radial fracture with tendon entrapment. Clinical Orthopaedics 124: 205–208

Mulder J D 1968 The results of 100 cases of pseudarthrosis in the scaphoid bone treated by the Matti-Russe operation. Journal of Bone and Joint Surgery 50B: 110–115

Munson G O, Gainor B J 1981 Percutaneous pinning of distal radius fractures. Journal of Trauma 21: 1032–1035

Murakami Y 1977 Dislocation of the carpal scaphoid. The Hand 9: 79–81

Murakami Y, Todani K 1981 Traumatic entrapment of the extensor pollicis longus tendon in Smith's fracture of the radius. Journal of Hand Surgery 6: 238–240

Müssbichler H 1961 Injuries of the carpal scaphoid in children. Acta Radiologica 56: 361–368

Myles J W 1978 A new device for the internal fixation of wrist fractures. Journal of the Royal Society of Medicine 71: 186–188

Nakamura R, Hori M, Horii E, Miura T 1984 Reduction of the scaphoid fracture with DISI alignment. Journal of Hand Surgery 12A: 1000–1005

Nakata R Y, Chard Y, Matiko J D, Frykman G K, Wood V E 1985 External fixators for wrist fractures: a biomechanical and clinical study. Journal of Hand Surgery 10A: 845–851

Neviaser R J 1983 Proximal row carpectomy for post-traumatic disorders of the carpus. Journal of Hand Surgery 8: 301–305

Nielsen P T, Hedeboe J 1984 Post-traumatic scapholunate dissociation detected by wrist cineradiography. Journal of Hand Surgery 9A: 135–138

Nisenfield F G, Neviaser R J 1974 Fracture of the hook of the hamate: a diagnosis easily missed. Journal of Trauma 14: 612–616

Norbeck D E, Larson B, Blair S J, Demos T C 1987 Traumatic longitudinal disruption of the carpus. Journal of Hand Surgery 12A: 509–514

Nyquist S R, Stern P J 1984 Open radiocarpal fracture–dislocations. Journal of Hand Surgery 9A: 707–710

O'Brien E T 1983 Acute fractures and dislocations of the carpus. Orthopedic Clinics of North America 15: 237–257

O'Brien E T 1984 Acute fractures and dislocations of the carpus. Orthopedic Clinics of North America 15: 237–257

O'Brien E T 1984 Fractures of the hand and wrist region. In: Rockwood C A, Wilkins K E, King R E (eds) Fractures in children. J B Lippincott, Philadelphia, pp 229–300

Ogunro O 1983 Fracture of the body of the hamate bone. Journal of Hand Surgery 8: 353–355

Ohshio I, Ogino T, Miyake A 1986 Dislocation of the hamate associated with fracture of the trapezial ridge. Journal of Hand Surgery 11A: 658–660

Okuhara T, Matsui T, Sugimoto Y 1982 Spontaneous rupture of flexor tendons of a little finger due to projection of the hook of the hamate. The Hand 14: 71–74

Older T M, Stabler E V, Cassebaum W H 1965 Colles' fracture: evaluation and selection of therapy. Journal of Trauma 5: 469–476

Ovesen J 1981 Shortening of the radius in the treatment of lunatomalacia. Journal of Bone and Joint Surgery 63B: 231–232

Palmer A K 1981 Trapezial ridge fractures. Journal of Hand Surgery 6: 561–564

Palmer A K 1987 Keinböck's disease. Journal of Hand Surgery 12B: 291–293

Palmer A K, Dobyns J H, Linscheid R L 1978 Management of post-traumatic instability of the wrist secondary to ligament rupture. Journal of Hand Surgery 3: 507–532

Palmieri T J 1982 The excision of painful pisiform bone fractures. Orthopaedics Review 11: 99

Panting A L, Lamb D W, Noble J, Haw C S 1984 Dislocations of the lunate with and without fracture of the scaphoid. Journal of Bone and Joint Surgery 66B: 391–395

Pardini A G 1984 Silastic arthroplasty for avascular necrosis of the carpal lunate. International Orthopaedics 8: 223–227

Pool C 1973 Colles' fracture. Journal of Bone and Joint Surgery 55B: 540–544

Porter M L, Stockley I 1986 Fracture of the distal radius: intermediate and end results in relation to radiological parameters. Journal of Bone and Joint Surgery 68B: 666

Pournaras J, Kappas A 1979 Volar perilunar dislocation. Journal of Bone and Joint Surgery 61A: 625–626

Primiano G A, Reef T C 1974 Disruption of the proximal carpal arch of the hand. Journal of Bone and Joint Surgery 56A: 328–332

Pring D J, Hartley E B, Williams D J 1987 Scaphoid osteosynthesis: early experience with the Herbert bone screw. Journal of Hand Surgery 12B: 46–49

Rand J A, Linscheid R L, Dobyns J H 1982 Capitate fractures. A long term follow-up. Clinical Orthopaedics 165: 209–216

Rask M R 1979 Carponavicular subluxation: report of a case treated with percutaneous pins. Orthopaedics 2: 134–135

Rauis A, Ledoux A, Thiebaut A, van der Ghinst M 1979 Bipolar fixation of fractures of the distal end of the radius. International Orthopaedics 3: 89–96

Rawlings D 1981 The management of dislocations of the carpal lunate. Injury 12: 319–330

Rayhack J M, Linscheid R L, Dobyns J H, Smith J H 1987 Post traumatic ulnar translation of the carpus. Journal of Hand Surgery 12A: 180–189

Reagan D S, Linscheid R L, Dobyns J H 1984 Lunotriquetral sprains. Journal of Hand Surgery 9A: 502–514

Ripperger R R, Cooney W P, Linscheid R L 1980 Distal pole scaphoid fractures. Orthopaedic Transactions 4: 18

Rose-Innes A P 1960 Anterior dislocation of the ulna at the inferior radio-ulnar joint. Journal of Bone and Joint Surgery 42B: 515–521

Rosardo A P 1966 A possible relationship of radio-carpal dislocation and dislocation of the lunate bone. Journal of Bone and Joint Surgery 48B: 504–506

Rosenthal D I, Schwartz M, Phillips W C, Jupiter J 1983 Fracture of the radius with instability of the wrist. American Journal of Roentgenology 141: 113–116

Rubinovich R M, Rennie W R 1983 Colles' fracture: end results in relation to radiologic parameters. Canadian Journal of Surgery 26: 361–363

Ruby L K, Stinson J, Belsky M R 1985 The natural history of scaphoid non-union. Journal of Bone and Joint Surgery 67A: 428–433

Rush L V 1954 Closed medullary pinning of Colles' fractures. Clinical Orthopaedics 3: 152–162

Russe O 1960 Fracture of the carpal navicular. Journal of Bone and Joint Surgery 42A: 759–768

Sadr B 1984 Sequential rupture of extensor tendons after a Colles' fracture. Journal of Hand Surgery 9A: 144–145

Sauneir J, Chamay A 1980 Volar perilunar dislocation of the wrist. Clinical Orthopaedics 157: 139–142

Scheck M 1962 Long-term follow-up of treatment of comminuted fractures of the distal end of the radius by transfixation with Kirschner wires and cast. Journal of Bone and Joint Surgery 44A: 337–351

Schoenecker P L, Gilula L A, Shively R A, Manske P R 1984 Radiocarpal fracture–dislocation. Clinical Orthopaedics 197: 237–244

Seidenstein H 1956 Two unusual dislocations at the wrist. Journal of Bone and Joint Surgery 38A: 1137–1141

Seiman L P 1972 Compound dislocation of the trapezium. Journal of Bone and Joint Surgery 54A: 1297–1300

Sherlock D A 1987 Traumatic dorsoradial dislocation of the trapezium. Journal of Hand Surgery 12A: 262–265

Siegel M W, Hertzberg H 1969 Complete dislocation of the greater multangular (trapezium). Journal of Bone and Joint Sugery 51A: 769–772

Siegert J J, Frassica F J, Amadio P C 1988 Treatment of chronic perilunate dislocations. Journal of Hand Surgery 13A: 206–212

Smaill G B 1965 Long term follow up of Colles' fracture. Journal of Bone and Joint Surgery 47B: 80–85

Soucacos P N, Hartefilakidis-Garofalidis G C 1981 Dislocation of the triangular bone. Journal of Bone and Joint Surgery 63A: 1012–1013

Southcott R, Rosman M A 1977 Non union of carpal scaphoid fractures in children. Journal of Bone and Joint Surgery 59B: 20–23

Stahl F 1947 On lunatomalacia. Acta Chirurgica Scandinavica 95 (suppl) 126

Stark H H, Jobe F W, Boyes J H, Ashworth C R 1977 Fracture of the hook of the hamate in athletes. Journal of Bone and Joint Surgery 59A: 575–582

Stark H H, Zemel N P, Ashworth C R 1981 Use of a hand-carved silicone rubber spacer for advanced Kienböck's disease. Journal of Bone and Joint Surgery 63A: 1359–1370

Stark A, Broström L A, Svartengren G 1986 Scaphoid non union treated with the Matti-Russe technique. Clinical Orthopaedics 214: 175–180

Stein A H 1971 Dorsal dislocation of the lesser multangular bone. Journal of Bone and Joint Surgery 53A: 377–379

Stein F, Siegel M W 1969 Naviculocapitate fracture syndrome. Journal of Bone and Joint Surgery 51A: 391–395

Stern P J 1981 Multiple flexor tendon ruptures following an old anterior dislocation of the lunate. Journal of Bone and Joint Surgery 63A: 489–490

Stern P J 1984 Transscaphoid–lunate dislocation; a report of two cases. Journal of Hand Surgery 9A: 370–373

Stewart H D, Innes A R, Burke F D 1984 Functional cast-bracing for Colles' fractures. Journal of Bone and Joint Surgery 66B: 749–753

Stewart H D, Innes A R, Burke F D 1985a Factors affecting the outcome of Colles' fracture: an anatomical and functional study. Injury 16: 289–295

Stewart H D, Innes A R, Burke F D 1985b The hand complications of Colles' fractures. Journal of Hand Surgery 10B: 103–106

Stewart M J 1954 Fractures of the carpal navicular (scaphoid). Journal of Bone and Joint Surgery 36A: 998–1006

Strickner M, Martinek H, Spängler H 1980 Post-traumatic pain in the ulnar part of the wrist joint. Journal of Bone and Joint Surgery 62B: 507

Stuart M J, Beckenbaugh R D 1987 Flexor digitorum profundus entrapment after closed treatment of a displaced Colles' fracture. Journal of Hand Surgery 12A: 413–415

Suman R K 1983 Unstable fractures of the distal end of the radius (transfixion pins and a cast). Injury 15: 206–211

Sumner J M, Khun S M 1984 Entrapment of the median nerve and flexor pollicis longus tendon in an epiphyseal fracture–dislocation of the distal radioulnar joint: a case report. Journal of Hand Surgery 9A: 711–714

Sundberg S B, Linscheid R L 1984 Kienböck's disease. Results of treatment with ulnar lengthening. Clinical Orthopaedics 187: 43–51

Tajima T 1966 An investigation of the treatment of Kienböck's disease. Journal of Bone and Joint Surgery 48A: 1649

Takami H, Takahashi S, Ando M 1982 Rupture of flexor tendon associated with previous fracture of the hook of the hamate. The Hand 15: 73–76

Taleisnik J 1980 Post-traumatic carpal instability. Clinical Orthopaedics 149: 73–82

Taleisnik J 1984 Triquetrohamate and triquetrolunate instabilities (medial carpal instability). Annales de Chirurgie de la Main 3: 331–343

Taleisnik J 1985 The wrist. Churchill Livingstone, Edinburgh

Taleisnik J, Watson H K 1984 Midcarpal instability caused by malunited fractures of the distal radius. Journal of Hand Surgery 9A: 350–357

Taylor A R 1969 Dislocation of the scaphoid. Postgraduate Medical Journal 45: 186–192

Taylor L J, Simonis R B, Moschos N 1985 Non union of the scaphoid: a prospective study of direct current stimulation. Journal of Bone and Joint Surgery 67B: 493–494

Therkelsen F, Andersen K 1949 Lunatomalacia. Acta Chirurgica Scandinavica 97: 503–526

Thomas F B 1957 Reduction of Smith's fracture. Journal of Bone and Joint Surgery 39B: 463–470

Thomas H O 1977 Isolated dislocation of the carpal scaphoid. Acta Orthopaedica Scandinavica 48: 369–372

Thomas A P, Birch R 1983 An unusual hamate fracture. The Hand 15: 281–283

Thomas E M, Tusan K W R, Browne P S H 1975 Fractures of the radius and ulna in children. Injury 7: 120–124

220   MEDICOLEGAL REPORTING IN ORTHOPAEDIC TRAUMA

Thompson G H, Grant T T 1977 Barton's fractures — reverse Barton's fractures. Clinical Orthopaedics 122: 210–221

Thomsen S, Falstei-Jensen S 1988 Rupture of the flexor pollicis longus tendon associated with an ununited fracture of the scaphoid. Journal of Hand Surgery 13A: 220–222

Trevor D 1950 Rupture of the extensor pollicis longus tendon after Colles' fracture. Journal of Bone and Joint Surgery 32B: 370–375

Trumble T, Bour C J, Smith R J, Edwards G S 1988 Intercarpal arthrodesis for static and dynamic volar intercalated segment instability. Journal of Hand Surgery 13A: 396–402

Uematsu A 1978 Intercarpal fusion for treatment of carpal instability. Clinical Orthopaedics 144: 159–165

Vahvanen V, Westerland M 1980 Fracture of the carpal scaphoid in children. Acta Orthopaedica Scandinavica 51: 909–913

Vance R M, Gelberman R H, Braun R M 1979 Chronic bilateral scapholunate dissociation without symptoms. Journal of Hand Surgery 4: 178–180

Vance R M, Gelberman R H, Evans E F 1980 Scaphocapitate fractures. Journal of Bone and Joint Surgery 62A: 271–276

Van der Linden A J 1986 Disk lesion of the wrist joint. Journal of Hand Surgery 11A: 490–497

Varodompun N, Limpivest P, Prinyaroj P 1985 Isolated dorsal radiocarpal dislocation; case report and literature review. Journal of Hand Surgery 10A: 708–710

Vaughan P A, Lui S M, Harrington I J, Mainstrelli G L 1985 Treatment of unstable fractures of the distal radius by external fixation. Journal of Bone and Joint Surgery 76B: 385–389

Vender M I, Watson H K, Wiener B D, Black D M 1987 Degenerative change in symptomatic scaphoid non union. Journal of Hand Surgery 12A: 514–519

Verdan C, Narakas A 1963 Fractures and pseudarthrosis of the scaphoid. Surgical Clinics of North America 48: 1083–1095

Viegas S F, Bean J W, Schram R A 1987 Trans-scaphoid fracture dislocations treated with open reduction and Herbert screw internal fixation. Journal of Hand Surgery 12A: 992–999

Villar R N, Marsh D, Rushton N, Greatorex R A 1987 Three years after Colles' fracture. Journal of Bone and Joint Surgery 69B: 635–638

Wagner C J 1956 Perilunar dislocations. Journal of Bone and Joint Surgery 38A: 1198–1207

Weber E R 1980 Biomechanical implications of scaphoid waist fracture. Clinical Orthopaedics 149: 83–89

Weber S C, Szabo R M 1986 Severely comminuted distal radial fracture as an unsolved problem: complications associated with external fixation and pins and plaster techniques. Journal of Hand Surgery 11A: 157–165

Weiss C, Laskin R S, Spinner M 1970 Irreducible trans-scaphoid perilunate dislocation. Journal of Bone and Joint Surgery 52A: 565–568

White R E, Omer G E 1984 Transient vascular compromise of the lunate after fracture-dislocation or dislocation of the carpus. Journal of Hand Surgery 9A: 181–184

Worland R L, Dick H M 1975 Transnavicular perilunate dislocations. Journal of Trauma 15: 407–412

8. The hand

P. G. Lunn

INTRODUCTION

Over 900 years ago King Canute, the Danish King of England from 1016 to 1035, drew up laws covering the principles of compensation for injuries (Bertelsen & Capener 1960). He stands out in history not only for his seaside exploits, which are well known, but also as one of the first people to have studied, in detail, the problems of assessing injuries and levels of compensation. In so doing he outlined the relative values of the individual digits of the hand and in fact his assessment bears a very close resemblance to those used in present times by the Department of Health and Social Security in the UK.

Approximately one-third of all injuries involve the upper extremity. The majority of these occur during the working years. In the USA upper limb injuries accounted for 90 million days of restricted activity at work and 60 million days lost from work in a single year (Kelsey et al 1980). The exact proportion of these injuries that will be involved in medicolegal proceedings is not known, but it is certainly a considerable number in the USA and results in a cost of $7 000 000 000 (approximately £4 billion) in indemnities for temporary and permanent disability. The medical costs and the loss of productivity resulting from time off work are not included in these sums. The assessment and prognosis given in a medicolegal report on a patient with a hand injury can therefore have very far-reaching effects, not only in terms of the future employment prospects of the patient, but also in financial terms to the individual, the employer, the insurance company and the community.

This chapter will attempt to cover the majority of the common hand injuries and conditions encountered in medicolegal reporting in the UK. It will highlight the important factors to be taken into account in the clinical assessment and formulation of an informed opinion of the degree of disability and in the prognosis for the future.

FORMULATION OF MEDICAL REPORTS

There are certain points worth emphasizing which relate to the way in which medicolegal reporting of a hand injury is carried out:

1. *Patient's details*: These include occupation and hand dominance.
2. *History*: It is important to know the mechanism of injury. Thus, if the hand was injured in a machine, it is necessary to know whether it was a sharp, blunt or crushing injury and whether or not there was any heat or other component to the injury.

   The details of treatment must be outlined, including any physiotherapy or occupational therapy.

   Duration of time lost from work should be recorded. It is also important to ascertain whether the patient returned to normal or light duties.
3. *Present situation*: This should include present symptoms and how they affect activity at work and at home.
4. *Clinical examination*: Concise findings of the examination of the injured part must be given, in such a way that solicitors and other medical experts can understand. Normal findings, where relevant, are also useful. Specific measurements can be helpful, but some measurements such as grip strength can be positively misleading if a standard grip meter is used. This measurement will only record what the patient wishes to convey as his grip strength; it is much more effective for the examiner to make his own assessment of strength on clinical grounds. (New devices are being developed with a view to obtaining objective measurements of grip strength but they are not yet generally available.) Diagrams and photographs are an effective means of demonstrating many of the physical findings.
5. *Investigations*: X-rays are frequently of value and may be used to describe the nature of the bony injury and any soft tissue swelling. They may also demonstrate pre-existing changes which may be relevant in relation to the present state of the patient and the possibility of future deterioration.
6. *Opinion and prognosis*: This is one of the main reasons why the solicitor requests the report so it is important to commit oneself and give positive views with percentages to indicate degree of disability. It may also be necessary to give an opinion on the mechanism of injury (there is sometimes inconsistency between the type of injury and the level of resulting disability), the response to treatment, and the length of time off work.

   It may be appropriate, in certain patients, to comment on the patient's level of motivation, bearing in mind the quotation from Seneca (4 BC–65 AD): 'It is a part of the cure to wish to be cured'. Sometimes this desire for a cure is tempered by a desire for recompense which can significantly alter the natural history of the healing process.

Long-term disability and any anticipated future complications should be included in this section of the report.

SOFT TISSUE INJURIES

Skin

Injuries to the skin may be either clean or contaminated, and either sharp or crushing in nature. A contaminated wound will not only require more intensive and prolonged treatment and therefore more time lost from work, but it is also more likely to result in a greater degree of scarring and fibrosis. There is therefore a higher risk of the development of an unsatisfactory result after such an injury and this can be reflected in a greater functional deficit. Similarly a crushing injury carries a greater risk of complications than a sharp injury. It is important therefore to include these factors in the history as well as the prognosis of a hand injury.

Prognosis

The two main problems which may occur after skin injuries are:

1. *Scar contracture*: This is likely to develop if a longitudinal scar extends across a flexor crease and is especially a problem in burns and crush injuries.
2. *Cosmetic disability*: The immature scar tissue is frequently discoloured and therefore may be much more unsightly at 2–3 months than at a year after injury. On the other hand, mature scars on extensor surfaces of joints, especially the elbow, can stretch and become unsightly.

Nerves

Nerve injury

Any injury to a nerve, other than a mild neuropraxia, will lead to some degree of permanent impairment in an adult. The commonest injury is a crush of the cutaneous nerves at the fingertip which may cause some degree of hypersensitivity to light touch, leading the patient to neglect this finger and transfer normal functions to an adjacent finger. This problem can often be alleviated by appropriate desensitization therapy which, although not curing the underlying hypersensitivity, may well enable the patient to retain the function of the affected finger for most tasks.

A partial or complete laceration of a nerve trunk will usually be explored and repaired surgically. The recovery of nerve function depends mainly on the type of nerve injured; a pure nerve such as a digital nerve which contains only sensory fibres will have the best result, while a mixed nerve such as the median or ulnar nerve will have a significantly poorer result.

The type of injury will also affect the outcome, so that a clean, sharp laceration will favour a good result whereas a contaminated crush injury is likely to lead to a poor result.

Results. As a rough guide it is reasonable to advise that the *best* possible outcome from a nerve injury (e.g. a sharp laceration to a digital nerve which is repaired under magnification as a primary procedure) can only be expected to give about 80% return of nerve function. In the case of a digital nerve this will mean that a very small area of the fingertip will have diminished sensation, and because of overlap from the adjacent digital nerve the overall disability will be slight. However, the ulnar side of the thumb-tip and the radial side of the index finger (and possibly middle finger) are the areas which will be associated with some disability if there is impairment of sensation because these are the most important sensory areas of the hand.

Division of the median nerve is more disabling than the ulnar nerve because it is the major sensory nerve to the hand. The level of disability can be assessed in various ways. It can be calculated roughly by assessing it as half the disability of the amputation of that part of the hand (Fig. 8.1), or more accurately using the chart devised by the American Academy of Orthopedic Surgeons, modified by Rank et al (Fig. 8.2).

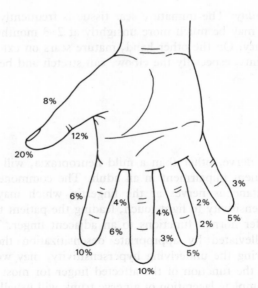

Fig. 8.1 Sensory impairment: relative value to the whole hand for total sensory loss of digit and comparative loss of radial and ulnar sides. Sensory loss is calculated at 50% that of amputation (from Swanson et al 1987, with permission)

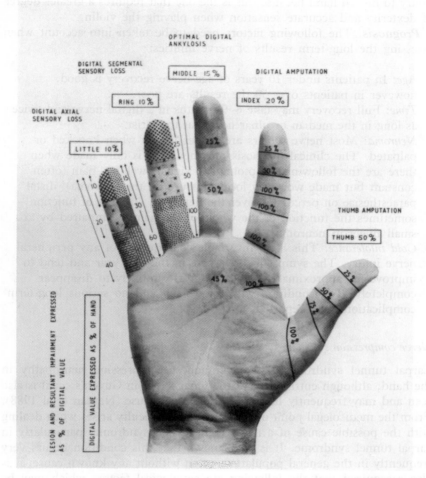

Fig. 8.2 Schematic illustration of a working basis for estimating the order of residual disability after hand injuries (from Rank et al 1973, with permission)

The percentage disability rating will depend on the opinion of the examining doctor who may well adjust the figure slightly in order to take into account the individual patient's requirements. For example, a bricklayer who has cold intolerance following a crush injury of the fingers will be considerably more disabled by this problem than a managing director or solicitor.

It is important to have some idea of what is involved in a patient's occupation or hobbies because this will obviously affect his level of disability. For example, a right-handed violinist will be more disabled by injury to his *left* hand because this is the one that requires a greater degree of dexterity and accurate sensation when playing the violin.

Prognosis. The following factors need to be taken into account when assessing the long-term results of nerve injuries:

1. *Age*: In patients under 10 years of age nerve recovery is good; however in patients over 50 the results are poor.
2. *Time*: Full recovery may take 6–9 months in a digital nerve and twice as long in the median or ulnar nerves at the wrist.
3. *Neuroma*: Most nerve repairs are tender locally when knocked or palpated. The clinical diagnosis of a neuroma is only made when there are the following symptoms and signs: swelling, pain (often constant but made worse by local pressure on the neuroma), distal paraesthesiae on percussion over the neuroma, and loss of function — sometimes the function of the whole of the hand is impaired by a small fingertip neuroma.
4. *Cold intolerance*: This is an invariable consequence of any peripheral nerve injury. The symptoms are worse in the first year and tend to improve for approximately 3 years but are unlikely to disappear completely. The condition will not worsen and no serious long-term complications are reported.

Nerve compression syndromes

Carpal tunnel syndrome is the commonest compression neuropathy in the hand, although entrapment of the ulnar nerve in Guyon's canal is also seen and may frequently have an occupational cause (Nathan et al 1988). From the medicolegal point of view the main difficulty arises when dealing with the possible cause of a nerve compression syndrome, particularly in carpal tunnel syndrome. It is well known that this condition occurs very frequently in the general population, often without any known cause; it is also recognized that the following are aetiological factors which may be associated with carpal tunnel syndrome (Leach & Odom 1968, Bleecker 1987):

1. Decreased cross-sectional area of the carpal tunnel, e.g. rheumatoid arthritis, trauma (wrist fracture), etc.
2. Increased volume of contents of the carpal canal, e.g. flexor tenosynovitis, fluid retention, especially associated with hormonal abnormalities such as pregnancy, menopause, diabetes, thyroid disorder acromegaly, etc.
3. Enlargement of the median nerve (rare).

The medical expert must decide whether the carpal tunnel syndrome has developed as a direct result of the patient's occupation or whether other aetiological factors are involved. The overall incidence of carpal tunnel syndrome is highest in females (in a ratio female:male of more than 2:1) between the ages of 40 and 60 years. If a patient is in this category or has one of the predisposing causes listed above it will be necessary to make a judgement on the relative importance of these factors and the type of work in relation to the development of the nerve compression syndrome. This is never easy. However, it may be helpful to give an assessment of the probability of the patient developing carpal tunnel syndrome if he had not been involved in his present occupation; is it greater or less than 50%, for instance? This will be a useful basis from which discussion may start with regard to the level of blame which can be attributed to an employer in so far as he is responsible for the nature of the work in which his employees are involved (see discussion in Chapter 19).

Compression of the ulnar nerve in Guyon's canal is a much less contentious issue and more commonly has a direct relationship to local trauma on the ulnar side of the hand (hypothenar hammer syndrome, etc.).

Results. Surgical decompression of the carpal tunnel gives good relief of symptoms when the compression has only been present for 6 months or less (Semple & Cargill 1969). Where there is a longer history, and where there is an occupational aetiology, the results are not so predictable. In occupational carpal tunnel syndrome some authorities therefore advocate alteration of the working conditions and a trial of conservative measures such as splintage and steroid injections as a first line of management (Eversmann 1988).

Similarly, the results of ulnar nerve decompression are good if there is only a short history, but less satisfactory if the compression has been present for over 6–12 months.

Prognosis. The factors associated with poor recovery following nerve compression are:

1. Long history.
2. Age: the older the patient, the longer will be the recovery period and the lower the chance of full recovery.
3. Systemic abnormalities, e.g. diabetes.

Tendons

Flexor tendon injuries are a well recognized source of short- and long-term problems. In the acute stage the tendon injury may be missed but if treated it should give a satisfactory result (Lister et al 1977). The exception to this is the injury in zone 2 which has a universally poor outlook (Fig. 8.3).

Extensor tendon injuries are generally easier to treat, heal quicker and have fewer complications than flexor tendon injuries. However, the main functional problem which may develop is a loss of flexion due to tenodesis of the extensor tendon which hinders gliding. If there is a loss of full

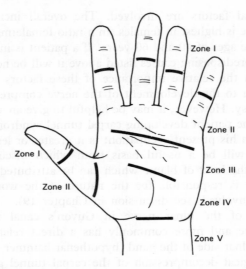

Fig. 8.3 Zone classification of flexor tendon injuries (from Leddy 1988, with permission)

extension of a finger this is unlikely to cause much functional deficit unless the extension loss is more than about 45°.

It is important to ascertain the mechanism of injury (i.e. sharp, crush, associated injuries, etc.) as this will have a significant bearing on the ultimate result.

Results.

Flexor tendons. As with any specialized surgery, the results depend on a number of factors including the type of injury, the timing of repair — primary repair within 1 week of injury appears to give better results — associated injuries, and in particular, the site of injury. The results of flexor tendon repair in zone 2 are predictably worse than at other sites (Amadio & Hunter 1987).

Strickland's review of the results of flexor tendon repairs is probably the best analysis of this subject (Strickland 1987, Strickland & Glogovac 1980, Strickland & Steichen 1982). It shows that the best outcome achieved in zone 2 in the published series is 65–80% excellent or good results. These results are from highly specialized units and therefore it is not unreasonable to suggest that the best results expected in zone 2 repairs from an 'average' treatment centre such as a district general hospital may well be nearer 50% satisfactory results.

Extensor tendons. Repair of extensor tendons results in a satisfactory outcome in the majority of cases. It is important to test flexion as well as extension in order to ensure that there is no tenodesis limiting flexion.

Prognosis.
Following primary tendon repair the long-term result can usually be assessed at 9–12 months after injury. If tenolysis is indicated it

is normally carried out between 3 and 9 months after the primary repair. If the repair fails and the tendon ruptures this can be treated either by direct secondary repair or tendon grafting. There is unlikely to be any significant alteration in the clinical situation in the long term once a steady state has been reached.

Ligaments

The collateral ligaments and volar plate of the proximal interphalangeal joints of the fingers and the metacarpophalangeal joint of the thumb are the most commonly injured ligaments in the hand. The majority of these injuries heal without significant long-term disability, although there may be some permanent thickening and swelling of the soft tissues around the affected ligament. Some injuries do result in long-term instability of the joint. However, as the ulnar collateral ligament of the thumb is particularly prone to this problem it is usually repaired surgically with good results. If surgery is required for instability of a proximal interphalangeal joint there is an increased risk of secondary joint stiffness developing.

Prognosis. A simple ligament injury which heals without any joint instability is unlikely to have any significant long-term complications. A joint which continues to dislocate is likely to develop osteoarthritic changes in the future.

Blood vessels

Vascular injuries usually result in some degree of cold intolerance in the affected part. Rarely, there may be claudication of the hand with vigorous activity if there has been a major arterial injury. In the rare instances when claudication does occur, atherosclerosis, smoking and diabetes are likely to be associated with deterioration in the patient's symptoms.

(Vibration white finger is a condition which probably involves neurological as well as vascular changes and is dealt with separately below.)

BONY INJURIES

Fractures should be classified into one of the following categories which will determine the type of outcome to be expected:

1. Closed or open (compound).
2. Metaphyseal or diaphyseal.
3. Intra- or extra-articular.
4. Avulsion.

Results and prognosis

1. Open fractures will take longer to heal and run the risk of infection. (Fractures in the hand normally heal within 3–4 weeks.)

2. Metaphyseal fractures heal more readily than diaphyseal fractures and there is a greater potential for moulding of the metaphysis, particularly in children.
3. Intra-articular fractures may require internal fixation. They often result in joint stiffness, at least temporarily, and in the long term may lead to osteoarthritis.
4. Avulsion fractures are often not important in so far as the bony injury is concerned, but will depend on the attachment which has caused the avulsion — usually a ligament or the profundus tendon. Persistent ligamentous laxity is likely to lead to osteoarthritic change in the future.

AMPUTATIONS

In general terms the hand may be regarded, from the functional point of view, as being made up of two main parts — the sensory side which comprises the thumb, index and middle fingers (the radial side), and the power side which comprises the ring and little fingers (the ulnar side; Littler 1960). An amputation on the radial side of the hand results mainly in impairment of sensation and fine, delicate activities. An amputation on the ulnar side of the hand mainly causes impairment of power grip.

Figure 8.2 gives values of the functional loss following amputation as a percentage of the function of the hand as a whole. Loss of length of the digit is not directly related to the functional deficit, so that amputation at the level of the distal interphalangeal joint — a loss of about a quarter of the length of the finger — results in about 50% loss of function of that digit. Similarly, amputation at the proximal interphalangeal joint level results in a 90–100% loss of function in that digit.

Results

The level of disability following an amputation of part or all of a digit must not be based solely on the level of amputation but should also take into account other factors which may warrant an increase in the percentage of disability.

Sensory changes such as numbness or hypersensitivity will impair function and cold intolerance is almost invariable; this is particularly disabling in people who work outside in all weathers.

A deformity of the fingernail can affect the function of a finger either because the nail curls over a shortened finger pulp or because a small spicule of nail remains following incomplete excision of the nailbed. This may be a painful situation, as the nail remnant gets caught on objects and can be torn or develop secondary infection.

Prognosis

The amputation stump of a finger has usually healed fully and reached a stable state by about 3–6 months after injury. If revision of the stump is required this is usually carried out during this time. The other surgical measures which may be required in the long term are excision of nail remnant and nailbed, excision or burying of a neuroma, or in some patients, complete revision by ray amputation. This is indicated in patients who have the 'gap hand' with complete amputation of the middle or ring fingers, leaving a gap which is not only cosmetically unsatisfactory but can also cause functional difficulties due to small objects falling out of the hand through the gap left by the amputated finger. The narrowing of the hand from ray amputation is associated with some decrease in grip strength and is therefore less likely to be of benefit in a manual labourer than in someone involved in a clerical occupation.

Other long-term complications are uncommon but the basic disability will obviously be permanent.

LESS COMMON CONDITIONS

Burns

The history is of great importance as the results and prognosis will vary considerably depending on whether the injury was caused by a simple scald from boiling water or an electrical burn; the latter injury has a much worse prognosis. Combination injuries such as the crush and burn from heated presses or rollers also have a poor prognosis.

Results

The cosmetic and functional aspects of the injury should be assessed. Cosmetic disability will depend on the site and extent of scarring as well as any secondary deformities such as joint contractures. The functional deficit will be related to the skin texture and sensitivity as well as joint and tendon mobility with any resulting loss of motion.

Prognosis

A skin graft may take a year or more to mature. The following complications may occur in the long term:

1. Contracture, which can cause secondary joint deformities and may require further surgery in the form of further skin cover or Z-plasty.
2. Splitting or fissuring of the grafted area, particularly in cold conditions. This mainly affects those involved in heavy manual outside work and may necessitate the use of protective gloves or, in severe cases, surgical revision of the graft by using a skin flap.

Injection injuries

High-pressure guns are widely used in industry and can cause severe injury due to penetration of the hand by fluids under pressure. Lubricants, paints, hydraulic solutions and other fluids may accidentally be injected subcutaneously, causing widespread toxic effects to the surrounding tissues.

Results

Stiffness is the main problem after these injuries because of the widespread fibrosis. However, this should be minimized by early surgical exploration, thorough lavage and debridement. Infection is often an early complication which can also increase the fibrotic response and will delay mobilization of the hand.

Most patients will require an intensive course of rehabilitation therapy before returning to work.

Prognosis

If the condition has been recognized and treated early, the patient may gradually regain full function in a matter of some weeks depending on the severity of the injury. Cases where the treatment has been delayed are likely to develop marked stiffness of the affected finger and, in some cases, if only one finger is involved and the disability is severe, amputation of the finger may be necessary to improve the function of the hand.

The clinical state of the hand has usually stabilized within 6 to 9 months of the injury and further deterioration would not be expected after that time.

Vibration white finger

This condition was recognized as an occupational disease by the Department of Health and Social Security in the UK in 1985. It was originally described in forestry workers who had used chain-saws for many years. It has also subsequently been described in other workers, including rock-drill operators and foundry workers. In the foundries it is the fettlers who are particularly at risk as they are constantly exposed to vibration through the use of powered grinding wheels to smooth down rough iron castings.

Results

The Taylor & Pelmear (1975) classification is at present accepted as the best means of recording the severity or staging of this condition. The assessment is based on the patient's symptoms as there are not yet any reliable objective criteria which can be used for staging, although a number of investigations have been made with this in mind. These include finger plethysmography, finger systolic pressure measurement, cold provocation tests and infrared thermography. However none of these has yet been found to be suitable for routine grading of this condition.

Prognosis

The natural history of this syndrome is not yet clearly known but it certainly appears that continued exposure to vibration results in progressive vasospastic symptoms over many years. It is uncertain whether there is an early stage when the symptoms are reversible and whether, in the worst cases, the condition can progress despite avoidance of the use of vibrating tools.

Cold conditions provoke symptoms, so affected patients may have to avoid working outside in winter or wear gloves to try and minimize the effects.

There have been no reports of serious vascular complications such as tissue necrosis or gangrenous changes occurring in affected digits, but compression of the median nerve at the wrist has been described in 30–60% of the reported series (Boyle et al 1988). Cystic changes in the carpal bones have been noted on X-rays of patients in some series but there is contention as to whether these are directly associated with the vibration or whether they are simply related to the age of the patients and the heavy manual work in which they are involved.

CONCLUSIONS

Ambrose Bierce (1842–1914) in his *Devil's Dictionary* defined the hand as: 'A singular instrument worn at the end of the human arm and commonly thrust into somebody's pocket'. In compiling a medicolegal report, the medical expert's opinion will often help determine whose pocket is going to supply the requisite compensation and how much compensation there will be.

As previously noted, it is also true that, as Seneca observed: 'It is part of the cure to wish to be cured'. Sadly, the present state of our system of compensation for personal injury is such that there is no incentive to be cured. In fact the incentive is to prolong and increase the disability as much as possible in order to gain the maximum financial benefit.

It behoves us therefore, as medical experts, to give fair and objective reports so that the well motivated patient who seeks to use his hands and return to work as quickly as possible does not lose his right to fair compensation. Equally, the malingerer should gain only his just deserts. Fortunately, there is now a greater awareness of the means of preventing hand injuries, although there is still a long way to go.

REFERENCES

Amadio P C, Hunter J M 1987 Prognostic factors in flexor tendon surgery in zone 2. In:
    Hunter J M, Schneider L H, Mackin E J (eds) Tendon surgery in the hand. C V Mosby,
    St Louis, pp 138–147
Bertelsen A, Capener N 1960 Fingers, compensation and King Canute. Journal of Bone
    and Joint Surgery 42: 390–392
Bierce A 1968 The Devil's dictionary. In Familiar medical quotations. Strauss M B (ed),
    Little Brown and Co., Boston
Bleecker M L 1987 Medical surveillance for carpal tunnel syndrome in workers. Journal of
    Hand Surgery 12A: 845–848
Boyle J C, Smith N J, Burke F D 1988 Vibration white finger. Journal of Hand Surgery
    13B: 171–176
Eversmann W W Jr 1988 Entrapment and compression neuropathies. In: Green D P (ed)
    Operative hand surgery, vol 2. 2nd edn. Churchill Livingstone, Edinburgh, pp 1423–1478
Kelsey J L, Pastides H, Kreiger N, Harris C, Chernow R A 1980 Upper extremity disorders.
    A survey of their frequency and cost in the United States. C V Mosby, St Louis
Leach R E, Odom J A 1968 Systemic causes of the carpal tunnel syndrome. Postgraduate
    Medicine 44: 127–131
Leddy J P 1988 Flexor tendons — acute injuries. In: Green D P (ed), Operative hand
    surgery. Churchill Livingstone, Edinburgh
Lister G D, Kleiners H E, Kutz J E 1977 Primary flexor tendon repair followed by
    immediate controlled mobilisation. Journal of Hand Surgery 2: 441–451
Littler J W 1960 The physiology and dynamic function of the hand. Surgical Clinics of
    North America 40: 259–266
Nathan P A, Meadows K D, Doyle L S 1988 Occupation as a risk factor for impaired
    sensory conduction of the median nerve at the carpal tunnel. Journal of Hand Surgery
    13B: 167–170
Rank B K, Wakefield A R, Hulston J T 1973 Surgery of repair as applied to hand injuries,
    4th edn. Churchill Livingstone, Edinburgh, p 376
Semple J C, Cargill A O 1969 Carpal tunnel syndrome. Results of surgical decompression.
    Lancet i: 918
Strickland J W 1987 Flexor tendon injuries. Part 5: Flexor tenolysis, rehabilitation and
    results. Orthopaedic Review XVI: 33–49
Strickland J W, Glogovac S C 1980 Digital function following flexor tendon repair in zone
    2. Journal of Hand Surgery 5: 537
Strickland J W, Steichen J B (eds) 1982 Functional recovery after flexor tendon severance
    in the finger: the state of the art. In Difficult problems in hand surgery. C V Mosby, St
    Louis
Swanson A B, Gorgan–Hagert C, Swanson G de G 1987 Evaluation of impairment in the
    upper extremity. Journal of Hand Surgery 12A No. 5 Part 2 908
Taylor W, Pelmear P L (eds) 1975 Vibration white finger in industry. Academic Press,
    London, pp xvii–xxii

FURTHER READING

Moberg E 1958 Objective methods for determining the functional value of sensibility in
    the hand. Journal of Bone and Joint Surgery 40: 454–476
Tubiana R 1985 The hand, vol II. W B Saunders, Philadelphia, pp 159–164

Results following lower limb fractures

Results following lower limb fractures

9. The hip

M. A. Foy

INTRODUCTION

Fractures and dislocations about the hip are common injuries. Their patterns vary with the mechanism and velocity of the trauma, and with the age and general health of the patient. The injuries themselves are so diverse that their classifications will be discussed within the individual sections rather than in this introduction.

ACETABULAR FRACTURES

The long-term results of acetabular fractures can become obscured within complex classifications of fracture patterns, as outlined by Judet et al (1964) and modified by Tile (1984). These classifications are vital to an understanding of the pathological anatomy, and to the planning of fracture management, but they do not provide clear guidelines for the prognosis. Within this section Judet's classification will be used. In assessing the prognosis of posterior wall fractures, the common association with hip dislocation is important. An apparently good result from the acetabular fracture may be prejudiced by subsequent avascular necrosis of the femoral head.

A clear and balanced approach to the management of acetabular fractures was presented in Tile's book, together with a critical review of the literature. He pointed out that spurious conclusions may be reached when results of methods of treatment of dissimilar fractures are compared. It is obviously quite unscientific to compare the results of conservative treatment of undisplaced acetabular fractures with the results of operative treatment of displaced fractures. Tile pointed out that the literature is full of such comparisons.

Prognostic factors

From the reports in the orthopaedic literature on the conservative and surgical management of acetabular fractures, it is possible to identify certain factors which directly affect the prognosis.

237

Residual acetabular displacement at the conclusion of treatment

This is the most critical factor in determining long-term results and is relevant to both conservative and operative treatment. If at the conclusion of treatment the acetabulum has been satisfactorily reduced then a good clinical result can be anticipated. In a series of 103 patients reported by Pennal et al (1980) there was residual displacement in 66 patients; 72% of these developed degenerative changes. Of the 37 patients with no residual displacement, only 30% developed degenerative changes. The clinical result in this series (based on the Toronto hip score) was significantly better in those cases without residual displacement. Those with no residual displacement had a mean Toronto hip score of 16.5 (indicating a good or excellent functional result), whereas those with residual displacement had a mean Toronto hip score of 14 (indicating a fair functional result). The mean follow-up in this series was more than 7 years.

It is not always possible to achieve a perfect anatomical reduction. The work of Hofmann et al (1984) and Matta et al (1985) suggested that as long as reduction to within 3 mm was achieved, the results were as good as if there was anatomical reduction, irrespective of whether the treatment was conservative or surgical.

A large series of patients with surgically treated acetabular fractures was presented by Letournel & Judet (1981). Of 170 patients with acetabular fractures treated by operation where a perfect reduction was obtained, 152 (90%) achieved a very good or good clinical result. Despite a perfect reduction, 12 (7%) of the patients in their series still developed osteoarthritis. Of the 72 patients with less than perfect reduction, 52 (72%) still had a very good or good result. The shortest follow-up in this group was 2 years.

In Hofmann et al's series (1984) of 38 patients with acetabular fractures, 12 were treated without operation. Of these, 6 were undisplaced or minimally displaced at the conclusion of treatment. Using the complex Harris hip score for assessment (Harris 1969), they had an average hip score of 96/100 (i.e. a very good result). Of the 6 patients with residual displacement at the conclusion of treatment, the average hip score was 59/100 (i.e. a fair result).

Heeg et al (1987) found that significantly better results could be expected if the weight-bearing dome of the acetabulum was reduced to within 2 mm by conservative methods.

Mayo (1987), in a recent review of acetabular fractures, stated; 'It now seems clear that loss of acetabular sphericity and articular steps of 2 to 3 mm or greater are poorly tolerated by the hip.'

Therefore residual displacement at the conclusion of treatment is an important prognostic factor. When there is a perfect or near perfect (within 2–3 mm) reduction, a good clinical result can be predicted in 85–90% of patients. When the final result falls outside these limits a good clinical result may be expected in about 70% of cases.

Comminution of the acetabular dome

Tile (1984) reported that the degree of comminution of the weight-bearing acetabular dome was important in determining the outcome of acetabular fractures. The results described by Pennal et al (1980) and Heeg et al (1987) confirm this. Pennal et al found that comminution of the acetabular dome resulted in post-traumatic arthritis in 84% of patients compared to a 46% incidence of post-traumatic arthritis in those without comminution.

Fracture type

The fracture type is less important than residual acetabular displacement in determining the long-term results. In the hands of experts, such as Letournel and Judet, very good and good clinical results were reported in over 80% of cases, whatever the fracture type, following operative treatment. They stressed that despite a 95% rate of perfect reduction of the posterior fractures, only 82% achieved a very good clinical result. This, they believed, was due to the occurrence of avascular necrosis of the femoral head in the posterior fractures, secondary to interference with the blood supply from an associated dislocation. Pennal et al (1980) pointed out that single-column fractures carried a better overall prognosis than two-column fractures, and that the T-fracture carried the worst prognosis of the two-column fractures.

Age of the patient

Pennal et al (1980) reported that patients over the age of 40 had significantly worse results following acetabular fractures. Letournel & Judet (1981) reported a 79% incidence of very good results in those aged under 40 but only a 62% incidence of very good results in those over 40. Tipton et al (1975) reported on 24 patients treated conservatively. Their results were assessed using the Harris hip score. The average score in those aged over 40 was 77, while in those under 40 it was 84. This difference is not statistically significant.

Associated injuries to the pelvic ring or femoral head

Pennal et al (1980) also identified certain other pelvic ring injuries associated with a poor result when combined with an acetabular fracture. They found that disruption of the pubic symphysis, a double vertical fracture (of the Malgaigne type) and an associated fracture, extending from the weight-bearing aspect of the acetabulum to the iliac crest, were all associated with a poorer result than would be expected from the acetabular injury alone. Similarly, Austin (1971), Rowe & Lowell (1961) and Tile (1984) pointed out that acetabular injuries with associated femoral head fractures have an increased risk of developing post-traumatic arthritis.

Incidence of osteoarthritis

It can be seen that the development of osteoarthritis depends upon:

1. The degree of residual acetabular displacement.
2. The degree of comminution of the weight-bearing dome.
3. The damage to the femoral head.
4. Associated pelvic ring disruption.

Letournel & Judet (1981) reported osteoarthritis in 16 of 244 (6.5%) patients treated operatively and subsequently reviewed. This is difficult to compare with Pennal et al's (1980) incidence of 56% degenerative change (58 out of 103 acetabular fractures). However, this brings us back to Tiles's (1984) point regarding the comparison of dissimilar cases.

Letournel & Judet (1981) have a separate category of post-operative osteophytosis which is present in 90 of their 244 hips. If this is added to their osteoarthritis group it brings the incidence to 43% (106 of 244 acetabular fractures), i.e. much closer to the figure reported by Pennal et al.

The different incidence may well be explained by the fact that all of Letournel & Judet's cases were treated operatively, compared with only 33% of Pennal et al's cases. Letournel & Judet commented that the long-term prognosis in their cases of osteophytosis must remain speculative.

Timing of medicolegal reports

From the medicolegal point of view, the time when these injuries stabilize is important. Rowe & Lowell (1961), Austin (1971) and Pennal et al (1980) all reported that the functional level 1 year after injury provided an accurate measure of the final outcome. This was well summarized by Lowell (1979), who suggested that:

A 1 year rule can be devised that allows considerable accuracy in predicting prognosis. Ninety-four per cent of patients rated excellent or good 1 year after injury will remain so. Ninety-one per cent of patients ultimately developing significant osteoarthritis or avascular necrosis will show at least early changes at the end of this same period, or will have failed to achieve good or excellent function.

Although the statistics and timing do not strictly fit into the '1-year rule', the long-term follow-up results presented in Letournel & Judet's book are interesting. Their patients, examined in 1971, were re-examined between 1976 and 1978. They reassessed 164 of the patients classified very good: 159 (97%) had remained very good. They were also able to reassess 28 patients classified as good. Only 14 (50%) remained good, but 8 (28.5%) had improved to very good.

Timing of return to work and leisure activities

Pennal et al (1980) found that 71% of their 103 patients returned to their original occupations. The average time lost from work was 11 months. Within this group, 34 patients were treated surgically, and 67% of these were able to return to their original occupations after an average time off work of 12 months (with a range of 3.5–26 months). The slight delay in return to work in the surgically treated group probably reflects the increased severity of the surgically treated injuries, together with the complications inherent in the surgery itself.

Austin (1971) followed up 25 patients for 4–20 years after their injury. Of these, 17 were treated conservatively and in none of these was an anatomical position obtained. Of the 8 who underwent open reduction, only 2 had an anatomical reduction, while 6 reductions were unsuccessful or incomplete. In this group 20 patients were able to follow their normal or equivalent occupations. Five (20%) had to change their jobs. Of the 19 who were involved in active pastimes, 8 (42%) had to modify their leisure activities.

Complications of surgical treatment

Tile (1984) pointed out that some of the late complications of acetabular fractures are inherent in the fracture (i.e. due to type, degree of displacement and degree of comminution), whereas others are a consequence of the treatment. Most of the results quoted in this section originate from centres with a special interest and expertise in acetabular fractures. Most orthopaedic surgeons will not treat enough acetabular fractures to develop such expertise. Indeed, Tile et al (1985) pointed out that the results of surgical treatment of acetabular fractures varied markedly with the skill of the surgical team.

Certain complications, such as venous thrombosis or infection, may occur after any operation. Other complications are specific to this type of surgery, such as sciatic nerve palsy and heterotopic ossification.

Sciatic nerve palsy

Letournel & Judet (1981) reported 34 post-operative sciatic nerve palsies in 302 patients (11.2%). Thirty of these occurred early, whereas four developed between the 14th and 19th day. Of the 30 patients with immediate post-operative palsies, 11 had not been examined adequately preoperatively. Therefore, some of these palsies may have been present before operation. As this happened in a centre of excellence, it is important to stress the early assessment of sciatic nerve function because of the obvious medicolegal implications.

The incidence of sciatic nerve palsy was 14% in 214 posterior approaches in this series. Letournel & Judet reviewed 27 of their patients with sciatic nerve palsies and found that 6 (22%) had totally recovered; 8 (30%) made a good recovery; 7 (26%) made a partial recovery; 4 (15%) retained a pure sensory deficit and 2 (7%) made no recovery. They concluded that; 'While serious, the prognosis of post-operative sciatic nerve palsy is not especially gloomy. Recovery takes place over a variable period. One case is still continuing to improve 3 years after operation.'

Tile et al (1985) reported 6 post-operative sciatic nerve palsies in 102 displaced acetabular fractures, of which 5 (83%) recovered fully. They also reported 16 cases of post-traumatic sciatic nerve palsy in their 102 cases, i.e. an incidence of 15%. Only 4 of these made a complete recovery, i.e. in this group of patients there is a 12% incidence of permanent nerve deficit as a result of injury. The degree of disability is not clear. This figure is similar to that quoted by Wilson (1982), who found a 10% incidence of permanent sciatic nerve paralysis in 40 patients.

Heterotopic ossification

Letournel & Judet (1981) reported heterotopic ossification in 61 of 302 patients (20%) while Tile et al (1985) found that it occurred in 18 of 102 cases (17.5%). It appeared early on the post-operative X-rays and matured 6–12 months after the operation. In the 61 cases reported by Letournel & Judet (1981), 39 (64%) suffered no significant clinical impairment, 8 (13%) developed slight limitation of movement and 14 (23%) had significant loss of movement. Significant loss of movement was associated with extensive calcification anteriorly or posteriorly.

The incidence of heterotopic ossification is considerably lower in the cases treated conservatively. Rowe & Lowell (1961) and Pennal and his colleagues (1980) reported an incidence of only 5% in their series.

Summary

1. Following acetabular fractures accurate prognosis may be given approximately 1 year after the injury. The functional level at that time is an accurate reflection of the final outcome.
2. Comminution of the superior weight-bearing surface of the acetabulum is a poor prognostic sign.
3. The type of acetabular fracture has some bearing on the end-result. Single-column fractures fare better than double-column fractures and T-fractures fare worst of all. In posterior fractures, where there is also hip dislocation, subsequent avascular necrosis of the femoral head may give rise to a poor result despite a good anatomical reduction.
4. Additional damage to the pelvic ring (through the pubic symphysis, iliac wing or sacroiliac joint) worsens the prognosis, as does associated femoral head fracture.

5. Patients over the age of 40 may fare worse than those under 40.
6. The most significant indicator of long-term prognosis is the amount of residual displacement of the articular surface at the conclusion of treatment. Residual displacement of greater than 3 mm is associated with a less satisfactory result.
7. There is a 10% incidence of permanent sciatic nerve deficit after acetabular fractures. The incidence of sciatic nerve deficit increases after operative treatment, particularly when a posterior approach is used. The prognosis of post-operative sciatic nerve palsy is good.
8. There is a small (5% or less) incidence of heterotopic ossification in conservatively treated patients. This increases to 20–30% following operation. Over 75% of these cases are either not impaired or have only minimal limitation of motion.

HIP DISLOCATIONS AND FEMORAL HEAD FRACTURES

Anterior dislocations

The two largest series of anterior dislocation of the hip were reported by Epstein (1980) and Brav (1962). There were 54 cases with a mean follow-up of 70 months in Epstein's series and 34 cases with a mean follow-up of 80 months in Brav's — 88 cases in all. The results were classified after Thompson & Epstein (1951), as shown in Table 9.1. The clinical results are shown in Table 9.2.

Table 9.1 Classification of results (Thompson & Epstein 1951)

Excellent
1. No pain
2. Full range of movements
3. No limp
4. No X-ray evidence of progressive changes

Good
1. No pain
2. A 75% range of hip movements
3. Slight limp
4. Minimal X-ray changes

Fair
Any one or more of the following:
1. Pain, but not disabling
2. Limited range of hip movements but no adduction deformity
3. Moderate limp
4. Moderate to severe X-ray changes

Poor
Any one or more of the following:
1. Disabling pain
2. Marked limitation of movement or adduction deformity
3. Redislocation
4. Progressive X-ray changes

Table 9.2 Clinical results following anterior dislocation of the hip

	Epstein (1980)	Brav (1962)	Combined series
Excellent	17	29	67 (76%)
Good	21		
Fair	11	5	21 (24%)
Poor	5		
Total	54	34	88

There was an overall incidence of excellent/good results of 76% and fair/poor results of 24%. There were 5 cases of avascular necrosis reported in the two series (6%). Epstein quoted an incidence of post-traumatic arthritis of 17% and an incidence of myositis ossificans of 4%. These occurred in patients with fair or poor results. Despite the relatively high incidence of satisfactory (excellent/good) results in Brav's series, only 10 (29%) had no trouble at all with the hip and only 19 (56%) felt that they could engage in all ordinary activities.

Posterior dislocations

Evaluation of the results following posterior dislocation of the hip is difficult because of the differing classifications used in reports of this condition. Thompson & Epstein (1951) classified their posterior dislocations into five types. Stewart & Milford (1954) suggested a modified classification. Brav (1962) combined Thompson & Epstein types II and III into his type II and Thompson & Epstein types IV and V into his type III. As the Thompson & Epstein classification is the most widely used and because Epstein (1980) has reported, in his monograph, the largest series of cases on record, this classification will be used here.

The five types of posterior dislocation according to Thompson & Epstein (1951) are:

Type I: Posterior dislocation without fracture.
Type II: Posterior dislocation with a large posterior acetabular rim fragment.
Type III: Posterior dislocation with comminution of the posterior acetabular rim.
Type IV: Posterior dislocation with a fracture of the acetabular rim and floor.
Type V: Posterior dislocation with fracture of the femoral head.

The series of Hunter (1969) and Upadhyay & Moulton (1981) will also be incorporated in the aggregated results. The latter report is particularly useful as it gives a much longer mean follow-up (12.5 years) than any other series.

Epstein (1980) assessed his results according to whether closed reduction, closed reduction followed by later open reduction or primary open reduction were employed. However, the results will be presented irrespective of the treatment employed as the numbers within these groups are small.

Type I posterior dislocation (Posterior dislocation without fracture or with minimal chip fracture of posterior acetabular rim.)
Only Epstein (1980) and Upadhyay & Moulton (1981) broke down the results into the four categories shown in Table 9.1. Table 9.3 shows the clinical results in 187 patients from these two series.

Table 9.3 Clinical results following type I posterior dislocation of the hip (from Epstein 1980 and Upadhyay & Moulton 1981)

Result	Number	%
Excellent	50	27
Good	77	41
Fair	24	13
Poor	36	19
Total	187	

If the cases of Brav (1962) and of Hunter (1969) are included (providing 323 cases in total), there are 237 cases which can be classified as excellent or good (73.5%) and 86 cases which are classified as fair or poor (26.5%).
As might be expected, there is a much higher chance of a poor clinical result if avascular necrosis of the femoral head occurs. The incidence of avascular necrosis varies from series to series. Table 9.4 shows the overall incidence to be approximately 16%.

Table 9.4 Incidence of avascular necrosis following type I posterior dislocation of the hip

Reference	Cases	Avascular necrosis
Epstein (1980)	134	20
Brav (1962)	110	24
Upadhyay & Moulton (1981)	53	3
Total	297	47 (16%)

Brav analysed the effect of avascular necrosis on the clinical result. A total of 85 patients had an excellent or good clinical result; only 5 of these (6%) had avascular necrosis. Of the 25 patients with a fair or poor clinical result, 19 (76%) had avascular necrosis.
Upadhyay & Moulton (1981) suggested that 26% of type I dislocations will ultimately develop osteoarthritis. They also commented that there

was an impression in the literature that type I injuries had few complications and always gave an excellent result. This does not appear to be the case, particularly when dislocation is complicated by avascular necrosis.

Type II posterior dislocations (Where a large posterior acetabular fragment is present.)

Table 9.5 Results following type II posterior dislocation of the hip (from Epstein 1980 and Upadhyay & Moulton 1981)

Result	Number	%	
Excellent	5	8%	Excellent/good 47%
Good	24	39%	
Fair	16	26%	Fair/poor 53%
Poor	17	27%	
Total	62		

Brav found that the incidence of avascular necrosis in types II and III dislocations was 25% (23 of 91 cases). As with the type I dislocations, there was a much greater chance of a fair or poor clinical result if avascular necrosis developed. Of 65 excellent or good results only 5 (7.7%) had avascular necrosis. Of 26 with fair or poor results 18 (69%) had avascular necrosis. It can be seen from these figures that Brav reports a higher incidence of excellent/good results in types II and III dislocations than either Epstein or Upadhyay & Moulton. The reason for this is not clear as the three reports used similar criteria for classifying their results. It is possible that Brav's methods were not quite so stringent as those of Epstein (listed in Table 9.1).

Type III posterior dislocations (Posterior dislocations with comminution of the posterior acetabular rim.)

The clinical results following type III posterior dislocations are shown in Table 9.6.

Table 9.6 Results following type III posterior dislocation of the hip (from Epstein 1980 and Upadhyay & Moulton 1981)

Results	Number	%	
Excellent	0	0%	Excellent/good 37%
Good	53	37%	
Fair	30	21%	Fair/poor 63%
Poor	60	42%	
Total	143		

   The incidence of avascular necrosis in types II and III dislocations is 25% according to Brav's figures. The presence of comminution of the posterior rim appears to worsen the outcome with a lower incidence of excellent, good and fair results and a higher incidence of poor results.

Type IV posterior dislocation (Posterior dislocation with fracture of the acetabular rim and floor.)

Epstein (1980) reported 69 patients with this injury, and the clinical results are shown in Table 9.7.

Table 9.7   Results following type IV posterior dislocation of the hip (from Epstein 1980)

Results	Number	%	
Excellent	0	0%	Excellent/good 23%
Good	16	23%	
Fair	18	26%	Fair/poor 77%
Poor	35	51%	
Total	69		

   The prognosis is significantly worse, with over half of the patients having a poor clinical result. Epstein reported 20 cases (29%) of avascular necrosis in this group.

Type V posterior dislocations (Posterior dislocation with fracture of the femoral head.)

This injury was reviewed and subclassified by Pipkin (1957) into four types. There are not enough cases reported in the literature to make the Pipkin subtypes important in predicting the outcome. Therefore these injuries will be considered as one group. Epstein et al (1985) reported 46 cases treated by closed reduction, closed followed by open reduction or primary open reduction. The overall results are shown in Table 9.8.

Table 9.8   Results following type V posterior dislocation of the hip (from Epstein et al 1985)

Results	Number	%	
Excellent	0	0%	Excellent/good 28%
Good	13	28%	
Fair	11	24%	Fair/poor 72%
Poor	22	48%	
Total	46		

These results show that this is an injury with a relatively poor prognosis. The figures also suggested that long-term results were better after primary open reduction than after conservative or delayed open reduction. Epstein (1980) only noted 11 (24%) cases of avascular necrosis in this group while Brav (1962) reported an incidence of 70% avascular necrosis in types IV and V dislocations. The reason for this discrepancy is not clear.

Time from injury to reduction of dislocation

Hougaard & Thomsen (1987) showed that reduction of posterior dislocations more than 6 hours after injury was associated with a significant increase in the incidence of avascular necrosis and osteoarthritis (Table 9.9). This suggests that reduction should be carried out within 6 hours unless contraindicated on other grounds.

Table 9.9 Development of osteoarthritis and avascular necrosis after posterior dislocation of the hip in relation to time of reduction (adapted from Hougaard & Thomsen 1987)

Time from injury to reduction	Number of patients	Osteoarthritis developed	Avascular necrosis developed
Less than 6 hours	83	25 (30%)	4 (5%)
More than 6 hours	17	13 (76%)	10 (58%)

Timing of medicolegal reports

It is difficult accurately to forecast a time when the results following these diverse injuries reach a plateau. Brav (1962) looked at 189 patients with dislocations that were symptomatic at the time of his study. In all, 81 (43%) stated that their hip complaints had been present since the time of injury. Of the remaining 108, 19 (10%) had onset of complaints 2–5 months after injury, 24 (13%) had onset of complaints 6–11 months after injury and 65 (34%) did not develop symptoms until 1 year or more after their injury. In 4 cases (2%) no symptoms were experienced until 5 years after injury.

Brav (1962) also pointed out that it may take up to 2 years to detect the radiographic changes of avascular necrosis. This should be borne in mind in the timing of medicolegal reports. Modern isotope and magnetic resonance imaging techniques may make it possible to assess the vascularity of the femoral head and consequent prognosis for the hip much earlier. After hip dislocation, final medical reports should probably be delayed for 18–24 months from the time of the injury.

Summary

1. After anterior dislocation of the hip there is a 76% chance of achieving an excellent or good clinical result.

2. Following type I posterior dislocation there is an excellent or good clinical result in 68% of patients. There is a 16% incidence of avascular necrosis, and the clinical result is likely to be worse if avascular necrosis develops.
3. Following type II posterior dislocations there is an excellent or good clinical result in 47% of patients. There is a 25% incidence of avascular necrosis, and the clinical result is significantly worse if avascular necrosis develops.
4. Following type III posterior dislocations there were no excellent results; good results were reported in 37% of patients.
5. Following type IV posterior dislocations there were no excellent results; good results were reported in only 23% of patients. The incidence of avascular necrosis was 29%.
6. Following type V posterior dislocations there were no excellent results; good results were reported in only 28% of patients. Epstein (1980) reported the incidence of avascular necrosis as 24%, while Brav (1962) reported the incidence as 70% in a combined series of types IV and V dislocations.
7. Final medicolegal reports may need to be delayed until 18–24 months after the injury.
8. The quoted results cannot be related to operative or non-operative management because the subgroups are too small.
9. The incidence of avascular necrosis and osteoarthritis is higher in posterior dislocations reduced more than 6 hours after the injury.

FRACTURES OF THE NECK OF THE FEMUR

Classification

Both intracapsular and extracapsular fractures of the upper femur will be considered in this section. The Garden system will be used to classify the intracapsular fractures, as follows:

Stage I: The abduction or impaction injury where the inferior cortex has not been completely breached.
Stage II: Complete fracture without displacement.
Stage III: Complete fracture with partial displacement.
Stage IV: Complete fracture with full displacement.

It can be difficult to distinguish stage I from stage II, and stage III from stage IV, and, as will be shown, both stage I and stage II can often be considered together from a prognostic viewpoint, as can stages III and IV.

Extracapsular or trochanteric fractures tend to be classified according to their stability rather than the situation of the fracture line. Stable fractures consist of two main fragments. Unstable fractures were defined by Dimon & Hughston (1967) as fractures where there is 'lack of continuity of bone cortex on the opposing surfaces of the proximal and distal fragments'. A lesser trochanteric fragment (including the calcar) or a separate posterior fragment will reduce stability, and in the more unstable injuries there may be four or more fragments. On this basis trochanteric fractures will be classified as stable or unstable.

Intracapsular fractures

There is a vast bibliography on the long-term results of intracapsular fractures of the femoral neck. The majority of these patients are elderly and have very osteoporotic bone which fractures with relatively minor trauma. For this reason medicolegal reports are not usually required in these cases. In patients under the age of 50 (unless there is osteoporosis secondary to conditions such as renal disease, steroid therapy or alcoholism), fractures of the neck of the femur are usually associated with severe trauma, and in this case medicolegal reports are often required.

It is not the brief of this book to examine the subtle differences in the results of many different treatment methods for intracapsular fractures of the femur in elderly patients. Nevertheless, the common complications and sequelae of these fractures in elderly patients will be reviewed, as the results do give clues to the outlook in younger patients. The differences in the nature of the trauma and the quality of the bone in those aged under 50 warrant their consideration as a separate group, and they will be reviewed later in this chapter.

There is still much controversy regarding the place of hemiarthroplasty versus reduction and internal fixation in displaced intracapsular fractures. The merits of various types of internal fixation techniques are also disputed. These issues will be addressed, but the two principal complications of avascular necrosis and non-union will be considered in more detail.

The most thorough appraisal of the results, and the factors influencing the results, following subcapital fractures was provided by Barnes et al (1976) in a prospective multicentre study prepared for the British Medical Research Council. Drennan Lowell (1980), in a comprehensive review of the results and complications of femoral neck fractures, pointed out that reports varied on the incidence of non-union and avascular necrosis rates. Union rates in the literature vary from 66 to 100%, while rates of avascular necrosis and late segmental collapse vary from 7 to 84%. These results require more detailed analysis, and as Barnes et al (1976) pointed out, there are many factors which contribute to the end-result. There are those over which the surgeon has no control, such as old age, female sex, osteoporosis and a Garden type III or IV fracture, and those over which the surgeon has a measure of control, i.e. acceptance of valgus or varus reduction, extreme retroversion or anteversion in reduction, positioning of the fixation device and timing of ambulation. These factors are considered in detail in the report by Barnes et al (1976).

The clinical results and complications in Garden stage I/II fractures and Garden stage III/IV fractures will be considered below.

Garden I/II fractures

Barnes et al (1976) reported on 295 stage I fractures (they classified 19 as stage II and did not report them as a separate group). The results are broken down according to sex and are summarized in Table 9.10. There was little difference between the rates of union in the two sexes. The union rate at 6 months is 153/248 (62%), at 12 months 220/237 (93%) and at 24 months 233/236 (99%).

Table 9.10 Rate of union related to time after injury in Garden I fractures (adapted from Barnes et al 1976)

Time after injury	Union	
	Female (n = 250)	Male (n = 45)
6 months	135/216 (62.5%)	18/32 (56%)
12 months	192/205 (93.5%)	28/32 (88%)
24 months	203/204 (99.5%)	30/32 (94%)

In the same paper the incidence of late segmental collapse was reported as 16% after 3 years' follow-up in Garden stage I fractures.

Banks (1962) provided another comprehensive review of intracapsular fractures, albeit with significantly fewer numbers (189 for whom the end-result was definable; 66 of these were Garden stage I or II). There was only a 1-year minimum follow-up. Banks found that 53 of 59 (90%) Garden stage I/II fractures healed with a good clinical result and the rate of avascular necrosis was 4/59 (7%). These results are very similar to those reported by Barnes et al (1976) at 12 months.

Garden stage III/IV

When the rate of union is considered following reduction and internal fixation in these fractures, there is little difference between stages III and IV. The union rates are broken down by Barnes et al according to sex and are summarized in Table 9.11.

Table 9.11 Rate of union related to time after injury in Garden III and IV fractures (adapted from Barnes et al 1976)

Time after injury	Union	
	Female (n = 988)	Male (n = 195)
6 months	117/811 (14%)	16/143 (11%)
12 months	360/747 (48%)	65/136 (48%)
24 months	458/728 (63%)	88/131 (67%)
36 months	474/722 (66%)	93/129 (72%)

The incidence of symptomatic avascular necrosis in these patients is important. Meyers (1985) pointed out that although avascular necrosis occurs frequently in ununited fractures, progress to late segmental collapse does not occur in these patients. Late segmental collapse only occurs when there is avascular necrosis in association with union of the fracture. Again, there is little difference between stage III and IV fractures in the Barnes series and the incidence of late segmental collapse is summarized in Table 9.12. It can be seen that there is a significantly higher incidence of late segmental collapse in females.

Table 9.12 Incidence of late segmental collapse in united Garden III/IV fractures (adapted from Barnes et al 1976)

Time after injury	Females	Males
12 months	38/360 (10.5%)	2/65 (3%)
24 months	105/458 (23%)	9/88 (10%)
36 months	131/474 (28%)	17/83 (18%)

Residual disability in patients with late segmental collapse is of profound importance in medicolegal reporting. Barnes et al (1976) referred to this in their report, and their findings are reproduced in Table 9.13. Overall, late segmental collapse was disabling in only 53 of 181 patients (29%) and in only 32 of these patients (18% of the total) was a salvage operation performed. In the remaining 128 patients with segmental collapse, the disability was functionally acceptable in 84 (46%) and asymptomatic in 44 (24%)

Table 9.13 Effect of late segmental collapse on residual disability in intracapsular fractures (from Barnes et al 1976 with permission of the Editor, Journal of Bone and Joint Surgery)

	Females	Males
Salvage operation performed	30 (18%)	2 (11%)
Disabling, but no operation performed	19 (21%)	2 (11%)
Functionally acceptable	77 (47%)	7 (39%)
Asymptomatic	37 (23%)	7 (39%)
Total	163	18

The paper from Barnes et al (1976) has been extensively quoted because it affords the most complete and thorough review available on the prognosis of intracapsular fractures of the femoral neck.

Mention should be made of the clinical results following insertion of endoprostheses in patients with displaced (Garden type III/IV) fractures. Patients with endoprostheses were specifically excluded from the Barnes series. Johnson & Crothers (1975) pointed out that the reported incidence of poor results after prosthetic replacement ranged from 12 to 33%. They followed up their patients with Austin Moore hemiarthroplasties for an average of $3\frac{1}{2}$ years. Similar reports were provided by Anderson et al (1964), Hinchey & Day (1964) and Whittaker et al (1972). The criteria for judging the subjective results in these series vary slightly in their complexity, but can be broadly classified into three groups, as follows:

Good: No pain or minimal pain. Can walk unsupported or with one stick.

Fair: Mild to moderate pain. May require two sticks or a walking frame.

Poor: Pain interfering with normal activities or severe pain. Confined to bed or house. Secondary operation may be required.

The results are summarized in Table 9.14. In the present context, there is little merit in comparing the detailed results of different endoprostheses following displaced fractures of the femoral neck. No single design is demonstrably superior.

Table 9.14 Clinical results following insertion of endoprostheses for displaced (Garden III/IV) fractures of the femoral neck

Series	Prosthesis used	Good	Fair	Poor
Johnson et al (1975)	Austin Moore	24	12	8
Anderson et al (1964)	Austin Moore/Thompson	28	4	1
Hinchey & Day (1964)	Austin Moore	67	8	8
Whittaker et al (1972)	Austin Moore/Thompson	65	36	12
		184	60	29
		(67%)	(22%)	(11%)

Extracapsular (trochanteric) fractures

The problems of non-union and avascular necrosis are infrequent in trochanteric fractures. An excellent review of the results following internal fixation of trochanteric fractures was provided in two separate papers by Steen Jensen et al (1980a, b). One dealt with the results in stable fractures, and one with the results in unstable fractures. In these reports they followed up 375 stable fractures and 1071 unstable fractures. Treatment was with one of four methods: McLaughlin nail-plate, Jewett nail-plate, sliding screw-plate or Ender nails. In the 375 stable fractures 349 (93%) united in the post-operative position. A further 7 (2%) united following secondary displacement. Technical failures of the implants were encountered in 19 patients (5%). No cases of non-union were reported. There was no significant difference between the fixation methods in terms of union or of technical failure. Re-operations were performed in 9 out of 252 patients (4%) with nail-plates or screw-plates. There was no significant difference between the methods. Re-operation was necessary in 9 out of 46 patients (20%) treated by Ender nailing, due to technical failure or distal nail migration, resulting in knee complaints. They concluded that in stable fractures the problems of obtaining union are minor, 'a fact which should encourage the use of simple methods of treatment'.

In unstable fractures they found that union in the post-operative position occurred in 43% (458/1071) of patients. In 208 out of 346 (60%) sliding screw fixations, union occurred after secondary displacement. Non-union was observed in 2 out of 293 patients (0.7%) using the McLaughlin nail-plate and 6 out of 309 patients (2%) using the Jewett nail-plate. There were no non-unions of the fractures treated with sliding screw-plates or Ender nails. The overall technical failure rate was 345 out of 1071 patients (32%). Of the failures, 154 out of 293 occurred after McLaughlin nail-plates, 147 out of 309 occurred after Jewett nail-plates and 23 out of 123 occurred after Ender nailing. Only 21 out of 346 sliding screw-plate fixations progressed to technical failure.

The authors concluded that sliding screw-plate fixation was the only suitable method of fixation for unstable intertrochanteric fractures because of its low failure rate and its low re-operation rate.

These findings were supported by Regazzoni & Reudi (1985) in a report on the AO dynamic hip screw. Regazzoni & Reudi reported an incidence of 0.5% (3/530) cases of avascular necrosis of the femoral head following trochanteric fractures.

Fractures of the femoral neck in adults under the age of 50

This group is singled out because there is more likelihood of litigation following femoral neck fractures in those aged under 50 due to the nature of the trauma involved. Klenerman (1985) pointed out that fractures in patients under 50 were rare because their bone was dense and therefore considerable violence was required to break it. However, in young adults with osteoporosis from an underlying condition such as steroid therapy, chronic renal failure or alcoholism, only slight trauma may be required to fracture the neck of the femur, and these cases behave like those in elderly patients. Klenerman (1985) suggested that the complications of intracapsular fractures of the femoral neck in young patients were higher than in the elderly.

The published results vary considerably, particularly in their assessment of the frequency of avascular necrosis and non-union. Protzman & Burkhalter (1976) reported a 59% incidence of non-union and an 86% incidence of avascular necrosis in 22 fractures in patients aged 22–40. Other reports, such as those of Kofoed (1982), Kulisch & Gustilo (1976), Askin & Bryan (1976) and Swiontkowski et al (1984), described a lower incidence of these complications than did Protzman & Burkhalter. All of these reports have adequate follow-up and criteria for avascular necrosis and non-union. The results are summarized in Table 9.15.

The Garden fracture classification is only clearly outlined in the work

Table 9.15 Incidence of avascular necrosis and non-union following intracapsular fractures of the neck of the femur in adults under the age of 50 (cases with associated medical problems and secondary osteoporosis excluded)

Reference	Number of cases	Avascular necrosis	Non-union
Protzman & Burkhalter (1976)	22	19	13
Kofoed (1982)	17	7	4
Kulisch & Gustilo (1976)	20	9	5
Swiontkowski et al (1984)	21	4	0
Askin & Bryan (1976)	16	3	3
	96	42 (44%)	25 (26%)

Table 9.16 Incidence of avascular necrosis and non-union according to Garden stage in patients under the age of 50

	Number	Avascular necrosis	Non-union
Garden stage I/II	14	2 (14%)	1 (7%)
Garden stage III/IV	40	12 (30%)	6 (15%)

of Swiontkowski et al, Kofoed, and Askin & Bryan. Protzman & Burkhalter (1976) commented that 'most were markedly displaced', but did not define the Garden stage for each patient. Analysis of the reports in which the Garden staging is clearly categorized has enabled the results in Table 9.16 to be produced.

These results merit emphasis of the following points:

1. They come from differing institutions with different approaches to documentation and treatment. The poorest results (Protzman & Burkhalter 1976) were compiled from seven military hospitals and a wide variety of fixation devices were used. The best results (Swiontkowski et al 1984) emanate from a single centre with a specific interest in trauma, where the fractures were treated as emergencies (within 8 hours of injury) and were fixed with 6.5 mm cancellous screws after adequate reduction.
2. Although Protzman & Burkhalter (1976) comment that most of their fractures were markedly displaced, this does not help in the interpretation of their results according to Garden staging. This undoubtedly causes a bias in the results in Table 9.16, for, if the Protzman & Burkhalter results could be included there would be a considerably higher incidence of avascular necrosis and non-union.
3. The question of the accuracy of reduction was addressed by Kofoed (1976). He found that when final reduction was good there was usually union without late segmental collapse (10 of 12 patients), whereas when there was malreduction (degree not specified), all 5 cases developed union with late segmental collapse.

An excellent follow-up study of intracapsular fractures in those aged under 50 was provided by Zetterberg et al (1982). Unfortunately 38% of the 108 patients had concomitant disease leading to osteoporosis, and these patients are not identified in their results. The complication rate in this group has therefore not been reported here.

One interesting observation the authors made concerned the working capacity of their patients. Of 48 patients who worked prior to their accident, only 27 (56%) were able to return to their former job; in other words, 44% had a reduced working capacity. In the military context, Protzman & Burkhalter (1976) found that only 1 of 21 patients with this injury was able to return to full duty.

Summary

1. In Garden stage I/II intracapsular fractures of the neck of the femur, union occurred in approximately 95% of patients at 12 months. Late segmental collapse occurred in 16% of cases at 3 years.
2. In Garden stage III/IV intracapsular fractures of the neck of the femur, union occurred in approximately 50% of patients at 12 months following reduction and internal fixation. By 24 months (with no further treatment) union occurred in 66–72% of patients.
3. In Garden stage III/IV intracapsular fractures of the neck of the femur, late segmental collapse occurred in 28% of women and 18% of men by 36 months. Late segmental collapse did not occur in the presence of non-union.
4. Although late segmental collapse occurred in 181 patients it was only disabling in 53 (29%). In 32 of these (i.e. 18% of the total number with late segmental collapse) a salvage procedure was performed.
5. Hemiarthroplasty was associated with good results in 67%, fair results in 22% and poor results in 11% with follow-up of over 3 years in an elderly population.
6. Stable intertrochanteric fractures of the femur united in 95–100% of patients irrespective of the type of implant used.
7. Unstable intertrochanteric fractures were associated with a small incidence of non-union (0–2%, depending on the selection of implant). There was a high risk of implant failure with unstable fractures, particularly with the McLaughlin nail-plate (53% failure) and the Jewett nail-plate (46% failure). The lowest rate of implant failure was associated with the sliding screw-plate (6% failure).
8. In patients under the age of 50 with intracapsular fractures of the neck of the femur but with no associated osteoporosis, the overall incidence of avascular necrosis was 44% and of non-union 26%. There was evidence that this could be reduced by early emergency treatment, accurate reduction and rigid internal fixation.

9. In patients under the age of 50 with intracapsular fractures of the neck of the femur, there was a 44% chance that their working capacity would be reduced as a result of the injury.

FRACTURES AND DISLOCATIONS ABOUT THE HIP IN CHILDREN

Fractures

Fractures of the proximal femur are much less common in children than in adults. Lam (1971) reviewed the world literature on the subject and found 652 reported cases. The most widely used classification of these fractures was described by Colonna (1929):

Type I: transphyseal
Type II: transcervical
Type III: basal cervical/cervicotrochanteric
Type IV: intertrochanteric

Some authors, such as Miller (1973) and Meyers (1985), have extended the classification to include subtrochanteric fractures. Subtrochanteric fractures will be considered in Chapter 10. Most of the reports of these fractures give only a 5–6-year follow-up, although reports by Canale & Bourland (1977) and Leung & Lam (1986) gave a mean follow-up of 17–18 years, which is of great relevance when providing medicolegal reports. The classification of long-term results into good, fair and poor follows the criteria described by Ratliff (1962), as shown in Table 9.17.

Table 9.17 Results of femoral neck fractures in children (after Ratliff 1962)

	Good	Fair	Poor
Pain	None or patient ignores it	Occasional	Disabling
Movement	Full or only terminal restriction	Over 50%	Less than 50%
Activity	Normal or patient avoids games	Normal or patient avoids games	Restricted
X-ray	Normal or some deformity of femoral neck	Severe deformity of femoral neck and mild avascular necrosis	Severe avascular necrosis; arthritis; ankylosis

Type I (transphyseal fractures)

As Meyers (1985), Miller (1973) and Ratliff (1962) pointed out, this diagnosis can only be made when there is a clear history of severe trauma; otherwise a diagnosis of slipped upper femoral epiphysis must be considered. There are insufficient numbers in the literature to allow comparison of different treatment methods. If there is severe displacement or associated hip joint dislocation the long-term results are poor. Canale & Bourland (1977) reported 5 such patients, all of whom developed avascular necrosis; 4 developed premature growth plate closure. The mean follow-up of those 5 patients was 30 years (range 18–43 years). Four had poor results, with severe arthritis or fibrous ankylosis, following avascular necrosis.

Miller (1973) reported 11 patients, but the follow-up was much shorter (mean 3 years). In the 3 patients with severe displacement there were 2 poor results and 1 fair result. He reported 5 cases with minimal displacement, whose ages ranged from 7 weeks to 22 months; all subsequently had normal hips with no problems at follow-up (mean 18 months).

Type II (transcervical fractures)

The most comprehensive review of these fractures was provided by Canale & Bourland (1977). They reported on 27 patients. There were 22 patients with displaced transcervical fractures with a mean follow-up of 19.5 years; their ages ranged from 2 to 16 years (mean 12.5). The majority (18) were treated by gentle closed reduction and fixation with Knowles pins. Fourteen (64%) developed avascular necrosis.

Ratliff (1962) described three distinct patterns of avascular necrosis and stated that it always appeared within 1 year of the injury. Four patients (18%) developed coxa vara (defined as a neck shaft angle of less than 135°). There were 2 cases of non-union (9%) and 16 patients (73%) suffered premature closure of the proximal femoral epiphysis; 4 (18%) required secondary operative procedures. At follow-up the result was good in 8 (36%) patients, fair in 7 (32%) and poor in 7 (32%).

In the 5 undisplaced transcervical fractures avascular necrosis, non-union and premature epiphyseal closure did not develop. There was 1 patient who developed coxa vara. At long-term follow-up the results were considered good in all 5 patients, and no secondary procedure had been performed.

The most important factor affecting the development of complications was the degree of displacement at the time of injury. Meyers (1985), Morrisey (1980) and Canale & Bourland (1977) pointed out that the incidence of avascular necrosis was related to displacement and the severity of the initial injury and was not influenced by the type of treatment. On the other hand Canale & Bourland reported that closure of the growth plate was more common when threaded pins which penetrated the growth plate were used.

Type III (basal/cervicotrochanteric fractures)

Lam (1971) reported a follow-up of 18 patients and Canale & Bourland (1977) reported 22. Of these 40 fractures, 28 (70%) were displaced. In the undisplaced cases, conservative treatment yielded universally good results with neither avascular necrosis nor growth plate closure occurring.

Considering the 28 cases with displacement, the complications were as listed in Table 9.18.

Table 9.18 Complications of displaced basal/cervicotrochanteric fractures in children (from Lam 1971, Canale & Bourland 1977)

Complication	Number	%
Avascular necrosis	10/28	36%
Coxa vara	15/28	54%
Premature growth plate closure	15/28	54%
Non-union	2/28	7%

The data in Table 9.18 require further expansion. Most patients with displaced fractures in Canale & Bourland's (1977) series were treated by manipulation and fixation (14 of 17), whereas all the 11 patients with displaced fractures in Lam's (1971) series were treated conservatively, with manipulation and plaster hip spica. Table 9.19 shows the complications related to the type of treatment.

Table 9.19 Complications of basal (cervicotrochanteric) fractures in children related to the use of internal fixation (from Lam 1971, and Canale & Bourland 1977)

Complications	Treatment without internal fixation (n = 14)	Treatment with internal fixation (n = 14)
Avascular necrosis	5 (36%)	5 (36%)
Premature growth plate closure	6 (43%)	9 (64%)
Coxa vara	11 (79%)	2 (14%)
Non-union	2 (14%)	0

From these results it appears that, as with transcervical fractures, the incidence of avascular necrosis is determined by the severity of the initial injury and is unaffected by the treatment. There was a higher incidence of premature growth plate closure in those cases undergoing internal fixation. Canale & Bourland (1977) recognized a high incidence of premature growth plate closure after penetration of the epiphysis with Knowles pins. There was a striking increase in the incidence of coxa vara in those cases treated without internal fixation. Lam (1971) recorded the degree of shortening in the 4 cases in which premature epiphyseal closure occurred. The ages of the children ranged from 7 to 15 years (mean 11 years) and the shortening ranged from 1.9 to 2.5 cm (mean 2.2 cm). Overall, Canale & Bourland (using Ratliff's 1962 grading) found that the long-term results of their displaced cervicotrochanteric fractures were 11 (65%) good, 3 (17.5%) fair and 3 (17.5%) poor. The follow-up in this group of children averaged 13.5 years.

Type IV (intertrochanteric fractures)

Meyers (1985) pointed out that fractures at the intertrochanteric level are the simplest and easiest of all children's hip fractures to treat. There is a low incidence of long-term problems and complications, and avascular necrosis is uncommon. Lam (1971) reported no avascular necrosis in his 13 intertrochanteric fractures; Canale & Bourland (1977) had 1 case (combined with premature epiphyseal fusion) in an undisplaced inter-trochanteric fracture treated with a hip spica. Jodoin et al (1980) reported no cases of avascular necrosis in 18 type IV fractures. Canale & Bourland (1977) described 4 displaced intertrochanteric fractures (2 treated by abduction hip spica and 2 by operation); 2 of these developed coxa vara and 1 showed premature growth plate closure (following delayed Jewett nailing). The mean follow-up in this group was 23.5 years (range 7–44 years). The long-term clinical results were good in 3 patients and fair in the other. There was no delayed union or non-union.

In the undisplaced fractures the results appeared uniformly good, other than in the case reported by Canale & Bourland.

Specific complications

Significance of initial displacement

In all types of undisplaced fractures there is a high percentage of good results irrespective of the treatment. In displaced fractures the results are

Table 9.20 Relationship of initial displacement to the final clinical result (from the combined work of Ratliff 1978, Lam 1971 and Canale & Bourland 1977)

Total fractures	290
Displaced	204
Undisplaced (or minimally displaced)	86
Displaced	
Good results	78 (38%)
Fair results }	
Poor results }	126 (62%)
Undisplaced (or minimally displaced)	
Good results	74 (86%)
Fair results	7 (8%)
Poor results	4 (4%)

much more variable. Table 9.20 shows the final clinical result related to initial displacement from the series of Ratliff (1978), Lam (1971) and Canale & Bourland (1977), comprising 191 patients. Those patients in Lam's series who presented late are excluded, and his cases with minimal displacement are grouped with the undisplaced fractures. In the displaced fractures the fair and poor results are grouped together since in the large series of 170 fractures reported by Ratliff (1978) the fair and poor results were not separated.

Avascular necrosis

Canale & Bourland (1977) and Ratliff (1978) carried out a detailed analysis of those 98 cases in their series which were complicated by avascular necrosis. In all, 89 (91%) were displaced at the time of injury. Radiographic evidence of avascular necrosis was noted at an average of 9 months following injury by Canale & Bourland. The long-term results in these patients are shown in Table 9.21. The average follow-up was 17 years. The authors described 7 patients within this group who showed radiological evidence of avascular necrosis with no evidence of remodelling. In 5 of these cases it was an average of 20 years before they complained of pain in the involved hip. The poor results in undisplaced fractures were all associated with severe avascular necrosis and, as Durbin (1959) pointed out, the prognosis must always be guarded, even in undisplaced fractures.

Table 9.21 Long-term results of 98 patients with avascular necrosis (from Canale & Bourland 1977, Ratliff 1978)

Result	n	%
Good	7	7%
Fair	35	36%
Poor	56	57%

Premature growth plate fusion

The relationship of premature growth plate closure to internal fixation has already been discussed. Canale & Bourland (1977) described 33 cases and attempted to correlate limb length discrepancy with premature closure of the subcapital femoral physis. Their results showed that there was a much higher incidence of significant shortening in patients with premature closure than those without. The 12 cases with shortening of more than 2 cm all had premature growth plate closure *and* avascular necrosis. Of 14 patients with less than 2 cm of shortening only 6 had both avascular necrosis and premature closure, while 8 had premature closure alone. Ratliff (1978) pointed out that premature closure may also occur in one of the growth plates of the knee on the side of the fracture. This compounds the shortening that may occur.

Coxa vara

A decrease in the neck shaft angle results in the hip operating at a mechanical disadvantage because there is upward displacement of the greater trochanter and shortening of the leg, resulting in a Trendelenburg gait. Lam (1971) felt that this was the commonest complication of hip fractures in children, but he believed that it was often compatible with a good clinical result. Ratliff (1978) reported an incidence of coxa vara of 15% (27 of 170) while Canale & Bourland (1977) reported an incidence of 21% (13 of 61). Canale & Bourland defined coxa vara as a neck shaft angle of less than 135°, whereas Ratliff (1978) defined it as a neck shaft angle of less than 120°. Of the 13 patients with coxa vara reported by Canale & Bourland, 4 (31%) had a good clinical result, 6 (46%) had a fair clinical result, and 3 (23%) a poor result.

Non-union

This complication occurred only in displaced fractures. In the series of both Canale & Bourland (1977) and of Ratliff (1978) there were 174 displaced fractures and non-union developed in 21 cases (12%).

Dislocations

The most comprehensive review of hip dislocations and their sequelae in both adults and children is Epstein's (1980) monograph, with a mean follow-up of 6.5 years in 51 dislocations in children.

The main points of prognostic interest after these injuries are:

1. The risk of developing avascular necrosis of the femoral head.
2. The long-term clinical results.

Anterior dislocations

Epstein (1980) reported follow-up of 7 anterior dislocations; 6 had excellent clinical results, while 1 had a good result (Table 9.1). There were no fair or poor results. Barquet (1982) reported an incidence of 13% (2 of 15) avascular necrosis in anterior dislocations reduced within 24 hours of injury. If anterior dislocations were reduced more than 24 hours after the injury then the incidence of avascular necrosis increased to 86% (6 of 7).

Posterior dislocations

In Epstein's (1980) series there were 38 simple posterior dislocations, with a mean follow-up of 6.5 years; 34 (89%) were associated with a good or excellent clinical result and 4 (11%) were associated with a fair result.

There are insufficient numbers of the other types of posterior dislocation to derive meaningful clinical results. The Pennsylvania Orthopaedic Society (1968) reported on the status at skeletal maturity of 44 children who had sustained posterior dislocation of the hip. They found that 16 had an imperfect clinical result; of these 16 children, 6 had associated fractures about the hip joint, 4 had reduction delayed beyond 24 hours, and 3 had developed avascular necrosis. They felt that these three features carried a high risk of a poor clinical result in children.

The incidence of avascular necrosis has been reported to be approximately 10 per cent by the Pennsylvania Orthopaedic Society (26 of 266 cases). Barquet (1982) has collected, both from his own practice and from the orthopaedic literature, 145 cases of avascular necrosis from a review of 1117 cases of traumatic hip dislocation in childhood. He felt that only in cases with a minimum of 2 years' clinical and radiological follow-up could avascular necrosis be confidently excluded. Using Barquet's strict criteria there are 145 cases of avascular necrosis in 412 cases with adequate follow-up (i.e. 35% incidence), whereas in the total group (145 from 1117) the incidence is approximately 13%. Barquet (personal communication) has recently claimed that he believes that the true incidence of avascular necrosis lies between 3 and 15% in dislocations that are reduced within 12 hours. Nowadays avascular necrosis can be diagnosed much earlier than 2 years from the time of the injury, particularly with the availability of isotope scanning and magnetic resonance imaging. However, many of the cases in the literature were reported before these facilities were available.

Barquet looked carefully at factors that may influence the development of avascular necrosis and reached the following conclusions:

1. There appears to be protection against avascular necrosis in children under the age of 6 years.
2. The severity of injury strongly influenced the result; in severe accidents the incidence of avascular necrosis was greater. The incidence was higher with an associated fracture.
3. The incidence of avascular necrosis was much lower when the dislocation was reduced within the first 24 hours after the injury.
4. The incidence of avascular necrosis was 11.5% in cases reduced within 24 hours. Barquet analysed the results within this period and found that the incidence in those cases reduced within 4 hours of injury was 6.25%; between 5 and 12 hours it was 12.8% and between 13 and 24 hours it was 13.5%.
5. Post-reduction immobilization appeared not to influence the development of avascular necrosis in posterior dislocation without fracture.
6. The interval from dislocation to weight-bearing appeared not to influence the development of avascular necrosis in posterior dislocation without fracture.

Summary

1. Transphyseal fractures of the hip are, in general, associated with a poor prognosis. Avascular necrosis is almost invariable if there is dislocation of the femoral head. Children under the age of 2 with minimal displacement tend to suffer no long-term problems.
2. Displaced transcervical fractures are associated with a poor prognosis. Undisplaced transcervical fractures are associated with a good prognosis (provided they do not displace during treatment).
3. Displaced cervicotrochanteric fractures are associated with good long-term clinical results in 65% of cases. The results vary according to the use of internal fixation; in particular, coxa vara is much more common in those treated without fixation. Premature growth plate closure is more common in those treated with internal fixation (Table 9.19). Undisplaced cervicotrochanteric fractures are associated with uniformly good results.
4. Intertrochanteric fractures are generally associated with a good long-term result.
5. A combination of avascular necrosis and premature growth plate closure carries a high risk of subsequent limb shortening.
6. According to Ratliff (1978), avascular necrosis always occurs within 1 year of injury. Canale & Bourland (1977) found radiological evidence of avascular necrosis at an average of 9 months after injury.
7. Avascular necrosis occurs in approximately 10% of posterior dislocations in children. The incidence may be as low as 6% if the dislocation is reduced within 4 hours of the injury.

REFERENCES

Anderson L D, Hamsan W R, Waring T L 1964 Femoral head prostheses: a review of 356 operations and their results. Journal of Bone and Joint Surgery 46A: 1049–1065
Askin S R, Bryan R S 1976 Femoral neck fractures in young adults. Clinical Orthopaedics 114: 259–264
Austin R T 1971 Hip function after central fracture dislocation: a long term review. Injury 3: 114–120
Banks H H 1962 Factors influencing the results in fractures of the femoral neck. Journal of Bone and Joint Surgery 44A: 931–964
Barnes R, Brown J T, Garden R S, Nicoll E A 1976 Subcapital fractures of the femur: a prospective review. Journal of Bone and Joint Surgery 58B: 2–24
Barquet A 1982 Avascular necrosis following traumatic hip dislocation in childhood: factors of influence. Acta Orthopaedica Scandinavica 53: 809–813
Brav E A 1962 Traumatic dislocation of the hip; army experience over a 12 year period. Journal of Bone and Joint Surgery 44A: 1115–1134
Canale S T, Bourland W L 1977 Fractures of the neck and intertrochanteric region of the femur in children. Journal of Bone and Joint Surgery 59A: 431–443
Colonna P C 1929 Delbet classification. In Fractures of the neck of the femur in children. American Journal of Surgery 6: 795
Dimon J H, Hughston J C 1967 Unstable trochanteric fractures of the hip. Journal of Bone and Joint Surgery 49A: 440
Drennan Lowell J 1980 Results and complications of femoral neck fractures. Clinical Orthopaedics 152: 162–172

Durbin F C 1959 Avascular necrosis complicating undisplaced fractures of the neck of the femur in children. Journal of Bone and Joint Surgery 41B: 758

Epstein H C 1980 Traumatic dislocation of the hip. Williams & Wilkins, Baltimore

Epstein H C, Wiss D A, Cozen L 1985 Posterior fracture dislocation of the hip with fractures of the femoral head. Clinical Orthopaedics 201: 9–17

Garden R S 1961 Low angle fixation in fractures of the femoral neck. Journal of Bone and Joint Surgery 43B: 647–663

Harris W H 1969 Traumatic arthritis of the hip after dislocation and acetabular fractures: treatment by mould arthroplasty. An end result study using a new method of evaluation. Journal of Bone and Joint Surgery 51A: 737–755

Heeg M, Oostvogel H J M, Klasen H J 1987 Conservative treatment of acetabular fractures. The role of the weight bearing dome and anatomic reduction in the ultimate result. Journal of Trauma 27: 555–559

Hinchey J J, Day P L 1964 Primary prosthetic replacement in fresh femoral neck fractures: a review of 294 consecutive cases. Journal of Bone and Joint Surgery 46A: 223–239

Hofmann A A, Dahl C P, Wyatt R W B 1984 Experience with acetabular fractures. American Journal of Trauma 750–752

Hougaard K, Thomsen P B 1987 Coxarthrosis following traumatic posterior dislocation of the hip. Journal of Bone and Joint Surgery 69A: 679–683

Hunter G A 1969 Posterior dislocation and fracture dislocation of the hip: a review of 57 patients. Journal of Bone and Joint Surgery 51B: 38–44

Jodoin A, Duhaime M, Labelle P, Morton D 1980 Fractures of the hip in children. Journal of Bone and Joint Surgery 62B: 128

Johnson J T H, Crothers O 1975 Nailing versus prosthesis for femoral neck fractures. Journal of Bone and Joint Surgery 57A: 686–692

Judet R, Judet J, Letournel E 1964, Fractures of the acetabulum: classification and surgical approaches for open reduction. Preliminary report. Journal of Bone and Joint Surgery 46A: 1615–1647

Klenerman L 1985 The young patient with a fractured neck of femur. British Medical Journal 290: 1928

Kofoed H 1982 Femoral neck fractures in young adults. Injury 14: 146–150

Kulisch S D, Gustilo R B 1976 Fractures of the femoral neck in young adults. Journal of Bone and Joint Surgery 58A: 724

Lam S F 1971 Fractures of the neck of the femur in children. Journal of Bone and Joint Surgery 53A: 1165–1179

Letournel E, Judet R 1981 Fractures of the acetabulum. Translated and edited by R A Elson. Springer-Verlag, Berlin

Leung P C, Lam S F 1986 Long-term follow up of children with femoral neck fractures. Journal of Bone and Joint Surgery 68B: 537–540

Lowell D 1979 External fixation: the current state of the art. Williams and Wilkins, Baltimore, p 119

Matta J M, Mehre D K, Roffi R 1985 Fractures of the acetabulum: early results of a prospective study. Clinical Orthopaedics 241–250

Mayo K A 1987 Fractures of the acetabulum. Orthopedic Clinics of North America 18.1: 43–57

Meyers M H 1985 Fractures of the hip. Chicago Year Book, Chicago

Miller W E 1973 Fractures of the hip in children from birth to adolescence. Clinical Orthopaedics 92: 155–188

Morrisey R 1980 Hip fractures in children. Clinical Orthopaedics 152: 202–210

Pennal G F, Davidson J, Garside H, Plewes J 1980 Results of treatment of acetabular fractures. Clinical Orthopaedics 151: 115–123

Pennsylvania Orthopaedic Society 1968 Final report of the scientific research committee on traumatic dislocation of the hip joint in children. Journal of Bone and Joint Surgery 590A: 79–88

Pipkin G 1957 Treatment of grade IV fracture–dislocation of the hip. Journal of Bone and Joint Surgery 39A: 1027–1042

Protzman R R, Burkhalter M D (1976) Femoral neck fractures in young adults. Journal of Bone and Joint Surgery 58A: 686–694

Ratliff A H C 1962 Fractures of the neck of the femur in children. Journal of Bone and Joint Surgery 44B: 528–542

Ratliff A H C 1978 Fractures of the neck of the femur in children. In: Lloyd-Roberts G C, Ratliff A H C (eds), Hip disorders in children. Butterworths, London, pp 165–199

Regazzoni P, Reudi T H 1985 The dynamic hip screw implant system. Springer-Verlag, Berlin

Rowe C R, Lowell D 1961 Prognosis of fractures of the acetabulum. Journal of Bone and Joint Surgery 43A: 30–59

Steen Jensen J, Sonne-Holm S, Tondevold E 1980a Unstable trochanteric fractures. A comparative analysis of four methods of internal fixation. Acta Orthopaedica Scandinavica 51: 949–962

Steen Jensen J, Tondevold E, Sonne-Holm S 1980b Stable trochanteric fractures. A comparative analysis of four methods of internal fixation. Acta Orthopaedica Scandinavica 51: 811–815

Stewart M J, Milford L W 1954 Fracture–dislocation of the hip. An end result study. Journal of Bone and Joint Surgery 36A: 315–342

Swiontkowski M, Winquist R A, Hansen S T 1984 Fractures of the femoral neck in patients between the age of 12 and 49 years. Journal of Bone and Joint Surgery 66A: 837–846

Thompson V P, Epstein H C 1951 Traumatic dislocation of the hip. A survey of 204 cases covering a period of 21 years. Journal of Bone and Joint Surgery 33A: 746–777

Tile M 1984 Fractures of the pelvis and acetabulum. Williams & Wilkins, Baltimore

Tile M, Kellam J F, Joyce M 1985 Fractures of the acetabulum: classification, management protocol and results of treatment. Journal of Bone and Joint Surgery 67B: 324–325

Tipton W W, D'Ambrosia R D, Ryle G P 1975 Non operative management of central fracture dislocation of the hip. Journal of Bone and Joint Surgery 57A: 888–893

Upadhyay S S, Moulton A 1981 The long term results of traumatic posterior dislocation of the hip. Journal of Bone and Joint Surgery 63B: 548–551

Whittaker R P, Abeshaus M M, Scholl H W, Chung S M K 1972 Fifteen years' experience with metallic endoprosthetic replacement of the femoral head for femoral neck fractures. Journal of Trauma 12: 799–806

Wilson J N 1982 Injuries of the hip. In: Watson Jones fractures and joint injuries. Churchill Livingstone, Edinburgh, p 931

Zetterberg G L, Irstam L, Anderson G B J 1982 Femoral neck fractures in young adults. Acta Orthopaedica Scandinavica 53: 427–435

10. The femur

M. A. Foy

INTRODUCTION

There is a considerable controversy concerning the merits of surgical and conservative treatment in all types of femoral fracture. Operative treatment of fractures is favoured where it is difficult to maintain reduction, e.g. displaced subtrochanteric fractures. Non-operative treatment is preferred where good results can be expected without surgery, e.g. in children.

In the sections within this chapter attempts will be made to consider the end-results in terms of both surgical and conservative treatment, where the appropriate information is available.

SUBTROCHANTERIC FRACTURES

There is no classification of subtrochanteric fractures that correlates well with prognosis. Boyd & Griffin (1949), Fielding et al (1974), Zickel (1976), Seinsheimer (1978) and Waddell (1979) have all suggested classifications. Velasco & Comfort (1978) and Delee (1984) rejected classification schemes for subtrochanteric fractures and recommended that each fracture should be assessed in terms of potential stability after internal fixation. As with fractures of the femoral neck, subtrochanteric fractures may be seen in two groups of patients — older patients suffering minor trauma to weakened bone and younger patients with normal bone who are subjected to high-velocity injury.

Delee (1984) pointed out that the two main problems arising from subtrochanteric fractures were malunion and delayed or non-union. The subtrochanteric area is composed mainly of cortical bone which may be comminuted in these fractures. The cortical bone vascularity and fracture surfaces are less than in the cancellous bone surfaces available in inter-trochanteric fractures. There are also large biomechanical stresses in the subtrochanteric region which may result in failure of internal fixation devices before bony union occurs.

Seinsheimer (1978) proposed a classification based on the number of major fragments and the location and shape of fracture lines. The classi-

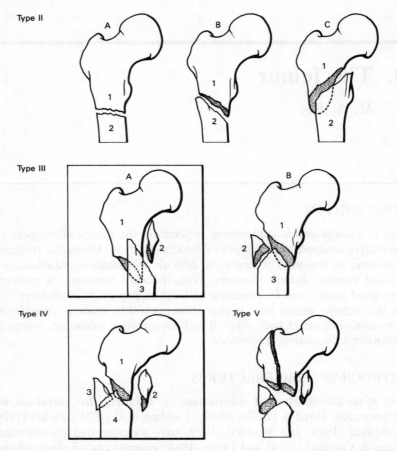

Fig. 10.1 Classification of subtrochanteric fractures (from Seinsheimer 1978, with permission)

fication is shown in Figure 10.1. It identifies two types of fracture, which, in Seinsheimer's (1978) series, were associated with all the implant failures and non-unions. These were his type IIIA (a three-part spiral fracture in which the lesser trochanter is part of the third fragment) and the type IV (a comminuted fracture with four or more fragments).

When Velasco & Comfort (1978) analysed their unsatisfactory results they found that 19 out of 22 (86%) had a medial defect of more than 2 mm, while in those with satisfactory results only 15 of 50 (30%) had a medial defect greater than 2 mm. Velasco & Comfort defined a satisfactory result as:

1. Full pre-injury activity or job status with slight or no pain.
2. Hip flexion of over 90° with less than 10° of rotational deformity.
3. No more than 10° varus.
4. Less than 1.25 cm of shortening.

The common feature throughout the various classifications is the import-ance of damage to the medial cortex of the femur and the less satisfactory results that occur if it is not reduced and stabilized to maintain a medial buttress.

Conservative treatment

The results of treatment in traction are fairly consistent in the literature, although the criteria for a satisfactory result vary slightly from series to series. Table 10.1 summarizes these results.

Table 10.1 Results of subtrochanteric fractures treated by traction

	Number of cases	Satisfactory	Unsatisfactory
Waddell (1979)	18	10	8
Velasco & Comfort (1978)	22	11	11
Seinsheimer (1978)	8	3	5
Watson et al (1964)	8	4	4
Total	56	28	28

The most common cause of an unsatisfactory result was a varus deformity in excess of 10° (13 out of 28 patients, i.e. 46%). Non-union or delayed union occurred in 5 out of 28 patients (18%) while shortening of more than 1.25 cm happened in 4 out of 28 patients (14%) and severe knee stiffness in 3 out of 28 patients (11%).

Delee et al (1981) described a treatment regime of preliminary traction followed by an ambulatory cast brace with a pelvic band for severely comminuted or open subtrochanteric fractures. In the 15 cases on which they reported they found no non-unions and 'no significant degree' of varus, rotation or shortening. They did stress that this treatment regime required exacting attention from the orthopaedic surgeon.

Surgical treatment

Most recent reviews of subtrochanteric fracture management advocate operative treatment. Trafton (1987) pointed out that there were significant complications after fixation with early hip implants such as the McLaughlin and Jewett devices. We will consider the results obtained following the use of devices commonly employed at the present time.

Compression hip screws

Reported results are good, and this may reflect the familiarity of the implant to most orthopaedic surgeons. Waddell (1979) reported 24 cases with 21 satisfactory results, 1 implant failure and 2 non-unions. Wile et al (1983)

reported 25 patients treated with a high-angle compression hip screw. There were no mechanical failures, delayed unions or non-unions. There were 2 instances of malunion in this series. Wile et al classified their fractures after Seinsheimer (1978) and found that the mean time to bony union was 3.6 months (range 1.3–6.9 months). In the series mentioned, the incidence of satisfactory results was 90% using the compression hip screw. Trafton (1987) reported that union without fixation failure was recorded in 95–100% of patients.

AO condylar blade plate

According to Trafton (1987) this is the only fixed-angle one-piece device that is still advocated for subtrochanteric fractures. Orthopaedic surgeons tend not to be as familiar with its use as they are with the compression hip screw. All authors emphasize the importance of reconstructing the medial cortical buttress when this device is used. In Waddell's (1979) series 40 patients were treated with the AO blade plate; 29 achieved a satisfactory result (72.5%). There were 7 implant failures and 4 non-unions requiring further surgical treatment.

Zickel nail

Reports on the success of the Zickel nail have varied from centre to centre. Trafton (1987) reported that there were satisfactory results in 90% of patients. Zickel (1976) reported a 3% non-union rate in 234 cases (Zickel et al 1985). Intra-operative complication rates have been reported to be as high as 20% by some groups (Winter et al 1979). Waddell (1979) reported unacceptable external rotation deformity in 8 of 10 patients on whom the Zickel nail was used. Removal of this implant after healing may be associated with a high complication rate.

Other implants

Fixed-angle nail plates have been extensively used in the past for subtrochanteric fractures, but as Delee (1984) pointed out, this method has met with mixed results. Condylocephalic (Enders) nails have been used but complications, particularly early loss of fixation, are common (Trafton 1987).

Problems with predicting prognosis in subtrochanteric fractures

There is insufficient uniformity in classification (although Seinsheimer's is the most widely quoted) to enable results following application of the various fixation devices to be accurately correlated. The advent of the interlocking nail and the dynamic condylar screw may change the techniques of fixation of these fractures, and it may be many more years before the situation is clear.

In Velasco & Comfort's (1978) series there were 50 fractures treated by operation, using the Jewett nail, the Massie nail, the AO blade plate and the Zickel nail. The results merit consideration as a general group as they were followed up using strict criteria for varus, shortening and rotational deformity. Of these, 39 patients (78%) achieved a good result while 11 (22%) achieved an unsatisfactory result. The reasons for the unsatisfactory results were varus deformity in 2 patients, shortening of more than 1.25 cm in 3 patients and non-union in 1 patient. Ten of the 11 failures (91%) occurred where there was a residual medial defect of more than 2 mm after fixation. In theory this medial defect may not be quite so critical with the compression/sliding hip screw — a device which was not used in this series.

The subtrochanteric fracture appears *par excellence* to be a condition where, if surgical treatment is contemplated, the prognosis is related to the familiarity of the surgeon with the implant to be used. The subtrochanteric fracture (particularly the Seinsheimer type IIIA and IV) is not a forgiving fracture. It is difficult, therefore, to formulate more than prognostic guidelines in this condition. Prospective trials, using accepted classifications, such as Seinsheimer's, are required to record accurate results and to clarify the prognosis. It should be recognized that each of the available implants may have advantages in certain types of subtrochanteric fracture, and implant selection should be made with reference to the fracture anatomy.

Summary

1. There is no accepted classification of subtrochanteric fractures that correlates well with prognosis.
2. The Seinsheimer type IIIA fracture (see Fig. 10.1) appears to be particularly associated with failure of internal fixation.
3. Traction results in satisfactory results in 50% of cases. The cases selected for traction in the series studied tended to be undisplaced or comminuted, such that a stable internal fixation could not be contemplated.
4. Operative treatment is favoured in the majority of cases but the choice of implant remains controversial. A high proportion of satisfactory results are reported with both the compression hip screw (90–100%) and Zickel nail (90%).

FEMORAL SHAFT FRACTURES

The treatment of fractures of the femoral shaft may be operative or non-operative. Non-operative treatment is still the method favoured by many orthopaedic surgeons while, at the other extreme, some orthopaedic surgeons feel that the advent of the interlocking nail has extended the indications for internal fixation.

Mooney & Claudi (1984) suggested that femoral fractures should be classified as simple, butterfly fragment and comminuted/segmental. The butterfly fractures can be further subdivided into single butterfly fragments, two butterfly fragments and those with three or more intermediate fragments.

There is a large volume of literature on femoral shaft fractures. However, only a small number of reports carefully assess the functional, anatomical and social results in detail. The most comprehensive review is Kootstra's (1973) monograph.

Problems arise with analysis of the results because definition of the femoral shaft is either not specified or varies from series to series. Kootstra defined the shaft as extending from the lower edge of the lesser trochanter to a line which parallels the joint space of the knee at a distance equal to the width of the condyles. A small number of subtrochanteric fractures may fall within this definition, but the meticulous follow-up of Kootstra's work is so important that this small potential bias is accepted in this chapter.

Delayed union

Opinions differ over the definition of delayed union. Kootstra (1973) and Dencker (1965) identified it in 104 of 741 patients with femoral shaft frac-had not been achieved by 8 months. Dencker applied a second criterion; he wrote of delayed union if the attending surgeon had to perform an operation within 8 months to accelerate union.

Kootstra described 84% of 261 fractures healed by 6 months in patients treated by conservative and operative methods. Winquist et al (1984) reported that 87% of 442 femoral fractures treated by intramedullary nailing were united by 3 months. Winquist et al are experienced and skilled proponents of closed intramedullary fixation of femoral fractures.

Kootstra (1973) identified delayed union in 16 of 261 patients and Dencker (1964) identified it in 104 of 741 patients with femoral shaft fractures. Aggregation of these figures (i.e. 120 of 1002 fractures) suggests an incidence of 12% for delayed union of femoral shaft fractures following a variety of treatments — traction, intramedullary nailing, AO plating and circlage wiring. Considering Dencker's second criterion for delayed union (see above) and its subjective nature, it may be that Kootstra's figure of 6% (16 of 261) is a clearer reflection of the incidence of delayed union in these fractures.

Kootstra used the radiological criteria of Charnley & Guindy (1961) to define osseous union: the presence of continuous bridging of bone at some part of the fracture, though not necessarily on all sides, combined with the absence of sclerosis. Figure 10.2 is reproduced from his work and clearly

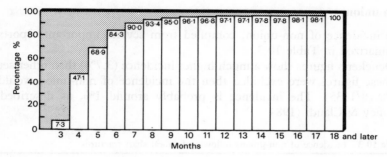

Fig. 10.2 Cumulative percentages of fracture unions per month (from Kootstra 1973, with permission)

Table 10.2 Comparison between three methods of treatment and their relation to delayed union (adapted from Kootstra 1973)

Month of union	Cumulative % united		
	Conservative	Intramedullary (K) nailing	AO plate
Third	13.4%	4.2%	5.4%
Sixth	92.7%	83.1%	70.2%
Eighth	95.1%	94.4%	86.5%

shows the cumulative percentages of fracture unions per month using this definition. Kootstra attempted to define factors which influenced the rate of union. Table 10.2 summarizes the duration of union following three different methods of treatment.

Although the rate of union at 8 months is lower following AO plating, this is not statistically significant. Kootstra also found no significant difference in the duration of union in open and closed femoral fractures. He found that the duration of union was significantly shorter in the age group 17–29 years when compared with those in the 30–70 years age group.

The criteria for osseous union outlined by Charnley & Guindy (1961) and used in Kootstra's work bear only limited relation to functional recovery. Rokkanen et al (1969) used functional results as the criteria for progress of fracture healing. In patients treated by operation they defined union according to the time elapsing between the accident and the time when the patient was able to walk without the aid of a stick, and subsequently to return to work. For patients treated conservatively, union was recorded as the time when immobilization was discontinued. Using this criterion all fractures had healed within 12 months of the accident. The work of Rokkanen et al is discussed in more detail in the section on social and occupational factors.

Non-union

The incidence of non-union, compiled from several important reports, is summarized in Table 10.3.

Dencker's figures show a much higher incidence (3.7%) than other series. If these figures were excluded then the incidence of non-union would be 0.6% (8/1335). The incidence is probably around 1%, as described by Mooney & Claudi (1984).

Table 10.3 Incidence of non-unions following femoral shaft fractures

Reference	Treatment	Non-unions
Dencker (1965)	Conservative/operative	31/837
Wickstrom et al (1968)	Intramedullary nailing	2/324
Rokkanen et al (1969)	Conservative/operative	0/154
Kootstra (1973)	Conservative/operative	1/261
Carr & Wingo (1973)	Conservative/operative	1/154
Winquist et al (1984)	Intramedullary nailing	4/442
Total		39/2172 (1.8%)

Refracture

Table 10.4 shows the incidence of refracture in four large series. The overall incidence is 3.9%. In Dencker's series, 17 of the 20 refractures occurred within a year of the original injury.

In addition to refracture in the first year after injury, refracture after removal of rigid internal fixation devices is a problem because the bone, under these circumstances, has been protected from functional stresses.

Of the 15 refractures in Kootstra's series, 9 occurred in 91 patients treated conservatively, 3 occurred in 43 patients treated by AO plating and 3 in 165 patients treated by intramedullary nailing. Hartmann & Brav (1954) and Seimon (1964) felt that approximately two-thirds of the refractures were avoidable. The avoidable cases occurred because of premature mobilization, carelessness of the patient or early removal of implants.

Table 10.4 Incidence of refracture following femoral shaft fractures treated by conservative and operative methods

Reference	Treatment	Refracture rate
Hartmann & Brav (1954)	Conservative/operative	12/135
Dencker (1964)	Conservative/operative	20/837
Seimon (1964)	Conservative/operative	21/476
Kootstra (1973)	Conservative/operative	15/300
Total		68/1748 (3.9%)

Femoral shortening

Shortening following femoral shaft fractures may be due to overlapping of the fracture fragments or to angular deformity. Assessment may be clinical or radiological. A myokinetic study by Morscher and Taillard (1965) showed that patients with 1 cm of shortening have a normal gait and many patients with 2 cm of shortening have a normal gait and are free of symptoms. With shortening in excess of 2 cm, which can be detected clinically, the gait is almost always disturbed.

Shortening in the lower limb is an important consideration as far as insurance companies assessing compensation following trauma are concerned. Shortening of 2 cm or more was found in 37 of 323 (11.5%) patients reported by Rokkanen et al (1969) and Kootstra (1973). Treatment was by traction, intramedullary nailing (open and closed) and AO plating. The results from these two series are summarized according to method of treatment in Table 10.5.

Table 10.5   Incidence of shortening >2 cm following femoral shaft fractures (from Rokkanen et al 1969, Kootstra 1973)

Method of treatment	Shortening > 2 cm	
	n	%
Conservative	23/81	28
Intramedullary nailing (open/closed)	13/209	6
AO plating	1/33	3.3
Overall	37/323	11.5

Kootstra found that 2 of 53 (3.8%) patients treated conservatively developed shortening of 5 cm. Of the 7 fractures in this series with shortening of 3 cm or more, 6 were comminuted and 1 was a spiral fracture with a butterfly fragment. Hardy et al (1979) reported a 31% incidence of shortening of more than 2 cm (i.e. similar to the conservative group shown in Table 10.5) in a series of 79 femoral shaft fractures treated by cast-bracing and early weight-bearing. Leg length in this series was assessed by scanogram, and the authors suggested that scanograms should be carried out routinely for medicolegal reasons. This is obviously a counsel of perfection and should not replace a full clinical assessment of the patient.

Angular deformities

Kootstra (1973) assessed varus, valgus and angular deformities in the sagittal plane in 232 patients with femoral shaft fractures. None of the patients with a varus deformity of less than 10° had symptoms referable to their deformity. Only 2 of 9 patients with varus deformity in excess of 15° were symptomatic. Varus deformity of 10° or more occurred in 11 of 63 patients

(17.5%) treated conservatively, 6 of 133 patients (4.5%) treated by intra-medullary nailing and in none of 36 patients treated by AO plating. The long-term effect of varus deformity of the femur on the knee joint is unclear.

There were 30 patients with measurable valgus deformities in Kootstra's series, but none were symptomatic. The greatest degree of valgus was 15°. Valgus of 10° or more was present in 3 of 63 patients (4.7%) treated conservatively, 8 of 133 patients (6%) treated by intramedullary nailing and in none of 36 patients treated by AO plating.

Recurvation was present in 64 of 232 patients (27.5%), but none were symptomatic. Recurvation of 10° or more was present in 6 of 63 patients (9.5%) treated conservatively, 5 of 133 patients (3.7%) treated by intra-medullary nailing and in none of 36 patients treated by AO plating. The opposite deformity of 'antecurvation' was less commonly found, but similarly gave no symptoms, even when it was 15° or more.

Rotational deformities

Nicod (1967) believed that significant clinical symptoms occurred with rotational deformities exceeding 20° and that external rotation deformities led to degenerative change in the lateral compartment of the knee joint, while internal rotation deformities led to degenerative changes in the medial compartment. Muller (1967) was of the opinion that rotational deformity in the femur could give rise to symptoms in the metatarsals and ankle joint.

Kootstra (1973) assessed 206 of his patients for rotational deformities. The findings are summarized in Table 10.6

Table 10.6 Frequency of rotational deformity exceeding 20° following femoral shaft fractures (adapted from Kootstra 1973)

Treatment	External rotation >20°	Internal rotation >20°
Conservative treatment	8/51 (15.7%)	2/51 (3.9%)
Intramedullary nailing	32/121 (26.4%)	4/121 (3.3%)
AO plating	1/34 (2.9%)	0/34

Rokkanen et al (1969) reported a lower incidence of rotational deformity in their series; the deformity exceeded 10° in 10–11% of fractures treated by intramedullary nailing and in 4% of those treated conservatively. These authors do not give any information on subsequent progress of these cases.

Kootstra (1973) assessed 23 patients with external rotation deformity of 20° and found that 8 (35%) were symptomatic, complaining of knee stiffness after walking, exertion fatigue in the leg and a tired feeling in the hip. There were assessments on 12 patients with external rotation deformity of 30° and 6 (50%) were symptomatic, complaining of fatiguability of the limb on exertion. Of 2 patients with an external rotation deformity of 40°; only

1 was symptomatic. In none of these patients (with a follow-up of from 2 to 11 years) was there radiological evidence of osteoarthritis of the knee or hip joint. One patient with a 50° external rotation deformity had unequivocal degenerative signs in the knee joint 8 years after the injury.

Of the 5 patients with internal rotation deformities of 20°, only 1 had symptoms of fatiguability of the leg; this patient had a co-existent valgus deformity. One patient with an internal rotation deformity of 30° suffered slight limitation of knee function, but was otherwise symptom-free. None of these patients had radiological evidence of osteoarthritis when assessed 2–11 years after injury.

Knee function

Laubenthal et al (1972) suggested that the average knee motion required for sitting is 93°; for climbing stairs it is 100°; for tying shoelaces it is 106° and for squatting to lift an object, it is 117°. Laros & Spiegel (1979) concluded, on the basis of this work, that 125° or more of knee flexion will be required to enable normal function; 110–124° will permit shoelace tying in most cases, while 100–109° of flexion will generally allow patients to sit comfortably and to climb stairs. Laros & Spiegel believed that less than 100° of knee flexion resulted in difficulty with sitting and significant functional loss.

Laros & Spiegel (1979) summarized the results in terms of knee flexion in 1003 femoral shaft fractures from the literature. Their findings are shown in Table 10.7.

Table 10.7 Range of knee flexion following various methods of treatment for femoral shaft fractures (adapted from Laros & Spiegel 1979)

	Knee flexion		
	0–90° Impaired function	91–120° Some impairment of function	>120° Normal function
Cast brace treatment	17%	37%	46%
Traction	17%	25%	58%
Open intra-medullary nailing	5.5%	94.5%	
Closed intra-medullary nailing	0	14%	86%
AO plating	0	6%	94%

Other reports do not consider range of knee movements in these precise terms and cannot be directly compared. Nichols (1963) found that a range of knee flexion greater than 90° was obtained less frequently after comminuted fractures (58%) than after simple (78%) or compound (60%) fractures, irrespective of whether the treatment was by traction or intramedullary nailing.

Social and occupational factors

In this section we will consider two factors — duration of unfitness to work and change of occupation. These factors are influenced not just by the type of fracture and its treatment but also by the nature of the patient's employment, the patient's age, associated injuries, the patient's personality and the labour market in general.

Duration of unfitness to work

As might be expected, hospitalization is less in those cases treated operatively compared to those treated non-operatively. Reviewing the work of Nichols (1963), Rokkanen et al (1969), Bilcher Toft & Hammer (1970) and Kootstra (1973), the mean duration of unfitness to work was approximately 9 months (with a range from 2 to 24 months) after femoral shaft fractures. Nichols (1963) and Kootstra (1973), found that patients were able to return to work approximately 2 months earlier (i.e after 7 months) following intramedullary nailing.

Carr & Wingo (1973) analysed the duration of unfitness to work according to fracture type. In simple, transverse or oblique fractures (72 patients treated by open (42) and closed (30) methods) the mean time for return to work was 9.5 months. In fractures with a butterfly fragment (33 patients treated by open (15) and closed (18) methods) the mean time for return to work was 10.5 months. In segmental or severely comminuted fractures (11 cases treated by open (5) and closed (6) methods) the mean time for return to work was 13.5 months.

Change of occupation

There is little information in the literature on the effect of a femoral shaft fracture on subsequent employability. Numerous factors affect occupation after femoral shaft fracture; the most important are the nature of the patient's job and the development of complications of the fracture or complications of its treatment. In a series of military personnel, Nichols (1963), reported that 28% of patients with femoral shaft fractures were subsequently invalided out of the service. Of this group 50% had fractures of the patella or tibia in the same limb.

Kootstra (1973) found that only 2 of 200 patients were unable to work after a femoral fracture, *solely* because of the femoral fracture, while 12 of 202 patients (6%) were unable to work because of associated injuries. Kootstra was only able to identify 5 out of 202 patients (2.5%) who had to change their occupation as a result of their femoral fracture. Moulton et al (1984) considered the influence of associated injuries in two matched series of femoral shaft fractures. They concluded that the presence of an associated injury increased the chance of permanent disability, as measured in terms of knee flexion less than 90°, shortening of more than 2.5 cm and angulation of more than 15°.

Summary

1. Delayed union, as defined by failure of full union to occur by 8 months, occurs in 6–12% of patients.
2. Non-union occurs in approximately 1% of femoral shaft fractures.
3. Refracture occurs in approximately 4% of femoral shaft fractures. The literature suggests that two-thirds of these are avoidable.
4. Shortening of 2 cm or more occurs in approximately 11% of patients with femoral shaft fractures. It is more common after conservative treatment (28%) than after intramedullary nailing (6%). Shortening in excess of 2 cm is usually associated with gait impairment.
5. Angular deformities, except where associated with shortening of more than 2 cm, were not usually symptomatic.
6. In Kootstra's (1973) series 40% of patients with external rotation deformities of 20° or more were symptomatic, while only 1 of the 5 patients with internal rotation deformities of 20° or more was symptomatic. In none of the patients with rotational deformities was there evidence of osteoarthritis of the knee joint (follow-up 2–11 years).
7. The incidence of impaired knee function (flexion less than 90°) is higher after conservative treatment (17%) than after operative treatment (0–5%).
8. The average time lost from work following a femoral fracture was 9 months. It was slightly less (7 months) in those patients who underwent operative treatment.
9. Following severely comminuted or segmental femoral fractures the mean time lost from work was 13.5 months.
10. Only 1% of patients were unable to return to work, while 2.5% were forced to change their job as a result of their femoral fracture.

SUPRACONDYLAR/INTERCONDYLAR FRACTURES

Hohl (1986) pointed out that fractures of the supracondylar and intercondylar regions of the femur inevitably lead to some functional sequelae ranging from loss of knee movement to instability, pain, weakness and traumatic arthritis. The AO classification (Muller et al 1979) is most commonly used to categorize these fractures.

Laros (1979) reviewed the literature up to that time on the clinical results following supracondylar fractures of the femur. He carefully analysed the available reports to enable comparison of results to be made from series to series. Results were graded as acceptable if they fell within the excellent–good–fair rating of Schatzker et al (1974), as follows:

Excellent
  Full extension

Flexion loss less than 10°
No varus, valgus or rotational deformity
No pain
Perfect joint congruity
Good
Not more than one of the following:
Loss of length not more than 1.2 cm
Less than 10° varus or valgus
Flexion loss not more than 20°
Minimal pain
Fair
Any *two* criteria from the good category

Failures (i.e. unacceptable results) were those with 90° or less flexion, varus or valgus deformity greater than 15°, joint incongruity and disabling pain, no matter how perfect the X-ray.

These figures give an indication of the *overall* incidence of acceptable results, but there are significant variations from series to series. The results of AO internal fixation are significantly better in experienced centres where the AO principles are rigidly adhered to, as pointed out by Schatzker & Lambert (1979). These authors also point out that even in centres of excellence if the AO principles are not rigidly adhered to the results are much less satisfactory. Some of the less satisfactory results of operative treatment analysed by Laros (1979) covered the period 1940 to 1960 when attitudes to open reduction and available implants were less sophisticated than those currently in use.

The overall incidence of acceptable results in 535 cases reviewed by Laros (1979) was 62%. The best results (100% acceptable) were reported by Schatzker (1979) following operative fixation with rigid adherence to AO principles. The worst results (31% acceptable) were reported by Neer et al (1967) following internal fixation using blade plates, Rush nails, plates and bolts and various combinations of wire, bolts and screws. The overall incidence of acceptable results was 64% of 254 patients treated operatively and 60% of 281 patients treated conservatively in this review. The overall incidence of non-union in this group of patients was 6% with no significant difference between operative and non-operative treatment.

Egund & Kolmert (1982) carried out a detailed analysis of the late results in 62 patients with distal femoral fractures. Their paper is worth referring to in an attempt to predict the future outlook for individual patients. Their conclusions were as follows:

1. The most significant predictor of osteoarthritis was a step in the articular surface exceeding 3 mm. The relationship of angular deformity to osteoarthritis was not clear.
2. Osteoarthritis most commonly affected the patellofemoral joint (14 of 62 cases: 22%) rather than the tibiofemoral joint (3 of 62 cases: 5%).

The patellofemoral joint requires careful assessment at follow-up and in medicolegal reports.

Behrens et al (1986) emphasized the importance of reconstructing the articular surface, and found a much lower incidence of osteoarthritis in articular fractures where there had been surgical reconstruction of the joint surface, compared to those treated non-operatively. However, their criteria for the diagnosis of osteoarthritis and degree of articular incongruity in the non-operatively treated cases are not described.

An overview of the situation suggests that two-thirds of the patients have acceptable results (as defined by Laros) following supracondylar fractures of the femur. However, in favourable circumstances, particularly with articular (intercondylar) fractures, strict application of AO principles can lead to a higher proportion of acceptable results. The literature suggests that patients with comminuted fractures do less well and that older patients with osteoporotic bone have less satisfactory long-term results. Seinsheimer (1980) found that patients aged 60 or over, regardless of fracture type or treatment, consistently achieved less knee flexion than those under 60.

Summary

1. The overall incidence of acceptable results (see text) following supracondylar or intercondylar fractures of the femur treated by a variety of methods is approximately 60%.
2. The most significant predictor of osteoarthritis is the congruity of the articular surface. Incongruity of more than 3 mm is associated with a significantly increased risk of osteoarthritis.
3. The patellofemoral joint requires careful assessment following supracondylar or intercondylar fractures of the femur, as osteoarthritis may occur there in up to 20% of cases.

FRACTURES IN CHILDREN

Subtrochanteric fractures

Velasco & Comfort (1978) reported on 10 subtrochanteric fractures in children. They were all treated conservatively and 8 out of 10 had good results. The 2 unsatisfactory results were due to a fixed rotational deformity in 1 child and shortening of 2.5 cm in another. They classed a good result as:

1. Full pre-injury activity achieved.
2. Minimal or no pain.
3. Hip flexion of 90° or more.
4. Rotational deformity of 10° or less.
5. Shortening of 1.25 cm or less

Ireland & Fisher (1975) described 20 subtrochanteric fractures in children; 19 were treated non-operatively. They found that angular or rotational deformity occurred but caused no functional problem. Three children (15%) had shortening in excess of 1.25 cm and this was felt to be a particular problem in older children. A 13-year-old female with 5 cm of shortening required a contralateral femoral shortening procedure.

Femoral shaft fractures

Staheli (1984) pointed out that length malunion was the most common problem in the management of femoral shaft fractures in children. The rate of overgrowth is related to the patient's age when the femoral fracture occurs. Growth stimulation is less predictable in infancy and most active between the ages of 2 and 10 (Ogden 1987). Staheli (1984) pointed out that shortening was more common in children over the age of 10. Figure 10.3 illustrates the rate of growth following a femoral fracture: growth stimulation is most active in the first 6 months after injury but may persist for 2 years or more.

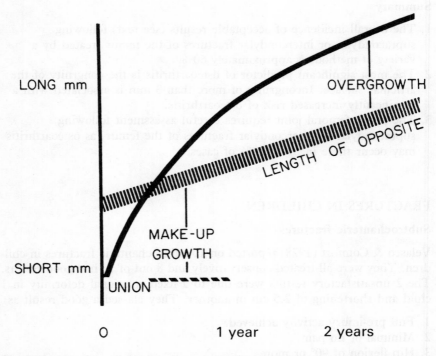

Fig. 10.3 Rate of growth following femoral shaft fracture in children. The fractured femur is initially short from overriding at union. Growth acceleration results in 'make-up' growth and in some cases overgrowth occurs (from Staheli 1984, with permission)

Shapiro (1981) found a mean femoral overgrowth of 0.92 cm in 74 patients with femoral shaft fractures, while Clement & Colton (1986) found an average overgrowth of 0.81 cm in 44 femoral shaft fractures. The latter authors found that overgrowth was more common in boys than girls. However, Staheli (1984) believed that as long as the leg lengths were within 1 cm of each other there would be no noticeable difference, while if there was a disparity of 1–2 cm it may be noticeable to the family but not the child. It is only if the leg length inequality exceeds 2 cm that both parents and child are aware of it.

There is no study encompassing all the interacting factors following the childhood femoral shaft fracture and relating these to leg lengths at skeletal maturity. Final leg length is a function of the age of the child, the type of fracture and particularly the degree of overlap accepted on traction during treatment of the fracture. The long-term effects of minor degrees of limb length inequality are not clear, but, as pointed out by Staheli (1984), it seldom produces structural scoliosis but may produce a slight asymmetry of gait and aggravate the common back pain problem of adult life. Malkawi et al (1986) reported an incidence of 2% (3 of 141) leg length inequality of over 1 cm in a group of patients followed for 2–10 years after treatment on skin traction.

Acceptable amounts of angular malunion in children's femoral fractures are controversial. Malkawi et al (1986) accepted 20° of initial angulation in the frontal (coronal) plane and 30° of initial angulation in the lateral (sagittal) plane in the expectation that remodelling would occur. Using the classification of Anderson (1967) that 0–5° of final angulation is excellent alignment, 5–10° of final angulation is satisfactory alignment and over 10° is unsatisfactory alignment, they found that 74% of their 141 cases had excellent alignment, 18% had satisfactory alignment and 8% had unsatisfactory alignment at final assessment 2–10 years after injury.

Brouwer et al (1981) considered the long-term incidence of rotational deformities following femoral shaft fractures in childhood, with a 27–32-year follow-up. They studied 50 cases and found a persistent rotational difference of more than 10° between the normal and the affected side in 6 cases, and in these cases it was asymptomatic. Moreover, in the long-term follow-up there was no evidence that persistent rotational deformity led to premature osteoarthritis.

Non-union or delayed union is very uncommon in childhood femoral fractures and as Blount (1955) pointed out, when they occur they are usually seen in patients who have had open procedures complicated by infection.

Epiphyseal damage can result from treatment. Anterior proximal tibial growth arrest with secondary recurvatum deformity has been reported following tibial skeletal traction (Van Meter & Branick 1980). Coxa valga can occur if intramedullary nailing is carried out in the child with an open greater trochanteric epiphysis (Staheli 1984).

Fractures involving the distal physis

Riseborough et al (1983) recognized that fracture separation of the distal femoral physis could lead to lower limb length discrepancy, angular deformity and reduced knee movement. It may also result in acute vascular or neurological injury. Ogden (1987) and Czitrom et al (1981) reported that growth at this physis contributes 40% to overall leg length.

Roberts (1984) believed that the prognosis for separation of the distal femoral physis was usually excellent. Czitrom et al (1981) reviewed 41 cases and found that results were good or excellent in 28 (68%). Good or excellent results implied minimal or no symptoms, minimal loss of motion, no ligamentous laxity, angular deformity of less than 5° and shortening of less than 1.5 cm.

Riseborough et al (1983) studied 66 children but did not feel that their incidence of complications was a true reflection because many were referred secondarily with growth problems. They reported that growth problems correlated well with the severity of the trauma. Growth problems were seen in each of the Salter–Harris groups (1963). They found that fractures in the age group 2–11 years were associated with the most severe trauma and the poorest prognosis. Injuries in patients over the age of 11 were usually caused by less extensive trauma — often sports injuries — and were associated with a lesser incidence of growth disturbance. Children under the age of 2 did not develop severe growth problems in this series.

Roberts (1984) reviewed the recent literature on this injury and found a 19% incidence of angular deformity greater than 5°, a 24% incidence of leg length discrepancy greater than 2 cm and a 16% incidence of knee stiffness (although the precise criteria for knee stiffness were not defined).

Controversy exists over the predictive value of the Salter–Harris classification. Czitrom et al (1981) found it useful, while Lombardo & Harvey (1977) felt that it was not valuable.

The final prognosis in these injuries is influenced by the mechanism and severity of injury, the amount of initial displacement, the adequacy of reduction, the classification of the injury and the time remaining to physeal closure.

Summary

1. Subtrochanteric fractures in children are usually managed conservatively and good results occur in over 80% of cases. The incidence of shortening in excess of 1.25 cm is approximately 13%.

2. Long-term results of femoral shaft fractures in children are usually good, with a 2% incidence of leg length inequality greater than 1 cm and an 8% incidence of angular deformity in excess of 10°. Rotational deformities in excess of 10° occurred in 12% of patients but were not symptomatic and did not appear to predispose the hip or knee joint to

premature degenerative change when followed for 27 to 32 years.
3. Approximately two-thirds of patients with injuries involving the distal femoral physis achieve good or excellent results (see text). Long-term results tend to be poorer in children aged between 2 and 11 years who sustain severe trauma.

SPECIAL GROUPS

Femoral shaft fracture with ipsilateral hip injury

Kootstra (1973) suggested that injury to the ipsilateral hip occurred in approximately 5% of femoral shaft fractures and stressed the importance of obtaining pelvic X-rays routinely in all cases of femoral shaft fractures.

Associated hip injuries may be of three types: proximal femoral fracture, acetabular fracture or hip dislocation. In Kootstra's series proximal femoral fracture occurred in 11 of 329 patients (3.4%) while acetabular fracture occurred in 5 of 329 patients (1.5%) and hip dislocation occurred in 1 of 329 (0.3%).

The additional variable of further injury with added treatment options and the small numbers of cases reported in the literature make it difficult to give clear prognostic guidelines. There is no doubt that the single most important factor is early recognition of the hip injury. Swiontkowski et al (1984) found that one-third of associated femoral neck fractures were missed at initial assessment. Dehne & Immermann (1951) found that 9 of 16 (56%) hip dislocations were missed at initial assessment when associated with a femoral shaft fracture. This correlates with Lyddon & Hartmann's (1971) observation that 50–54% of dislocations were initially unrecognized.

In these combined injuries prognosis has to be given on the basis of the individual injuries with due consideration made for the increased incidence of complications which may occur following late recognition of a hip dislocation or subcapital fracture (see Chapter 9).

Swiontkowski (1987) reviewed the orthopaedic literature and found 176 cases with proximal femoral fractures in association with femoral shaft fractures. He found an incidence of only 5% avascular necrosis of the femoral head, and suggested that this relatively low incidence occurred because the majority of energy causing the fracture was dissipated at mid-shaft level. This incidence may be falsely low, as the follow-up in some series was only 1 year and Swiontkowski suggested that the true incidence is probably 10–15%.

Femoral shaft fracture with fracture of the ipsilateral patella

Ipsilateral patellar fracture was found in 1.7% of Dencker's (1963) large series and 5.8% of Kootstra's (1973) series. Treatment methods are diverse (i.e. fixation versus patellectomy) and there are insufficient numbers to draw firm conclusions on the prognosis. The conclusion from Kootstra's work is that the results are less satisfactory when femoral shaft and patellar fracture are combined than when either occurs in isolation.

Femoral shaft fracture with fracture of the ipsilateral tibia

Again it is only possible to generalize on prognosis following combined tibial and femoral injuries because of the large number of variables involved and the small number of reports on the subject. Karlstrom & Olerud (1977) and Fraser et al (1978) reported follow-up on 87 patients using the same criteria for assessment of end-results, as shown in Table 10.8.

Table 10.8 Criteria for assessment of end-results in ipsilateral femoral and tibial fractures (after Karlstrom & Olerud 1977, with permission)

Criterion	Excellent	Good	Acceptable	Poor
Subjective symptoms from thigh or leg	Nil	Intermittent slight symptoms	More severe symptoms impairing function	Considerable impairment at rest
Subjective symptoms from knee or ankle joint	Nil	Same as above	More severe symptoms impairing function	Considerable impairment at rest
Walking ability	Unimpaired	Same as above	Walking distance restricted	Cane, crutches or other support
Work and sports	Same as before accident	Given up some sport; work as before accident	Change to less strenuous work	Permanent disability
Angulation, rotational deformity, or both	0	<10°	10–20°	>20°
Shortening	0	<1 cm	1–3 cm	>3 cm
Restricted joint mobility (hip, knee or ankle)	0	<10° at ankle <20° at hip, knee or both	10–20° at ankle 20–40° at hip, knee or both	>20° at ankle >40° at hip, knee or both

Both groups found that the worst results occurred in patients who had conservative treatment of both fractures, agreeing with the earlier work of Ratliff (1968). The 87 patients were divided into three groups according to their treatment.

Group I: both fractures rigidly internally fixed.
Group II: one fracture rigidly fixed; the other treated conservatively.
Group III: both fractures treated conservatively.

The mean follow-up of Karlstrom & Olerud (1977) was 2 years 9 months, while Fraser et al (1978) reported a mean follow-up of 5 years. Patients in group I were reported to be back at work in a mean time of 6 months by Karlstrom & Olerud and in 11 months by Fraser et al. Patients in group III returned to work in 15 and 21 months respectively in the two reports. The end-results in these patients are summarized in Table 10.9.

Table 10.9   End-results after ipsilateral femoral and tibial fractures in 87 patients reported by Karlstrom & Olerud (1977) and Fraser et al (1978). Results according to criteria of Karlstrom & Olerud (see Table 10.8)

	Excellent	Good	Acceptable	Poor
Group I (24)	7	8	8	1
Group II (31)	3	7	16	5
Group III (32)	0	9	13	8
Total (87)	10 (12%)	24 (28%)	37 (43%)	14 (16%)

The overall incidence of good or excellent results is 40%, with 62% good or excellent in group I and 28–33% good or excellent in groups II and III. Fraser et al (1978) pointed out that there was a higher incidence of chronic osteomyelitis in patients who had both fractures internally fixed.

Summary

1. Early recognition of ipsilateral hip injury requires a high level of clinical suspicion. The incidence of avascular necrosis of the femoral head following associated femoral neck fracture is probably 5–15%.
2. In ipsilateral femoral and tibial fractures the overall incidence of good/excellent results is 40% (see Table 10.9). Better results (62% good/excellent) were seen in patients who had internal fixation of both fractures.

REFERENCES

Anderson R L 1967 Conservative treatment of fractures of the femur. Journal of Bone and Joint Surgery 49A: 1371–1375
Behrens F, Ditmanson P, Hartleben P, Comfort T H, Gaither D W, Denis F 1986 Long term results of distal femoral fractures. Journal of Bone and Joint Surgery 68B: 848
Bilcher Toft M, Hammmer A 1970 Treatment of fractures of the femoral shaft. Acta Orthopaedica Scandinavica 41: 341
Blount W 1955 Fractures in children. Williams & Wilkins, Baltimore
Boyd H, Griffin L (1949) Classification and treatment of trochanteric fractures. Archives of Surgery 58: 853–866

Brouwer K J, Molenaar J C, Van Linge 1981 Rotational deformities after femoral shaft fractures in childhood: a retrospective study 27–32 years after the accident. Acta Orthopaedica Scandinavica 52: 81–89

Carr C W, Wingo C H 1973 Fractures of the femoral diaphysis: a retrospective study of the results and costs of treatment by intramedullary nailing and by traction and spica cast. Journal of Bone and Joint Surgery 55A: 690–700

Czitrom A A, Salter R B, Willis R B Fractures involving the distal epiphyseal plate of the femur. International Orthopaedics 4: 269–277

Charnley J, Guindy A (1961) Delayed operation in the open reduction of fractures of long bones. Journal of Bone and Joint Surgery 43B: 664

Clement D A, Colton C L 1986 Overgrowth of the femur after fracture in childhood: an increased effect in boys. Journal of Bone and Joint Surgery 68B: 534–536

Dehne E, Immermann E W 1951 Dislocation of the hip combined with fracture of the shaft of the femur on the same side. Journal of Bone and Joint Surgery 33A: 731–745

Delee J C 1984 Fractures and dislocations of the hip. In Rockwood C A Jr, Green D P (eds) Fractures in adults, vol 2, edn 2. J B Lippincott, Philadephia

Delee J C, Clanton T O, Rockwood C A Jr 1981 Closed treatment of subtrochanteric fractures of the femur in a modified cast brace. Journal of Bone and Joint Surgery 63A: 773–779

Dencker H M 1963 Fractures of the shaft of the femur. Orstadius Boktryckeri, Gothenborg

Dencker H M 1964 Refracture of the shaft of the femur. Acta Orthopaedica Scandinavica 35: 158

Dencker H M 1965 Shaft fractures of the femur: a comparative study of the results of various methods of treatment in 1003 cases. Acta Chirurgica Scandinavica 130: 173–184

Egund N, Kolmert L 1982 Deformities, gonoarthrosis and function after distal femoral fractures. Acta Orthopaedica Scandinavica 53: 963

Fielding J W, Cochran G, Van B, Zickel R E 1974 Biomechanical characteristics and surgical management of subtrochanteric fractures. Orthopedic Clinics of North America 5: 629–649

Fraser R D, Hunter G A, Waddell J P 1978 Ipsilateral fracture of the femur and tibia. Journal of Bone and Joint Surgery 60B: 510–515

Hardy A E, White P, Williams J 1979 The treatment of femoral fractures by cast brace and early walking: a review of 79 patients. Journal of Bone and Joint Surgery 61B: 151–154

Hartmann E R, Brav E A 1954 The problem of refracture in fractures of the femoral shaft. Journal of Bone and Joint Surgery 36A: 1071–1079

Hohl M 1986 Complications of treatment of fractures and dislocations of the knee. Ch 19, Section I: Complications of fractures. In: Epps C H Jr (ed) Complications in orthopaedic surgery, vol I. 2nd edn. J B Lippincott, Philadelphia, pp 537–556

Ireland D C R, Fisher R L 1975 Subtrochanteric fractures of the femur in children. Clinical Orthopaedics 110: 157–166

Karlstrom G, Olerud S 1977 Ipsilateral fracture of the femur and tibia. Journal of Bone and Joint Surgery 59A: 240–243

Kootstra G 1973 Femoral shaft fractures in adults: a study of 329 consecutive cases with statistical analysis of different methods of treatment. Van Gorcum, Assen, The Netherlands

Laros G S 1979 Supracondylar fractures of the femur: editorial comments and comparative results. Clinical Orthopaedics 138: 9–12

Laros G S, Spiegel P G 1979 Femoral shaft fractures: editorial comment and comparative results. Clinical Orthopaedics 138: 5–9

Laubenthal R N, Smidt G L, Kettelkamp D B 1972 A quantitative analysis of knee motion during daily living. Physical Therapy 52: 32

Lombardo S J, Harvey J P 1977 Fractures of the distal femoral epiphysis: factors influencing prognosis, a review of 34 cases. Journal of Bone and Joint Surgery 59A: 742–751

Lyddon D W Jr, Hartmann J T 1971 Traumatic dislocation of the hip with ipsilateral femoral fracture. Journal of Bone and Joint Surgery 53A: 1012–1016

Malkawi H, Shennak A, Hadidi S 1986 Remodelling after femoral shaft fractures in children treated by the modified Blount method. Journal of Paediatric Orthopaedics 6: 421–429

Mooney V, Claudi B F 1984 Fractures of the shaft of the femur. In: Rockwood C A Jnr,

Green D P (eds) Fractures in adults, vol 2. J B Lippincott, Philadelphia

Morscher E, Taillard W 1965 Beinlangenunterschiede. Karger, Basle

Moulton A, Upadhyay S S, Fletcher M, Bancroft G 1984 Does an associated injury affect the outcome of a fracture of the femoral shaft? A statistical analysis. Journal of Bone and Joint Surgery 66B: 285

Muller M E 1967 Vorwortin Posttraumatische Aschenfehlstellungen an den unteren Extremitaten. Hans Huber Verlag, Bern, pp 7–8

Muller M E, Allgower M, Schneider R, Willenegger H 1979 Manual of internal fixation: Techniques recommended by the AO group. 2nd edn, Springer Verlag, New York, Fig. 204, pp. 242–243

Neer C S, Grantham S A, Shelton M L 1967 Supracondylar fractures of the adult femur: a study of 110 cases. Journal of Bone and Joint Surgery 49A: 591–613

Nichols P J R 1963 Rehabilitation after fractures of the shaft of the femur. Journal of Bone and Joint Surgery 45B: 96–102

Nicod L 1967 Effets cliniques et pronostics des defauts d'axe du membre inferieur chez l'adulte, a la suite d'une consolidation vicieuse d'une fracture du membre inferieur. Posttraumatische Ashenfehlstellungen an den unteren Extremitaten. Hans Huber Verlag, Bern, pp 57–78

Ogden J A 1987 Pocket guide to pediatric fractures. Williams & Wilkins, Baltimore

Ratliff A H C 1968 Fractures of the shaft of the femur and tibia in the same limb. Proceedings of the Royal Society of Medicine 61: 906–908

Riseborough E J, Barrett I R, Shapiro F 1983 Growth disturbance following distal femoral epiphyseal fracture separations. Journal of Bone and Joint Surgery 65A: 885–893

Roberts J M 1984 Fractures and dislocations of the knee. In: Rockwood C A Jnr, Wilkins K E, King R E (eds) Fractures in children, vol 3. J P Lippincott, Philadelphia

Rokkanen P, Slatis P, Vankka E 1969 Closed or open intramedullary nailing of femoral shaft fractures? A comparison with conservatively treated cases. Journal of Bone and Joint Surgery 51B: 313–323

Salter R B, Harris W R 1963 Injuries involving the epiphyseal plate. Journal of Bone and Joint Surgery 45A: 587–622

Schatzker J, Lambert D C 1979 Supracondylar fractures of the femur. Clinical Orthopaedics 138: 77–83

Schatzker J, Horne G, Waddell J 1974 The Toronto experience with the supracondylar fracture of the femur 1966–1972. Injury 6: 113

Seimon L P 1964 Refracture of the shaft of the femur. Journal of Bone and Joint Surgery 46B: 32–39

Seinsheimer F 1978 Subtrochanteric fractures of the femur. Journal of Bone and Joint Surgery 60A: 300–306

Seinsheimer F 1980 Fractures of the distal femur. Clinical Orthopaedics 153: 169–179

Shapiro F 1981 Fractures of the femoral shaft in children. The overgrowth phenomenon. Acta Orthopaedica Scandinavica 52: 649–655

Staheli L T 1984 Fractures of the shaft of the femur. In: Rockwood C A Jnr, Wilkins K E, King R E (eds) Fractures in children, vol 3. J P Lippincott, Philadelphia

Swiontkowski M F 1987 Ipsilateral femoral shaft and hip fracture. Orthopedic Clinics of North America 18: 73–84

Swiontkowski M F, Hansen S T, Kellam J 1984 Ipsilateral fractures of the femoral neck and shaft: a treatment protocol. Journal of Bone and Joint Surgery 66A: 260–268

Trafton P G 1987 Subtrochanteric–intertrochanteric femoral fractures. Orthopedic Clinics of North America 18: 59–71

Van Meter J, Branick R 1980 Bilateral genu recurvatum after skeletal traction. Journal of Bone and Joint Surgery 62A: 837–839

Velasco R U, Comfort T H 1978 Analysis of treatment problems in subtrochanteric fractures of the femur. Journal of Trauma 18: 513–523

Waddell J P 1979 Subtrochanteric fractures of the femur: a review of 130 patients. Journal of Trauma 19: 582–592

Watson H K, Campbell R D, Wade P A 1964 Classification and complications of adult subtrochanteric fractures. Journal of Trauma 4: 457–480

Wickstrom J, Corban M S, Vise G T 1968 Complications following intramedullary nailing of 324 fractured femurs. Clinical Orthopaedics 60: 103–113

Wile P B, Panjabi M M, Southwick W O 1983 Treatment of subtrochanteric fractures with a high angle compression hip screw. Clinical Orthopaedics 175: 72–78

Winquist R A, Hansen S T Jr, Clawson D K 1984 Closed intramedullary nailing of femoral fractures: report of 520 fractures. Journal of Bone and Joint Surgery 66A: 529–539

Winter W G, Combs C R, Lewis N V 1979 Zickel subtrochanteric fracture fixation. Orthopedic Transactions 3: 256

Zickel R E 1976 An intramedullary fixation device for the proximal part of the femur. Journal of Bone and Joint Surgery 58A: 866–872

Zickel R E, Unis G L, Bercik R 1985 Subtrochanteric fractures of the femur. Orthopedic Transactions 9: 419

11. The knee

T. D. Bunker

INTRODUCTION

Prognosis following soft tissue injury of the knee is difficult for several reasons. The anatomy of the knee is extremely complex. Because the knee lacks bony congruity, stability has to be achieved by three means — the packing shape of the menisci, a complex system of ligaments, and a system of dynamic stabilizers in the form of musculotendinous units which cross the joint.

Any combination of injury to the menisci, the primary, and the secondary restraints of the knee may occur simultaneously. Fortunately certain patterns of injury are common and the long-term effects of these are known.

There has been a vast increase in our understanding of knee bio-mechanics, including the function of the primary and secondary restraints, and their modes of failure, and how this correlates with clinical symptoms and signs. For instance pivot shift was only rediscovered in 1972 (Galway et al 1972) and the role of anterior cruciate failure in pivot shift instability was debated until 1981 (Lipke et al 1981). Arthroscopy has brought about an increase in the accuracy of diagnosis following knee joint injury.

All these factors have contributed to changes in management, for instance from the philosophy of widespread meniscectomy to meniscal conservation. Such advances are bound to continue and this may mean that concepts and prognosis expounded within this chapter could well change over the next decade.

Surgical intervention itself changes the prognosis and adds to our knowledge so that the whole subject is continually evolving. Surin (1985) identified 341 publications on the treatment of the anterior cruciate in 7 years.

Finally knee function and radiographic changes are not directly related. This allows different interpretations to be made of certain classic texts, according to whether more emphasis is put upon knee function or radiographic appearance.

This chapter can only attempt to present the facts in an unbiased form and in such a manner as to help you whenever you have to make a prognosis upon any particular knee injury.

291

LIGAMENT INJURIES

Classification

In 1976 Hughston et al developed a classification of knee instability based on clinical examination. Instabilities are divided into straight and rotatory instability (Table 11.1).

Table 11.1   Hughston classification of knee instability (from Hughston et al 1976)

Instability	Test
Straight	
Medial	Abduction test
Lateral	Adduction test
Posterior	Posterior drawer sign (PDS)
Anterior	Anterior drawer sign (ADS)
Rotatory	
Anteromedial	Abduction stress at 30°
	ADS in external rotation
Anterolateral	Jerk test, pivot shift test
	Flexion rotation drawer sign (Noyes)
	ADS in neutral
Posterolateral	External recurvatum test
	Reversed pivot shift test
	Adduction stress at 30°

Straight instability

Medial instability. This is caused by a tear of the medial collateral ligament. It is demonstrated by a positive abduction stress test at 30° flexion. There is no rotation between the tibia and femur.

Lateral instability. This is caused by a tear of the lateral complex. It is demonstrated by a positive adduction stress test at 30° of flexion. There is no rotation between the femur and tibia.

Posterior instability. This is caused by a tear of the posterior cruciate and posterior capsule, in particular the posterior oblique ligament and the arcuate ligament. It is demonstrated by a positive posterior drawer with no rotation.

Anterior instability. This is caused by a tear of the anterior cruciate and is demonstrated by an anterior drawer sign with no rotation. If both anteromedial and anterolateral rotatory instability are present in combination there may be apparent, but not true, straight anterior instability.

Rotatory instability

Anteromedial rotatory instability. This is caused by a tear of the posteromedial corner, including the posterior oblique ligament, often accompanied by an anterior cruciate tear. It is demonstrated by a positive abduction stress test at 30°, and a positive anterior drawer test in external rotation.

Anterolateral rotatory instability. There is some debate as to the anatomical nature of this injury. Hughston et al (1976) stated that it is caused by a tear of the middle third of the lateral capsular ligament accentuated by an anterior cruciate tear; others state that it can occur after anterior cruciate tears alone (Fetto & Marshall 1979). It is demonstrated by the pivot shift test or one of its counterparts.

Posterolateral rotatory instability. This is caused by a tear of the arcuate complex.

Combined rotatory instability

Various combinations of rotatory instability may occur together, such as posterolateral and anterolateral, or anteromedial and anterolateral.

Injury to the medial collateral structures

Anatomy and function

The commonest injury to the knee is a valgus injury. The primary restraint to such a force is the medial collateral ligament. The secondary restraints are the posterior oblique ligament, the medial gastrocnemius tendon and the three tendons of the pes anserinus. The cruciates also act as secondary restraints.

Diagnosis

Isolated injury to the medial collateral ligaments is diagnosed by tenderness over the ligament and medial joint line opening with the knee flexed to 30°, to allow the posterior capsule to slacken. As more force is applied to the knee the posterior capsule, and in particular the posterior oblique ligament, will be torn and as the force continues one or both cruciate ligaments (usually the anterior) will be torn.

Natural history of medial collateral injury

Isolated tears of the medial ligament have a good prognosis. This was shown by Indelicato (1983) who followed isolated medial ligament tears where anterior cruciate damage had been excluded by arthroscopy. At 2 years 15 of 16 treated operatively, and 17 of 20 treated in plaster had an excellent result. These findings were confirmed by Sandberg et al (1987).

Anteromedial rotatory instability

The important papers on anteromedial rotatory instability were written by Hughston & Barrett (1983) and Jokl et al (1984).

Hughston & Barrett (1983). This is a retrospective, well documented, scientific paper on 93 knees with acute anteromedial rotatory instability with a 2–20-year follow-up. The medial collateral ligament was repaired in all patients but the anterior cruciate was not repaired.

Meniscectomy was found to be the major cause of a decrease in excellent and good objective findings. Anterior cruciate rupture did not progress to instability, nor did articular degeneration occur. A total of 94% were functionally capable of returning to their pre-injury sporting level, although only 71% chose to do so.

Hughston & Barrett stated that the key to success was restoration of the meniscus, posterior oblique ligament and semi-membranosus corner. Following repair 73% had satisfactory (excellent and good) objective ratings, and 89% had satisfactory subjective ratings. Even those who were objectively rated as fair or poor due to moderate laxity or arthritis had almost normal function through the dynamic stabilizers; this was the reason for the better subjective and functional results (Table 11.2).

Table 11.2 Results of anteromedial rotatory instability (from Hughston & Barrett 1983, with permission)

	Excellent	Good	Fair	Failure
Subjective	53	30 (89% satisfactory)	6	4
Objective	19	49 (73% satisfactory)	18	7
Functional	51	32 (89% satisfacotry)	5	5

In summary, Hughston & Barrett found it was not the anterior cruciate laxity which caused deterioration in the knee but failure of other secondary restraints.

Jokl et al (1984). Twenty-eight athletic patients with acute third-degree injuries to both the medial collateral ligament and the anterior cruciate ligament were treated conservatively and followed for 3 years. Twenty had a good or excellent result. Seventeen of the 24 sportsplayers (71%) returned to sports.

Lateral compartment instability

Anatomy and function

Lateral instabilities are less common than medial laxities but are more disabling (Hughston et al 1976). It is best to consider the lateral restraints as a complex — the lateral complex. Nicholas (1973) considered that there were four parts to the lateral complex — the iliotibial tract, popliteus tendon, lateral collateral ligament and the biceps femoris tendon. Hughston et al (1976) preferred to consider the lateral complex in thirds — the anterior third (capsule from patella to the iliotibial tract), middle third (iliotibial tract), and posterior third (the arcuate complex made up of the fibular collateral ligament, arcuate ligament and popliteus tendon).

Diagnosis

The commonest lateral instability is anterolateral rotatory instability; it is diagnosed by one of the forms of pivot shift test, and since most authorities — with the exception of Hughston — agree that it is mainly an event associated with anterior cruciate disruption, it is discussed below in the section on anterior cruciate ligament injury.

Posterolateral instability is caused by rupture of the arcuate complex; it is easily missed, misdiagnosed and mistreated. It is diagnosed by the external rotation recurvatum test, posterolateral drawer test or varus instability at 30° of knee flexion.

Natural history of posterolateral rotatory instability.

The important papers on this subject are by DeLee et al (1983) and Hughston & Jacobsen (1985).

DeLee et al (1983). These authors described 12 cases with a 7-year follow-up. At operation a tear was found in the arcuate complex in all cases. Primary operative repair resulted in a stable and functional knee in 8 of 11 patients. Eight participated in recreational sport and none had their daily lives interrupted by their knee. The results are shown in Table 11.3.

Table 11.3   Results of posterolateral rotatory instability (from De Lee et al 1983)

	Good	Fair	Poor
Subjective	8	3	0
Objective	8	2	1
Functional	7	3	1

Hughston & Jacobsen (1985). These authors followed up 95 cases for more than 2 years. Prior to referral, 71 had already had 112 unsuccessful operations. The patients complained of instability with the knee 'giving way backward', or hyperextending. Results are shown in Table 11.4.

Table 11.4   Results of posterolateral rotatory instability (from Hughston & Jacobsen 1985, with permission)

	Good	Fair	Poor
Subjective	78%	22%	0
Objective	85%	14%	1%
Functional	80%	16%	4%

Anterior cruciate ligament injury

Anatomy

The anterior cruciate ligament is made up of two main bundles of fibres, the anteromedial and posterolateral bundles. Norwood & Cross (1979) describe a further, intermediate bundle. Each bundle has a particular length, direction and function and because of this each may fail separately. The ligament originates from the posteromedial surface of the lateral femoral condyle, within the intercondylar notch and runs to insert into a depressed circular dimple in front of the anterior tibial spine. The ligament receives its blood supply from the middle geniculate artery and its nerve supply from the posterior articular branch of the posterior tibial nerve.

Function

The anterior cruciate ligament is the primary restraint to anterior subluxation of the tibia on the femur. It provides 86% of the total resisting force (Butler et al 1980); secondary restraint is provided by the collateral ligaments and posterior capsule. The hamstring tendons act as dynamic stabilizers against anterior tibial subluxation.

The anterior cruciate will elongate by 57% before ultimate failure (Noyes et al 1974), although it passes its elastic limit before this, and once deformation has occurred the function of the ligament will always be impaired.

The knee can withstand anterior subluxation forces of between 300 and 450 N depending on the degree of flexion during the test (Butler et al 1980). Generally the ligament is tightest in extension, but each bundle behaves differently, and each may tear individually. The posterolateral bundle is the largest and is tense in extension. The anteromedial band is tense both in extension and in flexion.

Diagnosis

Commonly anterior cruciate ligament ruptures occur during vigorous sport, often with the knee extended. Diagnosis depends on a history which includes an injury followed by a haemarthrosis, often accompanied by a popping sound and loss of function such that the patient was unable to continue playing. Noyes et al (1980) showed that 72% of patients with a traumatic haemarthrosis had anterior cruciate tears; 28% of those had a partial tear and 44% a complete tear.

Isolated anterior cruciate ligament ruptures are rare, accounting for only 8% of injuries. Usually anterior cruciate tears occur together with other damage: 26% are part of O'Donoghue's (1973) triad of anterior cruciate tear, medial meniscus tear and medial collateral ligament tear; 29% are anterior crucial tear and medial meniscal tear; 7% are torn anterior cruciate and both menisci; 11% are anterior cruciate and medial collateral ligament and 10% comprise other combined ligamentous and meniscal lesions (Alm et al 1976).

Once the secondary restraints give way the instability will become worse. In particular it will change from a straight instability to a rotatory instability, which may be either an anterolateral instability or an anteromedial instability. These rotatory instabilities are more significant from a prognostic point of view.

If the anterior cruciate ligament, the posteromedial corner and the posterolateral corner have been disrupted then a complex pattern of rotatory instability can occur with the tibia being extremely lax and subluxing anteriorly, anteromedially and also pivot shifting, that is, having anterolateral instability.

The natural history of anterior cruciate tears

The surgical literature shows a marked controversy over the long-term results of anterior cruciate rupture. A review suggests that there are two schools of thought.

The first states that injury to the anterior cruciate ligament is 'the beginning of the end' for the knee. This was first proposed by Feagan & Curl (1976), and has been restated by Fetto & Marshall (1980), and by Noyes et al (1983).

The second school of thought states that the 'anterior cruciate-deficient knee does not exist', and that indeed knees can have an absent anterior cruciate ligament with no functional disability and little or no objective instability (Hughston & Barrett 1983), and furthermore absence of an anterior cruciate neither precludes athletic participation nor causes meniscal tears, instability or progressive joint deformity.

Which school is right? In fact both are, for the controversy is based on semantics. Both agree that isolated anterior cruciate rupture rarely exists; rather, the problem is in identifying the degree of damage to the secondary restraints. Disagreement stems from comparison of dissimilar cases. Obviously if acute injuries (including mild partial tears) are compared with chronic symptomatic tears (total rupture with secondary restraints gone) it is not surprising that different results are obtained and different conclusions drawn.

Likewise, if anteromedial rotatory instability is compared with anterolateral rotatory instability it would not be surprising if the authors came to different conclusions, for it is agreed that most chronic instability symptoms are associated with pivot shifting, which by definition occurs with anterolateral, but not anteromedial, rotatory instability. Unfortunately this is what has happened in the literature.

It is not always possible to separate the dissimilar cases, since some papers contain both types. Perhaps it is more helpful to discuss the most important papers in the literature in detail, and then to try to identify unifying concepts of factors affecting prognosis. Anteromedial rotatory instability has been discussed with injuries to the medial collateral structures (see above), as it is mostly a feature of rupture of the semimembranosus corner and only half have an associated anterior cruciate tear (Hughston & Eilers 1973, O'Donoghue 1973).

Isolated anterior cruciate instability: the literature

McDaniel and Dameron (1980, 1983, 1987). These series have often been quoted as the 'gold standard' for the natural history of anterior cruciate ligament tears. Unfortunately, as the authors themselves point out, there are many inherent problems with the study. It was a 10-year retrospective assessment of knees which had had an arthrotomy for meniscal tear in the decade prior to 1973 (pivot shift was only rediscovered in 1972). One thousand arthrotomies were reviewed; of these, only 77 were thought to have an isolated anterior cruciate tear. A total of 53 of these 77 were reviewed: 39 had a complete tear and 14 a partial tear. Seventeen had classic anteromedial instability, 30 anterolateral instability, 14 combined instability and 2 had no rotatory instability. Unfortunately 43 of the 53 knees had a meniscectomy at the initial arthrotomy, and many of the radiographic changes are post-meniscectomy changes and not a consequence of the anterior cruciate tear (Table 11.6). The 10- and 14-year follow-ups included examination of the knee and the 18-year follow-up was carried out over the telephone.

Accepting these deficiencies in the study, this paper still has the longest follow-up in the literature. At 18 years 46% had no pain, 20% had pain only following an episode of instability, 30% had barometric aching and only 8% had a constant ache.

Fifty per cent had no instability, 38% had episodes less than once a month and the rest more than once a month.

Fifty per cent were still participating in strenuous sport at the 18-year follow-up (Table 11.7); although this was less than at 10 years, part of this reduction was due to age, lack of time and desire. These findings are illustrated in Figure 11.1.

Radiographic changes were thought to be secondary to meniscectomy rather than anterior cruciate deficiency.

Giove et al (1983). Twenty-four patients with anterior cruciate tears who had been treated by a vigorous muscle rehabilitation programme were reassessed to document their stability, strength and participation in sport. Nineteen had a positive anterior drawer in external rotation, 5 did not; 5 had a positive pivot shift and 19 did not. Thus it is possible that 19 had anteromedial rotatory instability and 5 had anterolateral rotatory instability, although it is stated in the paper that no *observable* rotational instability was detected. The authors went on to say that anterolateral rotatory instability may have been masked by hamstring anticipation. The affected knee was found to be as strong and mobile as the unaffected knee. There was no difference in radiological findings in the affected and unaffected knee.

In this athletic group 'success' as far as the patient was concerned was the ability to return to sport. All the subjects were actively engaged in sport at follow-up and 59% had returned to full participation. Return to sport varied according to the nature of that sport; sports requiring quick turns had the lowest level of return, with the exception of tennis. Swimming

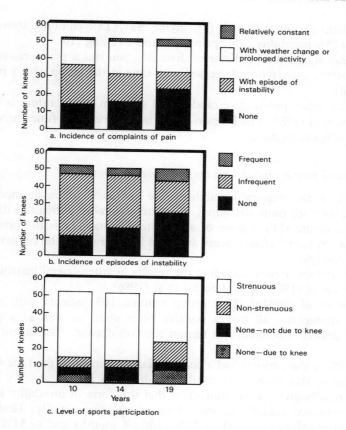

Fig. 11.1 Results for anterior cruciate-deficient knees: 18-year follow-up (from McDaniel & Dameron 1987)

appeared the easiest sport to return to, followed by golf, weight-lifting, cycling, running, tennis and skiing.

The authors concluded that the results were so good that surgery was not indicated for the primary management of anterior cruciate tears.

Sandberg et al (1987). This was an excellent controlled prospective study of 200 consecutive patients with an injury to either the anterior cruciate, medial collateral ligament or both, randomized to either surgical or non-surgical treatment. With or without surgery the results of medial collateral ligament injury were excellent.

There was no difference between surgical treament and non-operative treatment for anterior cruciate ligament injuries, except on two scores — the unoperated knees got better quicker, and the operated knees had less positive pivot shift signs.

Knee function was evaluated using the system of Lysholm and Gillquist

(1981); limp (5 points), stick (5), giving way (15), climbing stairs (10), squatting (5), instability (25), pain (25), and swelling (10).

The only significant predictor of dissatisfaction was a preoperative pivot shift. Patients' satisfaction decreased with time in the group with a positive pivot shift.

The only other prospective randomized study in the literature is that of Odensten et al (1985) which again found no difference in function with or without surgical treatment.

Anterolateral rotatory instability: the literature

Although lateral rotatory instabilities are not as common as medial instability, they are more disabling. They are also more difficult to diagnose and demonstrate. The feature of anterolateral instability is the pivot shift as the convex lateral tibial plateau subluxes forward under the convex lateral femoral condyle.

The important reports detailing the results in anterolateral instability are by Noyes et al (1983a,b) and Satku et al (1986).

Noyes et al (1983a). This group studied 103 patients with anterior cruciate disruption; all had a positive pivot shift, as well as a positive anterior drawer, Lachman and flexion rotation drawer. Assessment was at 5 years.

Only 7% of the patients had a correct diagnosis made at the time of their initial injury; this shows how subtle this diagnosis is.

Early results give a false impression that this form of instability is mild, as 82% returned initially to some form of sporting activity. However a significant re-injury occurred to 35% within 6 months and to 51% within a year. At 5 years only 35% were participating in strenuous sport.

Some 31% were disabled by just walking, 44% were disabled during daily activities and 74% during twisting or turning. A total of 30% had pain when walking, 47% experienced pain during sport and 69% had pain during strenuous sport. In all, 21% felt their knee giving way whilst walking, 33% whilst participating in sport and 65% during strenuous sport (Tables 11.5, 11.7).

Patients who had undergone menisscectomy had 2–4 times as much pain and swelling as those who had not.

Radiographic changes correlated with joint swelling but not pain. In this study radiographic changes were no more common in those who had under-

Table 11.5 Effects of anterolateral rotatory instability

	Symptomatic instability		Return to sport	
	Walking	Sport	Initial	Final (5–6 years)
Noyes et al (1983)	21%	33%	82%	35%
Satku et al (1986)	6%		63%	36%

Table 11.6 Radiographic changes of osteoarthritis following anterior cruciate injury

	Normal (%)	Minimal (%)	Moderate (%)	Severe %
'Isolated'				
McDaniel & Dameron (1980)	25	55	15	5
McDaniel & Dameron (1983)	13	55	23	9
Giove et al (1983)	38	38	18	6
Anterolateral				
Noyes et al (1983a)	54	25	19	2
Satku et al (1986)	89	11		

Table 11.7 Sporting activity following anterior cruciate injury

	No limit (%)	Reduced (%)	Nil (%)
McDaniel & Dameron (1983)	51	41	8
Giove et al (1983)	59	41	0
Noyes et al (1983)	11	71	18
Satku et al (1986)	46	/	/

gone meniscectomy than in those who had not. Radiographic changes, swelling and instability increased with length of time from injury.

Noyes et al (1983b). This study aimed to see whether physiotherapy rehabilitation and the use of a knee brace for activities could modify the poor natural history of anterolateral rotatory instability. Eighty-four patients with chronic anterior cruciate laxity and a positive pivot shift were studied.

It was found that one-third improved during therapy, one-third were unchanged and one-third became worse — Noyes' 'rule of thirds'. There was a wide spectrum of initial disability and it was not possible to predict the failures. In all, 12% required surgical repair and a further 21% were considering it.

Satku et al (1986). In this study, 97 anterior cruciate-deficient knees with a positive pivot shift were assessed at a mean of 6 years. This study agreed with Noyes et al that the initial good results were misleading in anterolateral instability. Although 63% initially returned to their sport, after 6 years 64% could not cope with the same level of sport. Some 58% had sustained damage to their menisci requiring meniscectomy after 6 years, and 6% had instability which interfered with activities of daily living (Table 11.5).

Posterior cruciate ligament injury

Anatomy and function

The posterior cruciate is a strong ligament, placed at the centre of the knee.

It originates from the lateral surface of the medial femoral condyle in the intercondylar notch and inserts into the posterior surface of the proximal tibia. It has two bands, posteromedial and anterolateral (Hughston et al 1980), and is strengthened by the meniscofemoral ligaments of Humphreys and Wrisberg.

The function of the posterior cruciate ligament is to prevent posterior subluxation of the tibia on the femur. Butler et al (1980) showed that it accounted for 95% of the passive posterior restraint of the knee. Both collaterals and the posterior capsule make up the secondary restraints, and the extensor mechanism acts as a strong dynamic restraint.

Diagnosis

Posterior cruciate injury usually occurs with a severe force applied to the front of the shin when the knee is flexed to a right angle — this is a common injury of motorcycle riders. The other method of injury is a fall from a height landing on the flexed knee, with the femur sliding forward on the tibia. Most authorities agree that the posterior drawer is always positive (Trickey 1968, Dandy & Pusey 1982). However Hughston et al (1980) stated that the posterior drawer may not be present and that the physician should rely on the sign of valgus opening or varus opening in extension.

Natural history of posterior cruciate injury

Posterior cruciate tears are rare; they account for only 8% of all ligament injuries to the knee (Lysholm & Gillquist 1981). Posterior instability is difficult to diagnose and may well have been underestimated in the past. The diagnosis is only made initially in 15% of cases (Dandy & Pusey 1982). Because of its rarity there have been few reports of the long term results in the literature, and most authorities can only muster a small number of cases.

Posterior cruciate tears: the literature

Trickey (1968). Thirteen of the 20 cases were avulsion fractures. Ten were treated surgically. The results are difficult to assess; most were left with a 10° fixed flexion contracture.

Torisu (1977). In this paper 21 cases were followed for 4 years: 12 were treated conservatively and 9 surgically; all had avulsion fractures. The results were satisfactory in all cases.

Hughston et al (1980). In this study there were 20 patients who underwent surgical repair. Good results were reported in 13, fair results in 4 and poor in 3. Fifteen knees also had a tear of the anterior cruciate. The authors stated that the unrepaired posterior cruciate was associated with poor results, but this was challenged by Hall (1980), who pointed out that this statement was based on historical results; it is also not in accord with Torisu (1977) or Dandy & Pusey (1982).

Dandy & Pusey (1982). Twenty patients were described; most were secondary referrals from other centres and therefore by definition symptomatic. Function bore no correlation to passive laxity. Eighteen felt that their symptoms did not warrant surgery. Fourteen had aching on long walks, 11 had pain on stairs and squatting, 9 had a sensation of the knee giving way on rough ground, 6 whilst coming down stairs and 4 on the flat, and 4 had swelling. Fourteen of the 17 who played sport returned to it. Results were graded as shown in Table 11.8.

Table 11.8 Results following posterior cruciate tear (from Dandy & Pusey 1982, with permission)

	Good (%)	Fair (%)	Poor (%)
Subjective	40	50	10
Objective	50	40	10
Functional	25	55	20

Ligament injury in children

Knee ligament disruption in children is extremely rare. This is because in the child the knee ligaments are strong in relation to the distal femoral physis and the proximal tibial physis. Because of this a severe injury to the skeletally immature knee usually leads to a physeal fracture and not to a ligament injury.

Clanton et al (1979) only managed to collect 9 cases. They stated that precise diagnosis in the child was difficult without an anaesthetic. Five children had avulsion of the tibial eminence. Despite repair all had objective laxity, although none were symptomatic. If meniscectomy was performed there was increased laxity.

Lipscombe & Anderson (1985) studied 24 anterior cruciate tears in adolescents. Fourteen of these patients had been referred with symptomatic instability; 8 of these complained of instability and 8 had had a re-injury. Of 17 of the patients in whom it was measured, 13 had a positive pivot shift. There were poor results if meniscectomy had been performed.

Knee dislocation

Dislocation of the knee is an extremely rare injury. Of 2 million case notes at the Mayo clinic, only 14 cases could be found. A review of 700 000 compensatable injuries by Kennedy (1963) only revealed 2 cases. The main form of dislocation is anterior displacement of the tibia; posterior dislocation is exceedingly rare as the extensor mechanism is so strong. Kennedy found on a cadaver model that anterior and posterior cruciate tears were common, but that the collaterals rarely tore but often stretched. Kennedy (1963) reviewed 22 cases and summarized that simple treatment leads to good results, but he found major vessel or nerve injury in one-half of cases. The bad results were associated with damage to the popliteal artery.

Meyers & Harvey (1971) reviewed 18 cases. There were 3 popliteal artery injuries, of which 1 required amputation. Six patients had peroneal nerve palsy; 4 were explored and of these, 3 had complete rupture of the nerve with extensive and irreparable traction injuries. Altogether the results were excellent in 1, good in 2, fair in 13 and poor in 2 (1 of whom was the amputee).

Summary

1. Knee injury is extremely common, particularly in young sporting adults.
2. Knee ligament injuries can be classified into straight and rotatory instability.
3. Isolated medial ligament injuries are common and tend to do well.
4. Lateral compartment injury is rare; with surgery 80% do well.
5. The anterior cruciate has been an enigma.
6. Anterior cruciate tears are often accompanied by medial ligament tears and medial meniscal tears.
7. There are two schools of thought on the long-term consequences of anterior cruciate tear — the 'beginning of the end' school, and the 'it'll be all right' school. These are discussed.
8. Anteromedial instability is common but not frequently disabling.
9. Anterolateral, although less common than anteromedial instability, has a worse prognosis. Disability increases with time. With muscle retraining one-third will get better, one-third stay the same and one-third get worse.
10. Anterior cruciate instability is made worse by meniscectomy.
11. Posterior cruciate injuries are rare and difficult to diagnose.
12. The long-term results following posterior cruciate tear are not as bad as had been previously thought.
13. Ligament injury in children is extremely rare as children tend to have physeal fractures instead.
14. Dislocation of the knee is extremely rare. One-half are associated with injury to the popliteal artery or peroneal nerve.

INJURIES TO THE MENISCUS

Introduction

Fairbank (1948) showed that degenerative radiological changes occurred in knees from which the meniscus had been excised. Up until this time meniscectomy had been considered a benign procedure, to such an extent that Sir Reginald Watson Jones (1956) wrote that the meniscus should be removed even if it looked normal. Over the last 30 years the critical function of the meniscus has been defined to the extent that in 1980 Goodfellow stated; 'the risks of removing a normal meniscus far exceed those of leaving a tear of the posterior third'.

Damage to the meniscus rarely occurs in isolation. In a detailed computerized study of 14 700 facts in 100 patients with meniscal tears, Bunker & Ackroyd (unpublished data) found 80 to have a second intra-articular pathology (25 cruciate tears, 34 tibial or femoral degeneration, 18 patellar degeneration, 2 loose bodies and 1 pathological plica). This incidence of second pathology confirmed the studies by Noyes et al (1980), Gillquist et al (1977) and DeHaven (1975). This means that there are no studies of 'pure' meniscal injury.

During the last decade arthroscopy has increased diagnostic accuracy, allowing more selective meniscal surgery. At the same time biomechanical research has shown the vital importance of the meniscus to knee joint function (Seedhom et al 1974), and biological research has shown the ability for peripheral repair of meniscal tears (Heatley 1980); this has been confirmed in man (Cassidy & Shaffer 1981, DeHaven 1981, Hamberg et al 1983). Even meniscal transplantation has now been reported in man.

All authors still agree that fresh traumatic tears through the body of the meniscus which are symptomatic and are affecting joint function will not heal and should undergo partial meniscectomy. This may be either arthroscopic or open.

The early results following surgery are summarized in Table 11.9. Hospital stay for arthroscopic partial meniscectomy averaged 1.3 days. A comparable stay for open partial meniscectomy was 3.3 days (Bunker & Ackroyd unpublished data). Patients were able to walk without a stick at

Table 11.9 Recovery following arthroscopic partial meniscectomy

Reference	Hospital stay (days)	Light work (days)	Heavy work (days)	Sport (days)
Bunker & Ackroyd (unpublished data)	1.3	19.7	37.2	57.4
Gillquist et al (1977)	1.7	20		71%*
Dandy (1981)	1.3	6.6	16.5	35.7
Tregonning (1983)	1.0	4.1	18.7	
Chana & Tubbs (1981)	1–4	10.7	20.8	88%*

*Percentage back at sport at 1 month.

6 days after arthroscopic meniscectomy and at 12 days for open partial meniscectomy. Return to light work was possible after 19.7 days in the arthroscopic group and after 32.9 days in the open group. Return to heavy work was possible after 37.2 days for the arthroscopic group and after 53.2 days for the open group. Return to sport was possible after 57.4 days for the arthroscopic group and 92.2 days for the open group (Bunker & Ackroyd unpublished data).

Long-term results after meniscectomy

There are many studies which show excellent early results following both open and arthroscopic meniscectomy; however, the late results tend to be more disappointing.

Gear (1967) examined the 10-year results of 50 open meniscectomies: 36% of patients were symptomatic and the commonest symptom was aching after use. Some 30% had a marked disability and this was more frequent with an associated lesion. In all, 62% had radiographic changes of osteoarthritis, of which 36% were symptomatic, and 26% asymptomatic (Table 11.10).

Table 11.10   Late results following meniscectomy

Reference	Radiographic changes of osteoarthritis	Symptomatic
Gear (1967)	62% (at 10 years)	36%
Johnston et al (1974)	74% (at 17.5 years)	55%
Tapper & Hoover (1969)		60%

Johnson et al (1974) examined 99 patients after open meniscectomy with a mean follow-up of 17.5 years. They excluded all patients with more than slight knee laxity. A total of 55% had an unsatisfactory result. Unsatisfactory results were more common in women. The results of lateral meniscectomy were worse than medial meniscectomy. Results were worse when there was anterior cruciate damage but not when there was associated medial collateral ligament injury. Damage to the articular cartilage did not influence the result. More than half had damage to the infrapatellar branch of the saphenous nerve causing sensory loss, which was irritating in 28%. In all, 74% showed one of Fairbank's (1948) radiographic changes and these changes were correlated with symptoms.

Tapper & Hoover (1969) examined 100 patients 10 years after open meniscectomy and questioned a further 100 by post. They found that 40% had a normal knee, 13% had a poor knee and the rest were in between. The younger patients and women had poorer results. There was no difference between partial and total meniscectomy. The greatest number of excellent knees occurred after excision of bucket handle tears alone. Meniscectomy was not found to preclude a man from working in highly physical occupations for a long period.

The commonest problems were effusions, weakness, pain and difficulty on kneeling. A quarter of the patients were unable to resume sports and a quarter stated that after 10 years their knees prevented them from doing some things that otherwise they would have liked to do.

Arthroscopic partial meniscectomy

Arthroscopic partial meniscectomy is still a relatively new procedure. There are no series in the world literature giving a 10-year follow-up. Dandy & Northmore Ball (1981) analysed 99 patients who had an average of 3-years follow-up. Knees without ligamentous injury had 90% excellent and good results and only 1 had a poor result. The bucket handle pattern of tear fared better than other patterns of tear, with 73% excellent results compared to 52% for the others. Results were worse in women and in the elderly. There was no statistical difference between medial and lateral arthroscopic meniscectomy. In only 2 patients did the knee interfere with their occupation.

It will take several more years before we are in a position to decide whether the long-term results of arthroscopic partial meniscectomy are superior to open meniscectomy. There is presently a body of opinion which states that the results of arthroscopic partial meniscectomy will be better than open meniscectomy. This is based on biomechanical theory, *but the facts are that the long-term results of partial and total meniscectomy are the same* (Tapper & Hoover 1969, Johnson et al 1974, Cargill & Jackson 1976).

Degenerative tears

Degenerative tears are extremely common (Smillie 1970): 60% of cadavers were found to have at least one meniscus with a cleavage tear (Noble & Hamblen 1975). The authors concluded that cleavage tears were so common in the elderly that they must usually be asymptomatic.

Cleavage tears initially appeared to be associated with arthritis in this study. However the finding that more than one-third of those with the worst arthritis had normal menisci and 18% of those with no arthritis had a cleavage tear did not add credence to a causal relationship as postulated by Frankel et al (1971). Fahmy et al (1983) concluded that there was no association between degenerative tears of the meniscus (cleavage tears) and osteoarthritis or vice versa.

PATELLAR FRACTURES AND DISLOCATIONS

Patellar fractures

Patellar fractures account for about 1% of all fractures. They usually require surgical treatment. The fracture may be caused by direct or indirect forces, and often by a combination of both.

Fractures may be classified into:

1. Undisplaced.
2. Transverse.
3. Comminuted.

Undisplaced fractures are unusual. Transverse fractures are the commonest type; they usually occur across the centre of the patella and displace leaving a gap in the extensor mechanism. Comminuted fractures are the result of more severe injury, often with direct trauma, and are becoming more common.

In general undisplaced fractures are treated in plaster for 6 weeks, transverse fractures are treated by internal fixation usually with a tension band technique, and comminuted fractures are treated by partial or total patellectomy.

Prognosis

Osteosynthesis with tension band wire

Transverse fractures. Aglietti (1984) reported 80 patients treated by tension band wiring; the results were evaluated by the Hospital for Special Surgery (HSS) knee score. In all, 40% had an excellent result, 45% good, 10% fair, and 5% poor. The patients with poor results had infection (1), pseudarthrosis (2) or pain (1).

A perfect reduction was obtained in 89% and there was a step or gap of over 2 mm in the rest. All had united at 60 days, with the exception of the 2 pseudarthroses. There was no correlation between degree of reduction and arthritis. Age had no influence on the results. Fractures near the ends of the bone did slightly better than mid-patellar fractures.

Muscle strength was normal in 72%. There was an extension lag in 4% and 59% had a full range of flexion. There was no pain in 79%, moderate pain in 21% and severe in 1 case.

Levack et al (1985) reported 30 patients followed for 6.2 years after treatment by osteosynthesis. Only 14 were treated by tension band wiring and of these, 7 were rated good, 5 fair and 2 poor. The results correlated with the quality of reduction and fixation. The failures in this group were due to pain and this correlated with degenerative changes seen on radiographs. Levack et al stated that it took 8 months to regain full strength following this procedure, and that results were optimum at this stage, whereas patients having undergone patellectomy continued improving for up to 2 years. The results are summarized in Table 11.11

Comminuted fractures. Dissatisfaction with patellectomy has led some authors to attempt osteosynthesis even in comminuted fractures. Böstman (1982) reviewed 21 patients. A step of 1–2 mm did not affect results, but 2 patients with a greater step were unsatisfactory. The 4 patients who had damage to the femoral condyles observed at surgery all had bad results.

Results after patellectomy

For 50 years the results of patellectomy have been controversial. The controversy started in 1937 when Brooke reported good results from patellectomy. Hey Groves could not believe such good results and personally examined 8 of Brooke's patients and had to agree with Brooke. However, 50 years on Hey Groves' initial doubts have been validated. Results are summarized in Tables 11.11 and 11.12. Only 50% of patients undergoing patellectomy will have an acceptable result.

Table 11.11 Results following surgery for patellar fractures

Reference	Percentage			
	Excellent	Good	Fair	Poor
Osteosynthesis				
Aglietti (1984)	40	45	10	5
Levack et al (1985)	0	50	36	14
Total	29	46	17	7
Patellectomy				
Aglietti (1984)	22	33	33	12
Levack et al (1985)	0	60	20	20
Wilkinson (1977)	23	39	0	39
Einola et al (1976)	0	21	64	15
Böstman (1982)	0	50	0	50
Mishra (1972)	17	53	20	10
Total	10	40	25	25

The main complaints following patellectomy are of weakness and instability, in contrast to osteosynthesis where the main complaint is pain (Levack et al 1985). It can take up to 2 years to regain full strength after patellectomy; the results tend to improve with time. This is confirmed by Duthie & Hutchinson (1958) and Einola et al (1976).

Weakness (Table 11.12). The greatest subjective complaint following patellectomy is weakness (Einola et al 1976, Levack et al 1985). Sutton et al (1976) measured the forces following patellectomy. The quadriceps force of the normal knee was found to be 143 kg; after partial patellectomy this dropped to 131 kg, and after total patellectomy to 78 kg. This was confirmed by Einola et al (1976) who found that in only a quarter of patients was the quadriceps force equal to or better than 75% of the undamaged knee. In particular, weakness led to difficulty when descending stairs.

Pain is less of a feature following patellectomy; however, aching on exercise was found in 43% of patients by Einola et al (1976).

Table 11.12   Poor results following patellectomy

	Percentage			
	Weakness	Stiffness	Pain	Osteoarthritis
Sutton et al (1976)	41	18		
Mishra (1972)	13	23	33	16
Einola et al (1976)	97	64	25	50

Osteoarthritis. Bruce & Walmsley (1942) found that patellectomy in the rabbit inevitably led to arthritis; this has led to vigorous debate in the subsequent literature. Wilkinson (1977) believed that there was no evidence of this inevitability in man. In Mishra's series (1972) 5 patients had femoral condylar arthritis, but the average age of these patients was 66 years. In Einola et al's (1976) series, only 4 of 18 cases where radiographs immediately following fracture were available (this was a 20-year follow-up and some of the original radiographs could not be traced) showed osteoarthritic changes. In 1 of these cases the changes had increased and 3 had appeared during the observation period, at 1, 4 and 10 years respectively.

Calcification of the tendon has often been noted following patellectomy. Wilkinson (1977) showed no correlation between calcification and results — a finding confirmed by Mishra (1972) and Einola et al (1976).

Patellar dislocation

Compared to recurrent dislocation of the patella there is a paucity of literature on acute traumatic dislocation and its sequelae. Predisposing abnormalities are said to be as follows:

1. Lateral insertion of the patellar tendon.
2. Excessive external tibial torsion.
3. Internal femoral torsion.
4. High patella (patella alta).
5. Shallow patellofemoral groove.
6. Weak patellar retinaculum.
7. Weak vastus medialis.
8. Genu valgum.
9. Genu recurvatum.
10. Hypermobile patella (Rockwood & Green 1975).

Many of these are abnormalities associated with recurrent dislocation.

Following acute dislocation it is difficult to calculate the risk of recurrence. Cofield & Bryan (1977) found that 27% of children with acute dislocation of the patella required further surgery.

Rorabeck & Bobechko (1976) showed that 5% of acute dislocations were associated with osteochondral fractures. In their series, 16% redislocated within 6 months. McManus et al (1979) confirmed this; they showed that 1 child in 6 developed recurrent dislocation, 2 in 6 had minor symptoms and the remainder were asymptomatic.

Radiographs cannot be used to predict those children who will develop recurrence as the majority have signs of patellofemoral dysplasia.

TIBIAL PLATEAU FRACTURES

Classification

Controversy still surrounds the management of tibial plateau fractures. Opposing views are held regarding the relative merits of closed or surgical treatment. It is not the intention to discuss here fracture management, but only to describe the results of treatment and those features which lead to good and poor results.

Most tibial plateau fractures occur as the result of a fall. One-third of fractures are caused by the bumper of a car hitting the side of the pedestrian's leg, which accounts for the old term of bumper or fender fracture. Roberts (1968) stated that the usual method of injury was a combination of axial loading and valgus, with the knee straight, causing the lateral femoral condyle to crush or split the lateral tibial plateau.

There are many ways of classifying tibial plateau fractures, as shown in Figure 11.2. The commonest classification is that of Hohl & Luck (1956):

  I: Undisplaced (24%).
 II: Local compression (26%).
III: Split compression (26%).
 IV: Total condylar depression (10%).
  V: Split (3%).
 VI: Comminuted (10%).

Assessment of results

Most papers use the modification of Hohl & Luck's (1956), grading system (Table 11.13) into excellent, good, fair and poor. Unfortunately, Hohl & Luck's classification of results is no longer acceptable in terms of modern fracture care. A knee with detectable degenerative change, excessive lateral laxity, or a range of movement of only 5–90° can no longer be called good, as it was in the 1950s. This should be noted by the present-day fracture surgeon called upon to make a prognosis on the results of tibial plateau fractures. Assessment of deformity by tomography or computerized tomography scanning is likely to necessitate a reappraisal of current concepts on the relationship between depression and outcome in the near future.

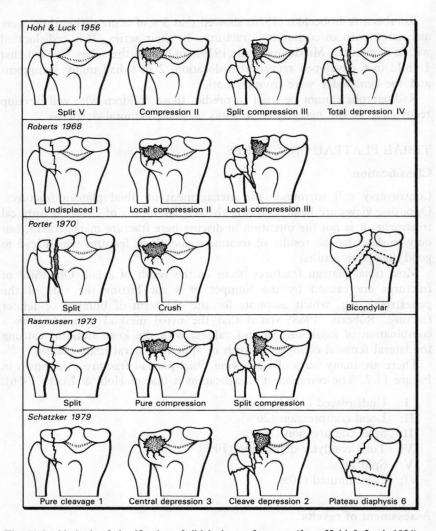

Fig. 11.2   Methods of classification of tibial plateau fractures (from Hohl & Luck 1956)

Prognostic factors

Age

Hohl & Luck (1956) found no significant difference between functional results and age. This finding was confirmed by Schatzker et al (1979).

Joint surface depression

There is still controversy as to whether residual joint surface depression

Table 11.13 Criteria used for grading 227 tibial condylar fractures (from Hohl & Luck 1956, with permission)

Anatomical grade

Excellent
(All of the following)
1. Normal valgus within 5°
2. Restoration of displacement within 3 mm
3. No degenerative joint changes

Good
(Not more than 1 of the following)
1. Valgus of more than 5°
2. Minimal degenerative joint changes

Fair
(Not more than 2 of the following)
1. Valgus deformity of more than 10°
2. Moderate degenerative joint changes
3. Lack of fracture reduction

Poor
(All of the following)
1. Moderate or severe degenerative joint changes
2. Lack of fracture reduction
3. Valgus deformity of more than 10°

Functional grade

Excellent
(All of the following)
1. Full extension of the knee
2. 120° range of motion or more
3. No abnormal abduction rocking
4. Normal strength and endurance
5. Occasional ache permissible

Good
(Not more than 1 of the following)
1. Lack of knee extension beyond 170°
2. Excessive lateral mobility
3. Mild aching each day
4. 90° total range of motion
5. Weakness or easy fatigue

Fair
(Not more than 2 of the following)
1. Lack of knee extension more than 170°
2. 75° range of motion
3. Discomfort for ordinary activity
4. Excessive lateral mobility

Poor
(Three or more of the following)
1. Lack of useful motion (less than 75°)
2. Unable to work
3. Pain in all activity
4. Excessive lateral mobility

seen on radiographs, corresponds with the actual cartilaginous surface of the tibia following plateau fracture. On the one hand Hohl & Luck (1956) created depressed tibial fractures in rhesus monkeys and showed both macroscopically and microscopically that the defect filled in with fibrocartilage. Similar observations have been made in humans with arthrography (Dovey & Heerfordt 1970) and arthrotomy (Maisel et al 1948, Reitel & Wade 1962). Drennan et al (1979) and Porter (1970) speculated that this infilling may account for good functional results in the face of radiographic abnormality. On the other hand, Schatzker et al (1979) stated that there was no evidence that articular defects could fill in.

Porter (1970) found a direct correlation between depth of depression and prognosis (Table 11.14). The results in cases with mild depression were good, whereas almost half of the patients with over 14 mm of depression had only fair or poor results. Porter also found that in patients with more than 10 mm of depression prognosis was related to the area of the plateau which had been depressed.

Table 11.14 Results of treatment related to depth of depression (from Porter 1970, with permission)

Depth	Acceptable	Unacceptable
Less than 10 mm	28	1
10–14 mm	15	6
More than 14 mm	10	8

Hohl & Luck (1956) found that the depth of radiographic depression was related to functional results; patients with under 1 cm of depression had 77% acceptable results (excellent or good by their standards), whereas those with over 1 cm had only 61% acceptable results.

Ligament damage

In general, joint instability following plateau fracture is caused by residual joint surface depression rather than ligament rupture. This may be because the forces which cause the fracture are compressive rather than distractive. This was confirmed experimentally on cadavers by Kennedy & Bailey (1968). The recorded incidence of ligament damage shows a wide scatter from 4 to 25%.

Rasmussen & Sorenson (1973) stated that collateral ligament and cruciate tears were of minor importance compared to bony deformity. Furthermore they felt that soft tissue fibrosis around the knee which occurred during fracture healing would produce ligamentous stability.

Porter (1970) detected anterior cruciate laxity in 6 of 138 patients under review; none had been noted primarily and only 1 was significant.

Roberts (1968) stated that 5 of 9 patients in whom rupture of the medial collateral ligament was diagnosed but not repaired, had unstable knees at follow-up. Schatzker et al (1979) stated that repair of ruptured collateral ligaments was essential for stability.

Meniscal injury

The incidence of meniscal injury varies from 17 to 85%. All authors agree that the meniscus should be preserved if at all possible. Schatzker et al (1979) found 16 meniscal tears in 70 patients: 14 of these tears were peripheral and could be repaired; only 2 were through the body of the meniscus. In one patient the fracture was irreducible due to interposition of the torn lateral meniscus.

Long-term results of tibial plateau fractures

Undisplaced fractures

Both Schatzker et al (1979) and Hohl & Luck (1956) reported 100%

excellent or good results following undisplaced fractures treated in plaster. Hohl & Luck's excellent and good results dropped to 90% if the knee was immobilized for more than 1 month. Anatomical results were between 97 and 100% excellent and good following undisplaced fracture.

Displaced fractures

As different classifications have been used in the major series it is more instructive to discuss each series in detail. Particular emphasis will be placed on the poor results in each series.

Hohl & Luck (1956). These authors reviewed 227 patients after 2–13 years using their criteria. In local depression fractures 70% had excellent or good function, despite the radiographs being acceptable in only 6%. Bony depression of over 1 cm caused a valgus deformity in 58% which reduced the level of excellent or good function to 61% in this group. Open reduction improved the appearance of the joint, as seen on radiographs, but did not improve the functional result.

In 1956 methods of internal fixation were not as refined as they are today. Hohl & Luck concluded that 1 cm of joint surface depression was an indication for surgery. A total of 79% of fractures with depression had excellent or good function.

Roberts (1968). He assessed 100 patients after 1–12 years: 81% of local compression fractures had excellent or good results. Poor results in this group were due to valgus deformity or stiffness. Of patients with more severe, unstable fractures, 74% had excellent or good results. Three infections occurred in the operated unstable fractures (an incidence of 12%). There were 2 peroneal nerve palsies and 1 amputation following popliteal artery damage.

Apley (1956). In this study, 60 patients were evaluated at 1–10 years by his functional method. There was no correlation between radiographic appearance and function; this was such a striking feature that Apley stated: 'Radiographs are irrelevant to treatment'. In all, 83% had excellent or good knees.

The same group was studied 8 years later and there was no deterioration in function. The patients were all treated by skeletal traction and early joint movement.

Porter (1970). Porter reviewed 68 patients at 3–13 years. Results were directly proportional to the area and depth of joint surface depression. Of those patients with less than 1 cm of joint surface depression, 97% had acceptable results. Patients with over 1 cm of depression had only 64% acceptable results (Table 11.4).

Rasmussen & Sorensen (1973). The 204 patients reviewed at an average of 7 years were assessed by these authors' own quantitative system. Although there was a slight difference between medial, lateral and bicondylar fractures, the results were not statistically significant ($p > 0.01$). In all, 87% of patients were rated excellent or good. There was a total lack of correlation between functional and anatomical results.

Burri et al (1979). These authors reviewed 278 patients who had been treated surgically, at an average of 2 years 8 months using stricter criteria than other series. Anatomical results were good but the price was poorer function. The results depended upon the surgeon; surgeons were classified as experienced if they had performed more than 7 procedures, inexperienced if less.

In the inexperienced group only 66% had excellent or good results. In this group there was a 15% infection rate; only 19% could walk over 10 km and 22% needed a stick to walk. Arthritis was present in 53–82%, but the definition of arthritis was not stated and may have been extremely strict.

In the experienced group results were much better — 97% good or acceptable — yet only 43% could walk over 10 km. The infection rate was only 0.7%.

Schatzker et al (1979). Seventy patients were functionally evaluated at 2 years 4 months. Less than half were treated by operation.

The split compression fractures had 66% excellent or good results. Joint surface depression of over 5 mm led to valgus malalignment and poor results.

In all, 80% of central depressed fractures were rated as excellent or good. The poor results were again due to valgus malalignment.

Medial plateau fractures had the worst results. They tended to occur in an older population with softer bone.

Although the surgically treated group were the worst fractures they had better functional results because of better stability and early movement.

Drennan et al (1979). These authors assessed 53 patients at an average of 4 years: 85% had excellent or good results. Of the 8 unsatisfactory results all had an unlimited walking distance, only 2 had slight pain and 2 had a fixed flexion deformity. Average flexion was 129° in the poor group. The poor results were attributed to valgus instability with an average valgus tibiofemoral angle of 12–25° (normal 7°).

Incidence of osteoarthritis in tibial plateau fractures

Rasmussen & Sorensen (1973) looked at this question in detail. They showed that there was a lack of correlation between functional and anatomical end-results (Fig. 11.3). They noted that many other studies confirmed this.

Rasmussen & Sorensen (1973) defined secondary osteoarthritis as narrowing of the joint space with or without subchondral sclerosis. A total of 26% were found to have typical changes of osteoarthritis at follow-up — although 2% of these had osteoarthritis before the injury and 2% had osteoarthritis in the other knee.

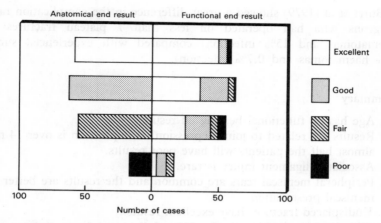

Anatomical end result   Functional end result

Excellent

Good

Fair

Poor

100   50   0   50   100

Number of cases

Fig. 11.3 Incidence of arthritis in tibial plateau fractures (from Rasmussen & Sorensen 1973, with permission).

There was a statistically significant difference between the incidence of osteoarthritis in bicondylar fractures (42%), medial fractures (21%) and lateral fractures (16%; $p < 0.01$). The incidence was also statistically correlated with alignment ($p < 0.01$). Normally aligned knees had a 13% chance of developing arthritis, valgus knees a 31% chance and varus knees a 79% chance.

Instability was also correlated with the development of osteoarthritis. Knees which were stable in extension had a 14% chance, and knees unstable in extension a 46% chance of developing osteoarthritis.

Rasmussen & Sorensen found no correlation between joint depression and radiological joint space narrowing or subchondral sclerosis. There was a link between condylar widening and osteoarthritis.

Osteoarthritis was found in 89% of patients with poor functional results, 53% with fair results and only 14% of those with excellent or good functional results.

Complications of surgery for tibial plateau fractures

Surgical repair of tibial plateau fractures requires great experience. Schatzker et al (1979) stated that it should be emphasized again and again that the results of poor open reduction are far worse than the results of poor non-operative treatment.

In the series of Schatzker et al the complication rate was 27% for those treated surgically. The most common complication was peroneal nerve palsy. It was not possible to say how many were iatrogenic, and all recovered. There were 2 infections at the graft donor site and 1 infection of the knee wound (7.3%).

Burri et al (1979) showed a great difference in the complication rate for surgeons who had operated on less than 7 plateau fractures (14% haematomas and 15% infection) compared with experienced surgeons (6% haematomas and 0.7% infection).

Summary

1. Age has no functional bearing on results.
2. Results are related to joint depression. If depression is over 14 mm, almost half the patients will have poor results.
3. Associated ligament injury is rare.
4. Peripheral meniscal tears are common and the results are better with meniscal preservation.
5. Undisplaced fractures have excellent results.
6. As judged by the old criteria, 70% of displaced fractures have excellent or good results.
7. Old criteria for assessment may not be relevant to modern practice and should be downgraded to allow for this.
8. Comparison between series is difficult.
9. Osteoarthritis is related to malalignment.

REFERENCES

Aglietti P 1984 In: Insall (ed) Surgery of the knee. Churchill Livingstone, London, pp 395–412
Alm A, Liljedahl S, Stromberg B 1976 Clinical and experimental evidence in reconstruction of the anterior cruciate ligament. Orthopedic Clinics of North America 7: 181–189
Apley A G 1956 Fractures of the lateral tibial condyle treated by skeletal traction and early mobilisation. Journal of Bone and Joint Surgery 38B: 699–707
Böstman O, Kiviluoto O, Nirhamo J 1982 Comminuted displaced fractures of the patella. Injury 13: 191–202
Brooke R 1937 The treatment of fractured patella by excision. British Journal of Surgery 24: 733–747
Bruce J, Walmsley R 1942 Excision of the patella. Journal of Bone and Joint Surgery 24: 311–325
Burri C, Bartzke G, Coldewey J, Muggler E 1979 Fractures of the tibial plateau. Clinical Orthopeadics 138: 84–93
Butler D L, Noyes F R, Grood E S 1980 Ligamentous restraints to anterior posterior drawer in the human knee. Journal of Bone and Joint Surgery 259–270
Cargill A, Jackson J P 1976 Bucket handle tear of the medial meniscus. Journal of Bone and Joint Surgery 58A: 248–251
Cassidy R E, Shaffer A J 1981 Repair of peripheral meniscal tears. American Journal of Sports Medicine 9: 209–214
Chana G S, Tubbs N 1981 Early results of arthroscopic surgery of the knee. 13: 227–229
Clanton T O, DeLee J C, Sanders B, Neidre A 1979 Knee ligament injuries in children. Journal of Bone and Joint Surgery 61A: 1195–1201
Cofield R, Bryan 1977 Acute dislocation of the patella. Results of conservative treatment. Journal of Trauma 17: 526

Dandy D J 1981 Arthroscopic surgery of the knee. Churchill Livingstone, Edinburgh
Dandy D J, Northmore Ball M D 1981 Long term results of arthroscopic partial
meniscectomy. Clinical Orthopaedics 167: 34–42
Dandy D J, Pusey R 1982 Long term results of unrepaired tears of the posterior cruciate
ligament. Journal of Bone and Joint Surgery 64B: 92–94
DeHaven K 1981 Peripheral meniscus repair. An alternative to meniscectomy. Orthopaedic
Transactions 5: 399–400
DeHaven K E, Collins H R 1975 Diagnosis of internal derangements of the knee. Journal
of Bone and Joint Surgery 57A: 802–810
DeLee J, Riley, Rockwood J 1983 Acute posterolateral rotatory instability of the knee.
American Journal of Sport Medicine 11: 199–207
Dovey H, Heerfordt F 1970 Tibial condyle fractures. Acta Chirurgica Scandinavica 137:
521
Drennan D B, Locher F G, Maylahn D J 1979 Fractures of the tibial plateau. Journal of
Bone and Joint Surgery 61A: 989–995
Duthie H L, Hutchinson J R 1958 The results of partial and total excision of the patella.
Journal of Bone and Joint Surgery 40B: 75–81
Einola S, Aho A J, Kallio P 1976 Patellectomy after fracture. Acta Orthopaedica
Scandinavica 47: 441–447
Fairbank T J 1948 Knee joint changes after meniscectomy. Journal of Bone and Joint
Surgery 30B: 664–670
Fahmy N R M, Williams E L, Noble J 1983 Meniscal pathology and osteoarthritis of the
knee. Journal of Bone and Joint Surgery 65B: 24
Feagan J A, Curl W W 1976 Isolated tears of the anterior cruciate ligament. American
Journal of Sports Medicine 4: 95–100
Fetto J F, Marshall J L 1979 The natural history and diagnosis of anterior cruciate ligament
insufficiency. Clinical Orthopaedics 147: 29–38
Frankel U M, Burstein A M, Brooks D B 1971 Biomechanics of internal derangement of
the knee. Journal of Bone and Joint Surgery 53A: 945–962
Galway R D, Beaupre A, MacIntosh D L 1972 Pivot shift, a clinical sign of anterior cruciate
instability. Journal of Bone and Joint Surgery 54B: 763
Gear M W 1967 The late results of meniscectomy. British Journal of Surgery 54: 270–272
Gillquist J, Hagberg P, Oretop N 1977 Arthroscopies in acute ligament injuries of the knee
joint. Acta Orthopaedica Scandinavica 48: 190–196
Giove T P, Miller S J, Garrick J G 1983 Non operative treatment of the torn anterior
cruciate ligament. Journal of Bone and Joint Surgery 65A: 184–192
Goodfellow J 1980 He who hesitates is saved. Journal of Bone and Joint Surgery 62B: 4–5
Hall F M 1980 Acute tears of the posterior cruciate ligament. Journal of Bone and Joint
Surgery 62A: 119
Hamberg P, Gillquist J, Lysholm J 1983 Suture of new and old peripheral meniscal tears.
Journal of Bone and Joint Surgery 65A: 193–197
Heatley F W 1980 The meniscus. Can it be repaired? Journal of Bone and Joint Surgery
62B: 397–402
Hey Groves E W 1920 The crucial ligaments of the knee joint. British Journal of Surgery
7: 505–515
Hohl M, Luck J V 1956 Fractures of the tibial condyle. A clinical and experimental study.
Journal of Bone and Joint Surgery 38A: 1001–1018
Hughston J C, Barrett G R 1983 Acute anteromedial rotatory instability. Journal of Bone
and Joint Surgery 65A: 145–153
Hughston J C, Eilers A F 1973 The role of the posterior oblique ligament in repairs of
acute medial ligament injuries of the knee. Journal of Bone and Joint Surgery 55A:
923–940
Hughston J C, Jacobsen K 1985 Chronic posterolateral instability. Journal of Bone and
Joint Surgery 67A: 351–359
Hughston J C, Andrews J R, Cross M J, Moschi A 1976 Classification of knee ligament
instabilities. Journal of Bone and Joint Surgery 58A: 159
Hughston J C, Bowden, Andrews J R, Norwood L A 1980 Acute tears of the posterior
cruciate ligament. Journal of Bone and Joint Surgery 62A: 438–450
Indelicato P A 1983 Non operative treatment of complete tears of the medial collateral
ligament. Journal of Bone and Joint Surgery 65A: 323–329

Johnson R J, Kettelkamp D B, Clark W, Leaverton P 1974 Factors affecting late results after meniscectomy. Journal of Bone and Joint Surgery 56A: 719–729

Jokl P, Kaplan N, Stovell P, Keggi K 1984 Non operative treatment of severe injuries to the medial and anterior cruciate ligaments of the knee. Journal of Bone and Joint Surgery 66A: 741–744

Kennedy J C 1963 Complete dislocation of the knee joint. Journal of Bone and Joint Surgery 45A: 889–903

Kennedy J C, Bailey W H 1968 Experimental tibial plateau fractures. Journal of Bone and Joint Surgery 50B: 1522

Levack B, Flannagan J P, Hobbs S 1985 Results of surgical treatment of fractures of the patella. Journal of Bone and Joint Surgery 67B: 416–419

Lipke J M, Janecki C T, Nelson C L et al 1981 The role of incompetence of the anterior cruciate ligament in anteromedial and anterolateral rotatory instability. Journal of Bone and Joint Surgery 63A: 954–959

Lipscombe A B, Anderson C 1985 Tears of the anterior cruciate ligament in adolescents. Journal of Bone and Joint Surgery 68A: 19–27

Lysholm J, Gillquist J 1981 Arthroscopic examination of the posterior cruciate ligament. Journal of Bone and Joint Surgery 63A: 363–366

Maisel B, Cornell N W 1948 Conservative treatment of fractures of the tibial condyles. Surgery 23: 591–598

McDaniel W J, Dameron T B 1980 Untreated ruptures of the anterior cruciate ligament. Journal of Bone and Joint Surgery 62A: 696–705

McDaniel W J, Dameron T B 1983 The untreated anterior cruciate ligament rupture. Clinical Orthopaedics 172: 158–163

McDaniel W J, Dameron T B 1987 Acute anterior cruciate ligament ruptures, is treatment really necessary? Seminars in Orthopaedics 1: 31–34

McManus F, Rang H, Heslin D J 1979 Acute dislocation of the patella in children. The natural history. Clinical Orthopaedics 139: 88–91

Meyers M H, Harvey J P 1971 Traumatic dislocation of the knee joint. Journal of Bone and Joint Surgery 53A: 16–29

Mishra U S 1972 Late results of patellectomy in fractured patella. Acta Orthopaedica Scandinavica 43: 256–263

Nicholas J A 1973 The five-one reconstruction for anteromedial instability of the knee. Journal of Bone and Joint Surgery 55A: 899–922

Noble J, Hamblen G 1975 The pathology of the degenerate meniscus lesion. Journal of Bone and Joint Surgery 57B: 180–186

Norwood L A, Cross M J 1979 Anterior cruciate ligament. American Journal of Sports Medicine 7: 23–26

Noyes F R, DeLucas J L, Torvik P J 1974 Biomechanics of anterior cruciate failure. Journal of Bone and Joint Surgery 56A: 236–253

Noyes F R, Bassett R W, Grood E S et al 1980 Arthroscopy in acute traumatic haemarthrosis of the knee. Journal of Bone and Joint Surgery 62A: 687–695

Noyes F R, Mooar P A, Matthews D S, Butler D L 1983a The symptomatic anterior cruciate deficient knee. Part 1. Journal of Bone and Joint Surgery 65A: 154–162

Noyes F R, Matthews D S, Mooar P A, Grood E S 1983 The symptomatic anterior cruciate-deficient knee, Part II. Journal of Bone and Joint Surgery 65A: 163–174

Odensten, Hamberg P, Nordin, Lysholm J, Gillquist J 1985 Surgical or conservative treatment of the acutely torn anterior cruciate ligament. A randomised study with short term follow up observations. Clinical Orthopaedics 198: 87–93

O'Donoghue D M 1973 Reconstruction for medial instability of the knee. Journal of Bone and Joint Surgery 55A: 941–955

Porter R B 1970 Crush fractures of the lateral tibial table. Journal of Bone and Joint Surgery 52B: 676–687

Rasmussen P S, Sorensen S E 1973 Tibial condylar fractures. Injury 4: 265

Reitel D B, Wade P A 1962 Fractures of the tibial plateau. Journal of Trauma 2: 337

Roberts J M 1968 Fractures of the condyles of the tibia. Journal of Bone and Joint Surgery 50A: 1505

Rockwood C A, Green D P 1975 Fractures. Lippincott, Philadelphia

Rorabeck C H, Bobechko W P 1976 Acute dislocation of the patella with osteochondral fracture. Journal of Bone and Joint Surgery 58B: 237–240

Sandberg R, Balkfors B, Nilsson B, Westlin N 1987 Operative versus nonoperative treatment of recent injuries to the ligaments of the knee. A prospective randomised study. Journal of Bone and Joint Surgery 69A: 1120–1126

Satku K, Kumar V P, Ngoi S S 1986 Anterior cruciate ligament, to council or to operate. Journal of Bone and Joint Surgery 68B: 458–461

Schatzker J, McBroom R, Bruce D 1979 The tibial plateau fracture. Clinical Orthopaedics 138: 94–104

Seedhom B B, Dowson D, Wright V 1974 The functions of the meniscus — a preliminary study. Journal of Bone and Joint Surgery 56B: 381–382

Smillie I S 1970 Injuries of the knee joint. E & S Livingstone, Edinburgh

Surin V 1985 Correspondence. Journal of Bone and Joint Surgery 67A: 1305–1306

Sutton F S, Thompson C U, Lipke J, Kettelkamp D B 1976 Effect of patellectomy on knee function. Journal of Bone and Joint Surgery 58A: 537–540

Tapper E M, Hoover N W 1969 Late results after meniscectomy. Journal of Bone and Joint Surgery 51A: 517–526

Torisu T 1977 Isolated avulsion fractures of the tibial attachment of the posterior cruciate ligament. Journal of Bone and Joint Surgery 59A: 68–72

Tregonning R J A 1983 Closed partial meniscectomy. Journal of Bone and Joint Surgery 65B: 378–382

Trickey E L 1968 Rupture of the posterior cruciate ligament. Journal of Bone and Joint Surgery 50B: 334–341

Watson Jones R 1956 Fractures and joint injuries. E & S Livingstone, Edinburgh

Wilkinson J 1977 Fractures of the patella treated by total excision. Journal of Bone and Joint Surgery 59B: 352–354

12. The tibia and fibula

M. A. Foy

INTRODUCTION AND CLASSIFICATION

The treatment of tibial fractures is controversial. There are two divergent schools of thought claiming equally good results: on the one hand, from operative treatment (Ruedi et al 1976, Allgower & Perren 1980), and on the other hand, from non-operative treatment with early weight-bearing (Sarmiento 1967, Brown 1974).

Ellis (1958b), Nicoll (1964), Johner & Wruhs (1983) and Waddell & Reardon (1983) showed that the severity of the injury was the major determinant of the prognosis. These authors, together with Leach (1984), showed that the anatomical site of the fracture in the tibia had no significant influence on the outcome. Therefore an anatomical classification of tibial shaft fractures is of no value in predicting prognosis.

Nicoll (1964) was the first orthopaedic surgeon to identify the 'personality of the fracture'. By this he meant the factors inherent in the fracture which would affect the prognosis, regardless of the method of treatment. He analysed the results in over 700 tibial fractures and identified four prognostic indicators:

1. The amount of initial displacement.
2. The degree of comminution.
3. The degree of soft tissue damage.
4. The presence of infection.

The first three factors are determined at the time of the injury, although a displaced fracture may reduce spontaneously or during transmission to hospital, and therefore displacement may not be appreciated at the initial assessment. Infection may result from contamination via the soft tissue wound or from surgical treatment.

In this chapter classification of tibial fractures will be made on the basis of injury severity, and not anatomical location, because of our concern with prognosis.

PROGNOSTIC FACTORS

Severity of injury

Leach (1984) believed that: 'a high energy force that causes an open tibial fracture with severe initial displacement, obvious comminution, and soft tissue injury with subsequent infection has the worst prognosis'.

Ellis (1958b) looked at the incidence, aetiology and types of residual disability in 343 tibial shaft fractures in 336 adults. The treatment in this group was conservative, with 65% treated in plaster, 33% by traction and only 2% by operation. The fractures were classified into three degrees of severity (Ellis 1958a):

1. *Minor*: undisplaced or angulated fragments (may be minor comminution or grade I compound wound).
2. *Moderate*: displaced fractures with minor comminution or grade I compound wound.
3. *Major*: displaced fractures complicated by major comminution or a major compound wound (grade II or III).

Delayed union (defined as clinical or radiological union not present by 20 weeks) occurred in 2% of minor severity injuries, 11% of moderate severity injuries and 60% of major severity injuries.

In Ellis's series, 86% of the patients had excellent clinical and anatomical results. Some 6% of the patients had shortening of 1–2 cm. This was usually of no consequence. Some 6% of the patients had limitation of ankle and/or foot movement and this proved to be a significant disability. This complication occurred in 1% of the minor severity fractures, 5% of the moderate severity fractures and 22% of the major severity fractures. Of 11 patients in this group who were engaged in heavy industry prior to their injury, only 2 were able to return to their former job.

Many of the reported series of tibial fractures describe the results only in terms of fracture healing and pay little attention to functional end-results. Follow-up by Ellis ranged from 1 to 6 years and he drew some important conclusions on functional end-results.

Other factors related to the severity of the injury are displacement, comminution and soft tissue injury.

Displacement

The prognostic significance of initial displacement is controversial. Leach (1984) felt that the amount of initial displacement was the best predictor of bony healing. Johner & Wruhs (1983) believed that displacement was an unreliable factor because reduction might occur prior to X-ray examination.

Nicoll (1964) looked at the effect of displacement on fracture healing. In closed undisplaced fractures with no comminution, 91% were healed within

20 weeks. In closed displaced fractures with no comminution, 73% were healed within 20 weeks. In this series treatment was conservative and delayed union was three times more common in displaced fractures.

Weissman et al (1966), in a series of 140 patients, found that increasing displacement caused delayed union. The tibial shaft fractures with no displacement or displacement of less than one-fifth of the shaft diameter united in an average of 3 months; those with complete displacement of the shaft took on average 6 months to unite.

It appears that the degree of displacement is one of the indicators of the severity of the injury. It is directly related to fracture union, but there is no evidence that displacement per se affects the long-term clinical result.

Comminution

Leach (1984) pointed out that fractures with comminution took longer to heal than those without. Comminution is another feature of high-velocity injury. Nicoll (1964) found an 18% incidence of delayed union in patients without comminution compared with a 30% incidence where comminution was present.

There are no figures directly correlating comminution and final clinical result; however, as with displacement, comminution is associated with injuries of greater severity and, consequently, less satisfactory results.

Soft tissue injury

Nicoll (1964) found that the incidence of joint stiffness was almost three times greater where there was a moderate or severe soft tissue injury. He also found that the incidence of delayed union was 18% where there was no wound or only a minor wound compared to an incidence of 37% where there was a moderate or severe wound.

Johner & Wruhs (1983) reported their results in a group of patients treated operatively. They found twice as many cases of non-union and five times as many cases of osteomyelitis after open than after closed tibial fractures. These facts again emphasize the effect of injury severity on the early and late clinical results.

Fibular fracture

There have been conflicting opinions on the effect of an associated fibular fracture on the prognosis. Nicoll (1964), Weissman et al (1966) and Hoaglund & States (1967) thought that absence of a fibular fracture was associated with a better prognosis because the injury was associated with less severe trauma. However, Teitz et al (1980), in a group of 23 patients over the age of 20, found a 26% incidence of delayed or non-union and a 26% incidence of varus malunion of the fractured tibia when the fibula was intact.

Leach (1984) concluded that the available evidence indicated that the tibial fracture with an intact fibula was associated with a more favourable prognosis because it indicated less initial displacement and soft tissue damage. This view is supported by most of the large reports in the literature.

Patient's age

Age appears to have little effect on the prognosis of tibial fractures occurring in patients over the age of 16 (Ellis 1958a, Nicoll 1964, Hoaglund & States 1967, Leach 1984).

Sites of the fracture

Fracture site appears to have little influence on the prognosis (Ellis 1958a, Weissman et al 1966, Leach 1984). Allum & Mowbray (1980) found a higher incidence of delayed union for fractures occurring at the junction of the upper and middle third of the tibia. Union by 20 weeks occurred in only 40% of these patients, compared with 65–85% healing by 20 weeks in fractures at other sites. Nicoll (1964) found a slightly increased rate of delayed union in fractures of the middle third of the tibia. The rate of delayed union was slightly lower in the lower third of the tibia.

Sepsis

Karlstrom & Olerud (1974) examined 15 reports from the orthopaedic literature in order to estimate the incidence of infection after tibial fractures. They found that closed fractures treated by closed methods rarely became infected (incidence 0–0.19%). Closed fractures treated by semi-open methods, e.g. percutaneous cerclage or closed intramedullary nailing, also had a low incidence of infection (0.48–0.98%). Closed fractures treated by open methods became infected in 1.4–3.8% of cases. Ruedi et al (1976) reported 3 cases of osteomyelitis in 323 patients (0.9%) with closed tibial fractures treated by dynamic compression plating according to AO techniques.

Karlstrom & Olerud (1974) found that the frequency of infection in open fractures treated by closed methods ranged from 6 to 17%. Patients with open fractures treated by internal fixation developed infection in 1–17% of cases where the fixation was non-stable and 3–7.6% where the fixation was stable. Ruedi et al (1976) reported an 11.6% incidence of infection after internal fixation of open fractures. Nine of these cases healed in an average of 10 months.

Nicoll (1964) believed that if infection developed it heralded a poor prognosis. He found that it increased the incidence of delayed union and non-union to 60%. Leach (1984) noted that infection in association with non-union was disastrous and always resulted in long-term disability.

Summary

1. The most important prognostic indicator is the severity of the initial injury ('the personality of the fracture' according to Nicoll).
2. The presence of a fibular fracture, the age of the patient and the site of the fracture appear to have little influence on the prognosis.
3. If infection occurs it is associated with a poorer prognosis in terms of healing and long-term clinical result.

CONSERVATIVE TREATMENT COMPARED WITH OPERATIVE TREATMENT

There is little merit in a detailed comparison of operative and non-operative treatment. Advocates of non-operative treatment have claimed a high percentage of satisfactory results (Sarmiento 1967, Brown 1974, Sarmiento & Latta 1981). Supporters of operative treatment have also reported a high percentage of satisfactory results (Ruedi et al 1976, Allgower & Perren 1980).

The 'personality' of the fracture is the important determinant of the end-result. Good personality fractures (low-energy injuries with little displacement, minimal comminution and minimal soft tissue injury) will do well with all forms of treatment. Poor personality fractures (high-energy injuries with marked displacement, severe comminution and severe soft tissue injury) will do less well irrespective of the method of treatment.

Plaster immobilization

The clinical results from Ellis (1958b) have already been discussed above. They show that 86% of 343 patients with tibial fractures treated by plaster immobilization or traction followed by plaster immobilization achieved excellent functional and anatomical results. There was a higher incidence of complications in the injuries of moderate and major severity (poor personality fractures), as discussed above.

Nicoll (1964) reported a 26% incidence of significant stiffness in tibial fractures treated by immobilization in plaster. Significant stiffness was. defined as:

Knee: Any loss of extension. Loss of more than 10° of flexion.
Ankle: Loss of more than 25% flexion or extension.
Subtalar joint: Loss of more than 25% inversion or eversion.

Within this group of patients Nicoll found that one-third (9% of the total) had severe, disabling stiffness. This was defined as:

Knee: Loss of 15° or more of extension. Loss of more than 30° of flexion.
Ankle: Loss of more than 50% flexion or extension.
Subtalar joint: Loss of more than 50% inversion or eversion.

Table 12.1 Incidence of significant stiffness after tibial shaft fracture treated by plaster immobilization (adapted from Nicoll 1964)

	Incidence of significant stiffness
Good personality fractures (type 1)	11/18 (12.5%)
Fractures tending toward good personality (types 2, 3, 4)	13/67 (19.5%)
Fractures tending toward poor personality (types 5, 6, 7)	28/71 (39.5%)
Poor personality fractures (type 8)	10/15 (66.5%)

See text for definition of personality types and of significant stiffness.

The frequency of significant joint stiffness can be related to fracture personality, as shown in Table 12.1. Nicoll divided the tibial fractures into 8 groups based on the presence of displacement (D), comminution (C), and a wound (W). Each factor was assigned as nil or slight (N) or moderate or severe (S). This gave 8 personality types:

1. ND, NC, NW
2. ND, NC, SW
3. ND, SC, NW
4. SD, NC, NW
5. ND, SC, SW
6. SD, NC, SW
7. SD, SC, NW
8. SD, SC, SW

Type 1 fractures ought to have a good personality. Types 2, 3 and 4 are categorized here as 'tending toward good personality', as they only have one S factor. Types 5, 6 and 7 are categorized here as 'tending toward poor personality' as they have two S factors. Type 8 ought to have a poor personality.

Nicoll (1964) also assessed residual deformity in 671 of the patients in this series: 58 (8.6%) had significant residual deformity. Significant deformity was defined as varus/valgus angulation, anterior/posterior bowing or rotational deformity in excess of 10° in any of these planes. In addition, shortening of more than 2 cm was assessed as significant deformity.

Weissman et al (1966) reported a perfect clinical recovery in 90% of 140 patients with tibial shaft fractures treated by long leg casts and delayed weight-bearing.

From the work of Ellis (1958b), Nicoll (1964) and Weissman et al (1966) it appears that, overall, conventional plaster immobilization resulted in satisfactory anatomical and functional results in 75–90% of patients with tibial shaft fractures.

Functional bracing with early weight-bearing

The importance of early weight-bearing was not emphasized in the work of Ellis or Nicoll. It was reported in 1961 by Dehne et al. Later Sarmiento (1967), Brown (1974) and Sarmiento & Latta (1981) confirmed the benefit of functional bracing with early weight-bearing.

Sarmiento & Latta (1981) produced a detailed anatomical analysis of the results in 733 tibial fractures. However, they did not give a breakdown of the functional results in these patients.

Operative treatment

Enthusiastic supporters of rigid internal fixation have reported very good results after operative treatment of fractures of the tibial shaft. Ruedi et al (1976) reported a series of 418 patients: 98% of the closed fractures were rated very good or good (normal or minimal symptoms) when reviewed after 1 year. Of open fractures, 88% were rated very good or good after 1 year.

The most thorough appraisal of the results after internal fixation of tibial shaft fractures was made by Johner & Wruhs (1983). They followed 291 fractures in 285 patients; 97% were followed for up to 8 years. The authors classified the results as shown in Table 12.2. In this group, 67% were treated by plating, 30% by intramedullary nailing and 3% with an external fixator.

Table 12.2   Criteria for evaluation of final results after tibial shaft fractures (from Johner & Wruhs 1983 with permission)

	Excellent (left = right)	Good	Fair	Poor
Non-union, osteitis, amputation	None	None	None	Yes
Neurovascular disturbances	None	Minimal	Moderate	Severe
Deformity				
Varus/valgus	None	2–5°	6–10°	>10°
Anteversion/recurvation	0–5°	6–10°	11–20°	>20°
Rotation	0–5°	6–10°	11–20°	>20°
Shortening	0–5 mm	6–10 mm	11–20 mm	>20 mm
Mobility				
Knee	Normal	>80%	>75%	<75%
Ankle	Normal	>75%	>50%	<50%
Subtalar joint	>75%	>50%	<50%	
Pain	None	Occasional	Moderate	Severe
Gait	Normal	Normal	Insignificant limp	Significant limp
Strenuous activities	Possible	Limited	Severely limited	Impossible

Johner & Wruhs (1983) described a complex morphological classification comprising 9 groups representing increasing degrees of comminution and differing modes of injury. The detailed results are too extensive to reproduce here. The final results were reported as excellent in 41% of patients, good in 45%, fair in 9% and poor in 5%.

Analysis of these results showed that the lowest incidence of excellent/good results occurred in bending fractures with several butterfly fragments (75% excellent/good), segmental fractures (68% excellent/good) and crush fractures (50% excellent/good).

The average time before return to work in this series was 155 days (range 79–227 days). Some 5% of the patients subsequently had their disability assessed at 20% or less, while 2% had their disability assessed at over 20% for employment purposes.

The authors found a marked difference in the results after open than after closed fractures. Excellent or good results were reported in 88% of closed fractures but in only 71% of open fractures. Inability to work also differed markedly; it averaged 129 days in closed fractures and 246 days in open fractures.

The report by Johner & Wruhs (1983) is worth consulting before preparing a medicolegal report on a tibial shaft fracture treated by internal fixation. These authors described a large number of patients with a detailed follow-up of up to 8 years.

The results again emphasize the importance of the personality of the fracture. Expert internal fixation carried out according to AO principles is still associated with less satisfactory results after high-energy injuries with significant comminution and soft tissue damage.

Summary

1. Treatment of tibial fractures in a long leg plaster with delayed weight-bearing is associated with satisfactory anatomical and functional results in 75–90% of cases.
2. Enthusiasts of internal fixation have claimed good or excellent results in 85–95% of cases.

Note: The criteria for 'satisfactory anatomical and functional results' and 'good or excellent' results, as discussed above, differ and are therefore not directly comparable from treatment method to treatment method.

SPECIFIC COMPLICATIONS

Delayed union/non-union

In the context of this chapter, delayed union is defined as a tibial fracture where bony union has not occurred by 20 weeks.

Nicoll (1964) found that 78% of 674 fractured tibias had united by 20 weeks. These fractures were treated in long leg plasters and no emphasis was placed on early weight-bearing. Nicoll showed quite clearly that the incidence of delayed union (and non-union) increased with moderate to severe displacement (36%) and moderate to severe comminution (30%).

If Nicoll's results are broken down according to fracture personality, then the figures shown in Table 12.3 are obtained. The higher frequency of delayed union and non-union in the poor personality fractures is shown.

Table 12.3 Incidence of delayed union and non-union after tibial fractures treated by plaster immobilization (adapted from Nicoll 1964)

	Incidence of delayed union and non-union
Good personality fractures (type 1)	24/254 (9%)
Fractures tending toward good personality (types 2, 3, 4)	40/197 (20%)
Fractures tending toward poor personality (types 5, 6, 7)	58/157 (37%)
Poor personality fractures (type 8)	17/44 (39%)

See p. 328 for definition of personality types.

Ellis (1958a) made similar observations in a series of 343 tibial fractures; 85% had united by 20 weeks. The incidence of delayed union was 2% in the minor severity injuries, 11% in the moderate severity injuries and 60% in the major severity injuries (see p. 324 for Ellis's definition of severity). Treatment of patients in this group was similar to that in Nicoll's (1964) series.

Ruedi et al (1976) reported a 3% incidence of delayed union in closed fractures, and a 7% incidence of delayed union in open fractures. All fractures were treated by AO dynamic compression plating. In the same series, the incidence of non-union was 1% in closed fractures and 5% in open fractures.

Johner & Wruhs (1983) described 283 tibial shaft fractures (both open and closed) and reported a 1% incidence of non-union. All fractures in this group were treated operatively by dynamic compression plating, intramedullary nailing or, rarely, external fixation.

Sarmiento & Latta (1981) reported less than 1% non-unions in a large series of 733 open and closed tibial shaft fractures treated by early weight-bearing and functional bracing.

Malunion

Malunion of tibial shaft fractures can result in:

1. Angular deformity.
2. Rotational deformity.
3. Shortening.

There is no general agreement on what constitutes a 'significant' mal-union. Leach (1984) believed that angulation greater than 5° in any plane was unacceptable.

Olerud (1971) showed that rotational deformity, even when relatively moderate, may cause significant functional problems. He also pointed out that most reports of results after tibial fractures fail to address this problem.

Sarmiento (1967) believed that shortening of 8 mm or less as a result of a tibial shaft fracture was of no clinical or functional significance.

Angular deformity

Nicoll (1964) found that 9% of 671 patients with conservatively treated tibial fractures had angular deformities of over 10°. A third of these patients had abnormal varus/valgus angulation and a third had angular deformities in both the sagittal and coronal planes.

Johner & Wruhs (1983) reported a 9% incidence of residual varus or valgus angulation of 5° in their group of 283 patients with tibial shaft fractures. They also noted a 2.5% incidence of anteroposterior angulation of 10°. The patients in this group were treated almost exclusively by rigid internal fixation.

Rotational deformity

Most reports fail to consider this problem. Leach (1984) believed that external rotation was better tolerated than internal rotation.

Nicoll (1964) found only 2 patients with a rotational abnormality of over 10° (0.3%) in 671 conservatively treated patients. Gamble et al (1972) described a 3% incidence of rotational deformity in a series of tibial fractures treated by plaster fixation and early weight-bearing.

Shortening

Nicoll (1964) reported a 2.5% incidence of shortening of over 2 cm in 671 tibial shaft fractures treated by plaster immobilization. Ellis (1958a) reported a 5.5% incidence of shortening of between 13 and 19 mm in a group of 343 patients treated by similar methods. Weissman et al (1966) found a 3% incidence of shortening of over 1 cm in 140 patients treated in plaster.

Supporters of early weight-bearing (Dehne et al 1961, Sarmiento 1967) believed that physiological shortening allowed impaction and this favoured early union. Sarmiento reported an average shortening of 6.4 mm, with a maximum of 2 cm, in his patients treated by functional bracing with early weight-bearing.

Johner & Wruhs (1983) described a 1.4% incidence of shortening of 5 mm in 283 patients treated almost exclusively by rigid internal fixation.

Compartment syndrome/ischaemic contracture

Nicoll (1964) believed that ischaemic problems were rarely associated with tibial shaft fractures. Owen & Tsimboukis (1967) were of the opinion that they occurred more commonly and often passed un-noticed.

Leach (1984) and Tile (1987) outlined the importance of early diagnosis and recognition of compartment syndromes. They stressed the importance of prompt treatment in the prevention of ischaemic muscle damage.

Nicoll (1964) found only 5 patients with ischaemic contracture in 671 tibial shaft fractures (0.75%). Ellis (1958b) found 9 patients with this problem in 225 tibial shaft fractures (4%). Ellis was specifically looking for ischaemic contracture and this may explain the higher incidence in his series. Two-thirds of the patients with ischaemic contractures had sustained major severity injuries. Seven of the 9 limbs with ischaemic contracture had marked limitation of ankle and foot movement. Clawing of the toes was observed in 7 patients, hallux flexus in 6 and equinus deformity in 3 patients.

The true incidence probably lies between these two authors' figures; it is likely to be closer to Ellis's figure of 4% as he was specifically looking for the sequelae of ischaemia in his patients.

Karlstrom & Olerud (1974) believed that open treatment of the fracture, together with suction drainage, provided prophylaxis against ischaemic damage.

Joint stiffness

This may be a cause of significant morbidity after a tibial shaft fracture. Nicoll (1964) reported that 9% of his patients had disabling joint stiffness. He defined disabling stiffness as loss of more than 50% movement compared to the normal side. This mainly affected the ankle and subtalar joints, although 3 cases of disabling knee stiffness were recorded. Table 12.1 relates stiffness to the personality of the fracture.

Ellis (1958b) found a 2.5% incidence of reduced knee flexion and a 6% incidence of reduced ankle flexion after tibial shaft fractures. In the group with ankle stiffness 11 had heavy jobs and only 2 were able to return to work as a consequence of their stiff ankles. The incidence of significant stiffness was greater as the severity of the fracture increased.

Ruedi et al (1976) described 6 cases with reduced movement of 20–30° in 323 patients with closed tibial fractures treated by AO plating (2%). The incidence of reduced movement rose to 8% in open fractures in this group of patients. Assessment in this series took into account total reduced movement in knee, ankle and subtalar joints.

Refracture

The incidence of refracture has been reported as 3% in tibial fractures treated in plaster (Chrisman & Snook 1968).

Ruedi et al (1976) reported a 0.5% incidence of refracture after AO plating in 388 patients. However, higher refracture rates have been reported after AO plating; these have ranged from 1.9 to 6% (Solheim 1960, Karlstrom & Olerud 1974).

Post-phlebitic syndrome

Recent reports have highlighted the importance of the post-phlebitic syndrome after fractures of the tibia (Aitken et al 1987, Wolfe 1987). Wolfe found that post-phlebitic symptoms occurred more commonly after tibial fractures than after femoral fractures. He also found that this syndrome was less common in patients under the age of 25.

Aitken et al (1987) emphasized the medicolegal importance of this condition. They particularly stressed that it may take 5–10 years before significant clinical features of chronic venous insufficiency develop. They described other reports which revealed an increasing incidence of post-phlebitic limbs with the passage of time — 13, 35 and 39% at 3, 9 and 14 years respectively, following tibial shaft fractures. The authors advise patients and their legal representatives to be cautious in settlement of personal injury claims following tibial shaft fractures. It may be that an early 'full and final settlement' will leave the patients with no redress if a post-phlebitic limb should develop later.

In the series of Aitken et al (1987), 11 of 60 limbs (18%) had clinically disabling post-phlebitic symptoms, including venous ulceration. In this group of patients there were both femoral and tibial shaft fractures.

Summary

1. Delayed union occurs in 15–22% of tibial shaft fractures treated by plaster immobilization without early weight-bearing.
2. Delayed union occurs in approximately 3% of closed tibial fractures and approximately 7% of open tibial fractures treated by dynamic compression plating.
3. Non-union occurs in 1–5% of tibial fractures treated by internal fixation.
4. There is a 1–4% incidence of ischaemic contracture following tibial shaft fractures.

5. The post-phlebitic syndrome may be a clinically significant factor after tibial shaft fracture. It may take 5–10 years for symptoms to develop fully.

TIBIAL FRACTURES IN CHILDREN

Proximal tibial physis

Ogden (1987) pointed out that this fracture was uncommon because of the local anatomy, particularly the anterior overhang of the tibial tuberosity. Neer & Horwitz (1965) described an incidence of 0.8% in 2500 consecutive physeal fractures.

The two largest series reporting injuries to the proximal tibial physis were from Shelton & Canale (1979) and Burkhart & Peterson (1979). Shelton & Canale described follow-up to skeletal maturity in 28 physeal injuries in 27 patients. Burkhart & Peterson reported 26 injuries; 5 of these were compound lawnmower injuries and all 5 had a uniformly poor prognosis.

Shelton & Canale (1979) classified their results as satisfactory or unsatisfactory. A result was considered unsatisfactory if any of the following was present:

1. Leg length discrepancy of 2.5 cm or more.
2. Angular deformity of more than 7°.
3. Incongruity of the joint with secondary traumatic arthritis or pain.
4. Neurovascular compromise with resultant loss of function in the limb.

Treatment of patients in these two groups consisted of cast immobilization in the Salter–Harris (1963) types I and II injuries and open reduction and internal fixation for displaced Salter–Harris types III and IV injuries (Salter & Harris 1963). Average follow-up was 7 years in the patients reported by Shelton & Canale (1979) and 2.5 years in Burkhart & Peterson's (1979) series. Nine of the 49 patients in these series had unsatisfactory results according to Shelton & Canale's criteria: an incidence of 18%.

The lawnmower injuries reported by Burkhart & Peterson (5 cases) had a very poor prognosis. Four of the patients developed significant angulation (12–30°) and 2 developed leg length discrepancy of over 3.5 cm. One case developed osteomyelitis after open reduction and internal fixation and 1 a severed peroneal nerve. All results were unsatisfactory.

In these two series the Salter–Harris classification was not a reliable predictor of growth disturbance. Indeed, in Shelton & Canale's series all of the 7 patients exhibiting growth abnormalities were Salter–Harris type I or II injuries. Roberts (1984) believed that this was due to longitudinal compression causing damage to the deeper proliferative zone of the growth plate in these cases.

Tibial tuberosity fractures/avulsions

Ogden et al (1980) reported 15 fractures of the tibial tuberosity in 14 adolescents. Hand et al (1971) reported 7 avulsion fractures in adolescents.

Ogden et al concluded that complications were rare after this injury, and that the theoretical possibility of the subsequent development of genu recurvatum appeared unlikely, since most of these injuries occurred when the physis of the tuberosity was undergoing normal closure.

Both of these reports stressed the importance of accurate reduction if the tibial tuberosity was displaced.

Bolesta & Fitch (1986) reported similar experience with 15 tibial tubercle avulsions. All patients were able to return to full activity, including sports, when reviewed 3 months or more after injury.

Tibial shaft fractures

Blount (1955) believed that the treatment of fractures of the tibia in children was gratifying because they had a short healing time, a low complication rate and there were no cases of non-union or delayed union, if surgery was omitted. Allum & Mowbray (1980) confirmed the rapid healing of tibial fractures in children. Weissman et al (1966) reported normal function and absence of subjective complaints in 60 children under the age of 16 following tibial shaft fractures.

Hansen et al (1976) described the subjective and objective findings in 85 children under 15 years of age at 2 years after their tibial shaft fracture. Six patients (7%) experienced pain after major exertion. The authors did not find any gait abnormalities and observed symmetrical hip, knee and ankle movements in all patients. They found restriction of subtalar movements in 2 patients (2%).

Swaan & Oppers (1971) believed that the capacity for children to correct angular deformity diminished with increasing age. However, even in the youngest age groups angular correction did not exceed 5°. Hansen et al (1976) estimated that the overall spontaneous correction of angular deformity in tibial fractures in children was 13.5%. They concluded that more than 10% correction should not be expected after the conclusion of treatment.

Dias (1984) summarized the literature on the potential for the tibia to correct angular malalignment in children. He concluded that the maximum angulation that should be accepted during treatment was 10° of recurvatum and 5° of varus or valgus.

There is general agreement that rotational deformity in the tibia will not correct spontaneously (Blount 1955, Dias 1984).

Leg length discrepancy is not a major problem following tibial fractures in children (Dias 1984). Swaan & Oppers (1971) found that the younger the child at the time of the tibial fracture, the greater the chance for tibial overgrowth.

Fractures of the proximal tibial metaphysis in children may develop undesirable consequences and need to be carefully monitored (Rang 1974, Dias 1984); in particular, they may develop valgus angulation. The incidence of this complication is unclear. Jordan et al (1987) reviewed the possible aetiologies and concluded that valgus angulation was due to an increased vascular response causing an asymmetric growth stimulation of the medial metaphysis of the proximal tibia.

Summary

1. Over 80% of children with injuries to the proximal tibial epiphysis achieve a satisfactory result.
2. Complications are rare after injuries to the tibial tuberosity in adolescents.
3. Most children with tibial shaft fractures achieve a normal clinical result. Even in young children, the evidence suggests that angular correction of more than 5–10° does not occur.

REFERENCES

Aitken R J, Mills C, Immelman E J 1987 The post-phlebitic syndrome following shaft fractures of the leg. A significant late complication. Journal of Bone and Joint Surgery; 69B: 775–778
Allgower M, Perren S M 1980 Operating on tibial shaft fractures. Unfallheilk/Traumatology 83: 214–218
Allum R L, Mowbray M A S 1980 A retrospective review of the healing of fractures of the shaft of the tibia with special reference to the mechanism of injury. Injury 11: 304–308
Blount W P 1955 Fractures in children, 3rd edn. Williams & Wilkins, Baltimore
Bolesta M J, Fitch R D 1986 Tibial tubercle avulsions. Journal of Paediatric Orthopaedics 6: 186–192
Brown P W 1974 Early weight bearing treatment of tibial shaft fractures. Clinical Orthopaedics 105: 165–178
Burkhart S S, Peterson H A 1979 Fractures of the proximal tibial epiphysis. Journal of Bone and Joint Surgery 61A: 996–1002
Chrisman O D, Snook G A 1968 The problem of refracture of the tibia. Clinical Orthopaedics 60: 217–219
Dehne E, Metz C W, Deffer P, Hall R 1961 Non-operative treatment of the fractured tibia by immediate weight bearing. Journal of Trauma 1: 514–535
Dias L S 1984 Fractures of the tibia and fibula. In: Rockwood C A Jr, Wilkins K E, King R E (eds) Fractures in children, vol 3. J B Lippincott, Philadelphia
Ellis H 1958a The speed of healing after fracture of the tibial shaft. Journal of Bone and Joint Surgery 40B: 42–46
Ellis H 1958b Disabilities after tibial shaft fractures. Journal of Bone and Joint Surgery 40B: 190–197
Gamble W E, Clayton M L, Leidholt J D, Cletsher J O 1972 Complications following treatment of tibial fractures with weight bearing. Journal of Bone and Joint Surgery 54A: 1343
Hand W L, Hand C R, Dunn A W 1971 Avulsion fractures of the tibial tubercle. Journal of Bone and Joint Surgery 53A: 1579–1583
Hansen B A, Greiff J, Bergmann F 1976 Fractures of the tibia in children. Acta Orthopaedica Scandinavica 47: 448–453
Hoaglund F T, States J D 1967 Factors influencing the rate of healing in tibial shaft fractures. Surgery, Gynecology and Obstetrics 124: 71–76

Johner R, Wruhs O 1983 Classification of tibial shaft fractures and correlation with results after rigid internal fixation. Clinical Orthopaedics 178: 7–25

Jordan S E, Alonso J E, Cook F F 1987 The aetiology of valgus angulation after metaphyseal fractures of the tibia in children. Journal of Paediatric Orthopaedics 7: 450–457

Karlstrom G, Olerud S 1974 Fractures of the tibial shaft: a critical evaluation of treatment alternatives. Clinical Orthopaedics 105: 82–115

Leach R E 1984 Fractures of the tibia and fibula. In: Rockwood C A, Green D P (eds) Fractures in adults, vol 2. J B Lippincott, Philadelphia

Neer C S, Horwitz B S 1965 Fractures of the proximal humeral epiphyseal plate. Clinical Orthopaedics 41: 24–31

Nicoll E A 1964 Fractures of the tibial shaft. A survey of 705 cases. Journal of Bone and Joint Surgery 46B: 373–387

Ogden J A 1987 Pocket guide to paediatric fractures. Williams & Wilkins, Baltimore

Ogden J A, Tross R B, Murphy M J 1980 Fractures of the tibial tuberosity in adolescents. Journal of Bone and Joint Surgery 62A: 205–214

Olerud S 1971 Kan fotledsfunktionen forbattras genom korrektion av fellakt underbensfraktur? Nordist Medicin 86: 876

Owen R, Tsimboukis B 1967 Ischaemia complicating closed tibial and fibular shaft fractures. Journal of Bone and Joint Surgery 49B: 268

Rang M 1974 Children's fractures. J B Lippincott, Philadelphia

Roberts J M 1984 Fractures and dislocations of the knee. In: Rockwood C A Jr, Wilkins K E, King R E (eds) Fractures in children, vol 3. J B Lippincott, Philadelphia

Ruedi T, Webb J K, Allgower M 1976 Experience with the dynamic compression plate (DCP) in 418 recent fractures of the tibial shaft. Injury 7: 252–265

Salter R B, Harris W R 1963 Injuries involving the epiphyseal plate. Journal of Bone and Joint Surgery 45A: 587–622

Sarmiento A 1967 A functional below-the-knee cast for tibial fractures. Journal of Bone and Joint Surgery 49A: 855–875

Sarmiento A, Latta L L 1981 Closed functional treatment of fractures. Springer-Verlag, Berlin

Shelton W R, Canale S T 1979 Fractures of the tibia through the proximal tibial epiphyseal cartilage. Journal of Bone and Joint Surgery 61A: 167–173

Solheim K 1960 Disabilities after shaft fractures of the bones of the leg. A clinical and radiographic follow-up study of 131 patients after approximately 15 years. Acta Chirurgica Scandinavica 119: 280

Swaan J W, Oppers V M 1971 Crural fractures in children. Archivum Chirurgicum Neerlandicum 23: 259–272

Teitz C C, Carter D R, Frankel V H 1980 Problems associated with tibial fractures associated with intact fibulae. Journal of Bone and Joint Surgery 62A: 770–776

Tile M 1987 Fractures of the tibia. In: Schatzker J, Tile M (eds) The rationale of operative fracture care. Springer-Verlag, Berlin

Waddell J P, Reardon G P 1983 Complications of tibial shaft fractures. Clinical Orthopaedics 178: 173–178

Weissman S L, Herold H Z, Engelberg M 1966 Fractures of the middle two-thirds of the tibial shaft. Journal of Bone and Joint Surgery 48A: 257–266

Wolfe J H N 1987 Post-phlebitic syndrome after fractures of the leg. British Medical Journal 295: 1364–1365

13. The ankle

M. A. Foy

INTRODUCTION

Buhr & Cooke (1959) found that ankle fractures accounted for 11% of all fractures. Willenegger (1961) and Phillips et al (1985) reported that the ankle was the most commonly injured weight-bearing joint.

Ankle fractures may follow falls, sporting injuries and road traffic accidents. They may be the subject of personal injury litigation. There is controversy regarding the tolerance of the ankle joint to minor degrees of incongruity. The indications for internal fixation of ankle fractures are controversial. Some orthopaedic surgeons hold the view that internal fixation has a pivotal role in the management of many ankle fractures. Others disagree, arguing that internal fixation is rarely indicated.

In this chapter an attempt will be made to clarify these issues when assessing the results.

LIGAMENT INJURIES

Injuries to the lateral ligament complex of the ankle joint are diverse. There is no reliable information on the incidence of instability, or on the potential for the ankle to develop osteoarthritis.

Current treatment policy of lateral ligament injuries has been outlined by Lightowler (1984). Recurrent instability of the ankle joint may follow lateral ligament rupture. It has not been possible to identify the incidence of recurrent instability following these injuries. The incidence is related to the severity of the initial injury, and also to the method and duration of treatment.

Coltart (1951), Harrington (1979), Glasgow et al (1980) and Bauer (personal communication) suggested that long-term chronic lateral instability of the ankle joint may lead to osteoarthritis. This was said to be due to unbalanced loading of the medial joint space. Harrington (1979) reported on 36 patients with lateral ligament instability which had been present for at least 10 years. X-ray examination and arthroscopy revealed arthritic changes in all cases.

339

No statistics can be given for the risk of developing osteoarthritis from the present published reports. However, the available evidence suggests that there may be a tendency for osteoarthtitis to develop in chronic lateral ligament instability.

Isolated injury to the medial ligament is much less common than isolated lateral ligament injury. Chronic medial ligament instability is rare. Medial ligament injuries tend to occur as part of more complex ankle fracture patterns, particularly abduction injuries.

Summary

1. Injuries to the lateral ligament are common. They may lead to ankle instability. There is evidence to suggest that chronic instability may predispose the ankle joint to develop osteoarthritis.
2. Isolated injuries to the medial (deltoid) ligament are uncommon. They rarely lead to long-term problems.

ANKLE FRACTURES

Classification

The most comprehensive and widely used classification of ankle fractures is the genetic system described by Lauge-Hansen (1948). He assigned double names to each fracture type. The first part defined the position of the foot, and the second defined the direction of the injuring force. There have been criticisms of this classification, but it is the most useful one in terms of prognosis. Four major groups were defined:

1. Supination–adduction fractures.
2. Supination–eversion (external rotation) fractures.
3. Pronation–abduction fractures.
4. Pronation–eversion (external rotation) fractures.

Details of this classification are given in Figures 13.1–13.4. The injuries occur in stages, as shown. These stages reflect the progressive severity of the injury.

In 1949 Danis described a classification which was later used by Weber (1972). In this classification, fractures were divided into three groups, A, B and C, according to the level of the fibular fracture and its relationship to the tibiofibular syndesmosis. This classification has been adopted by the AO group and is widely recognized.

The Danis–Weber classification is not detailed enough to make it valuable in the prediction of prognosis. This view is supported by the work of Niethard & Plaue (1977), Zenker & Nerlich (1982) and Bauer (1985). Cedell (1967), for example, described the frequency of post-traumatic arthritis in stage II supination–eversion fractures as 2.6%, compared to an incidence of 23.5% for stage IV supination–eversion fractures. This differ-

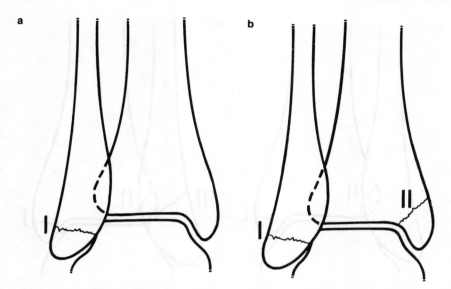

Fig. 13.1a Stage I supination–adduction injury with a lateral malleolar fracture below the ankle joint (or a lateral ligament injury). **b** Stage II supination–adduction injury with a vertical or oblique fracture through the medial malleolus

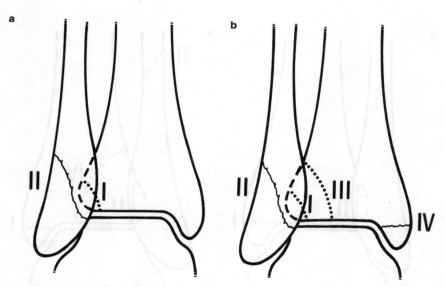

Fig. 13.2a Stage I and II supination–eversion injury. Stage I is an injury to the anterior tibiofibular ligament with either a bony avulsion or in-substance rupture. Stage II is an oblique fracture of the fibula at the level of the joint. **b** Stage III and IV supination–eversion injury superimposed on Figure 13.2a. Stage III is a fracture of the posterior tibial malleolus. Stage IV is a 'pull-off' fracture through the medial malleolus or a deltoid ligament rupture

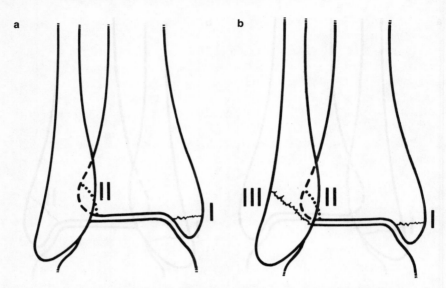

Fig. 13.3a Stage I and II pronation–abduction injury. Stage I is an avulsion fracture of the medial malleolus. Stage II is an injury to the anterior tibiofibular ligament. **b** Stage III pronation–abduction injury superimposed on Figure 13.3a. This is a short oblique fracture of the fibula just above the level of the ankle joint

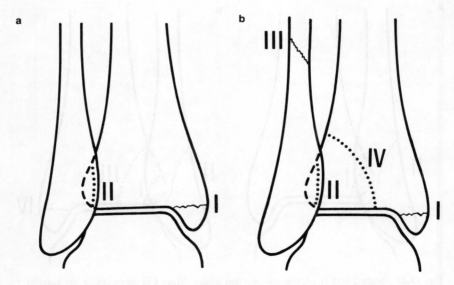

Fig. 13.4a Stage I and II pronation–eversion injuries. Stage I is an avulsion fracture of the medial malleolus. Stage II is an injury to the anterior tibiofibular ligament. **b** Stage III and IV pronation–eversion injury superimposed on Figure 13.4a. Stage III is a torsional fracture of the fibular shaft, well above the level of the ankle joint. Stage IV is a fracture of the posterior tibial malleolus

ence in the severity of the injuries would not have been easily recognized from the Danis–Weber classification.

Assessment of the end-results of ankle fractures may be difficult. Phillips & Spiegel (1979) reported that the correlation between X-ray appearances and clinical symptoms was often poor. Difficulties arose in comparing results following open reduction and closed manipulation because the adequacy of reduction was not defined. Phillips & Spiegel summarized the problem well: 'The degree of tolerance permissible between an *exact* anatomic reduction and an *acceptable* or *adequate* reduction remains undefined'.

Incidence of osteoarthritis

According to Phillips & Spiegel (1979), although the ankle is the most frequently injured weight-bearing joint, it has the lowest incidence of degenerative joint disease. In medicolegal reporting the risk of the patient developing post-traumatic osteoarthritis is of importance in the assessment of damages.

It is difficult accurately to predict the risk of a patient developing osteo-arthritis after an ankle fracture. Wilson (1984) reported that it occurred in 20–40% of ankle fractures 'regardless of the method of treatment'. This is still a controversial issue. There is agreement between orthopaedic surgeons that an anatomical reduction should be the aim of treatment. Controversy surrounds the influence of open reduction and internal fixation, compared to successful closed manipulation, on the incidence of osteoarthritis.

The only prospective randomized trial which attempted to answer this question was reported by Phillips et al (1985). They studied grade IV supination–eversion and pronation–eversion fractures and used a complex scoring system to assess their results. Their criteria for a satisfactory closed reduction are shown in Table 13.1. The only significant difference between open reduction with internal fixation and closed manipulation was seen in the adequacy of reduction, based on radiographic measurements. When

Table 13.1 Criteria for a satisfactory closed reduction of an ankle fracture (from Phillips et al 1985, with permission)

1. Medial clear space not more than 2 mm wider than the space between the tibial plafond and the dome of the talus

2. Less than 2 mm of displacement of the medial malleolus in any direction

3. Less than 2 mm of lateral displacement of the distal end of the fibula at the fracture

4. Less than 5 mm of posterior displacement of the distal end of the fibula

5. Less than 25% of the anteroposterior length of the tibial articular surface, as seen on the lateral radiograph, included in the posterior fracture fragment, or less than 2 mm of displacement of a posterior fragment that includes more than 25% of the anterior–posterior length of the articular surface

reduction was satisfactory, there was no significant difference in the clinical results or in the incidence of osteoarthritis.

Bauer (1985) reviewed 27 reports in the orthopaedic literature, and found that the frequency of post-traumatic arthritis ranged from 18 to 86% in patients treated conservatively, and from 7 to 70% in patients treated by internal fixation. Colton (personal communication) pointed out that this may reflect unfairly on the operatively treated patients because the methods of internal fixation in some of the quoted series would be unacceptable when judged by current standards.

Minor degrees of osteoarthritis may cause no symptoms. There is more agreement regarding the occurrence of subjective symptoms following ankle fractures. Bauer (1985) reported that after 7 years approximately one-third of patients with supination–eversion fractures (Danis–Weber B) complained of residual discomfort. Magnusson (1944), Klossner (1962) and Cedell (1967) described similar results, with no difference between operative and conservatively treated patients.

There are many variables influencing the development of osteoarthritis following ankle fractures. The conclusions from the orthopaedic literature are unclear and frequently contradictory. The report from Phillips et al (1985) attempted to clarify the situation. Unfortunately only 51% of their patients returned for follow-up. They were unable to prove that open reduction and internal fixation were superior to adequate manipulative treatment, as defined in Table 13.1, in terms of clinical results and development of osteoarthritis.

It is only possible to emphasize those factors which make the development of osteoarthritis more likely. In current orthopaedic practice Wilson's (1984) assessment of a 20–40% incidence, irrespective of treatment, is reasonable.

Factors influencing the development of osteoarthritis

Severity of initial injury

The studies of Cedell (1967), Niethard & Plaue (1977), and Zenker & Nerlich (1982) found a good correlation between the development of osteoarthritis and the number of single lesions, as reflected in the Lauge-Hansen (1948) stages.

The presence of a posterior tibial fragment indicates a more severe injury. Olerud (1981) pointed out that a posterior tibial fragment, even if radiographically well reduced, 'implies a substantially increased risk of arthritis, and thus a poorer prognosis'. Bauer (1985) described 12 other scientific reports supporting this view. In the Lauge-Hansen (1948) classification the presence of a posterior tibial fragment reflects a later stage in the injury sequence, usually stage III or IV. Neithard & Plaue (1977) found that even the smallest flake fragment posteriorly doubled the rate of post-traumatic arthritis.

Lindsjo (1981) considered the clinical and radiological results in 174 patients with posterior tibial fragments. The clinical results were poorer when there was a large articular fragment. Arthritis occurred in 34% of patients with a posterior articular fragment, but in only 17% of patients with a posterior non-articular fragment. If the articular fragment was not anatomically reduced, then the incidence of arthritis was 44%. All the patients in this study were surgically treated using AO principles. The criteria for a diagnosis of arthritis were based on reduction of the joint space as described by Magnusson (1944) and, later, Cedell (1967).

A posterior tibial fragment indicates a more severe injury and a greater risk of developing osteoarthritis.

The posterior tibial fragment occurring in these stage III and IV injuries should not be confused with the much less common isolated fracture of the posterior tibial margin which follows hyperplantarflexion injuries. These isolated injuries have a good prognosis (Bauer personal communication).

Adequacy of the reduction

Lindsjo (1981) reported a series of over 300 ankle fractures treated by open reduction and internal fixation. On the post-operative X-rays residual displacement was assessed. Lindsjo paid particular attention to the presence of small displaced fragments, incongruity between the articular surfaces, irregularity of the articular surface and articular surface defects. He found that there was a significant difference in the clinical results between accurately reduced fractures and inadequately reduced fractures. This is illustrated in Table 13.2.

Table 13.2 The adequacy of reduction related to the treatment result (from Lindsjo 1981, with permission)

	Excellent–good results (%)
Accurately reduced fractures (n = 217)	86.6
Inadequately reduced fractures (n = 89)	68.5

Lindsjo (1981) defined osteoarthritis in terms of reduction of the joint space of the ankle. He found a statistically significant relationship between the degree of arthritis and the clinical result: this is shown in Table 13.3.

Bauer (1985) supported the view that accurate reduction led to a better clinical result. He found that this opinion was supported in 23 other publications dealing with the results of ankle fractures.

There is strong evidence and opinion to support the accurate reduction of ankle fractures. This improves the long-term results. When considering long-term clinical results, and the development of osteoarthritis, there is no

Table 13.3 Relationship of osteoarthritis of the ankle joint to clinical result (from Lindsjo 1981, with permission)

	Frequency of excellent–good clinical results (%)
No arthritis	82
Slight joint space narrowing	76
Joint space reduced to at least half	42
Joint space virtually eliminated	0

conclusive evidence that satisfactory open reduction and internal fixation are better than satisfactory closed manipulation.

Age and sex of patient

Lindsjo (1981) found that the worst overall results — in both clinical and radiographic terms — occurred in females aged from 45 to 64 years. Beauchamp et al (1983) reported that patients over the age of 50 had less satisfactory results after displaced ankle fractures.

Radiographic indicators

Residual displacement on X-ray, and its implications for prognosis, has already been discussed.

Phillips et al (1985) considered several radiographic measurements in an attempt to find a reliable predictor of satisfactory and unsatisfactory results. The only reliable indicator proved to be the talocrural angle, as described by Sarkisian & Cody (1976). This is shown in Figure 13.5. Two lines are drawn, one between the tips of the malleoli and one parallel to the tibial plafond, on an anteroposterior X-ray in internal rotation (the mortise view). A perpendicular is taken from the line of the tibial plafond. The talocrural angle is the superomedial angle, where the perpendicular intersects the line joining the tips of the malleoli.

The normal range of the talocrural angle in adults is $83 \pm 4°$. The difference in the angle between two ankles in a normal individual is less than $2°$. Phillips et al (1985) classified a difference of over $5°$ as abnormal, because this was the smallest angle that they could reliably measure. They found significantly better overall results when the talocrural angles were within $5°$ of each other. Sarkisian & Cody (1976) proposed that fibular rotation led to shortening and this altered the talocrural angle.

Other radiographic measurements have been studied, but have not proved to be reliable predictors of prognosis.

Time taken for arthritis to develop

This is an important consideration when deciding on the timing of medicolegal reports. Willenegger (1961) and Lindsjo (1981) found that the

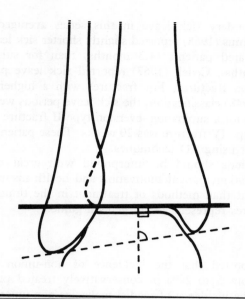

Fig. 13.5 The talocrural angle as described by Sarkisian & Cody (1976). One line is drawn parallel to the tibial plafond and a second between the tips of the malleoli on a true anteroposterior (mortise) X-ray. The talocrucal angle is the superomedial angle subtended when a perpendicular is dropped from the line parallel to the plafond (see text for further details)

majority of arthritic change occurred in the first 12–18 months from injury. Lindsjo (1981) examined his patients at mean periods of 18 months and 4 years from their injury. There was no significant difference in the incidence of osteoarthritis at these times. Between these two follow-up appointments, both subjective and objective results tended to improve rather than deteriorate.

It is wise to delay a final medical report until 18 months after the ankle fracture. If osteoarthritis is going to develop, radiographic evidence should be apparent at this stage. Symptoms and signs are more likely to improve than deteriorate after 18 months.

Social/occupational factors

Lindsjo (1981) considered the functional results in 305 patients treated surgically according to AO principles. In all, 90% were able to continue in the same occupation; 82% were able to continue sports and other physical activities at the same level. There was no significant difference in working, sports and walking capacity between male and female patients.

Lindsjo (1981) found that sick leave following operative treatment of ankle fractures ranged from 13 to 18 weeks. He also assessed further sick leave, usually associated with implant removal. The combined duration of primary and secondary sick leave in this series averaged 22.5 weeks. Solonen & Lauttamus (1968) reported slightly shorter sick leave periods for conservatively treated patients (4.3 months) than for surgically treated patients (4.5 months). Cedell (1967) reported sick leave periods for 355 supination–eversion fractures. For fractures with a higher grade in the Lauge-Hansen (1948) classification, the sick leave periods were longer. The average sick leave for a supination–eversion type II fracture was 14 weeks, while that for a type IV fracture was 20 weeks. These patients were treated surgically, but not using AO techniques.

Sick leave periods should be interpreted with great caution. Social conditions, occupation, patient motivation and health insurance are probably more relevant than methods of treatment in the timing of return to work. These figures represent a very general guide.

Non-union

Bauer (1985) reported that the incidence of non-union of the medial malleolus was from 5 to 20% in conservatively treated patients. Wilson (1984) reported the incidence of medial malleolar non-union as 10–15% in conservatively treated patients. Lindsjo (1981) reported only 1 non-union of the medial malleolus in 314 fractures treated operatively by AO techniques (0.3% incidence). Opinions vary regarding the significance of a medial malleolar non-union. Mendelsohn (1965) and Sneppen (1971) suggested that non-union did not influence the long-term prognosis. Cox & Laxson (1952) suggested that non-union predisposed to the development of osteoarthritis.

Non-union of the lateral malleolus is rare. Bauer (1985) reported the incidence to be around 0.1%. He found no lateral malleolar non-unions in 51 patients treated surgically and 200 patients treated conservatively. Lindsjo (1981) found 1 lateral malleolar non-union in 314 fractures treated operatively.

Summary

1. The incidence of osteoarthritis after ankle fractures is probably 20–40%.
2. When there is anatomical reduction of the ankle fracture, and this is maintained until healing, both internal fixation and closed treatment show similar clinical results and similar risks of developing osteoarthritis.
3. Approximately one-third of patients experience discomfort in their ankle when followed up for 5 years or more. This occurs equally in both operatively and non-operatively treated patients.
4. The presence of a posterior tibial fragment represents a more severe injury, in terms of the Lauge-Hansen classification. It is associated with an increased risk of developing arthritis.

5. The talocrural angle (Fig. 13.5) is the only reliable radiographic indicator of prognosis.

6. Final medical reports should be delayed until 18 months after ankle fractures. If osteoarthritis is going to develop, radiographic evidence should be apparent at that time.

TIBIAL PLAFOND/PILON FRACTURES

Pilon fractures are usually classified according to Ruedi & Allgower (1969). They recognized three fracture types, as shown in Figure 13.6.

Bone (1987) reported that in experienced hands, open reduction and internal stabilization with plate fixation gave the best results for this difficult fracture. Dillin & Slabaugh (1986) offered a cautionary warning on the hazards of inexperienced surgeons operating on these fractures.

Ruedi (1973) reported good and excellent functional results in 74% of patients treated operatively, according to the principles of the AO group (Muller et al 1979).

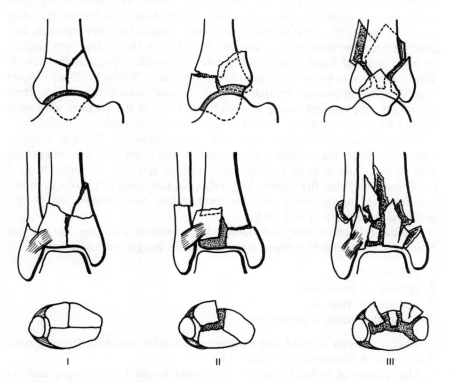

Fig. 13.6 AO classification of pilon fracture. I, fissure fracture without significant displacement; II, fissure fracture with significant articular incongruity; III, compression fracture with displacement of the weight-bearing cancellous segments of the metaphysis (from Muller et al 1979, with permission).

In 1979 Ruedi and Allgower assessed a group of 75 patients in a city hospital to see if these results were reproducible. These patients were treated according to AO principles. At an average of 6 years post-operatively, 80% of the patients were able to use the injured limb normally. Only 15% complained of disability or discomfort. Some 5% underwent arthrodesis for severe osteoarthritis. Over half (54%) of the patients went back to playing sport, and 63 patients (84%) had returned to the same job. Twelve patients (16%) had to find a new job as a result of their injury, some with lower income. Objective assessment revealed normal movement or restriction of movement of less than 10° in 69% of patients.

Ovadia & Beals (1986) reviewed 145 fractures of the tibial plafond. Mean follow-up was 57 months, with a minimum of 24 months. These authors extended the classification into 5 groups. Their types I and II are equivalent to Ruedi & Allgower's type I; their type III is equivalent to Ruedi & Allgower's type II, and their types IV and V correspond to Ruedi & Allgower's type III, as shown in Figure 13.6.

Results of rigid internal fixation (80 cases) were compared to results of other treatment (65 cases). The final clinical results of treatment by open reduction and rigid internal fixation were better than those treated by other methods. Some 35 (54%) of the 65 fractures treated by other methods had good or excellent final clinical results; 59 (74%) of the 80 fractures treated by rigid internal fixation achieved a good or excellent final clinical result. This difference is statistically significant. Ovadia & Beals (1986) also found that 55 (69%) of patients treated by rigid internal fixation returned to their pre-injury employment, compared with 28 (43%) of the patients who were treated by other methods. This difference is also statistically significant.

An excellent clinical result was defined by Ovadia & Beals as follows: absence of pain; the patient had returned to the same job; the patient was able to carry out normal recreational activities and had no limp. A good result indicated that the patient had mild pain following strenuous exercise, had returned to the same job, had undertaken mild moderation of recreational activities and had no limp.

Ovadia & Beals (1986) considered the variables affecting the clinical results. They found that there were four main prognostic indicators:

1. Fracture type.
2. Quality of reduction.
3. Treatment method.
4. Associated medical problems.

Ovadia & Beals showed that prognosis correlates well with fracture type. This point is illustrated in Figure 13.7.

The quality of reduction is closely related to the fracture type and the method of treatment. Better reduction was obtained in type I and II (Ruedi & Allgower's type I) fractures and in those fractures treated by rigid internal fixation. The quality of the reduction correlated well with the

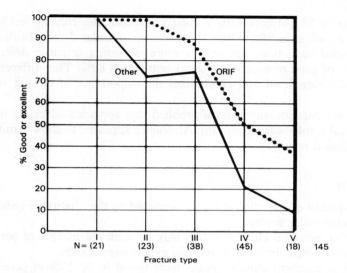

Fig. 13.7 Correlation of pilon fracture type with prognosis (from Ovadia & Beals, with permission). (ORIF, open reduction internal fixation)

Table 13.4 Classification of reduction of tibial plafond fractures (from Ovadia & Beals 1986, with permission)

	Good	Fair	Poor
Malleolus			
Lateral	Anatomical or <1 mm displacement	2–5 mm displacement	>5 mm displacement
Medial	<2 mm displacement	2–5 mm displacement	>5 mm displacement
Posterior	Proximal displacement	Proximal displacement	Proximal displacement
Mortise widening	<0.5 mm	0.5–2 mm	>2 mm
Talus			
Tilt	<0.5 mm	0.5–1 mm	>1 mm
Displacement	<0.5 mm	0.5–2 mm	>2 mm

clinical result. Of the patients whose reduction was rated as good using Ovadia & Beals's criteria (shown in Table 13.4), 89% had an excellent or good final clinical result. All of the 18 patients who had a poor reduction also had a poor final clinical result.

Another variable related to fracture reduction was the presence of a gap in the articular surface. One or more gaps in the articular surface, measuring 1–4 mm on the post-reduction X-ray, were identified in 35 of 83 patients who were otherwise judged to have a good reduction. In this subgroup of 83 patients with a good reduction, the clinical results were good or excellent in 98% where there was no articular defect. In the group with a good reduction, but one or more persisting articular defects, the incidence of good or excellent clinical results was 80%. This difference was statistically significant and emphasizes the importance of closing articular defects.

The only concomitant medical problem that appeared adversely to affect the clinical results was alcoholism. Alcoholics appeared to show significantly worse clinical results.

Summary

1. The quality of the clinical result is related to the quality of reduction of the articular surface.
2. Good or excellent clinical results may be achieved in 75% of patients treated by rigid internal fixation in experienced hands.
3. Good or excellent clinical results were found in 50–55% of patients treated by a variety of methods, other than rigid internal fixation.

ANKLE FRACTURES IN CHILDREN

Spiegel et al (1978) analysed 184 patients with epiphyseal fractures of the distal end of the tibia and fibula. They reported significant skeletal complications in 14% of patients. The majority of the complications (23/26) involved the tibial growth plate. The authors identified three risk groups according to the likelihood of developing shortening, angular deformity or joint incongruity. The risk groups are defined in Table 13.5. The fracture types refer to the classification of Salter & Harris (1963).

There are four types of complication which may follow ankle fractures in children — angular deformity, rotational deformity, leg length discrepancy and joint surface incongruity.

Table 13.5 Risk of development of skeletal complications following distal epiphyseal injuries of the tibia and fibula (from Spiegel et al 1978)

Risk	Type of fracture
Low risk (6.7% incidence of complications)	Type I and II fibular fractures Type I tibial fractures Type III and IV tibial fractures with less than 2 mm displacement Epiphyseal avulsions
High risk (32% incidence of complications)	Type III and IV tibial fractures with more than 2 mm displacement Juvenile Tillaux fractures Triplane fractures Comminuted epiphyseal fractures
Unpredictable risk (16.7% incidence of complications)	Type II tibial fractures

Angular deformity

This may result from asymmetrical growth plate closure or malunion.

Dias (1984) considered that varus deformity was the commonest angular deformity associated with asymmetric closure of the tibial growth plate. He reviewed 101 Salter–Harris type III and IV fractures from the literature and found that varus deformity occurred in 14%. He stated that varus deformity was rarely associated with a Salter–Harris type II fracture. Spiegel et al (1978) identified 5 cases in their series, with over 5° of varus angulation due to asymmetric growth plate closure. Two of these were Salter–Harris III fractures, but the others were Salter–Harris II. The authors found that only 1 patient, with varus angulation of 15°, required additional surgical treatment.

Dias (1984) reported that valgus deformity was uncommon following asymmetric growth plate closure. Spiegel et al (1978) found only 1 case with significant valgus deformity (15°). This occurred in a Salter–Harris type II fracture which was inadequately reduced and subsequently developed asymmetric growth plate closure. Dias (1984) pointed out that complete arrest of the distal fibular growth plate could lead to fibular shortening and valgus deformity. Spiegel et al (1978) described 21 cases of Salter–Harris type I and II fractures of the fibula. Three type I fractures developed premature closure of the fibular growth plate, 2 with shortening. However, none had angular deformities.

Rotational deformity

Rotational deformity is uncommon following ankle fractures in children. Cooperman et al (1978) reported follow-up on 12 children with triplane fractures. Three of these patients had external rotation deformity of 5–10°. Spiegel et al (1978) did not describe rotational deformity in their follow-up series.

Leg length discrepancy

Dias (1984) reported that leg length discrepancy occurred in 10–30% of patients with injuries to the distal tibial growth plate. Chadwick & Bentley (1987) described growth retardation in 8 out of 28 (29%) children with distal tibial growth plate injuries. Spiegel et al (1978) described 17 patients (9%) with growth retardation of 0.4–1.3 cm in their series of 184 children.

The incidence of leg length discrepancy is related to the Salter–Harris fracture type, as shown in Table 13.6. In the majority of these cases the shortening was less than 2 cm and required no treatment.

Joint surface incongruity

Joint surface incongruity is determined partly by the nature of the injury

Table 13.6 Leg length discrepancy following injuries of the distal tibial epiphysis: relationship to Salter–Harris classification (from Spiegel et al 1978 and Chadwick & Bentley 1987)

	Cases with shortening	Number of cases	%
Salter–Harris type			
I	1	28	3.5
II	11	78	14
III	3	45	6.5
IV	6	11	54
V	1	2	50
Triplane fractures	3	20	15
Total	25	184	13.5

and partly by the approach to treatment. There is evidence from Lindsjo's work (1981) that articular incongruity predisposes to osteoarthritis in adults. Spiegel et al (1978) demonstrated that there was a higher incidence of skeletal complications when articular steps of 2 mm or more were present.

Summary

1. Significant skeletal complications occur in approximately 15% of children with epiphyseal fractures of the distal end of the tibia and fibula. Risk groups related to fracture type have been identified by Spiegel et al (1978) (see Table 13.5).
2. Growth arrest may be delayed following epiphyseal injury. Follow-up should continue for at least 1 year before a final prognosis is given.
3. Varus deformity occurs more commonly than valgus deformity as a complication of ankle fractures in children.
4. Leg length discrepancy occurs in 10–30% of children with injuries to the distal tibial growth plate. It appears to be more common after Salter–Harris type IV injuries. In the majority of cases, it is less than 2 cm and requires no treatment.

REFERENCES

Bauer M 1985 Ankle fractures: with special reference to post-traumatic arthrosis. MD Thesis, Lund University, Malmo.
Beauchamp C G, Clay N R, Thexton P W 1983 Displaced ankle fractures in patients over 50 years of age. Journal of Bone and Joint Surgery 65B: 329–332
Bone L B 1987 Fractures of the tibial plafond. Orthopedic Clinics of North America 18: 95–104
Buhr A J, Cooke A M 1959 Fracture patterns. Lancet, vol I, March 14: 531–536
Cedell C 1967 Supination — outward rotation injuries of the ankle. Acta Orthopaedica Scandinavica (suppl) 110

Chadwick C J, Bentley G 1987 The classification and prognosis of epiphyseal injuries. Injury 18: 157–168

Coltart W D 1951 Sprained ankle. British Medical Journal ii: 957–961

Cooperman D R, Spiegel P G, Laros G S 1978 Tibial fractures involving the ankle in children: the so-called triplane epiphyseal fracture. Journal of Bone and Joint Surgery 60A: 1040–1046

Cox F J, Laxson W W 1952 Fractures about the ankle joint. American Journal of Surgery May: 674–679

Danis R 1949 Théorie et pratique de l'osteosynthèse. Desouer et Masson, Liège

Dias L S 1984 Fractures of the tibia and fibula. In: Rockwood C A Jr, Wilkins K E, King R E (eds) Fractures in children, vol 3. J B Lippincott, Philadelphia

Dillin L, Slabaugh P 1986 Delayed wound healing, infection and non union following open reduction and internal fixation of tibial plafond fractures. Journal of Trauma 26: 1116–1119

Glasgow M, Jackson A, Jamieson A M 1981 Instability of the ankle after injury to the lateral ligament. Journal of Bone and Joint Surgery 62B: 196–200

Harrington K D 1979 Degenerative arthritis of the ankle secondary to long standing lateral ligament instability. Journal of Bone and Joint Surgery 61A: 354–361

Klossner O 1962 Late results of operative and non operative treatment of ankle fractures. Acta Chirurgica Scandinavica (suppl) 293

Lauge-Hansen N 1948 Fractures of the ankle. Analytic–historic survey as the basis of a new experiment, roentgenologic and clinical investigations. Archives of Surgery 56: 259–317

Lightowler C D R 1984 Injuries to the lateral ligament of the ankle. British Medical Journal 289: 1274

Lindsjo J 1981 Operative treatment of ankle fractures. Acta Orthopaedica Scandinavica 52: (suppl) 189

Magnusson R 1944 On the late results in non operated cases of malleolar fractures. A clinical, roentgenological, statistical study: I fractures by external rotation. Acta Chirurgica Scandinavica (suppl) 84

Mendelsohn H A 1965 Non union of malleolar fractures of the ankle. Clinical Orthopaedics 42: 103–118

Muller M E, Allgower M, Schneider R, Willenegger H 1979 Manual of internal fixation. Springer Verlag, Berlin

Neithard F V, Plaue R 1977 Das lintere tibiakantenfragment als prognostisches kriterium. Archiv für Orthopaedische und Unfallchirurgie 87: 213–221

Olerud S 1981 Foreword to operative treatment of ankle fractures. Acta Orthopaedica Scandinavica 52 (suppl) 189

Ovadia D N, Beals R K 1986 Fractures of the tibial plafond. Journal of Bone and Joint Surgery 68A: 543–551

Phillips W A, Spiegel P G 1979 Evaluation of ankle fractures: non operative v operative. Clinical Orthopaedics 138: 17–20

Phillips W A, Schwartz H S, Keller C S et al 1985 A prospective randomised study of the management of severe ankle fractures. Journal of Bone and Joint Surgery 67A: 67–78

Ruedi T 1973 Fractures of the lower end of the tibia into the ankle joint: results 9 years after open reduction and internal fixation. Injury 5: 130–134

Ruedi T, Allgower M 1969 Fractures of the lower end of the tibia into the ankle joint. Injury 1: 92–99

Ruedi T, Allgower M 1979 The operative treatment of intra-articular fractures of the lower end of the tibia. Clinical Orthopaedics 138: 105–110

Salter R B, Harris W 1963 Injuries involving the epiphyseal plate. Journal of Bone and Joint Surgery 45A: 587–622

Sarkisian J S, Cody S W 1976 Closed treatment of ankle fractures: a new criterion for evaluation — a review of 250 cases. Journal of Trauma 16: 323–326

Sneppen O 1971 Treatment of pseudarthrosis involving the malleolus: a post operative follow up of 34 cases. Acta Orthopaedica Scandinavica 42: 201–216

Solonen K A, Lauttamus L 1968 Operative treatment of ankle fractures. Acta Orthopaedica Scandinavica 39: 223–237.

Spiegel P G, Cooperman D R, Laros G S 1978 Epiphyseal fractures of the distal end of the tibia and fibula. Journal of Bone and Joint Surgery 60A: 1046–1050

Weber B G 1972 Die verletzunger des oberen sprunggelenkes. Aktuelle probleme in der chirurgie. Band 3. Verlag Hans Huber, Bern

Willenegger H 1961 Die behandlung der luxationsfrakturen des oberen sprunggelenkes nach biomechanischen gesichtspunkten. Helvetica Chirurgica Acta 28: 225–239

Wilson F C 1984 Fractures and dislocations of the ankle. In: Rockwood C A Jr, Green D P (eds) Fractures in adults, vol II. J B Lippincott, Philadelphia

Zenker H, Nerlich M 1982 Prognostic aspects in operated ankle fractures. Acta Orthopaedica and Trauma Surgery 100: 237–241

14. The foot

M. A. Foy

INTRODUCTION

It has been estimated in the USA that of every 300 men working in heavy industry, 15 working days are lost per month as a result of foot problems. Of these lost days, 65% result from trauma (Hillegass 1976). The National Safety Council (1972) estimated that over 500 million dollars were paid in compensation in 1971 in the USA as a result of work-related leg and foot injuries.

Fractures and ligamentous injuries involving the foot are common. Injuries of the hindfoot have been covered fairly well in the orthopaedic literature and the prognosis following these injuries is reasonably clear.

Reports on the results of injuries to the midfoot and forefoot are less comprehensive. There is less agreement on the classification of these injuries. These factors make it much more difficult to predict the prognosis after injuries affecting the midfoot and forefoot.

CALCANEAL FRACTURES

The calcaneus is the most commonly fractured tarsal bone. As long ago as 1908, Cotton & Wilson believed that: 'ordinarily speaking, the man who breaks his heel bone is "done", so far as his industrial future is concerned'.

There is still a great deal of controversy regarding the classification, management and prognosis of calcaneal fractures. Wilson (1982) assessed 1172 calcaneal fractures from the orthopaedic literature. A total of 75% were intra-articular and 25% were extra-articular. This ratio is typical of other large reported series.

When classifying calcaneal fractures it is important to try to separate those injuries with a good prognosis from those with a poor prognosis. Essex-Lopresti (1952), in his classic paper, emphasized the difference between extra-articular fractures, which tend to do well, and fractures involving the subtalar joint, which have a poorer prognosis.

Heckman (1984) suggested classification of extra-articular fractures into five groups (anterior process, tuberosity, medial process, sustentaculum tali and body) and intra-articular fractures into four groups (undisplaced,

357

tongue fractures, joint depression/thalamic fractures and comminuted fractures). The tongue fractures and joint depression fracture patterns were described by Essex-Lopresti (1952). He recognized them as two distinct subtypes in the intra-articular group. In both types the secondary fracture line arises from or near to the 'crucial angle' of Gissane.

Extra-articular fractures

Essex-Lopresti (1952) followed up 47 patients with extra-articular fractures. All were able to return to work, and 92% did so within 6 months. A total of 93% had no symptoms or only trivial symptoms. He also found that those cases treated by early mobilization returned to work quicker than those treated in plaster.

Nade & Monahan (1973) found that the average time lost from work was 7–8 weeks. Over 80% of patients in this group had no long-term symptoms.

Rowe et al (1963) followed up 68 patients with extra-articular fractures. The length of follow-up ranged from 1 to 20 years. They used a scoring system to evaluate their results. Patients were treated by a variety of surgeons and a variety of methods. The authors found that 93% of patients had excellent or good results. There were no poor results.

Degan et al (1982) reported 25 patients with avulsion fractures of the anterior process of the calcaneus. Eighteen of these patients were successfully treated by plaster immobilization. Seven patients subsequently underwent excision of the anterior fragment for symptomatic non-union. In 4 of these cases the diagnosis had been missed for between 4 and 24 months. Five of the 7 patients were relieved by excision of the fragment. The 2 patients who had the diagnosis delayed longest (22 and 24 months respectively) were not relieved of symptoms by operation. The authors pointed out that even in the conservatively treated patients who had a successful result, full recovery sometimes took 6–12 months.

Fractures of the posterior tuberosity are relatively uncommon. Rowe et al (1963) reported this injury in 6 (4%) of their 146 patients. All 6 patients had good or excellent results following closed or open reduction. Lowy (1969) pointed out that the practice of classifying these injuries into 'beak' fractures and avulsion fractures is probably unnecessary. His dissections, together with the work of Korn (1942), showed that the insertion of the calcaneal tendon may cover a variable portion of the posterior aspect of the calcaneus. Therefore, avulsion may be the causative mechanism for fractures of any part of the calcaneal tuberosity.

Rowe et al (1963) and Heckman (1984) showed that fractures of the medial tuberosity and sustentaculum tali were rarely associated with long-term symptoms. Heckman (1984) pointed out that rarely non-union of the sustentaculum may occur and may require excision.

Rowe et al (1963) described 30 patients with fractures of the body of the calcaneus not involving the joint. In all, 90% of these cases were rated excellent or good at follow-up.

Heckman (1984) commented that all extra-articular fractures tend to do well. However, aching pain associated with changes in the weather can be expected to occur for 12–18 months after the injury.

Intra-articular fractures

Approximately 75% of calcaneal fractures are intra-articular. No single method of treatment is suitable for all these fractures. The percentage of satisfactory (excellent or good) clinical results is difficult to define. The numbers of successfully treated cases reported in the literature are often not comparable from series to series. This is because quality of reduction and subsequent functional results are frequently poorly defined.

Undisplaced intra-articular fractures have a good prognosis. Thoren (1964) reviewed 13 cases; all achieved excellent or good results. Essex-Lopresti (1952) found excellent or good results in 84% of 32 patients with undisplaced fractures.

The results following displaced intra-articular fractures can be broadly classified into three groups from the work of Lindsay & Dewar (1958), Lance et al (1963), Rowe et al (1963), Thoren (1964) and Pozo et al (1984):

1. *Excellent/good*: The patient felt that the foot was entirely normal or experienced only minor symptoms.
2. *Fair*: The patient could resume previous or similar work but had to limit recreational activities. There was moderate pain and swelling.
3. *Poor*: The patient continued to suffer moderate to severe pain and had limited employability. Patients requiring major secondary surgery are included in this group.

If those patients treated by primary subtalar arthrodesis and internal fixation are excluded, then 210 of 338 patients (62%) achieved an excellent or good result. Lindsay & Dewar (1958) and Pozo et al (1984) did not distinguish clearly between the fair and the poor results. The other authors made this distinction, and 47 of 234 patients (20%) had a fair result and 57 of 234 (24%) a poor result. These figures are unbalanced because the

Table 14.1 Results after non-operative treatment of displaced intra-articular fractures of the calcaneus

	Number of cases	Excellent/ good	Fair	Poor
Pozo et al (1984)	21	17	4	
Lindsay & Dewar (1958)	83	63	20	
Thoren (1964)	75	43	18	14
Rowe et al (1963)	62	32	15	15
Lance et al (1963)	97	55	14	28
Total	338	210/338 (62%)	47/234 (20%)	57/234 (24%)

two studies which did not categorize fair and poor results showed the highest incidence of good and excellent results (Table 14.1).

Lindsay & Dewar (1958) reported an average follow-up of 8 years in their patients. The average time before symptoms stabilized was 18 months, and 15% of their patients required 3 years or more for stabilization of their symptoms.

Sources of residual disability and timing of medicolegal reports

It has been shown by Essex-Lopresti (1952), Nade & Monahan (1973) and Lindsay & Dewar (1958) that it may take 18–36 months for symptoms to reach a plateau following intra-articular fractures of the calcaneus. McLaughlin (1963) summarized the main problems that may occur:

1. *Pain*: This may arise from subtalar osteoarthritis, peroneal tendonitis, calcaneofibular abutment due to bulging of the lateral wall of the calcaneus, heel pain secondary to plantar fasciitis or a bony spur and, rarely, nerve entrapment.
2. *Deformity*: Broadening of the heel, which may lead to calcaneofibular abutment as described above. Thoren (1964) found that broadening (measured with a caliper below the tip of the lateral malleolus) in excess of 1 cm occurred in approximately 50% of intra-articular fractures. He found a correlation between broadening of the heel and functional result. If broadening of the heel was less than 1 cm, 84% of patients (37 of 44) achieved a good or excellent result. If there was broadening of 1 cm or more, only 46% (21 of 46) patients achieved a good or excellent result. These results refer to a comparison with the normal heel.
3. *Stiffness*: This results from fibrous ankylosis or osteoarthritis in the subtalar joint.
4. *Persistent swelling*.

In view of the time taken for symptoms to reach a plateau, final medicolegal reports should not be given until at least 2 years after the injury.

Prognostic factors

Fracture classification

The important feature in the classification is the degree of intra-articular displacement. Extra-articular fractures and undisplaced intra-articular fractures have been shown to have a relatively good prognosis. Displaced intra-articular fractures have been shown to fare less well. There is no evidence to suggest that tongue fractures have a worse prognosis than joint depression fractures.

Thoren (1964) assessed the results in patients who had been treated conservatively. The degree of displacement of the posterior articular facet was classified as moderate or considerable. Of 40 patients, 34 (85%) with moderate displacement achieved a good or excellent result. Only 9 of 35 patients (26%) with considerable displacement achieved a good or excellent result. This difference is not quantifiable, but emphasizes the important effect of displacement on the prognosis.

Essex-Lopresti (1952) showed the importance of restoring joint congruity in displaced intra-articular fractures. Of 52 patients, 36 (70%) achieved a good clinical result after a successful reduction of the joint surface. Only 6 of 28 patients (21%) achieved a good result when the attempted reduction was unsuccessful.

Residual displacement is therefore a reliable indicator of long-term prognosis.

Residual deformity

This has been discussed in the previous section. Widening of the heel by more than 1 cm is associated with a worse prognosis. This is due to loss of calcaneal height and hence is linked to malreduction of the joint.

Age

Essex-Lopresti (1952) and Vestad (1968) suggested that patients over the age of 50 did not do as well as those under 50 following surgical treatment. Thoren did not confirm this finding.

Time to weight-bearing

Weight-bearing too early can convert a minimally displaced fracture into a more severely displaced fracture with a poorer prognosis. Lance et al (1963) described 14 patients in whom this occurred. They found that it did not occur if weight-bearing was delayed until 8 weeks after the injury.

Heel pad atrophy

Lance et al (1963) pointed out that when heel pad atrophy was present, it was usually associated with a poor prognosis.

Summary

1. Extra-articular fractures of the calcaneus are associated with a good long-term prognosis in over 90% of cases.
2. Undisplaced intra-articular fractures of the calcaneus are associated with a good long-term prognosis in over 90% of cases.
3. Displaced intra-articular fractures of the calcaneus are associated with a good or excellent long-term prognosis in approximately 60% of cases.

4. Residual symptoms may take 18–36 months to settle completely. In symptomatic patients, final medicolegal reports should not be given until at least 2 years after the injury.

FRACTURES AND DISLOCATIONS ABOUT THE TALUS

Fractures of the neck of the talus

The most widely used classification of talar neck fractures was described by Hawkins (1970). This classification is useful in the prediction of prognosis. Hawkins recognized three fracture types:

Type I: Undisplaced fracture of the talar neck.
Type II: Displaced fracture of the talar neck with subtalar joint subluxation.
Type III: Displaced fracture of the talar neck with dislocation of the body of the talus from both the subtalar and ankle joints.

The frequency and severity of complications are directly proportional to the degree of displacement of the fracture. The main complications are delayed union, malunion, avascular necrosis of the body of the talus and osteoarthritis of the subtalar and ankle joints. Heckman (1984) pointed out that all the recent reviews of this subject concluded that the best results occurred when prompt anatomical reduction of the fracture was achieved and maintained. Comfort et al (1985) and Szyszkowitz et al (1985) supported this view.

Delayed union/non-union

Hawkins (1970), Peterson et al (1977) and Lorentzen et al (1977) considered the frequency of delayed and non-union in their patients. In these three series there were 216 patients with talar neck fractures and 14 examples of delayed or non-union (6%). Peterson et al (1977) defined delayed union as occurring when there was no evidence of healing at 6 months. The results from these reports are broken down according to Hawkins's classification in Table 14.2.

Table 14.2 Incidence of delayed union or non-union in talar neck fractures (from Hawkins 1970, Peterson et al 1977 and Lorentzen et al 1977)

Hawkins type	Delayed or non-union	Number of fractures	%
I	1	68	1.5
II	7	96	7
III	6	52	11.5
Total	14	216	6

Malunion

Tile (1987) felt that malunion was of greater clinical significance than avas-cular necrosis in talar neck fractures. He pointed out that the consequence of malunion was chronic subluxation of the subtalar joint, leading to secondary degenerative arthritis and altered foot mechanics.

Malunion occurred in 18 of the 123 patients described by Lorentzen et al (1977). Fifteen of these cases occurred in the 53 type II fractures (28%). Canale & Kelly (1978) found 18 malunions in 71 talar neck fractures. Most of the malunions occurred in type II fractures.

The incidence of malunion reflects the approach to treatment. The inci-dence of malunion and its sequelae ought to be less in patients in whom the fractures are reduced and internally fixed.

Avascular necrosis

This is a common complication of talar neck fractures, although it is not always associated with disabling symptoms. Table 14.3 illustrates the inci-dence of avascular necrosis from six series (401 patients in all).

Table 14.3 Incidence of avascular necrosis following talar neck fractures (Hawkins' 1970 classification)

	Number of cases (avascular necrosis in brackets)			Follow-up (years)
	Type I	Type II	Type III	
Peterson et al (1977)	8 (0)	19 (3)	9 (3)	6
Lorentzen et al (1977)	54 (2)	53 (13)	16 (11)	2
Hawkins (1970)	6 (0)	24 (10)	27 (20)	not known
Norgrove Penny & Davis (1980)	5 (0)	11 (2)	11 (11)	6
Canale & Kelly (1978)	15 (2)	30 (15)	23 (19)	13
Coltart (1952)	37 (0)	38 (12)	15 (14)	not known
Total	125 (4)	175 (65)	101 (78)	
	[3%]	[37%]	[77%]	

Hawkins (1970) described a radiographic sign, usually present at 6–8 weeks after injury, which enables avascular necrosis to be recognized. The appearance of subchondral osteoporosis at this stage was said to exclude avascular necrosis. Heckman (1984) felt that this was the best radiographic indicator of viability of the talar body. Canale & Kelly (1978) described 23 patients who had subchondral osteoporosis 6–12 weeks after injury; only 1 (4%) developed avascular necrosis. These authors had 26 patients without subchondral osteoporosis and 20 (77%) developed avascular necrosis. This demonstrated that Hawkins' sign was a useful, although not infallible, prognostic indicator.

Table 14.4   Evaluation of results using Hawkins' (1970) criteria

	Points
Pain	
None	6
After activity	3
Continuous	0
Limp	
Absent	3
Present	0
Ankle range of motion	
Full	3
Limited	2
Fused	1
Fixed deformity	0
Subtalar range of motion	
Full	3
Limited	2
Fused	1
Fixed deformity	0
Excellent result	13–15
Good result	10–12
Fair result	7–9
Poor result	6 or less

Not all patients with avascular necrosis experience disabling symptoms. Most series evaluate results according to Hawkins' criteria (Table 14.4).

Table 14.5 shows the final results in 60 patients with avascular necrosis of the talus. In all, 28% had a good or excellent clinical result. Canale & Kelly (1978) described better results in patients who had a positive Hawkins' sign and were treated by prolonged avoidance of weight-bearing. Norgrove Penny & Davis (1980) did not agree that prolonged avoidance of weight-bearing improved the prognosis.

Table 14.5   Results in patients with avascular necrosis after talar neck fractures (Hawkins' 1970 criteria)

	Number of cases with avascular necrosis	Excellent	Good	Fair	Poor
Hawkins (1970)	24	1	2	12	9
Norgrove Penny & Davis (1980)	13	0	2	3	8
Canale & Kelly (1978)	23	4	8	5	6
Total	60	5	12	20	23
		28%		72%	

Osteoarthritis

This may affect the ankle joint, the subtalar joint or both. It commonly, but not invariably, follows avascular necrosis.

Table 14.6 shows the incidence of osteoarthritis in the ankle and subtalar joints in the 123 patients followed up by Lorentzen et al (1977). The follow-up in this series was from 7 to 73 months (average 22 months). A quarter of the patients had arthritis involving both joints. These figures broadly correspond with those published in other reports.

Table 14.6 Incidence of osteoarthritis following fractures of the talar neck (from Lorentzen et al 1977)

Hawkins type	Number of patients	Ankle joint arthritis	Subtalar joint arthritis
I	54	8 (15%)	13 (24%)
II	53	19 (36%)	35 (66%)
III	16	11 (69%)	10 (63%)
Total	123	38 (31%)	58 (47%)

Clinical results

The most widely applied classification of clinical results is the points system described by Hawkins in 1970 (Table 14.4). This system is heavily weighted for pain, and an excellent result can only be achieved when pain is absent. Table 14.7 incorporates the clinical results from the work of Hawkins (1970), Peterson et al (1977) and Norgrove Penny & Davis (1980).

Table 14.7 Clinical results in 108 talar neck fractures (from Hawkins 1970, Peterson et al 1977 and Norgrove Penny & Davis 1980)

Hawkins type	Number of patients	Excellent	Good	Fair	Poor
I	18	7	6	4	1
		72%		28%	
II	48	7	11	12	18
		35.5%		62.5%	
III	42	2	8	16	16
		24%		76%	

It has already been shown, in the section on avascular necrosis, that the clinical results are significantly worse if avascular necrosis develops. However, over one-quarter of the patients with avascular necrosis still had a satisfactory (excellent or good) clinical result (Table 14.5).

Syszkowitz et al (1985) and Grob et al (1985) described operative treatment of displaced talar fractures. Unfortunately classification of the fractures and assessment of the results differed from the series already described in which conservative treatment predominated, i.e. plaster immobilization, closed reduction/plaster immobilization or open reduction/ plaster immobilization.

There are insufficient numbers to allow comparison of differing methods of operative treatment or the influence of rigid fixation and early mobilization on the long-term outcome.

Fractures of the body of the talus

Fractures of the body of the talus are much less common than fractures of the neck. The most extensive review of these injuries was by Sneppen et al (1977). They described 31 patients who suffered shearing fractures (17), compression fractures (10) or crush fractures (4) of the body of the talus. Eight patients (26%) developed avascular necrosis of the talus. This occurred in 3 of the 4 crush fractures.

Nineteen of these patients (61%) developed osteoarthritis of the ankle joint, subtalar joint or both. Only 11 patients (35%) were able to return to their previous job. Twelve (39%) were forced to obtain lighter work and 8 (25%) were unable to continue working due to their persisting disability. All of these patients were assessed by the Directorate of Employment Accident Insurance in Copenhagen, in order to quantitate their disability. They all had a significant level of disability, and in 17 (55%) it was assessed at over 12%.

Manipulation and plaster immobilization were the commonest method of treatment in this group. The final results were not related to the degree of residual displacement; Szyszkowitz et al (1985) hoped that better results might be possible in experienced hands, with open reduction and internal fixation of displaced articular fractures.

The careful assessment in Sneppen's et al's (1977) series of patients is very valuable in providing guidelines to the prognosis. The length of follow-up in this series was relatively short — from 9 to 76 months, with an average of 23 months.

Coltart (1952) described 22 cases of fractures of the body of the talus with only 1 case of avascular necrosis. The classification and assessment of talar body fractures in Coltart's series were not as detailed as in Sneppen et al's series. Kenwright & Taylor (1970) described 6 patients with fractures of the talar body in a series of 58 patients with major talar injuries. Two of these patients developed avascular necrosis.

Peripheral fractures of the talus

Head of the talus

This is a rare fracture. Coltart (1952) found 6 cases in 228 injuries of the talus, and Kenwright & Taylor (1970) found 2 cases in 58 talar injuries, indicating an incidence of approximately 3% of all talar injuries.

There are not enough cases of talar head fractures reported to enable meaningful conclusions to be drawn. Both of the patients reported by Kenwright & Taylor (1970) regained full function; however neither of these patients had comminuted fractures.

Heckman (1984) described talonavicular arthritis as a potential complication of this type of injury.

Lateral process of the talus

Hawkins (1965) and Mukherjee et al (1974) reported the two largest series of these injuries, with 13 patients in each study. In Hawkins's series the injury was missed at the initial assessment in 6 of the 13 patients. The treatment was conservative in this group. Seven of the patients had no symptoms and normal function 8 weeks after injury. The other 6 still had pain 6 months after the injury and 3 required an operation; in 2 patients this consisted of excision of the fragment and in the other subtalar fusion. The other 3 patients had pain, but it was not of sufficient severity to merit surgical treatment.

Mukherjee et al (1974) argued that Hawkins's patients had received inadequate treatment. Their results suggested that early excision or reduction of the lateral process, if it was displaced or comminuted, produced better results. Of the 12 patients that they were able to follow up, 7 were symptom-free at an average of 14 months after the injury. Two were awaiting subtalar fusion and 3 had mild discomfort.

Analysis of these results suggests that 50–60% of patients do well, irrespective of the treatment. Some 20–25% have persistent discomfort sufficient to warrant surgery at 6–18 months from the injury and 20–25% have mild symptoms not severe enough to merit operation at this time.

Posterior process of the talus

The posterior process has both a medial and lateral tubercle. The tubercles are separated by a groove in which the flexor hallucis longus tendon runs. Wilson (1982) pointed out that a fracture of the posterior process can be distinguished from the os trigonum by its irregular outline and by the presence of tilting of the fractured process. Heckman (1984) reported that fractures occur more commonly in the lateral tubercle than in the medial tubercle. He also emphasized the importance of correlating the clinical and radiological findings. He observed that an X-ray of the contralateral ankle might be helpful in difficult cases, because the os trigonum, when present, was bilateral in 60% of cases.

There are no large reported series of patients with problems following this injury. Heckman (1984) found several reports in the literature describing un-united persistently symptomatic fractures of the lateral tubercle of the posterior process. These cases usually responded to excision of the un-united fragment.

Osteochondral fractures of the dome of the talus

These injuries may occur on the medial or lateral side of the talar dome. Berndt & Harty (1959) classified osteochondral fractures as follows:

Type I: Compression fractures (they may not become visible on X-ray until resorption takes place).
Type II: Incomplete fracture.
Type III: Complete fracture without displacement.
Type IV: Complete fracture with displacement.

Pettine & Morrey (1987) described follow-up on 71 osteochondral fractures in 68 patients. The average length of follow-up was 7.5 years. They adopted a simple classification of their results:

Good: No symptoms.
Fair: Symptoms but little limitation of daily activities.
Poor: Symptoms interfered with or prevented daily activity.

They found that 75% of patients still complained of some pain and 22% had pain all the time. They also found that most patients stabilized approximately 1 year after definitive treatment; this is important when deciding on the timing of medicolegal reports.

Pettine & Morrey's (1987) results are shown in Table 14.8. Most of the patients treated by operation had excision of the osteochondral fragment; only 5 had the fragment re-attached. These results indicate a significantly poorer prognosis for type III and IV fractures.

Table 14.8   Results of treatment in osteochondral fractures of the talus (adapted from Pettine & Morrey 1987)

Type of fracture (Berndt & Harty 1959)	Number of patients	Results					
		With operation			Without operation		
		Good	Fair	Poor	Good	Fair	Poor
I	5	0	0	0	3	1	1
II	17	2	0	1	11	2	0
III	27	6	4	4	3	5	5
IV	17	2	2	7	0	0	6

Dislocation about the talus

Subtalar dislocation (peritalar dislocation)

This occurs more commonly to the medial than the lateral side. Wilson (1982) reported that avascular necrosis seldom occurred and the results were usually satisfactory.

Review of the results in 62 patients reported by Dunn (1974), Christensen et al (1977), Monson & Ryan (1981) and Delee & Curtis (1982) shows that the outcome is not always satisfactory (Table 14.9). The incidence of avascular necrosis is approximately 5%, but osteoarthritis of the ankle or subtalar joint occurred in over half of the patients.

Table 14.9 Incidence of avascular necrosis and osteoarthritis after subtalar dislocations

Reference	Number of patients	Medial	Lateral	Avascular necrosis	Osteoarthritis
		dislocation			
Dunn (1974)	7*	5	1	1	N/A
Christensen et al (1977)	30	26	4	2	19
Monson & Ryan (1981)	8	7	1	0	5
Delee & Curtis (1982)	17*	12	4	0	7
Total	62	50	10	3 (5%)	31/55 (56%)

*One anterior and one posterior dislocation included.

Table 14.10 Subjective results after subtalar dislocation

	Number of patients	Good	Fair	Poor	Follow-up
Dunn (1974)	7	4	2	1	15 months
Christensen et al (1977)	30	9	16	5	23 months
Monson & Ryan (1981)	8	3	4	1	28 months
Delee & Curtis (1982)	17	8	6	3	35 months
Total	62	24 (39%)	28 (45%)	10 (16%)	26 months

The subjective symptoms in these patients are shown in Table 14.10. The criteria are based upon the level of pain:

Good: No pain.
Fair: Mild pain, or pain only when walking on uneven ground.
Poor: Severe pain.

The average follow-up in these patients was only 26 months.

The results appear to be worse in patients with compound injuries, associated fractures and lateral dislocations. Delee & Curtis (1982) found that when subtalar dislocations occurred as a result of a simple inversion injury the results were uniformly good. They found that the results were significantly worse in the high-velocity injuries with compound dislocation and intra-articular fractures.

Total dislocation of the talus

Heckman (1984) reported that most of these injuries were compound and that the results were often devastating. Dettenbeck & Kelly (1969) described 9 cases and found that permanent infection occurred in 8. Talectomy and tibiocalcaneal fusion were required in these cases. Coltart (1952) described similar experience with 9 total dislocations of the talus.

The results after this injury are certainly poor, and Wilson (1982) suggested that in those cases where the dislocation is reduced, the incidence of avascular necrosis is over 50%.

Summary

1. Delayed or non-union of talar neck fractures occurs in approximately 6% of cases.
2. Avascular necrosis occurs in approximately 3% of Hawkins type I talar neck fractures, 37% of type II fractures and 77% of type III fractures. The presence of subchondral osteoporosis 6–12 weeks after the injury (Hawkins' sign) is a useful indicator of the vascularity of the talus.
3. Some 28% of patients with talar neck fractures who develop avascular necrosis may still have a good or excellent clinical result.
4. Osteoarthritis more commonly involves the subtalar joint than the ankle joint after talar neck fracture (see Table 14.6).
5. Avascular necrosis develops in about one-quarter of patients with talar body fractures.
6. Of patients with talar body fractures, 60% develop osteoarthritis of the ankle, subtalar joint or both.
7. In all, 50–60% of patients with fractures of the lateral process of the talus have a satisfactory result; 20–25% either have mild pain not requiring surgery or have symptoms warranting excision of the fragment.
8. Type III and IV osteochondral fractures of the talar dome have a poor prognosis (see Table 14.8).
9. Osteoarthritis develops in over half the patients with a subtalar dislocation. Of these patients, 60% continue to experience moderate or severe pain.
10. Total dislocation of the talus is associated with a poor long-term prognosis.

MID-TARSAL FRACTURE DISLOCATIONS

The most comprehensive review of these injuries was made by Main & Jowett (1975). They described the treatment and results in 73 patients. It is interesting that in 30 of these patients (41%) the diagnosis was delayed because of lack of awareness of the injury or because of inadequate X-rays.

Main & Jowett (1975) divided the injuries into five types based on the direction of the causative violence — the direction of violence does not materially affect the prognosis. Their results are analysed according to the type of injury in Table 14.11. Fracture sprains are characterized by flake fractures of the dorsal margins of the talus or navicular and of the calcaneus and cuboid.

The results are classified after Main & Jowett (1975):

Excellent: No symptoms or signs.
Good: Trivial symptoms and signs insufficient to impair function.
Fair: Residual symptoms and signs with some disability.
Poor: Marked symptoms and limitation of function, with subsequent arthrodesis or a request for further treatment from the patient.

Table 14.11   Results after injury to the mid-tarsal joint (adapted from Main & Jowett 1975)

Injury	Number	Excellent	Good	Fair	Poor
Fracture sprains	20	13 (65%)	5 (25%)	2 (10%)	0
Fracture dislocations	32	1 (3%)	6 (19%)	13 (41%)	12 (37%)*
Dislocations (including swivel dislocations)	10	1 (10%)	5 (50%)	1 (10%)	3 (30%)*
Crush fractures	4	0	1 (25%)	3 (75%)	0
Isolated navicular fractures	5	4 (80%)	1 (20%)	0	0

* Of the patients with poor results, 11 underwent mid-tarsal or triple arthrodesis.

Main & Jowett (1975) noted a much higher incidence of poor results where a closed reduction failed to improve the position. Unfortunately the length of follow-up was not specified in this report.

There are insufficient numbers of patients in this series to infer that one treatment method is better than another. However, better results appear to be associated with accurate reduction maintained until healing occurred.

Kenwright & Taylor (1970) reported a better experience with mid-tarsal dislocation. Eight of their 10 cases had a good or excellent result.

Summary

1. Some 90% of fracture sprains in the mid-tarsal region are associated with an excellent or good clinical result.
2. Only 20% of fracture dislocations in the mid-tarsal region are associated with an excellent or good clinical result.
3. Isolated dislocations, including swivel dislocations, are associated with an excellent or good result in 60–80% of patients.

TARSOMETATARSAL FRACTURE DISLOCATIONS

There is controversy regarding the importance of accurate reduction of these injuries. Key & Conwell (1956), Wilpulla (1973), Wilson (1972), Hardcastle et al (1982), Myerson et al (1986) and Arntz & Hansen (1987) were all agreed that treatment of these injuries should aim for anatomical reduction in order to achieve better results. Brunet & Wiley (1987) agreed that anatomical reduction should be the aim, but pointed out that poor reduction was often associated with good function.

The classification of these injuries follows that suggested by Quenu & Kuss in 1909, and has been used in the majority of the reports mentioned above. Quenu & Kuss described three injury types, as shown in Figure 14.1:

1. Total incongruity.
2. Partial incongruity.
3. Divergent.

Myerson et al (1986) and Brunet & Wiley (1987) both saw no correlation between the type of dislocation and the subsequent result. However, closer analysis of Brunet & Wiley's patients revealed that half of the group with total incongruity had functionally unsatisfactory results; this compares with

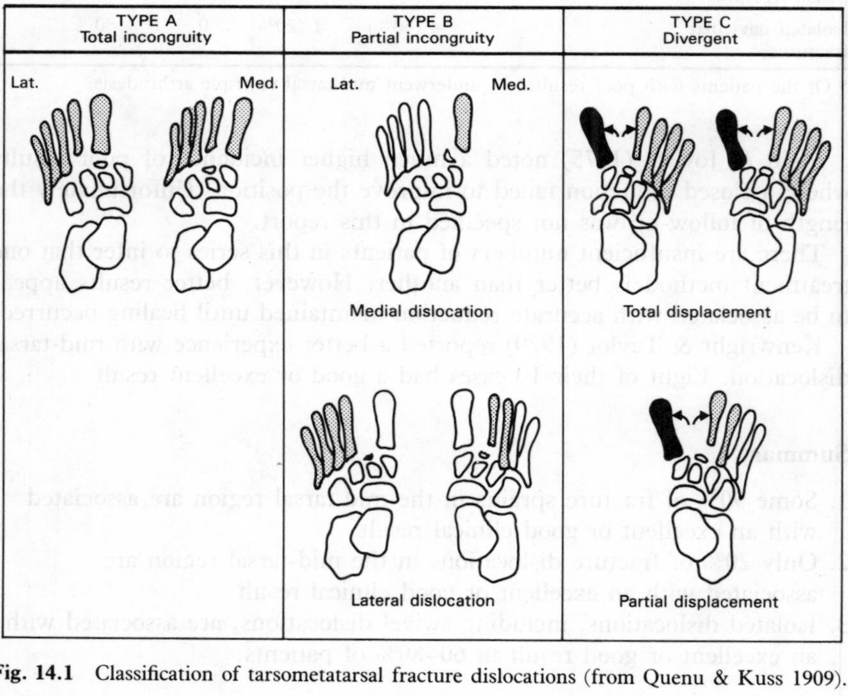

Fig. 14.1 Classification of tarsometatarsal fracture dislocations (from Quenu & Kuss 1909).

Table 14.12 Clinical results after tarsometatarsal fracture dislocations

Reference	Number of patients	Good	Fair	Poor	Mean follow-up
Wilpulla (1973)	26	9	9	8	5 years
Hardcastle et al (1982)	68	46	16	6	18 months–12 years
Myerson et al (1986)	55	27	13	15	4.2 years
Total	149	82 (55%)	38 (25%)	29 (20%)	

only 1 unsatisfactory result in 23 patients with partial incongruity. The clinical results from these series comprising 132 patients are shown in Table 14.12. Over half of the patients achieved good results. The criteria in these three groups were broadly as listed below:

Good: No pain (or trivial pain), could stand on tiptoe, normal gait and no deformity.

Fair: Moderate pain on activity, difficulty standing on tiptoe, a limp.

Poor: Marked continuous pain, inability to stand on tiptoe, limp and deformity.

The longest follow-up was reported by Brunet & Wiley (1987); it averaged 15 years. Unfortunately the subjective results reported by these authors are not strictly comparable with those given in Table 14.12. In Brunet & Wiley's series, 27 out of 33 patients (approximately 80%) felt either no pain or trivial pain. These authors found that symptoms usually progressed to a stable level after 3 months to 5 years (average 1.3 years). This is an important consideration for the timing of medicolegal reports.

In all the cases mentioned so far, there was a preponderance of patients with partial incongruity (type B fracture dislocation) and treatment was by a variety of methods ranging from plaster immobilization to open reduction and internal fixation. Myerson et al (1986) carefully analysed their results from three treatment groups — closed reduction and plaster immobilization; closed reduction and percutaneous wire fixation and open reduction and internal fixation. Using the painful foot centre (PFC) scoring system, they found an increased point score with both percutaneous pinning and open reduction and internal fixation, indicating a better clinical result. The maximum point score possible was 100, and the patients in these three groups achieved mean values of 57, 67 and 75 respectively.

Myerson et al also described a small group of 5 patients in whom the diagnosis was missed. The results in this group were significantly worse, with a mean PFC score of 45. This careful analysis certainly supports the view that treatment should aim for anatomical reduction.

Brunet & Wiley (1987) pointed out that they had 10 patients with persistent widening of the gap between the base of the first and second metatarsals. This ranged from 4 to 10 mm as measured on anteroposterior X-ray. They felt that this persistent gap had little bearing on the final result as far as pain and function were concerned.

Myerson et al (1986) carefully assessed this radiological parameter. In those of their patients rated as good, the average width between the first and second metatarsal base was 2.9 mm (range 2–5 mm). In those patients rated fair and poor, the average width was 5.8 mm (range 5 to 14 mm). Myerson et al's findings suggest that a persistent gap of more than 5 mm between the base of the first and second metatarsals may lead to a less satisfactory clinical result. Obviously, this parameter does not apply to total incongruity (type A) fracture dislocations.

Osteoarthritis is relatively common after these injuries. It does not always cause significant symptoms. Brunet & Wiley (1987) observed arthritis in 25 of 32 patients (78%). This was mild in all cases. Only 20–25% of patients with osteoarthritis had symptoms which affected their work or social activities. In view of the length of follow-up in this series, these figures are of considerable value in predicting the prognosis, and also in assessing the effect of osteoarthritis after these injuries.

Brunet & Wiley also pointed out that 76% of their patients were able to return to their original job (10 had been labourers and 16 were involved in office or clerical work). The other patients were forced to seek lighter work due to persistent foot discomfort.

Summary

1. Over half of the patients with tarsometatarsal fracture dislocations have a good long-term result.
2. The long-term results cannot be correlated with fracture type, although there is some evidence that type A (total incongruity) injuries may fare worse.
3. Symptoms reach a stable level at an average of 1.3 years after injury. Final medicolegal reports should probably not be given until 18 months after injury.
4. The results appear to be better in those cases where accurate reduction is achieved and maintained.
5. Osteoarthritis is common after these injuries (78% in Brunet & Wiley's series with a 15-year follow-up). However, only 20–25% of these patients had a significant functional problem.

METATARSAL AND PHALANGEAL INJURIES

Metatarsal fractures

These injuries usually follow direct violence, such as a heavy object falling on the foot. They may also occur after indirect trauma, as a result of a twisting injury.

Metatarsal shaft injuries

Spector et al (1984) followed up 12 patients with lesser metatarsal shaft fractures. Their therapeutic aim was to achieve anatomical reduction, early mobilization and full function. They evaluated the results using a scoring system based on pain, walking distance, activities, limp and X-ray appearances, modified from La Tourette et al (1980). The maximum point score was 50; 40–50 was rated good to excellent, 33–40 was rated fair and 0–33 was rated poor. Eight patients (67%) were rated good to excellent and 4 (33%) were rated fair. Length of follow-up was not specified.

Joplin (1958) reported excellent results in 26 (76%) of 34 patients with metatarsal fractures.

Heckman (1984) was of the opinion that displacement of fractures of the second, third or fourth metatarsals in the coronal plane was usually of no consequence. However, he believed that displacement in the sagittal plane was a cause for concern, because prominence of the metatarsal head on the sole or dorsum of the foot could lead to significant morbidity.

Fractures of the base of the fifth metatarsal

These fractures may be divided into two types — those involving the tuberosity (usually avulsion fractures) and those involving the proximal part of the shaft distal to the tuberosity (the Jones fracture). Jones (1902) described this injury in his own foot.

Dameron (1975) pointed out that the prognosis in avulsion fractures was excellent, with union occurring in 2 months in 99% of patients. In the other patient there was a non-union but it was asymptomatic.

Dameron drew attention to the fact that the Jones fracture was a more troublesome injury. He reported 20 cases and found that 12 (60%) united in 2–12 months and 3 within 21 months with conservative treatment. Five (25%) required a surgical procedure to achieve union. Not all non-unions in this series were asymptomatic.

Kavanaugh et al (1978) described 23 patients with Jones fractures. Follow-up in these patients averaged 3.5 years. The history and clinical picture in 40% of the patients in this group suggested a stress fracture. Approximately half of these fractures had not united 6 months after injury.

Torg et al (1984) reported 43 patients with Jones fractures and were able to follow them up for an average of 40 months. Twenty-five of these fractures were acute injuries; the others were delayed or non-unions. Ten of the acute fractures were treated with immobilization and early weight-bearing; only 4 (40%) of these went on to uneventful union. The other patients required surgery for symptomatic delayed or non-union. The other 15 patients were treated by plaster immobilization and non-weight-bearing; 14 (43%) healed uneventfully and the other patient required surgical treatment for a symptomatic non-union. The authors recommended that acute Jones fractures should be treated in a below-knee, non-weight-bearing plaster for 6 weeks.

Metatarsophalangeal disorders

Traumatic dislocations of these joints are much less common than those occurring as a manifestation of degenerative disease. Heckman (1984) was of the opinion that most of these injuries healed well, causing little long-term disability. There are no reports which contradict this view.

Interphalangeal dislocations

This is a more frequent injury than metatarsophalangeal dislocation. Reduction is usually easy. Wilson (1982) pointed out that in fracture dislocations exact reduction was unnecessary in the lesser toes but was desirable in the hallux. Again, there are no long-term results reported in the literature.

Phalangeal fractures

Heckman (1984) believed that displaced intra-articular fractures in the hallux should be reduced. He described painful non-union as an uncommon complication of these injuries. There is no mention in the literature of any significant long-term complications after lesser phalangeal fractures.

Sesamoid fractures

Both Wilson (1982) and Heckman (1984) described persistent discomfort as a complication of this uncommon injury. The precise incidence is unknown and when it occurs careful excision of the affected sesamoid is required. Elleby & Marcinko (1985) reported that it was not unusual to have to resort to surgical excision of the fractured sesamoid.

Wilson (1982) listed the major features used in the differentiation of a bipartite sesamoid from a fracture. The radiological features indicative of a fracture are separation of the fragments, irregular edges of the fragments and callus formation.

TRAUMATIC PARTIAL AMPUTATIONS OF THE FOOT

Millstein et al (1988) reported a series of 118 amputations in 113 patients following trauma. Follow-up ranged from 1 to 68 years, with a mean of 16 years. In this series there were in addition 49 patients whose partial amputation was considered a failure and later revised to a Symes or below-knee amputation.

The amputations were classified as digital, transverse and longitudinal. Transverse amputations were classified as metatarsophalangeal if all toes were removed, transmetatarsal, Lisfranc and Chopart. Longitudinal amputations were in the sagittal plane and involved resection of either the medial or lateral side of the foot.

The authors devised a grading system based on foot pain, the quality of the stump, functional disability and employment status. The results were graded as follows:

Good: Same (or similar) employment as before accident. No restriction of function or gait. No ulceration or pain.

Fair: Change of occupation required. Moderate pain. Recurrent callosities and shoe modifications. Restriction of function.

Poor: Persistent pain. Severe limitation of function and gait. Recurrent ulceration. Unable to work or had retired prematurely.

The results are shown in Table 14.13. Those patients who required revision of the stump did so because of complete inability to tolerate the partial-foot amputation. Revision in these cases was to a Symes or below-knee amputation.

Table 14.13 Outcome of 167 partial traumatic amputations of the foot (adapted from Millstein et al 1988)

Initial level of amputation	Number	Revised	Good	Fair	Poor
Digital	34	5 (15%)	14 (41%)	7 (21%)	8 (23%)
Transverse					
Metatarsophalangeal	13	4 (31%)	4 (31%)	5 (38%)	0
Transmetatarsal	54	15 (28%)	11 (20%)	17 (32%)	11 (20%)
Lisfranc	20	5 (25%)	7 (35%)	7 (35%)	1 (5%)
Chopart	23	14 (61%)	6 (26%)	3 (13%)	0
Longitudinal					
Medial	12	6 (50%)	4 (33%)	2 (17%)	0
Lateral	11	0	5 (45%)	4 (36%)	2 (19%)
Total	167	49 (29%)	51 (30%)	45 (27%)	22 (13%)

In those patients not requiring revision surgery, 43% were rated good, 38% were rated fair and 19% were rated poor.

Patients with a good result returned to work within 9 months of injury. Those with poor results who were able to return to work took 17 months.

The authors found that preservation of length in the foot did not give a better clinical result. They believed that it was more important to obtain well covered, innervated skin flaps, preferably from plantar skin.

Summary

1. In a large group of patients suffering traumatic partial amputation of the foot, 29% required revision surgery, 30% had a good clinical result, 27% had a fair clinical result and 13% had a poor clinical result.

FOOT INJURIES IN CHILDREN

Fractures of the calcaneus

Schanz & Rasmussen (1987) and Schmidt & Weiner (1982) showed that extra-articular fractures of the calcaneus were commoner than intra-articular fractures in children. There were 133 children in these two series; 63% sustained extra-articular fractures and 37% intra-articular fractures. This is in contrast to the situation in adults (see p. 357). Neither of these series provides information on the long-term results. However, Schmidt & Weiner (1982) concluded that calcaneal fractures had a benign prognosis in children.

Schanz & Rasmussen (1986) looked at the prognosis of displaced intra-articular fractures in children. They re-examined 15 children at an average of 12 years from their injury. They were all treated conservatively and no attempt was made to improve the position of the fracture. None of the patients had any functional problems. Nine had slight inconvenience and deformity as a result of their injury. All had heel-broadening and reduction of Bohlers angle on X-ray. The authors concluded that the prognosis in children was better than in adults.

Wiley & Profitt (1984) reviewed 34 calcaneal fractures in 32 children, and concluded that the outlook in these fractures was favourable. However, their follow-up averaged only 33 months.

Thomas (1969) reported 5 children with calcaneal fractures; 4 involved some degree of displacement of the articular surface of the subtalar joint. All had a satisfactory clinical result.

Matteri & Frymoyer (1973) reported 3 infants aged 16–30 months with this fracture, and concluded: 'This injury in our limited follow-up has produced minimum disability in comparison to fractures of the calcaneus in adults'. They added that longer-term follow-up was needed to confirm whether this injury in the very young was really benign.

Marti (1980) suggested that displaced intra-articular fractures of the calcaneus should be reduced and internally fixed. The 3 patients described by him were 12–15 years of age. It may be that a more aggressive approach is indicated in severely displaced fractures in adolescents.

Ogden (1987) mentioned the possibility of growth arrest and subtalar arthritis as potential complications of calcaneal fractures in children. There is no evidence in the orthopaedic literature to suggest that these complications occur commonly.

Talar fractures

Gross (1984) described avascular necrosis as the most significant complication of a fracture of the talus in a child. Marti (1980) outlined the risk of avascular necrosis developing after various types of talar fractures (Fig. 14.2).

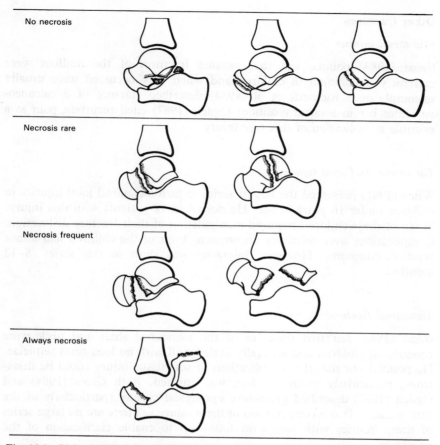

No necrosis

Necrosis rare

Necrosis frequent

Always necrosis

Fig. 14.2 Risk of avascular necrosis in various types of fracture of the talus in children (from Weber et al 1980, with permission).

Letts & Gibeault (1980) reported 3 cases of avascular necrosis in 13 children with undisplaced fractures of the neck of the talus. Canale & Kelly (1978) described 2 similar cases in a group of 5 children with undisplaced talar neck fractures. These figures suggest a 28% incidence of avascular necrosis in Hawkins type I fractures of the neck of the talus in children. This is higher than the incidence in similar fractures in adults (see Table 14.3).

Of the 3 children reported by Letts & Gibeault (1980) who developed avascular necrosis, 2 were under 2 years of age. Both of these children developed flattening of the talus with marked ankle stiffness. The length of follow-up was not specified.

There is not enough information available in the orthopaedic literature to give any meaningful prognostic information about other types of talar fractures.

Other fractures

Mid-tarsal injuries

Gross (1984) pointed out that isolated fractures of the midfoot were extremely uncommon in children and when they occurred were usually uncomplicated. Richards et al (1984) described fracture of a calcaneo-navicular bar in a tarsal coalition; Ogden (1987) cited recurrent pain as a possible complication of this rare injury.

Tarsometatarsal joint injuries

Wiley (1981) presented the largest series of tarsometatarsal joint injuries in children under 16 years of age. He described 18 patients with this injury. Seven of these children required manipulation of their fracture dislocation. Complications were relatively uncommon. Four of the children had minor residual symptoms. However, follow-up was short in this series (8–12 months).

Metatarsal fractures

Gross (1984) felt that fractures of the metatarsal shaft and neck were common in children and generally healed well with no long-term sequelae. He pointed out that the complications of soft tissue injury could be disastrous, particularly when the foot was crushed. Both Gross (1984) and Ogden (1987) described premature epiphyseal closure (particularly of the first metatarsal) as a complication of these injuries. There are no large series of these injuries with long-term follow-up to enable clarification of the prognosis.

When metatarsal fractures occur as a result of crushing injuries, complications are more likely to arise from the soft tissue and vascular injury rather than the bony injury.

Avulsion fractures of the base of the fifth metatarsal are relatively common in children. They should be differentiated from the Jones fracture (see above). Ogden (1987) described non-union as a possible complication of these injuries. There are no figures available on the incidence of this potential complication in children.

Summary

1. Calcaneal fractures in children are associated with a good long-term prognosis.
2. Undisplaced (Hawkins type I) fractures of the neck of the talus are associated with a higher risk of avascular necrosis than similar fractures in adults.

3. The long-term results of fractures of the midfoot and forefoot in children are ill defined. It is difficult to give a clear prognosis in these injuries, other than on an empirical basis.

REFERENCES

Arntz C T, Hansen S T 1987 Dislocations and fracture-dislocations of the tarso-metatarsal joints. Orthopedic Clinics of North America 18: 105–114
Berndt A L, Harty M 1959 Transchondral fractures of the talus. Journal of Bone and Joint Surgery 41A: 988–1020
Brunet J A, Wiley J J 1987 The late results of tarso-metatarsal joint injuries. Journal of Bone and Joint Surgery 69B: 437–440
Canale S T, Kelly F B 1978 Fractures of the neck of the talus: long term evaluation of 71 cases. Journal of Bone and Joint Surgery 60A: 143–156
Christensen S B, Lorentzen J E, Krogsoe O, Sneppen O 1977 Subtalar dislocation. Acta Orthopaedica Scandinavica 48: 707–711
Coltart W D 1952 Aviators astragalus. Journal of Bone and Joint Surgery 34B: 545–567
Comfort T H, Behrens F, Gaither D W, Denis F, Sigmond M 1985 Long term results of talar neck fractures. Clinical Orthopaedics 199: 81–87
Cotton F J, Wilson L T 1908 Fractures of the os calcis. Boston Medical and Surgical Journal 159: 559–565
Dameron T B 1975 Fractures and anatomical variations of the proximal portion of the fifth metatarsal. Journal of Bone and Joint Surgery 57A: 788–792
Degan T J, Morrey B F, Braun D P 1982 Surgical excision for anterior process fractures of the calcaneus. Journal of Bone and Joint Surgery 64A: 519–524
Delee J C, Curtis R 1982 Subtalar dislocation of the foot. Journal of Bone and Joint Surgery 64A: 433–437
Dettenbeck L C, Kelly P J 1969 Total dislocation of the talus. Journal of Bone and Joint Surgery 51A: 283–288
Dunn W A 1974 Peritalar dislocation. Orthopedic Clinics of North America 5: 7–17
Elleby D H, Marcinko D E 1985 Digital fractures and dislocations. Clinics in Pediatry 2: 233–245
Essex-Lopresti P 1952 The mechanism, reduction technique and results in fractures of the os calcis. British Journal of Surgery 39: 395–419
Grob D, Simpson L A, Weber B G, Bray T 1985 Operative treatment of displaced talus fractures. Clinical Orthopaedics 199: 88–96
Gross R H 1984 Fractures and dislocations of the foot. In: Rockwood C A, Wilkins W E, King R E (eds) Fractures in children, vol 3. J B Lippincott, Philadelphia
Hardcastle P H, Reschauer R, Kutscha-Lissberg E, Schoffman W 1982 Injuries to the tarso-metatarsal joint. Journal of Bone and Joint Surgery 64B: 349–356
Hawkins L G 1965 Fracture of the lateral process of the talus: a review of 13 cases. Journal of Bone and Joint Surgery 47A: 1170–1175
Hawkins L G 1970 Fractures of the neck of the talus. Journal of Bone and Joint Surgery 52A: 991–1002
Heckman J D 1984 Fractures and dislocations of the foot. In: Rockwood C A, Green D P (eds) Fractures in adults, vol II. J B Lippincott, Philadelphia
Hillegass R C 1976 Injuries to the mid foot. In: Bateman J E (ed) Foot science. W B Saunders, Philadelphia
Jones R 1902 Fracture of the base of the fifth metatarsal bone by indirect violence. Annals of Surgery 35: 697–700
Joplin R J 1958 Injuries of the foot. In: Cave C F (ed) Fractures and other injuries. Year Book Publishers, Chicago
Kavanaugh J H, Brower T D, Mann R V 1978 The Jones fracture revisited. Journal of Bone and Joint Surgery 60A: 776–782
Kenwright J, Taylor R G 1970 Major injuries of the talus. Journal of Bone and Joint Surgery 52B: 36–48
Key J A, Conwell H E 1956 The management of fractures, dislocations and sprains, 6th edn. C V Mosby, St Louis

Korn R 1942 Der bruch durch das lintere obere drittel des fersenbeines. Achiv für Orthopädische und Unfall-Chirurgie 41: 789

Lance E M, Carey K J Jr, Wade P A 1963 Fractures of the os calcis: treatment by early mobilisation. Clinical Orthopaedics 30: 76–90

La Tourette G, Perry J, Patzakis M J 1980 Fractures and dislocations of the tarso-metatarsal joint. In: Bateman J E, Trott A W (eds) The foot and ankle. Brian C Decker, New York

Letts R M, Gibeault D 1980 Fractured talus in children. Foot and Ankle 1: 74–77

Lindsay W R N, Dewar F P 1958 Fractures of the os calcis. American Journal of Surgery 95: 555–575

Lorentzen J E, Bach Christensen S, Krogsoe O, Sneppen O 1977 Fractures of the neck of the talus. Acta Orthopaedica Scandinavica 48: 115–120

Lowy M 1969 Avulsion fractures of the calcaneus. Journal of Bone and Joint Surgery 51B: 494–497

Main B J, Jowett R L 1975 Injuries of the mid-tarsal joint. Journal of Bone and Joint Surgery 57B: 89–97

Marti R 1980 Fractures of the talus and calcaneus. In: Weber B G, Brunner C, Freuler F (eds) Treatment of fractures in children and adolescents. Springer-Verlag, New York

Matteri R E, Frymoyer J W 1973 Fracture of the calcaneus in young children. Journal of Bone and Joint Surgery 55A: 1091–1094

McLaughlin H L 1963 Treatment of late complications after os calcis fractures. Clinical Orthopaedics 30: 111–115

Millstein S G, McCowan S A, Hunter G A 1988 Traumatic partial foot amputation in adults: a long term review. Journal of Bone and Joint Surgery 70B: 251–254

Monson S T, Ryan J R 1981 Subtalar dislocation. Journal of Bone and Joint Surgery 63A: 1156–1158

Mukherjee S K, Pringle P M, Baxter A D 1974 Fracture of the lateral process of the talus: a report of 13 cases. Journal of Bone and Joint Surgery 56B: 263–273

Myerson M S, Fisher R T, Burgess A R, Kenzora J E 1986 Fracture dislocation of the tarso-metatarsal joints: end results correlated with pathology and treatment. Foot and Ankle 6: 225–242

Nade S, Monahan P R W 1973 Fractures of the calcaneum. A study of the long term prognosis. Injury 14: 200–207

National Safety Council 1972 Accident facts, pp 23–29. In: Kleiger B Work related injury of the foot and ankle, pp 254–256, Foot Science (ed. J E Bateman), W B Saunders, Philadelphia

Norgrove Penny J, Davis L A 1980 Fractures and dislocations of the neck of the talus. Journal of Trauma 20: 1029–1037

Ogden J A 1987 Pocket guide to paediatric fractures. Williams & Wilkins, Baltimore

Peterson L, Goldie I F, Irstam L 1977 Fractures of the neck of the talus: a clinical study. Acta Orthopaedica Scandinavica 48: 696–706

Pettine K A, Morrey B F 1987 Osteochondral fractures of the talus. A long term follow up. Journal of Bone and Joint Surgery 69B: 89–92

Pozo J L, Kirwan E O'G, Jackson A M 1984 The long term results of conservative management of severely displaced fractures of the calcaneus. Journal of Bone and Joint Surgery 66B: 386–390

Quenu E, Kuss G 1909 Etude sur les luxations du metatarse. Revue Chirurgicale 39: 231–336, 720–791, 1093–1134

Richards R R, Evans J G, McGoey P F 1984 Fracture of a calcaneo-navicular bar: a complication of tarsal condition. Clinical Orthopaedics 185: 220–221

Rowe C R, Sakellarides H T, Fasman P A, Sorbie C 1963 Fractures of the os calcis: a long term follow up study of 146 patients. Journal of the American Medical Association 184: 920–923

Schanz K, Rasmussen F 1986 The prognosis of displaced intra-articular fractures of the calcaneus in children. Acta Orthopaedica Scandinavica 57: 471

Schanz K, Rasmussen F 1987 Calcaneal fractures in the child. Acta Orthopaedica Scandinavica 58: 504–506

Schmidt T L, Weiner D S 1982 Calcaneal fractures in children: an evaluation of the nature of the injury in 56 children. Clinical Orthopaedics 171: 150–155

Sneppen O, Bach Christensen S, Krogsoe O, Lorentzen J 1977 Fractures of the body of the talus. Acta Orthopaedica Scandinavica 48: 317–324

Spector F C, Karlin J M, Scurran B L, Silvani S L 1984 Lesser metatarsal fractures: incidence, management and review. Journal of the American Pediatry Association 74: 259–264

Szyszkowitz R, Reschauer R, Seggl W 1985 Eighty-five talus fractures treated by ORIF with 5 to 8 years of follow up. Study of 69 patients. Clinical Orthopaedics 199: 97–107

Thomas H M 1969 Calcaneal fracture in childhood. British Journal of Surgery 56: 664–666

Thoren O 1964 Os calcis fractures. Acta Orthopaedica Scandinavica (suppl) 70: 1–116

Tile M 1987 Fractures of the talus. In: Schatzker J, Tile M (eds) The rationale of operative fracture care. Springer Verlag, Berlin

Torg J S, Baldvinis F C, Zelko R R, Pavlov H, Peff T C, Das M 1984 Fractures of the base of the fifth metatarsal distal to the tuberosity. Journal of Bone and Joint Surgery 66A: 209–214

Vestad E 1968 Fractures of the calcaneum. Open reduction and bone grafting. Acta Chirurgica Scandinavica 134: 617–625

Weber B G, Bruner C, Freuler F 1980 Treatment of fractures in children and adolescents. Springer-Verlag, New York, p 375

Wiley J J 1981 Tarso-metatarsal joint injuries in children. Journal of Paediatrics Orthopaedics 1: 255–260

Wiley J J, Profitt A 1984 Fractures of the os calcis in children. Clinical Orthopaedics 188: 131–138

Wilpulla E 1973 Tarso-metatarsal fracture-dislocation. Acta Orthopaedica Scandinavica 44: 335–345

Wilson D W 1972 Injuries of the tarso-metatarsal joints. Journal of Bone and Joint Surgery 54B: 677–686

Wilson D W 1982 Fractures of the foot. In: Klenerman L (ed) The foot and its disorders. Blackwell, Oxford

Results following fractures of the axial skeleton

15. The pelvis

M. A. Foy

INTRODUCTION

A satisfactory classification of pelvic fracture patterns is fundamental to any attempt to interpret complications and long-term results. Generally, pelvic fractures may be classified into stable and unstable types. The Pennal classification (Pennal & Sutherland 1961, Pennal et al 1980) was an important contribution to a logical understanding of pelvic fractures. It utilized easily reproducible X-ray views (such as a standard anteroposterior view of the pelvis, a pelvic inlet view and a pelvic outlet view at 90° to the inlet view).

This classification has been modified by Tile (1984, 1988) as shown in Table 15.1. Tile made the point that there was a spectrum of stability, and if the anteroposterior or lateral compression force was of sufficient severity, then the posterior sacroiliac ligamentous complex may be disrupted, resulting in an unstable situation. Macdonald (1980) pointed out that pelvic ring distortion at the time of impact may be gross, but some pelvic injuries (particularly symphysis pubis and sacroiliac injuries) may spontaneously reduce during transfer of the patient to hospital, and the severity of the original injury may not be appreciated on X-ray assessment. These factors cause difficulties in assessing the severity of pelvic injuries and hence predicting prognosis.

Table 15.1 Classification of pelvic ring disruption (after Tile 1988)

Type A:	*Stable*
	A1: Fractures of the pelvis not involving the pelvic ring.
	A2: Stable, minimally displaced fractures of the pelvic ring.
Type B:	*Rotationally unstable, vertically stable*
	B1: Anteroposterior compression (open-book)
	B2: Lateral compression (ipsilateral)
	B3: Lateral compression (contralateral)
Type C:	*Rotationally and vertically unstable (Malgaigne)*
	C1: Unilateral
	C2: Bilateral
	C3: Associated with acetabular fracture

Tile's modification of the Pennal classification combines two inter-related factors, namely, stability and direction of the injuring forces. A brief look at the fracture patterns which follow these injury mechanisms may help in relating them to prognosis. For a detailed interpretation of fracture patterns the reader is referred to Tile (1984).

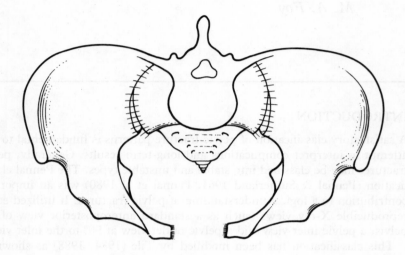

Fig. 15.1 The open-book disruption

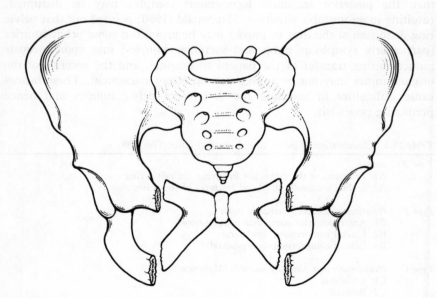

Fig. 15.2 Isolated four-rami (butterfly or straddle) fracture

Anteroposterior compression

There are two typical injuries which follow anteroposterior compression:

1. The open-book disruption (Fig. 15.1).
2. The isolated four-rami (straddle or butterfly) fracture (Fig. 15.2).

The degree of symphyseal separation in open-book disruptions may be divided into those with less than 2.5 cm (Tile's stage I) and those with more than 2.5 cm (Tile's stage II). If the anteroposterior compression force contains a shearing element then the posterior ligaments may be disrupted, resulting in a vertically unstable fracture.

Four-rami fractures may also result from a lateral compression or vertical shearing force; Tile believed that this was a more common cause.

Lateral compression

A lateral compression force may cause several types of injury. Most will be stable because the lateral compression force causes impaction of the posterior pelvic complex leaving the posterior ligaments intact. The common injury patterns are:

1. Ipsilateral anterior and posterior injury (Fig. 15.3).
2. Contralateral (bucket handle) type (Fig. 15.4).

In the ipsilateral injury there may be fractures of the pubic rami or a locked symphysis anteriorly. In the contralateral injury the lateral compressive force is combined with a rotatory element and the anterior injury is combined with a posterior lesion on the opposite side.

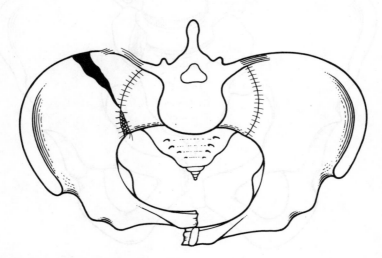

Fig. 15.3 Lateral compression injury: ipsilateral pattern

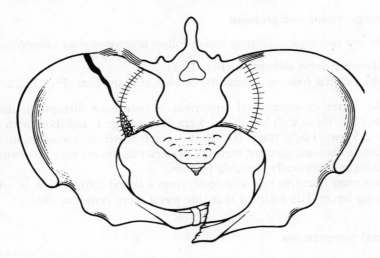

Fig. 15.4   Lateral compression injury: contralateral pattern

Vertical shear

This fracture pattern was originally described by Malgaigne (1855) and consists of two vertical fractures, separating at one side of the pelvis, and a middle fragment comprising the hip joint as shown in Figure 15.5. The anterior lesion involves either both pubic rami or the pubic symphysis and

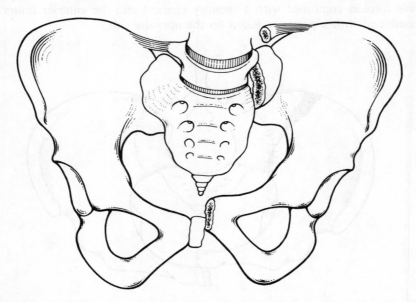

Fig. 15.5   Vertical shear pattern as described by Malgaigne (1855)

is associated with massive disruption through the sacrum, ilium or the sacroiliac joint. This fracture is always grossly unstable in both rotational and vertical planes.

In summary, two important considerations affect the long-term results of these fractures:

1. The degree of displacement and hence instability within the pelvic ring.
2. The associated injuries caused by the pelvic disruption which may in themselves have predictable complication rates. These will be discussed later.

The role of computerized tomography (CT) scanning in the evaluation of major pelvic injuries has been described by Gill & Bucholz (1984) and Dalinka et al (1985), and in the future CT scanning may have a more important role in the classification and perhaps the assessment of prognosis in fractures of the pelvis.

One further point concerns attitudes to the treatment of displaced pelvic fractures. In 1930 Noland & Conwell reported that excellent functional results were frequent in cases in which a good anatomical position was by no means achieved. More recently, Watson Jones (1962) commented that excellent results were often found even when considerable displacement persisted. However, Letournel (1978) and Bucholz (1981) stated that the accuracy of reduction of major fracture dislocations of the hemipelvis appeared to be of central importance in the avoidance of late disability from these injuries. Certainly there is a trend, as with many other fractures, towards accurate reduction and stabilization of pelvic fractures at the present time. In the assessment of sequelae of displaced fractures the accuracy of reduction will be taken into account whenever possible.

STABLE PELVIC FRACTURES

The surgeon is likely to be confronted either by a patient who has a clearly definable fracture pattern for which a prognosis is sought, or by a problem whose future outlook is in question. Therefore the principal mechanisms of injury will be considered first, in this and the next two sections, followed by a discussion of specific complications.

Avulsion fractures

These are uncommon but well recognized injuries. They occur at the anterior superior iliac spine, the ischial tuberosity and the iliac crest. They usually follow sudden strong muscle contraction. One report by Metzmaker & Pappas (1985) of 24 cases of pelvic avulsion fractures reported excellent results in 22 patients (92%). An excellent result was defined as a full return to pre-injury fitness within 4 months. One patient returned to pre-injury fitness but took longer than 4 months and the other patient complained of an intermittent dull aching sensation 1 year after avulsion of the ischial apophysis.

There are sporadic reports of cases with poor results following avulsion fractures but unfortunately the size of the patient population from which these poor results are drawn is unknown and therefore the incidence of unacceptable results cannot be accurately determined. Barnes & Hinds (1972) reviewed the English language literature on ischial apophyseal avulsions and of the 39 cases reviewed by them, 27 (68%) did not unite while 10 (26%) underwent late excision for disabling pain. However, this is a highly selective group and the size of the total patient population from which these cases came is unknown.

Schlonsky & Olix (1972) carefully assessed two ischial tuberosity avulsions for more than 2 years following conservative treatment. The end-result was thigh-wasting of 1 or 2 cm and diminution of hamstring power by over 20% in both cases. Both patients were asymptomatic in their everyday life but their athletic ability had declined significantly. Irving (1964) reported a case of exostosis formation after traumatic avulsion of the anterior inferior iliac spine and this caused a limp and difficulty in running, and the exostosis required excision. Goodwin (1959) described myositis ossificans as a late complication of avulsion of the anterior inferior iliac spine. An accurate incidence of these complications is unknown but they must be extremely uncommon. There are no reports of poor results following iliac crest or anterior superior iliac spine avulsions.

Stable fractures of the pubic rami

The work of Gertzbein and Chenoweth (1980) demonstrated, using Tc 99 mm methylene diphosphonate bone scans, that even in apparently isolated fractures of the pubic ramus there was disruption elsewhere in the pubic ring, usually in the acetabulum or sacroiliac regions. This probably explains the discomfort that patients with pubic rami fractures experience in the hip and low back. This work shows that there is more to these simple, stable fractures than is at first apparent.

In 207 cases of 'isolated' pubic rami fractures reported by Connolly & Hedberg (1969), Dunn & Morris (1968) and Peltier (1965), only one long-term complication was reported — a non-union of two undisplaced pubic rami fractures. Connolly & Hedberg reported 1 urinary tract injury in their series of 82 unilateral pubic rami fractures, but the precise nature of the injury is not indicated. Levine & Crampton (1963) in a series which included 251 patients with pubic rami fractures, both stable and unstable, reported 2 cases of bladder rupture where only 3 pubic rami were fractured. Stress fractures of the pubic rami have been reported by Pavlov et al (1982) and Meurman (1980) and sporadically by other authors. Pavlov et al reported 12 cases, all of which occurred in the inferior pubic ramus near to the pubic symphysis. There were two complications, namely delayed union and refracture. Both of these problems occurred in patients who continued running despite pain and the fracture eventually healed after a period of rest.

Iliac wing fractures

In the reports of Connolly & Hedberg (1969), Dunn & Morris (1968) and Peltier (1965), there were 32 iliac wing fractures in a total of 497 pelvic fractures, giving an overall incidence of 6.5%. These fractures cause lower abdominal tenderness and rigidity, making exclusion of intra-abdominal injury difficult. There is no report of any long-term disability from this injury.

Summary

1. The incidence of excellent results following pelvic avulsion fractures is over 95%. Poor results, although very uncommon, seem to be particularly associated with avulsion of the ischial tuberosity.
2. Stable fractures and stress fractures of the pubic rami are rarely associated with long-term disability.
3. Iliac wing fractures are not associated with long-term disability.

ROTATIONALLY STABLE/VERTICALLY UNSTABLE PELVIC FRACTURES

Anteroposterior compression fractures (Figs 15.1, 15.2)

The work of Peltier (1965), Dunn & Morris (1968) and Tile (1984) suggested an incidence of 18% for these injuries (90 of 497 pelvic fractures). This excludes avulsion injuries, acetabular fractures and pathological fractures.

Tile, in his series of 248 pelvic fractures, carried out the most careful and well documented assessment of the results in the literature, and to a large extent we must be guided by these results. Tile's results were tabulated by a point system heavily weighted towards pain, with lesser scores for malunion, leg length discrepancy and non-union. Of 29 patients in Tile's series with anteroposterior compression injuries, 17 (59%) were free of pain, 11 (38%) had moderate pain while 1 (3%) had severe pain. Mean follow-up was 45 months in these patients. The results were not broken down into types of symphyseal disruption or to identify isolated straddle fractures.

Tile (1984) pointed out that even in stage I injuries (i.e. less than 2.5 cm of separation of the symphysis pubis) there may be prolonged and signifi-cant pain and tenderness in the region of the pubic symphysis. Holdsworth

(1948) reported that symphyseal pain often took up to 2 years to settle completely.

Sarkin (1976) reported, at the South African Orthopaedic Association, 79 cases of symphyseal separation in black Africans. These patients were treated by 6 weeks non-weight-bearing. He found no permanent disability. Dunn & Morris (1968) described treatment of 6 cases in a pelvic sling. The patients were subsequently mobilized between 5 and 6 weeks from injury; 2 redisplaced, leading to persistent sacroiliac discomfort. Dunn & Morris also described 10 patients with straddle fractures who were treated conservatively; none of these patients suffered permanent disability.

Madsden et al (1983) reported a series of obstetric patients with a history of pelvic fracture. Of the 3 patients who developed problems, attributable to their pelvic injury during confinement, 2 were due to redisplacement of the pubic symphysis. This is an important consideration when preparing medicolegal reports on the prognosis of symphyseal disruptions in women of childbearing age.

The differences in the reported results of anteroposterior compression injuries are difficult to explain. All the patients reported by Tile (1984) were involved in major high-energy injuries. The results in Tile's patients are comprehensive in that all patients were interviewed, examined and X-rayed at follow-up review. The incidence of post-injury pain in these patients has already been mentioned and the overall incidence of satisfactory results was 21 of 29 (72%), with 8 of 29 (28%) unsatisfactory results.

Lateral compression fractures (Figs 15.3, 15.4)

A lateral compression force causes marked inward rotation of the affected side of the pelvis. Many of these injuries leave the posterior ligaments intact and are vertically stable.

Tile's (1984) figures suggest that this is the commonest type of pelvic injury mechanism. Other series fail to recognize clearly and categorize this mechanism of injury and their figures are therefore difficult to interpret. Tile classified 183 (75%) of the pelvic fractures as lateral compression injuries. According to his rigorous criteria, 132 (72%) of these cases achieved a satisfactory result, while 51 (28%) had an unsatisfactory result. Tile looked specifically at pain following lateral compression injuries and found that 64% had no pain at all, 33% had moderate pain and 3% had severe pain.

Summary

1. Anteroposterior compression injuries are associated with persisting moderate or severe pain in approximately 40% of cases. The overall incidence of unsatisfactory results is approximately 28%.
2. Lateral compression injuries are associated with persisting moderate or

severe pain in approximately 36% of patients. The overall incidence of unsatisfactory results is approximately 28%.

ROTATIONALLY AND VERTICALLY UNSTABLE PELVIC FRACTURES (Malgaigne Fractures)

The double vertical fractures have received much more attention in the literature than other types of unstable pelvic fracture. A study of the published reports reveals that some of these injuries are in fact severe anteroposterior or lateral compression injuries with associated major posterior disruption leading to vertical instability. However, the end-result in these circumstances is a rotationally and vertically unstable hemipelvic segment and the prognostic implications are the same.

The work of Noland & Conwell (1933), Peltier (1965) and Dunn & Morris (1968) suggested that the incidence of double vertical fractures was 8% in 374 pelvic fractures. Slatis & Huittenen (1972) suggested that the incidence of vertical shear fractures was in the region of 20% from their own series and an extensive literature review, while Tile (1984) reported 34 cases in his series of 248 high-energy pelvic fractures — an incidence of 14%. The reason for this apparent disparity is that the report by Slatis & Huittenen included severe anteroposterior and lateral compression injuries with their double vertical fractures.

Slatis & Huittenen (1972) reported on 163 double vertical fractures with a long-term follow-up on 65. When they considered patients of working age without major complicating injuries, 43% returned to work within 16 weeks, 74% returned to work within 24 weeks and 97% returned to work within 1 year of the injury.

Karaharju & Slatis (1978) described follow-up on 13 patients with double vertical fractures treated by external fixation using a trapezoid compression frame. The average time for return to work was 5–6 months. The longest period lost from work was 8 months. The authors felt that the incidence of low back pain and impaired gait was reduced by this method of treatment.

Slatis & Huittenen (1972) noted that recovery was more rapid where displacement was minimal; where displacement was present, recovery was related to the nature of the posterior injury. Symptoms resulting from dislocation of the sacroiliac joint took much longer to settle than fractures adjacent to the joint. Follow-up examination (1–7 years after injury) on 65 patients revealed an unexpectedly high incidence of late sequelae. Persistent dislocation of the hemipelvis secondary to unsatisfactory reduction gave rise to a limp, problems with walking and oblique inclination of the pelvis on sitting. Over half of these patients complained of chronic low back pain on the affected side in the region of the sacroiliac joint. There was no disabling pain in the pubic area even with wide separation of the symphysis or displaced pubic rami fractures.

Holdsworth (1948) had earlier reported similar findings in 50 patients with Malgaigne-type unstable fractures. Holdsworth reported a mean follow-up of 5 years and described a satisfactory result as the ability to return to pre-accident work or similar heavy work (in the case of women the ability to return to full household chores). He traced 42 cases and the results are shown in Table 15.2.

Table 15.2   End-results in 42 double vertical fractures (adapted from Holdsworth 1948)

	Total	Able to return to heavy work	Painful
Fracture or dislocation of the pubis with:			
Sacroiliac joint dislocation	27	12	15
Fracture of the sacrum or ilium adjacent to joint	15	13	2

These results confirm that the nature of the posterior injury is important in determining the prognosis. Only 44% of patients with sacroiliac dislocations were able to return to heavy work while 87% of those with fractures adjacent to the sacrum and ilium were able to do so. All patients in this series complained of pubic pain but in each case it had disappeared 2 years after injury. Holdsworth (1948) appeared to be satisfied with the position achieved after conservative treatment with traction, and weight-bearing was delayed for 12 weeks.

Lander (1984) confirmed that posterior disruption of the sacroiliac joint is associated with a poor prognosis. In his series of 31 sacroiliac disruptions treated conservatively, 15 were followed up for a mean period of 5.3 years. Thirteen (87%) complained of persistent low back pain, 3 (20%) had to change their occupation, 8 (53%) had difficulty with low or hard chairs and 3 (20%) had difficulty climbing stairs. He concluded that long-term disability follows traumatic sacroiliac disruption.

According to Langloh et al (1972) from a series of 24 double vertical fractures with posterior sacroiliac disruption, improvement may occur up to 12 months after injury and therefore a final prognosis should be deferred until this time.

Tile (1984) found that 14 (41%) of his 34 patients had a satisfactory result, while 20 (59%) had an unsatisfactory result. In terms of pain, 13 (38%) were pain-free while 15 (44%) experienced moderate pain and 6 (18%) suffered severe pain. Similar results were reported by Semba et al (1983), in a critical analysis of 30 patients with conservatively treated Malgaigne fractures followed for 2 to 12 years. They found that only 11 of the patients were symptom-free (37%) at follow-up.

Summary

1. The most significant indicator of long-term disability is the nature of the posterior injury. Sacroiliac dislocations fare much worse than fractures of the sacrum or ilium.
2. Symptoms may improve up to 12 months from injury and a final assessment should not be made before this time.
3. Double vertical fractures are associated with persisting moderate or severe pain in approximately 62% of cases. The overall incidence of unsatisfactory results is 59%.

SPECIFIC COMPLICATIONS

Neurological complications

The most comprehensive reviews of the subject were provided by Patterson & Morton (1961) and Huittenen & Slatis (1971). The incidence of neurological complications is unclear. Patterson & Morton found the overall incidence to be 1.2% in a series of 809 pelvic fractures, while Huittenen & Slatis felt that the incidence was 10–12%. Huittenen & Slatis found a much higher incidence in double vertical fractures with 31 of 68 (46%) showing signs of nerve damage. In all cases in both series there was a significant posterior injury, either fractured sacrum or sacroiliac dislocation.

Patterson & Morton (1961) considered the final results in 10 patients with neurological injury. Six were assessed as good, since final disability was minimal and their original heavy occupation was resumed. Of the 4 others, 1 had persisting incontinence of urine as a result of neurological injury while the others had poor results. Considering the neurological lesion in isolation, in no patient (even those where the final disability was minimal) did the neurological lesion recover fully. In this series the mean follow-up was 18 months.

Huittenen & Slatis (1971) found that the neurological signs affected all nerve roots from L4 to S5, with L5 and S1 being most commonly involved. Of the 31 cases with evidence of nerve injury 22 had motor signs and 26 had sensory signs; 17 had both motor and sensory signs. The follow-up was 1–5 years and even in those followed up for 5 years the authors found that the nerve lesion had not fully recovered.

Summary

1. Neurological injuries occur more commonly when there is dislocation of the sacroiliac joint or fracture of the sacrum.
2. The prognosis following neurological injury is poor; in no case did the neurological lesion recover completely.

Tile (1984) analysed the factors resulting in unsatisfactory results in his patients. Of 104 unsatisfactory results, the commonest factor was unacceptable pain in 69 (66%). Leg length discrepancy of over 2 cm accounted for 9 unsatisfactory results. Permanent nerve damage accounted for 12 unsatisfactory results and urethral symptoms for 6. These factors, together with the influence of pelvic fracture on subsequent pregnancy, will be considered in more detail.

Urological injury and impotence

The urological injuries directly associated with pelvic fracture are rupture of the bladder and rupture of the urethra. Urethral rupture is by far the most serious of these injuries because of the high incidence of serious complications, namely stricture, incontinence and impotence.

The incidence of haematuria following pelvic fractures was 33% based on 623 cases reported by Noland & Conwell (1933), Flaherty et al (1968) and Slatis & Huittenen (1972). The incidence of significant bladder or urethral injury was much less, as shown in Table 15.3. The overall incidence of significant urological injury following pelvic fracture is in the region of 10%.

Table 15.3   Reported incidence of urological injuries in 1158 patients

Reference	Pelvic fractures	Urological injury		
		Bladder ruptures	Urethral ruptures	Bladder and urethral ruptures
Noland & Conwell (1930)	125	22	9	
Levine & Crampton (1963)	425	8	5	1
Peltier (1965)	138	14	4	
Dunn & Morris (1968)	111	8	3	
Slatis & Huittinen (1972)	163	9	4	3
Colapinto (1980)	196	17	10	
Total	1158	78 (6.7%)	35 (3%)	4 (0.3%)

Colapinto (1980) observed in his series of 196 patients that all the urethral ruptures occurred in men. There were 96 female patients in this series, some with severe pelvic fractures, but none sustained a urethral rupture.

Froman & Stein (1967) believed that it was difficult to correlate fracture patterns with urological injury because of the complex forces involved. However, Kaiser & Farrow (1965), Flaherty et al (1968) and more recently Mitchell (1984) pointed out that straddle fractures cause over 50% of urethral injuries, while the rest are associated with various patterns of instability.

The incidence of urethral stricture is difficult to predict with any accuracy because it depends upon precise knowledge of the original injury and on the subsequent management of the injury. Controversy still exists amongst urologists over the place of early surgery and the role of conservative management in the treatment of urethral ruptures.

However if the urethra has been completely disrupted, an attempt should be made to re-establish its continuity by formal surgical exploration (Heyes et al 1983, Patterson et al 1983).

Kaiser & Farrow (1965) reported a careful follow-up of 22 cases of rupture of the bladder or urethra caused by pelvic fracture with a minimum follow-up of 4 years. Of the 6 patients with a ruptured bladder who survived, the only long-term complication was a bladder calculus which was removed, leading to an uneventful recovery and a transient perineal fistula. These authors treated their urethral ruptures by a modified conservative method of realignment and approximation of the divided urethra, suprapubic catheterization of the bladder and drainage of the prevesical space. Of the 8 cases who survived, 7 had complete recovery with no sequelae. One patient developed a fistula and a stricture. Mitchell (1984) pointed out that the outlook for patients with urethral strictures is better today with the use of the optical urethrotome.

The incidence of incontinence following urethral injury is unknown. Incontinence can also be caused by damage to the S2, S3 outflow at the sacral foraminae. Morehouse & Mackinnon (1969) believed that the statistics on incontinence were inadequate, but of 10 patients referred to them for urethroplasty for urethral stricture, 7 were incontinent.

Impotence is a source of considerable personal embarrassment to the male patient and also, according to Mitchell (1984), is 'the most severe disability in the eyes of the court'. Recently more attention has been paid to this problem in the orthopaedic and urological journals. The incidence of impotence following a pelvic fracture is related to:

1. The severity of the urethral injury.
2. The nature of the pelvic fracture.
3. The age of the patient.

The severity of the urethral injury

King (1975) reported impotence in 13 of 31 cases with urethral injury (43%) and 3 of 59 cases without urethral injury (5%). King defined impotence as the inability to produce an erection, failure to achieve orgasm, failure to ejaculate and retrograde ejaculation. Similar observations were made by Chambers & Balfour (1963), who followed up 31 patients with pelvic fracture and urological injury; 8 of the 17 (47%) with partial or complete rupture of the posterior urethra were permanently impotent.

A very important medicolegal consideration is the incidence and timing of the return of potency. Gibson (1970) in a report of 35 patients with a fractured pelvis with urethral rupture identified 13 cases of permanent impotence (35%) and 8 cases (22%) where potency returned up to 19

Table 15.4 Incidence of permanent and temporary impotence following urethral injury

Reference	Urethral injury (n)	Permanent impotence (n)	Temporary impotence (n)
Chambers & Balfour (1963)	17	8	7
Gibson (1970)	35	13	8
Total	52	21 (40%)	15 (28%)

months after injury. A similar experience was reported by Chambers & Balfour (1963): 7 of their 31 cases reported loss of potency for 4 months to 4 years, with a mean of 19 months. These findings are summarized in Table 15.4. The figures from King's paper are not included, as duration of follow-up was not specified.

The nature of the pelvic fracture

King (1975) noted that fracture patterns were broadly similar in potent and impotent patients. The major difference was the presence of disruptions of the pubic symphysis in 5 of the 16 (31%) impotent men compared with similar disruptions in only 15 of 90 (17%) potent men.

The age of the patient

Mitchell (1984) reported that in his series of 23 patients, of those under the age of 30 all but 1 recovered normal potency while of those over the age of 30, less than 50% recovered a normal, full and sustained erection.

Summary

1. Significant urological injury occurs in approximately 10% of unstable pelvic fractures.
2. Permanent impotence occurs in approximately 40% of patients with posterior urethral injury and unstable pelvic fracture.
3. Final prognosis on impotence should be withheld for at least 2 years in patients with posterior urethral injury and unstable pelvic fracture, as potency may return in up to 28%.
4. Impotence may occur in 5% of patients with unstable pelvic fractures and no urethral injury.

Non-union and delayed union

There are only three reports in the literature concerning non-union of pelvic fractures. Hundley (1966) described 20 cases of symptomatic non-union in 141 pelvic fractures. Pennal & Massiah (1980) reported on 32 cases of established non-union and 10 cases of delayed union in pelvic fractures. Tile (1984) described 8 cases of non-union in his series of 248 pelvic fractures. These figures suggest that the incidence of non-union lies between 3% and 14%. Tile pointed out that non-union was more common in double vertical fractures and this was supported by analysis of the figures of both Hundley (1966) and Pennal & Massiah (1980). These showed that 56% of the non- and delayed unions occurred in double vertical fractures, as shown in Table 15.5.

Table 15.5 Incidence of non-union and delayed union in rotationally and vertically unstable fractures

	Total number of unstable fractures	Total number of non-union and delayed unions	Number of non-unions in rotationally and vertically unstable fractures
Hundley (1966)	141	20	18
Pennal & Massiah (1980)	?	42	17
Total		62	35 (56%)

In Pennal & Massiah's series the average time at diagnosis of delayed union or non-union was 9 months from the time of injury and the commonest presenting symptoms were pain and a limp. Of their 42 patients, 18 underwent operation which consisted of bone grafting and stabilization in 14, onlay graft in 2 and excision of bone fragment in 2. Their final results are shown in Table 15.6.

Table 15.6 Final disability assessment in non-union and delayed union of pelvic fractures (from Pennal & Massiah 1980, with permission)

Result	Group	
	Operative	Non-operative
Returned to pre-injury occupation	11	5
Returned to sedentary occupation	7	10
Permanently totally disabled	0	7
Permanently disabled by 50%	0	2
Total	18	24

Summary

1. Non-union and delayed union occur most commonly in double vertical fractures. The overall incidence is 3–14%.
2. The best results in terms of functional outcome occurred in patients treated with bone grafting and stabilization for their non-unions.

Malunion

Tile (1984) considered that minor degress of malunion causing leg length inequality of less than 1 cm were common after major pelvic disruption. He believed that a smaller number of patients were left with significant malunions with leg length discrepancy of over 2 cm or with major rotational deformities of the pelvis. He quoted an overall incidence of 5%. Malunion is not always associated with pain.

Effect on subsequent pregnancy

There are important medicolegal implications of the effect of the fracture on future confinement when young women sustain unstable pelvic fractures. Watson Jones (1982) reported that problems with pregnancy were uncommon, and that even major deformities of the pelvic inlet were not incompatible with natural childbirth. Noland & Conwell (1933) reported 1 patient out of 44 women who required caesarean section because of impairment of the pelvic outlet.

Madsden et al (1983) have followed up 34 females with pelvic fractures through pregnancy. Ten of the patients had increased or recurrent pain throughout pregnancy; 27 had uncomplicated vaginal deliveries; including 13 patients with displaced pelvic fragments. Of the 7 patients with complications, in only 3 cases could the complications be attributed to the previous pelvic fracture. Two developed re-disruption of the pubic symphysis and one underwent caesarean section because vaginal delivery was felt to be too dangerous.

Summary

1. Some 9% of patients (3 of 34) suffered complications of childbirth as a result of their pelvic fracture.
2. In all, 29% of patients (10 of 34) suffered increased or recurrent pelvic pain during pregnancy.

OTHER GROUPS

Sacral and coccygeal fractures

Isolated sacral fractures are uncommon. Sacral fractures usually occur as part of a more complex pelvic disruption. Fountain et al (1977) found 6 isolated sacral fractures in a group of 184 patients admitted with pelvic fractures — an incidence of 3%. All of the fractures involved S1, S2 or S3. All patients had evidence of urinary retention, a decrease in anal tone or both. Five of the 6 failed to improve and underwent sacral laminectomy and decompression. All of these patients improved over a 4–6-month period and no long-term disability was recorded.

It is generally felt that isolated sacral fractures cause no long-term problems; however, Foy (1988) reported on 16 cases with a mean 5.5-year follow-up. Two of these patients required excision of un-united low transverse sacral fractures. Of the remaining 14, only 6 (36%) were symptomfree; 7 (50%) complained of mild or moderately severe pain (sacrodynia) at the site of their fracture and 1 (7%) complained of severe pain related to the site of the fracture. Two (14%) had evidence of persistent neurological dysfunction. In a report by Hazlett (1980) of 50 cases of sacral fracture, only 1 case of malunion was reported.

Coccygeal pain may be a source of persistent morbidity. There is often a history of trauma to the sacrococcygeal region. Torok (1974) reported that trauma was responsible in over 70% of the patients. Pyper (1957) reported a history of trauma to the coccyx in 14 of 28 cases (50%). In this group there was evidence of coccygeal fracture in only 1 case. All of the cases in Pyper's series underwent coccygectomy and 89% showed either marked improvement or complete relief of symptoms. Unfortunately no study has followed up a group of patients with post-traumatic coccygeal pain to assess the chance of a painful disabling coccydynia.

Summary

1. Isolated sacral fractures may give rise to long-term symptoms, particularly pain at the site of the fracture (sacrodynia). This occurred in 57% of patients in one small series of 14 patients.
2. The subject of coccydynia and its relationship to trauma remains unclear.

Pelvic fractures in children

The most comprehensive study of this subject was reported by Torode & Zieg (1985). Their specific aim was to determine the incidence of bony complications in children with pelvic fractures, and to formulate a classification bearing some relationship to the final outcome. They described 141 children with ages ranging from 2 to 17 years. Eleven of their patients died (a mortality of 8%), leaving 130 patients available for clinical review. They found the Pennal classification difficult to apply to children and suggested an alternative which essentially differentiated between stable and unstable injuries.

Torode & Zieg recognized an increased incidence of iliac wing fractures in children when compared to adults. In their series there were 18 cases (an incidence of 13% compared to the incidence of 6.5% reported in adults earlier in this chapter). One patient with an iliac wing fracture also sustained a urethral injury. The authors noted that in the long term, iliac wing fractures — even those associated with injury to the iliac apophysis — did not cause any significant functional problems. Two patients appeared to have delayed ossification of the iliac apophysis, but at follow-up 2 years after the injury there was no significant difference between the two sides.

In their stable group of fractures (68 cases) Torode & Zieg (1985) identified 2 cases of delayed union of pubic rami fractures (incidence 3%). These fractures subsequently healed 1 year after injury. They noted that generally even displaced pubic rami fractures and gross displacement of the pubic symphysis were associated with good healing and no long-term symptoms. The better prognosis for symphyseal disruptions in children was explained in terms of the separation of the bone–cartilage interface and avulsion of a sleeve of periosteum, while in adults there is disruption of the fibrocartilaginous symphysis. Therefore, in the child, healing involves filling in with bone derived from the cartilaginous growth plate and periosteum. Torode & Zieg reported 1 urethral injury and 1 bladder injury in this group.

In the children with unstable pelvic fractures (40 cases) there were 13 bony complications (an incidence of 32%). These included 8 cases of nonunion of the pubic rami, 3 cases of premature closure of the triradiate cartilage, malunion of an acetabular fracture and 1 closure of the sacroiliac joint. There were 5 urethral injuries and 3 bladder ruptures in this group. It was not possible to correlate the results following operative and nonoperative treatment as only 3 of the 40 cases underwent operative stabilization.

Macdonald (1980) reported similar results to Torode & Zieg in a series of 15 displaced pelvic fractures in children. Follow-up ranged from 6 to 24 years in Macdonald's series. Five of the 15 patients (33%) had residual symptoms and significant radiological changes.

Torode & Zieg (1985) reported 7 urethral injuries (an incidence of 6%). Mitchell (1984) pointed out that it was particularly difficult to give a prognosis on the future fertility of a boy who sustained a fractured pelvis and a ruptured urethra. There are no long-term follow-up studies to assess potency and fertility in adult life following these injuries. Kelalis et al (1976) described 7 boys with urethral rupture who were subsequently all potent; 4 of the subjects had married and of these, 3 had fathered children.

Summary

1. Unstable pelvic fractures in children are associated with a 30–40% incidence of bony complications.
2. Pelvic fractures in children are associated with a 6% incidence of urethral injury. The long-term prognosis is unclear, but the work of Mitchell (1984) and Kelalis et al (1987) revealed an optimistic outlook when considering a small number of patients.

REFERENCES

Barnes S T, Hinds R B 1972 Pseudotumour of the ischium. A late manifestation of
   avulsion of the ischial epiphysis. Journal of Bone and Joint Surgery 54A: 645–647
Bucholz R W 1981 The pathological anatomy of Malgaigne fracture dislocation of the
   pelvis. Journal of Bone and Joint Surgery 63A: 100–404
Chambers H L, Balfour J 1963 The incidence of impotence following pelvic fractures with
   associated urinary tract injury. Journal of Urology 89: 702–703
Colapinto V 1980 Trauma to the pelvis; urethral injury. Clinical Orthopaedics 151: 46–55
Connolly W B, Hedberg E A 1969 Observations on fractures of the pelvis. Journal of
   Trauma 9: 104–111
Dalinka K D, Arger P, Coleman B 1985 CT in pelvic trauma. Orthopedic Clinics of North
   America 16: 471–480
Dunn A W, Morris H D 1968 Fractures and dislocations of the pelvis. Journal of Bone and
   Joint Surgery 50A: 1639–1648
Flaherty J J, Kelley R, Burnett B et al 1968 Relationship of pelvic bone fracture patterns to
   injuries of the urethra and bladder. Journal of Urology 99: 297–300
Fountain S S, Hamilton R D, Jameson R M 1977 Transverse fractures of the sacrum. A
   report of 6 cases. Journal of Bone and Joint Surgery 59A: 486–489
Foy M A 1988 Morbidity following isolated fractures of the sacrum. Injury 19: 379–380
Froman C, Stein A 1967 Complicated crushing injuries of the pelvis. Journal of Bone and
   Joint Surgery 49B: 24–32
Gertzbein S D, Chenoweth D R 1980 Occult injuries of the pelvic ring. Clinical
   Orthopaedics 151: 202–207
Gibson G R 1970 Impotence following fractured pelvis and ruptured urethra. British
   Journal of Urology 42: 86–88
Gill K, Bucholz R W 1984 The role of computerised tomographic scanning in the
   evaluation of major pelvic fractures. Journal of Bone and Joint Surgery 66A: 34–39
Goodwin M A 1959 Myositis ossificans in the region of the hip joint. British Journal of
   Surgery 46: 547
Hazlett J W 1980 Fractures of the sacrum. Journal of Bone and Joint Surgery 62B: 130–131
Heyes E E, Sandler C M, Corriere J N 1983 Management of the ruptured bladder
   secondary to blunt abdominal trauma. Journal of Urology 129: 946
Holdsworth F W 1945 Dislocation and fracture-dislocation of the pelvis. Journal of Bone
   and Joint Surgery 30B: 461–466
Huittenen V M, Slatis P 1971 Nerve injury in double vertical pelvic fractures. Acta
   Chirurgica Scandinavica 138: 571–575
Hundley J M 1966 Un-united unstable fractures of the pelvis. Journal of Bone and Joint
   Surgery 48A: 1025
Irving M H 1964 Exostosis formation after traumatic avulsion of the anterior inferior iliac
   spine. Journal of Bone and Joint Surgery 46B: 720–722
Kaiser T F, Farrow F C 1965 Injury of the bladder and prostatomembranous urethra
   associated with fracture of the bony pelvis. Surgery, Gynecology and Obstetrics 120:
   99–112
Karaharju E, Slatis P 1978 External fixation of double vertical pelvic fractures with a
   trapezoid compression frame. Injury 10: 142–145
Kelalis P P, King L R, Belman A B 1976 Clinical paediatric urology. Saunders, Philadelphia
King J 1975 Impotence after fractures of the pelvis. Journal of Bone and Joint Surgery
   57A: 1107–1109
Lander R O 1984 Sacro-iliac injuries. Journal of Bone and Joint Surgery 66B: 611
Langloh N D, Johnson E W, Jackson C B 1972 Traumatic sacro-iliac disruptions. Journal
   of Trauma 12: 931–953
Letournel E 1978 Pelvic fractures: annotation. Injury 10: 145–148
Levine J I, Crampton R S 1963 Major abdominal injuries associated with pelvic fractures.
   Surgery, Gynecology and Obstetrics 116: 223–226
Macdonald G A 1980 Pelvic disruptions in children. Clinical Orthopaedics 151: 130–134
Madsden L V, Jensen J, Christenson S T 1983 Parturition and pelvic fracture. A follow up
   of 34 obstetric patients with a history of pelvic fracture. Acta Obstetrica Gynaecologica
   Scandinavica 62(6): 617–620

Malgaigne J F 1855 Double vertical fractures of the pelvis. Reproduced and translated in Clinical Orthopaedics 151: 8–11, 1980

Metzmaker J N, Pappas A M 1985 Avulsion fractures of the pelvis. American Journal of Sports Medicine 13: 349–358

Meurman K O A 1980 Stress fractures of the pubic arch in military recruits. British Journal of Radiology 53: 521–524

Mitchell J P 1984 Urinary tract trauma. Wright, Bristol

Morehouse D D, MacKinnon K J 1969 Urological injuries associated with pelvic fractures. Journal of Trauma 9: 479–494

Noland L, Conwell H E 1930 Acute fractures of the pelvis. Treatment and results in 125 cases. Journal of the American Medical Association 94: 174–179

Noland L, Conwell H E 1933 Fractures of the pelvis. A summary of treatment and results attained in 185 cases. Surgery, Gynecology and Obstetrics 56: 522–525

Patterson D E, Barrett D M, Myers R P, Deweerd J H, Hall B B, Benson R C 1983 Primary management of urethral injuries. Journal of Urology 29: 573

Patterson F P, Morton K S 1961 Neurologic complications of fractures and dislocations of the pelvis. Surgery, Gynecology and Obstetrics 112: 702–706

Pavlov H, Nelson T L, Warren R F, Torg J S, Burstein A H 1982 Stress fractures of the pubic ramus. Journal of Bone and Joint Surgery 64A: 1020

Peltier L F 1965 Complications associated with fractures of the pelvis. Journal of Bone and Joint Surgery 47A: 1060–1069

Pennal G F, Massiah K A 1980 Non union and delayed union of fractures of the pelvis. Clinical Orthopaedics 151: 124–129

Pennal G F, Sutherland G O 1961 Fractures of the pelvis. Motion picture in the American Academy of Orthopedic Surgeons film library

Pennal G F, Tile M, Waddell J P, Garside H 1980 Pelvic disruption; assessment and classification. Clinical Orthopaedics 151: 12–21

Pyper J B 1957 Excision of the coccyx for coccydynia: a study of 28 cases. Journal of Bone and Joint Surgery 39B: 733–737

Sarkin T L 1976 Injuries of the pelvis. Journal of Bone and Joint Surgery 58B: 396

Schlonsky J, Olix M L 1972 Functional disability following avulsion fracture of the ischial epiphysis. Journal of Bone and Joint Surgery 54A: 641–644

Semba R T, Yasukawa K, Gustilo R B 1983 Critical analysis of results of 53 Malgaigne fractures of the pelvis. Journal of Trauma 23: 535–537

Slatis P, Huittenen V-M 1972 Double vertical fractures of the pelvis: a report on 163 patients. Acta Chirurgica Scandinavica 138: 799–807

Tile M 1984 Fractures of the pelvis and acetabulum. Williams & Wilkins, Baltimore

Tile M 1988 Pelvic ring fractures: should they be fixed? Journal of Bone and Joint Surgery 70B: 1–2

Torode I, Zieg D 1985 Pelvic fractures in children. Journal of Paediatric Orthopaedics 5: 76–84

Torok G 1974 Coccygodynia. Journal of Bone and Joint Surgery 56B: 386

Watson Jones R 1962 Comment following presentation of a paper on pelvic fractures at a meeting of the British Orthopaedic Association 1961. Journal of Bone and Joint Surgery 44B: 216

16. The spine

S. I. Esses and T. J. Dowling

CERVICAL SPINE INJURIES

FRACTURES

The overwhelming majority of fractures in the cervical spine can be successfully treated either in a halo or with surgical stabilization. The two instances in which the outcome is less successful are unrecognized instability and unrecognized fractures.

There have been many attempts to classify cervical spine injuries. Most fracture classifications rely on the mechanism of injury. This, unfortunately, has very little prognostic significance. Stability is the most important prognostic factor in fractures of the cervical spine. For this reason, we do not present a classification but recommend that every cervical spine injury should be carefully analysed in terms of stability. If there is any doubt as to the integrity of the cervical spine column, then the criteria of White et al (1975) may be used.

White and his colleagues carried out a biomechanical analysis of 8 cadaveric cervical spines to assess stability below C2. They defined clinical stability as the ability of the spine to limit its pattern of displacement under physiological loads so as not to damage or irritate the spinal cord or nerve roots.

Their conclusions were that the adult cervical spine is unstable or on the brink of instability when any of the following conditions is present:

1. All of the anterior elements (the posterior longitudinal ligament and all structures anterior to it) or all of the posterior elements (everything posterior to the posterior ligament) are destroyed or unable to function.
2. There is more than 3.5 mm of horizontal displacement of one vertebra in relation to an adjacent vertebra, measured on lateral X-rays (plain or flexion–extension films).
3. There is more than 11° of rotational difference to that of either adjacent vertebra, measured on a plain or flexion–extension lateral X-ray.

Rorabeck et al (1987) reviewed 26 patients with unilateral facet dislocation. Those patients in whom the diagnosis was made early were treated by reduction with traction or operative reduction and fusion. All of these patients were pain-free at follow-up. In contrast to this, 70% of patients who were allowed to heal in the displaced position had disabling pain at follow-up.

Bohlman (1979) reviewed 300 patients with fractures and dislocations of the cervical spine. In 90 cases a diagnosis was delayed from 2 days to 6 months and in 10 patients a diagnosis was delayed between 6 and 18 months. As outcome is dependent upon early management, it is essential that a thorough and careful evaluation of the cervical spine should be made in the Accident and Emergency department. Woodring & Goldstein (1982) showed that 85% of fractures of the articular processes are not evident on plain films. It is suggested therefore that other imaging techniques should be used in the full assessment of cervical spine injuries, including computerized tomography (CT) scanning, multidirectional tomography and dynamic X-rays.

Careful follow-up of all neck injuries is essential. Over 25% of patients with simple cervical compression fractures develop late spinal instability. Mazur & Stauffer (1983) showed that almost all these patients are severely disabled because of pain.

SOFT TISSUE INJURIES

General considerations

The cervical spine may be subjected to forces in multiple directions because of its anatomical configuration with a fixed weight at one end (the head) and its anchorage to the body at the other. This exposes soft tissue structures to numerous stresses which can result in injuries of varying degrees and complexities. The direction and magnitude of force, muscular tone, and structural integrity of the various soft tissue components all play a role in the development of cervical spine injuries. With hyperextension of the neck, there is no natural limit to displacement as there would be with hyperflexion where the chin comes to rest on the chest or on lateral flexion where the head is eventually buttressed by the shoulder. Both neck tone and posture also have an influence on the type and extent of neck injury sustained. There is a significant difference when the patient is bracing himself for an expected head-on collision compared to a sudden impact from behind.

Anatomical considerations include elasticity of various structures as well as their structural integrity. The ligamentum flavum is elastic up to the point of rupture but elongates less and ruptures under less stress with advancing age. The interspinous ligaments in the cervical region are thin and translucent and one or more of them may frequently be absent (Hollinshead 1982).

The prognosis may be related not only to the type of injury sustained, but also to the time of its detection and its eventual treatment.

Types of injury

Cervical injuries may be defined by location, i.e. upper or lower cervical, by direction of the force, i.e. hyperextension or hyperflexion, or as injury to specific structures defined by strain, sprain or disc injuries. On examining upper cervical injuries, a rupture of the transverse ligament is a purely ligamentous injury of the C1–C2 complex. There is no effective non-operative treatment that will successfully stabilize the C1–C2 junction. It has been reported that there are no residual symptoms after C1–C2 surgical fusion has been performed (Levine & Edward 1986).

Of the lower cervical injuries, the major ones include unilateral or bilateral facet subluxation or dislocations. A closed reduction with traction and halo immobilization generally leads to a 5–7% incidence of later instability (American Academy of Orthopedic Surgeons 1984). In one review of patients with unilateral facet dislocation of the cervical spine, all patients in whom the dislocation was reduced with traction were pain-free and had full motion and no instability with a follow-up averaging a little over 3 years. All patients who underwent an open reduction and fusion were also pain-free at follow-up. Seven of 10 patients who were allowed to heal in a displaced position had disabling pain at follow-up. Of these 26 patients reviewed, 12 had isolated unilateral facet dislocation (Rorabeck et al 1987).

Hyperextension injuries

Hyperextension or whiplash injuries may result from direct trauma to the front of the head but are usually indirect, i.e. rear-end collisions. Residual symptoms can be expected in 12–45% of these patients. These include intermittent neckache, stiffness and occasional radicular pain (Griffin 1987). If shoulder pain and hand and arm pain are present, even slower progress may be noted, with only 37% of patients being asymptomatic after an average of 7 weeks (Greenfield & Illfield 1977). This may also be true with upper back and intrascapular pain.

A poor prognosis has also been related to reversal of the normal lordotic cervical curve, as well as restricted range of motion at one level on flexion–extension radiographs (Hohl & Hopp 1978, Cervical Spine Research Society 1983, Hohl 1984). A better recovery has been recorded in men. At an average of 7 years post-injury, 39% of patients had degenerative disc disease at one or more levels as compared to 6% in a matched control population (Cervical Spine Research Society 1983).

Complaints of dizziness generally indicate a severe extension sprain with muscle rupture. After 1 week of bedrest most patients continue to be symptomatic for another 6 weeks. Patients who are still symptomatic 6 weeks after injury can be expected to have complaints for 6 months to a year. Blurred vision and tinnitus are both of no prognostic significance (Hohl 1984).

The standard treatment for a whiplash injury has been soft collar immobilization in conjunction with oral anti-inflammatory agents. A wide variety of therapeutic regimens have been reported in the literature. One study noted that traction therapy led to a slower recovery compared to patients treated without it. The patients treated in traction generally had a worse result (Greenfield & Illfield 1977). A randomized study of 61 patients compared standard treatment with early active mobilization (Mealy et al 1986). At 8 weeks post-injury it was found that those patients treated with early mobilization had less pain and a better range of motion than did the controls.

In cases where there is interspinous and capsular facet soft tissue injury, it is important to apply the criteria of White et al (1975) to ascertain whether there is significant instability. In over 30% of cases where instability can be demonstrated, long-term disability can be predicted (Griffin 1987).

Disc injuries with root involvement rarely result from whiplash injuries (Hohl 1984). Athletic injuries to the disc in most cases respond satisfactorily to a simple collar and traction treatment. It was suggested in one study (Kumano & Umcyama 1986) that if radicular signs and symptoms were present then 5 months were necessary before return to full sporting activities should occur; 60% of these patients had some residual symptoms after their initial treatment.

Cervical strains

Cervical strains are defined as a tearing or stretching of a musculotendinous unit beyond its physiological limit (American Academy of Orthopedic Surgeons 1984). Occasionally they precipitate a chronic pain syndrome which may last for several years. Strains may be graded into four categories:

1. *Grade I* strain is a partial strain. There is no deficit in the ligament and there is no evidence of instability.
2. *Grade II* strain is a deficit in the ligament without instability. These stable injuries should be braced in an extended position and assessed at 2–3 months to rule out late instability.
3. *Grade III* strain is a complete tear of the ligament with instability and with possible subluxable facet joints.
4. *Grade IV* strains are complete dislocations.

If there is no fracture associated with these injuries, they tend to heal poorly and there is a high percentage of late instability (American Academy of Orthopedic Surgeons 1984). If the injury is a purely ligamentous one it will not heal fully, even with prolonged rigid immobilization, unless there is a spontaneous anterior interbody fusion (Bohlman 1979). Bohlman reviewed 229 cervical spine injuries involving C3 to C7 and noted that 33 patients developed late instability following non-operative treatment. Of these, 21 were flexion injuries with torn posterior ligamentous complexes and 12 were hyperextension injuries of an osteoarthritic spine with longitudinal ligament and disc disruption (Epps 1978).

CERVICAL SPINE INJURIES IN CHILDREN

Patterns of injuries in children, especially those under the age of 8, tend to be different from those in adults. This is probably due to head size relative to the rest of the body, as well as to the more elastic nature of soft tissue structures (Hollinshead 1982, Hill et al 1984). The diagnosis of severe ligamentous injuries of the cervical spine in children may easily be missed if appropriate high-quality X-rays are not obtained (Pennecot et al 1984).

With atlanto-occipital dislocations, immobilization has been shown to be successful in children, although the small number of cases reviewed precludes definite conclusions as to the best method of treatment for this injury (Bundens et al 1984). A report of 3 cases noted that acute traumatic rotatory dislocation of the atlanto-occipital joint could be successfully treated conservatively by reduction and bracing (Khoury et al 1984). A 10-year review of 122 paediatric patients hospitalized with neck injuries noted 48 patients with a diagnosis of cervical strain. They were treated with bedrest, with or without a soft collar and with or without analgesics. Of these 48 patients, only 1 went on to develop subsequent instability (Hill et al 1984).

THORACOLUMBAR SPINAL INJURIES

STABLE FRACTURES

More than 80% of fractures in the thoracic and lumbar spine are stable using the classification of Holdsworth (1963) or Dennis (1983). There are, however, very few studies in which the long-term outcome of these injuries has been assessed. It is generally thought that compression fractures of the thoracic and lumbar spine have a good prognosis particularly if there is less than 40% compression. This opinion appears to be misguided in view of two studies. In 1973, Young analysed the notes of 623 patients and interviewed 116 patients who had sustained a compression fracture. He found that about 75% of patients with stable fractures of the thoracic and lumbar vertebral bodies continued to have pain. As a result of these symptoms, 25% of patients were considered partially or completely incapacitated. There was no demonstrable correlation between the severity of symptoms and radiological findings.

These findings are similar to those reported by Day & Kokan (1977). They studied 142 patients with compression fractures and concluded that persistent back pain is not uncommon. In contrast to Young's study, these authors found that severe compression of the vertebral body, comminution, and disc space narrowing adjacent to the fracture site were factors more likely to be associated with persistent pain.

BURST FRACTURES

Burst fractures result from axial loading. Historically these fractures have been treated non-operatively, but there is increasing enthusiasm for operative stabilization and decompression. McEvoy & Bradford (1985) compared the results of operative and non-operative management of burst fractures of the thoraco-lumbar spine. Only 3 of 31 patients treated with early surgery were disabled at follow-up averaging more than 3 years. This differed from those patients treated non-operatively in that 5 of 15 patients were disabled and had not returned to work.

These results are similar to those reported from Quebec (Judoin et al 1985) in which there was a clear tendency for patients who had been treated surgically to ambulate earlier and to have less pain at follow-up. Thus, the prognosis for those patients treated operatively was significantly better than those treated non-operatively. There is, however, a significant risk associated with surgical stabilization, ranging from 10 to 20%. Burst fractures are usually associated with retropulsed bony fragments causing compromise of the spinal canal. There is no correlation between the degree of canal compromise and the neurological status of the patient. It remains controversial as to whether decompression of the spinal canal should be carried out. Clearly, there is a potential risk of late neurological symptoms as a result of spinal stenosis but this is not quantifiable.

OTHER UNSTABLE FRACTURES

The late sequelae of unstable injuries in the thoracic and lumbar spine are primarily those of increasing spinal deformity and late pain. Soreff et al (1982) showed that there is less residual deformity in patients treated operatively. These data are comparable to those of Jacobs et al (1980). Operative treatment also allows earlier ambulation and may avoid many of the complications associated with recumbency. In the review by Jacobs et al, complications were reduced from 18% in the recumbent group, to 7% in the Harrington rod group.

SOFT TISSUE INJURIES

Generally, 6 weeks to 2 months is usually enough for soft tissue structures to heal. However, 10% of back injuries do not resolve within 2 months (American Academy of Orthopedic Surgeons 1984). Most current reviews and studies state that 90% of patients with low back symptoms are better after 3 months regardless of specific treatment and that 50–60% are better in less than 1 week (Day & Kokan 1977, American Academy of Orthopedic Surgeons 1984).

The problem in treating soft tissue injuries of the thoracolumbar regions is defining the aetiology of the pain. There are nerve fibres capable of transmitting pain present in the lumbodorsal fascia, supraspinous and infraspinous ligaments, the periosteum, anterior and posterior longitudinal ligaments, posterior annular fibres, layers of the ligamentum flavum, the intervertebral joint capsule, as well as the blood vessels and muscles (Wyke 1970, White & Panjabi 1978).

According to Frymoyer et al (1987), current research suggests that in only 0.05% of cases do X-rays provide evidence for diagnosis, prognosis and treatment. CT scans and myelograms reveal high false positive rates in 20–30% of asymptomatic subjects (Scientific Approach to the Assessment and Management of Activity-related Spinal Disorders 1987). One study demonstrated that normal males had as much as 8 mm translation at the L4–L5 segment on flexion–extension radiographs (Mouley 1987).

Anatomical studies of the lumbar region have shown significant structural variations. The intraspinous ligaments, intact in children, have been demonstrated to have deficits after the age of 20, especially at the L4–L5 and L5–S1 spaces. With increasing age there is degeneration and frequent discontinuity of these ligaments, especially in the lower three interspaces. Disc development continues up to the third decade but after that time there is a decreased fluid content with fibrous degenerative changes in the nucleus pulposus. The degenerative changes in the annulus also parallel this time sequence (Hollinshead 1982).

According to Macnab (1977), direct blows to the back as well as falls are extremely rare as aetiological factors in persisting backache. He stated that 3 weeks was the usual period of time for full recovery for myofascial sprains or strains. He noted that these myofascial injuries were generally seen in a younger population, while an older population usually sustained posterior joint strains. Nachemson (1985) noted that patients with low back pain and/or sciatica of greater than 6 months' duration have only a 40% chance of successful rehabilitation. When the pain lasts for longer than 1 year, their probability of successful rehabilitation is approximately 15%.

Weber (1983) reported on patients with a proven herniated nucleus pulposus; 80–90% of both surgically and non-surgically treated patients were asymptomatic at 4 years. Less than 2% of either group were symptomatic at 10 years. Patients with shear or flexion–distraction-type injuries of their spine are considered unstable. If they are not surgically stabilized they may develop neurological deficits and/or structural deformities, which include kyphosis or scoliosis or a combination of both (American Academy of Orthopedic Surgeons 1984).

Paediatric considerations

Unlike adults, patients under 20 years of age usually do not have idiopathic back pain and a firm diagnosis is possible in approximately 60% of these patients (American Academy of Orthopedic Surgeons 1984). In the paediatric population, patients with disc herniations frequently relate a history of trauma. Patients in this age group tend not to have any neurological deficit (Giroux & Leclereq 1982). In a study of 33 patients under 19 years of age with a documented lumbar disc herniation, 10 reported onset of symptoms after trauma. The others gave no history of a specific traumatic incident, but all were active in sports and therefore subjected to a variety of injuries. Follow-up in this group of patients ranged from 2 to 17 years. All 10 patients who were treated conservatively returned to full activity levels, with only 1 patient complaining of mild recurrent back pain. Of the surgically treated patients, 8 were noted to have good results; 3 reported a recurrence of symptoms and 1 had no improvement (Zamani & MacEwen 1982). However, in another series of surgically treated patients all were noted to have good results (Giroux & Leclereq 1982).

In a separate series of 43 patients who were 21 years of age or less and were treated surgically for lumbar disc protrusion, 10% required re-operation within 3 years. The others had satisfactory to excellent results, with a follow-up range from 4 to 30 years (Fisher & Sander 1981).

FRACTURES IN CHILDREN AND ADOLESCENTS

Spinal fractures are less common in children and adolescents than in adults. There are two distinct differences in the long-term prognosis between these two populations. In unstable fractures, there is a spontaneous progression of deformity in young patients. This is probably as a result of direct damage to the epiphyseal plate. Progressive displacement has been documented even in stable flexion injuries. For this reason, early reduction and fusion are recommended.

The second difference between adults and children is that the incidence of post-traumatic pain is very small in children. In a review by McAfee & Bohlman (1985), only 3 of 42 children had pain at the level of their injury at follow-up. This was only mild and intermittent.

Summary

1. Most thoracolumbar fractures are stable. Unstable fractures may be best managed operatively.
2. Fractures in children can lead to progressive spinal deformity.
3. Most soft tissue injuries in the thoracolumbar spine resolve without late sequelae, regardless of treatment, in 6–8 weeks. In cases where the duration of pain is more than 6 months, the likelihood of successful rehabilitation is low.

REFERENCES

American Academy of Orthopedic Surgeons 1984 Orthopedic knowledge update I and II home study syllabus. American Academy of Orthopedic Surgeons, Chicago
Bohlman H H 1979 Acute fractures and dislocations of the cervical spine: an analysis of 300 hospitalised patients and review of the literature. Journal of Bone and Joint Surgery 61A: 119
Bundens D A, Rechtine G R, Bohlman H H 1984 Upper cervical spine injuries. Orthopaedic Review 13: 556
Cervical Spine Research Society. The cervical spine. J B Lippincott, Philadelphia, p 282
Day B, Kokan P 1977 Compression fractures of the thoracic and lumbar spine from compensable injuries. Clinical Orthopaedics 124: 173
Dennis F 1983 The three column spine and its significance in the classification of acute thoracolumbar spine injuries. Spine 8: 817
Epps C H Jr 1978 Complications in orthopaedic surgery. J B Lippincott, Philadelphia
Fisher R G, Sander R L 1981 Lumbar disc protrusion in children. Journal of Neurosurgery 54: 481–483
Frymoyer J W et al 1987 Spine radiographs in patients with low back pain: an epidemiological study in men. Journal of Bone and Joint Surgery 66A: 1048–1055
Giroux J C, Leclereq T A 1982 Lumbar disc excision in the second decade. Spine 7: 168–170
Greenfield J, Illfeld F W 1977 Acute cervical strain: evaluation and short term prognostic factors. Clinical Orthopaedics 122: 196–200
Griffin P P (ed) 1987 Instructional course lectures. American Academy of Orthopedic Surgery, St Louis, p 503
Hill S A, Miller C A, Kosnik E J, Hunt W E 1984 Pediatric neck injuries. A clinical study. Journal of Neurosurgery 60: 700–706
Hohl J, Hopp E 1978 Soft tissue injuries of the neck II. Factors influencing prognosis. Abstracted Orthopaedic Trauma 2: 29
Hohl M 1984 Soft tissue injuries of the neck in automobile accidents. Journal of Bone and Joint Surgery 56A: 1675–1687
Holdsworth R W 1963 Fractures, dislocations and fracture–dislocation of the spine. Journal of Bone and Joint Surgery 45B: 6
Hollinshead W H 1982 Anatomy for surgeons, vol 3. Harper & Row, Philadelphia, p 3
Jacobs R R, Ascher M A, Snider R K 1980 Thoracolumbar spinal injuries. A comparative study of recumbent and operative treatment in 100 patients. Spine 5: 463
Judoin A, Dupuis P, Fraser M, Beamont P 1985 Unstable fractures of the thoracolumbar spine: 10 year experience at Sacré-Coeur hospital. Journal of Trauma 25: 197
Khoury G Y, Clark C R, Gravett R W 1984 Acute traumatic rotatory anatomical dislocation in children. A report of 3 cases. Journal of Bone and Joint Surgery 66A: 774–777
Kumano K, Umcyama T 1986 Cervical disk injuries in athletes. Archives of Orthopedic and Trauma Surgery 105: 223–226
Levine A M, Edward C C 1986 Treatment of injuries in the C1–C2 complex. Orthopedic Clinics of North America 17: 31–44
Macnab I 1977 Backache. Williams & Wilkins, Baltimore
Mazur J M, Stauffer E A 1983 Unrecognised spinal instability associated with seemingly 'simple' cervical compression fractures. Spine 8: 687

McAfee P C, Bohlman H H 1985 Complications following Harrington instrumentation
    for fractures of the thoracolumbar spine. Journal of Bone and Joint Surgery 67A: 672
McEvoy R D, Bradford D S 1985 The management of burst fracture of the thoracic and
    lumbar spine: experience in 53 patients. Spine 10: 631
Mealy K, Brennan H, Fenelon G C 1986 Early mobilisation of acute whiplash injuries.
    British Medical Journal 292: 656–677
Mouley V 1987 Where is the pain coming from? Spine 12: 754–759
Nachemson A L 1985 Advances in low back pain. Clinical Orthopaedics 200: 266–278
Pennecot G F, Leonard P, Peyrot DesGashols S, Hardy Jr, Pouliquen S C 1984 Traumatic
    ligamentous instability of the cervical spine in children. Journal of Pediatric
    Orthopaedics 4: 339–345
Rorabeck C H, Rock M G, Hawkins R J, Bourne R D 1987 Unilateral facet dislocation of
    the cervical spine. An analysis of the results of treatment in 26 patients. Spine 12: 23–27
Scientific Approach to the Assessment and Management of Activity-related Spinal
    Disorders. Spine 12
Soreff J, Axdorph G, Bylund P, Odeen J, Olerud S 1982 Treatment of patients with unstable
    fractures of the thoracic and lumbar spine: a follow up study of surgical and
    conservative treatment. Acta Orthopaedica Scandinavica 53: 369
Weber H 1983 Lumbar disc herniation. A controlled prospective study with 10 years
    observation. Spine 8: 131–140
White A A, Johnson R M, Panjabi M D, Southwick W O 1975 Biomechanical analysis of
    clinical instability in the cervical spine. Clinical Orthopaedics 109: 85–95
White A A, III, Panjabi M 1978 Clinical biomechanics of the spine. J B Lippincott,
    Philadelphia
Woodring J H, Goldstein S J 1982 Fractures of the articular processes of the cervical spine.
    American Journal of Radiology 139: 341
Wyke B 1970 The neurological basis of thoracic spine pain. Rhema Physical Medicine 10:
    356
Young M H 1973 Long-term consequences of stable fractures of the thoracic and lumbar
    vertebral bodies. Journal of Bone and Joint Surgery 55B: 295
Zamani M A, MacEwen G D 1982 Herniation of the lumbar disc in children and
    adolescents. Journal of Pediatric Orthopaedics 12: 528–533

17. Traumatic spinal cord injury

J. R. Silver and L. A. Frankland

INTRODUCTION

Traumatic spinal cord injuries have been known for thousands of years; the first account was given by the ancient Egyptians. They recognized that the patients invariably died within a few days of injury and felt it was a condition not to be treated. This high mortality remained throughout ancient times, the middle ages and until comparatively recently. During the First World War when medicine and surgery had reached quite a high stage of development, virtually all the patients with spinal injuries died from pressure sores and ascending urinary tract infection within weeks of injury. With the advent of the Second World War came the setting up of spinal centres, where the patients were all congregated together and all aspects of their treatment were supervised by one doctor. This was combined with better bladder management and better understanding of the importance of regular turning. Patients then began to survive the initial injury and to leave hospital.

Initially the specialty developed in the UK under the influence of Sir Ludwig Guttmann in 1944, as a result of the casualties from the fighting in Europe.

During the last 45 years centres have been set up throughout the world. Initially the patients were treated by a variety of doctors — neurosurgeons, orthopaedic surgeons, neurologists and urologists — but with the increasing development of skills and services, spinal injuries became recognized as a specialty in its own right. There are now consultants in spinal injuries in the UK who devote themselves exclusively to the management of patients with spinal cord injuries. They hold an appropriate higher training accreditation which is recognized by the Royal Colleges of Physicians and Surgeons.

Patients with spinal injury are now being resuscitated in intensive care units and transferred within hours, by helicopter or ambulance, to an appropriate spinal injury centre. As a result of this rapid transfer, better understanding of the management of patients and the evolution of treatment, the immediate mortality has been reduced but the patients are

417

surviving with severe disabilities. The long-term problems remain — returning the patient to society, finding suitable work and housing to enable the patient to lead an independent, integrated existence. In order to live in society the patient with spinal injury requires an understanding of his needs and suitable provisions for them, as clearly someone who is confined to a wheelchair will be unable to use stairs or resume work at heights or as a jockey. However with suitable treatment, retraining, provision of care and adaptations to housing he can resume a useful, happy, productive life.

Head injuries and spinal injuries are among the most expensive cases in terms of compensation. Figures in excess of £1 million are now commonplace. This money is largely given to compensate for loss of earnings and the amount of care required to allow the person to live in society. Consequently, determination of the natural history of the condition, the ability to return to work with appropriate retraining, the development and subsequent treatment, prevention of complications, and the prognosis largely govern the amount of compensation allocated.

GUIDELINES GOVERNING COMPENSATION

There are four areas which determine the compensation awarded:

1. Loss incurred directly as a result of the accident; damage to clothes, travelling to hospital by the family, damage to car and loss of earnings.
2. Pain and suffering.
3. The present condition.
4. What the future holds; the prognosis and natural history of the condition.

Direct loss

The doctor is not going to be concerned with this loss; it is easily computed by the patient's legal advisers. The doctor may be asked to sign a certificate to verify that the patient was confined to hospital and unable to follow his normal occupation.

Pain and suffering

There is a difference here between British and American practice. In the UK there is no provision for distinguishing between pains; how can you compare the pain of blindness with the pain of a mother losing a child? As such, under the British legal system an arbitrary sum is allocated for this and the doctor will not be asked to advise, since this is more of a philosophical and moral question.

The present condition and future outlook

The doctor is concerned with the patient's present condition and future outlook and whether it will change. If it is likely to improve the damages will be reduced; if it is likely to deteriorate greater damages will accrue because more care is necessary.

Satisfactory settlement of the case is a major factor in returning patients to society. Little research has been done but the following studies, from general accident cases, show that the reports do not always produce the required information on which the lawyers can base a reasonable settlement.

Cornes (1987) in a study of 818 settled claims found that in most cases the effects of the injury, treatment and recovery were adequately dealt with. However in the majority of cases information about the patients' social situation was inadequate, and may have had an adverse effect on the assessment of their compensation requirements. The median time from accident to settlement was 29 months.

Lee & Aitken (1984) found that orthopaedic surgeons predicted only 48% of the surgical and psychosocial problems that occurred after surgery. This study indicated the importance of repeated assessment at intervals in order to overcome the inaccuracy of prediction.

In common with other cases, the consultant treating the patient will usually give the report on the patient's behalf because he knows the patient, is aware what future treatment is planned and has an understanding of the various sequelae and consequences of spinal injuries. Other opinions may be requested on the patient's behalf when there is doubt about the extent of the knowledge of the doctor treating the patient. For example, if a patient with a spinal injury has sustained a fractured wrist as part of his injuries, then the risks of arthritis or stiffness or the need for osteotomy should be assessed by an orthopaedic surgeon and a report requested. If the patient has difficulty in emptying his bladder with recurrent urinary tract infection then the views of a urologist should be requested.

Settlement of these cases involves such large sums of money that the insurance company or the solicitors for the other side will often require their own expert to see the patient to ascertain whether the reports and the views expressed are acceptable.

CONTENT OF REPORT

It is necessary for the court to know not only how the patient is now, but whether his disability will increase or his need for care will change in the future. This will depend on an accurate examination and history of the injury. Previous medical conditions such as alcoholism, heavy smoking, drug addiction or suicide attempts are unlikely to be improved by spinal injury and will have an adverse effect upon the future management. The housing situation and care arrangements must also be considered, as must the effect of the injury upon his physical state and how it has changed from normal. The following points must be discussed, assessed and analysed:

> motor power, ambulation, need for wheelchair, preservation of sensation, presence of pressure sores, presence or absence of spasms, type and nature of pain, bowels and bladder management, sexual function, future and present housing needs, method of transport, need for physiotherapy, previous work, possibilities of obtaining work, independence, need for care, how that care is to be provided, implications upon the family and upon the children, self-esteem of the patient, time spent in bed with illnesses, mental state, change in lifestyle, ability to have holidays, immediate and remote risks, need for special equipment and life expectancy.

Clearly, to discuss all these things in detail would involve writing a textbook on spinal injuries but certain points must be emphasized.

General examination

It is *vital* that the patient should be examined within 6 months of the court hearing. The practice of going to court with stale reports, some 3 or 4 years old, is to be deplored as the patient's condition can rapidly deteriorate. When the doctor is called to substantiate his opinions it is embarrassing to be confronted with a patient covered with pressure sores which have developed since the time of the last examination. Such points can only be brought out in court to the patient's and doctor's detriment unless the best information is available. The practice of submitting reports based on a study of the case notes is to be deplored since it relies on the accuracy of another doctor's examination, and this doctor may be inexperienced. Frequently errors are copied from one set of notes to another and from one report to another.

It is desirable to see the patient at home so that adaptations can be inspected, their suitability commented on and further changes requested. The carers should be interviewed and such telltale signs as empty alcohol bottles and tensions within the family noted.

Physical examination

It is necessary to be able to perform an accurate and comprehensive examination of the nervous system. This normally means that the doctor must have done a neurological house job and preferably a registrar job in neurology, since, almost without exception, the following features, which could affect the prognosis, are ignored even by specialists.

Head injury

It is almost impossible to fracture the cervical spine without sustaining a head injury. Approximately 50% of admissions to a spinal unit are tetraplegic and the presence of head injury with spinal injury is frequently overlooked. The patient's rehabilitation can be impaired because of difficulty in concentrating, aggression, forgetfulness and impairment of intellect. This must be taken into account and amplified by psychiatric, psychological and psychometric assessments, reports from previous employers and the general practitioner and interviews with the spouse.

Motor power

The patient *must* be examined. Unfortunately one is often confronted with reports submitted from a study of the notes or, if the patient has been seen at home, he has not been examined or has been examined in a wheelchair. It may seem self-evident but motor power cannot be evaluated unless a patient is undressed; the shoulder muscles and the posterior muscles are almost invariably ignored. In cauda equina lesions the glutei and soleus muscles are frequently not examined because they are on the posterior aspect and their paralysis is ignored.

Reflexes

For aesthetic reasons a vital reflex, the anal reflex, is usually omitted. This is a most important indicator of bladder function and predictor of the return of bladder activity.

Sensation

The sensory examination may well only be carried out in a perfunctory manner and the ascent of sensory loss in post-traumatic syringomyelia is frequently missed. Sensory sparing, which may be around the anus in cauda equina lesions, is again frequently missed and the sacral segments are not examined for aesthetic reasons.

Pressure sores

Unless the patient is examined and all dressings removed the presence of pressure sores might be missed since the patient may be ashamed or unwilling to disclose these sores.

Bladder

In the past, life expectancy was entirely governed by the function of the urinary tract and for this reason we will elaborate on the subject. There are two aspects — the social problem and the effect on the life expectancy. In females it is impossible to fit a satisfactory appliance and it is almost invariable for paraplegic women to be incontinent of urine, having to change their clothes several times a day. This is extremely embarrassing and yet the women make light of it and do not complain unless specifically asked. If they have a permanent indwelling catheter this will lead to dilatation of the urethra, requiring a urinary diversion. In contrast, males can have a satisfactory device but the presence of a collecting device and leg bag is embarrassing and hinders sexual activity.

In both sexes the presence of defective emptying leads to ascent of infection which will involve the kidneys and can shorten the patient's life expectancy. Evaluation of these matters is clearly a subject for the specialist; assessment by a urological surgeon and renal physician is required and extensive investigation in the form of X-rays, ultrasound tests, urine cultures, clearance studies and blood estimations will need to be carried out.

Bladder function should be evaluated neurophysiologically because it enables an opinion to be given regarding the use of a sacral nerve root stimulator. These matters are clearly for ultraspecialists in neurosurgery and urology but they do change the patient's outlook, and can transform a patient's life from one of dribbling incontinence to independence. As the implants are expensive their discussion is a matter of importance and the necessity and cost of such treatment, which is not available under the National Health Service, should be discussed.

Sexual function

This aspect is almost totally ignored. Considering what a dominant factor this is, it should be discussed in full and not purely in mechanical terms. The women may be able to have children but will need extra care in looking after them. The effect of pregnancy upon a tetraplegic patient is a specialist subject as the patient may develop severe infections and autonomic dysreflexia. Although women with spinal injuries are fertile they may well have total loss of appreciation and, due to anaesthesia, spasms and incontinence; the sexual act may thus be impossible or totally distasteful. On the other hand, the male may well be infertile but may be able to achieve intercourse. Skilled advice is needed to evaluate sexual function.

Social and psychological problems

These problems are vast and cannot be adequately dealt with in a chapter of this size. Housing is a major problem in everyone's lives. Although the population in this country has remained static, social changes have meant that people no longer live at home until they get married. Young people often move into smaller housing units, such as flats. People may have had a satisfactory flat before injury, but it may be totally unsuitable when they are paralysed.

Early provision of suitably modified or purpose-built accommodation is a major factor in trying to return any patient to society. This may well be available in a compensation case by means of an interim payment and can transform the rehabilitation programme. The courts accept that the patient should have proper housing, paid for privately, and this cannot be provided by the state. Figure 17.1 illustrates the complex problems of organizing rehousing. Clearly the patient will require ground floor accommodation or a lift and this is an area where specialist reports by architects may be needed. The doctor may well be asked to comment on the suitability of the adaptations, and any omissions should be discussed.

Provision and facilities for care

Some patients, such as paraplegic patients, can be completely independent and while they require no care it is not desirable for them to live on their own. It may take them a long time to get their clothes and equipment together, which might preclude them from going to work, and it is desirable that they should have some assistance. On the other hand, high tetraplegic patients with C4 transections require total care and cannot be left on their own for more than a short period. Some 50% of admissions to a spinal unit are tetraplegics. Who provides the care and how is it to be provided? This is a complex issue. There are nursing agencies, the family, children, neighbours, district nurses, twilight schemes and local authorities. It has been suggested that a manager should be employed to co-ordinate all these agencies.

In general, after the Second World War patients with spinal injuries were accommodated in hostels like large boarding schools, where they could live with a certain amount of support and go out to work. Things have now progressed and people expect to live as normal members of society. In the past it has been assumed that the family would provide care on discharge from hospital. This is not necessarily the best solution; in fact, surveys have shown that it is probably the worst solution. The decision whether the family should care for the spinal injured person requires advice from social workers, interviews with the family and accurate assessment of how much care is needed to look after the patient at home. At current rates it may cost £12 000 per nurse per year to look after a tetraplegic at home, and several nurses may be required so many thousands of pounds may be needed for continuing care. How this is to be achieved is a matter for specialist discussions with the nursing agencies.

Prognosis and life expectancy

Thus far we have concentrated on the patient's present state, which may be assessed by examination. The questions the doctor is most often asked

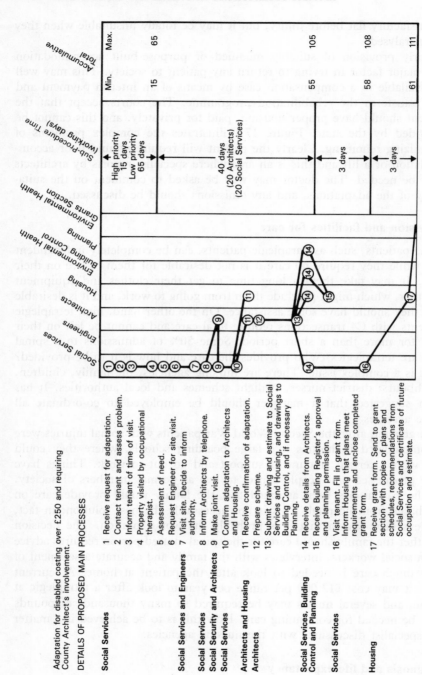

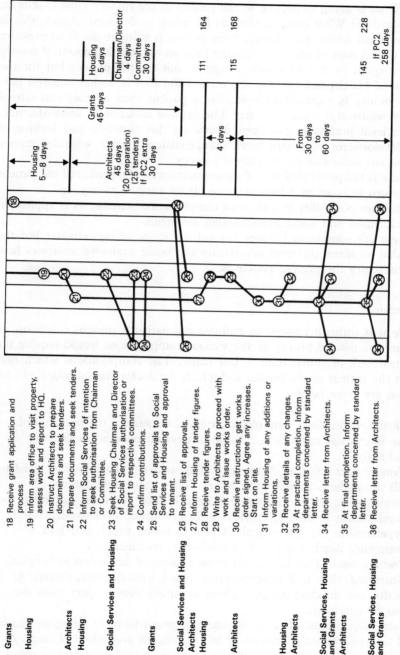

Fig. 17.1 Details of main processes involved in the adaptations required for disabled persons (from Cardiff City Council, with permission)

are: 'What is going to happen to the patient in the future? How long is he going to live? What complications is he going to develop?' Again, this is an enormous subject but clearly, if the patient is going to die from pressure sores within days of the court hearing then an enormous amount of money will be spent by the insurance company, not for the patient but for the benefit of his dependants. On the other hand if it is underestimated how much money is required to look after a patient then he may run out of money whilst still requiring care. The present situation is unsatisfactory.

The legal profession has been discussing this situation and looking at the development of a structured compensation scheme whereby money is paid out according to the patient's needs.

There is the possibility that if a complication can be predicted the patient can return to court at a later stage to obtain further money.

A further possibility is a no-fault compensation scheme, as is applied in New Zealand and some Scandinavian countries.

These are complicated issues beyond the scope of this chapter but the fact that so many different approaches are being evaluated indicates how unsatisfactory the present system is.

Prognosis

While it is difficult enough to evaluate the patient's present condition, to predict the natural history or the various complications would require not one textbook of spinal injuries but many. The complications which may affect the patient in the future, and which the doctor should address in his report, are given below:

1. *Chest complications*: Tetraplegic patients, because of the paralysis of the intercostal muscles, are liable to develop pneumonia and die suddenly.
2. *Urinary tract infection*: Acute ascending urinary tract infections used to kill the patients rapidly after injury. These have been largely eliminated in the acute stage but are still liable to occur. Later on, the development of stones, amyloid disease, chronic pyelonephritis and hypertension are all recognized complications which can lead to premature death and can be modified by treatment.
3. *Pressure sores*: This is the commonest cause of admission to hospital. Untreated, they lead to septicaemia, penetration of bone, chronic ill health and amyloid disease. There are many causes apart from the loss of sensation.
4. *Cystic degeneration*: The development of post-traumatic syringomyelia is ill understood but it does occur in a significant proportion of cases. As many as 5% of patients develop it, and it may lead to ascending sensory loss and progression of paralysis. Treatment is still unsatisfactory and is being modified.

Life expectancy

This is the question most frequently posed and depends on the patient's present state; age; level and completeness of the lesion, what treatment the patient is undergoing, and whether the patient has got or is likely to develop complications. The most important of these have been mentioned. It is necessary to compare the population of paraplegic patients with a matched normal population to calculate risk.

Life expectancy is an area of guesswork and bargaining and few accurate figures are available. Previously all patients died within a few weeks. Latterly it has been clear that patients are surviving for much longer. A few patients have lived from the time of the First World War. These patients invariably had non-interference with their bladders or rapidly discontinued catheters, since life expectancy then was governed by the development of ascending urinary tract infection.

With improved methods of treatment the mortality has been reduced. Until the Second World War, veterans died rapidly of pressure sores. With better understanding of the development of sores this risk has been reduced, but it is still a major cause of admission to hospital and there is always a risk of the patient dying of sores and the late development of amyloid disease. Death may also occur with the development of respiratory failure in the high tetraplegic patient, as paralysis of the intercostal muscles enables secretions to accumulate and pneumonia to develop. There is an increased risk of suicide, cancer and cystic degeneration.

These major causes of death reduce life expectancy. The only way that this can be calculated is by comprehensive evaluation of all the patients passing through a spinal unit; the causes of death should be correlated with the level of the lesion, complications and bladder function. These patients should be compared with a similar population in the same country at the same time. As yet no comparison exists for the UK.

There are enormous areas of controversy here, such as, does a patient who becomes tetraplegic at the age of 20 and has lived to the age of 40 have the same life expectancy as a person who becomes tetraplegic at the age of 40? Such questions can only be answered by further research, which is currently under way. A tetraplegic does have a worse life expectancy than a paraplegic but much depends on how carefully a patient looks after himself and how well he is motivated.

WHO SHOULD GIVE THE REPORT?

Who should give a report on a spinal injury case? The first point is that in general the number of reports asked for depends upon the cost of the case. Thus with a very minor injury (a sprained wrist) which may be settled for under £1000 the insurance company will not necessarily go to the expense of obtaining a report from its own doctor and may be satisfied with a report from the general practitioner. In cases of greater complexity, the hospital consultant treating the patient will be asked to report. Where cases are of the greatest complexity and sums of up to £1 million are awarded, then reports will be requested from many specialists, particularly where there are contentious issues. In general, the courts listen to and take account of the doctor who is treating the patient because he is familiar with the patient's condition, has treated the patient from the outset and will have planned future treatment. He is responsible for the patient's care and as such the judge will listen to him. It is common that when reports have been submitted the insurance company will ask another doctor to see the patient. In spinal cases this is now almost invariably a spinal consultant who will have an understanding of the natural history of the condition and the complications. Other specialists may be called in to give reports — a urological surgeon on the bladder management, a neurosurgeon on the syringomyelia, a plastic surgeon on the pressure sore management. An orthopaedic surgeon may well be requested to give a report on such aspects as the management of the initial fracture or the management of the spinal fracture, and whether it is unstable and needs fixation. He may also be asked to comment on the possibility of arthritis developing as a result of fractures, management of associated fractures, development of osteoporosis and management of complications such as contractures and the need for tendon release.

It may be that the spinal patient will have been admitted in the first instance to an accident unit and then transferred to a spinal centre within days. Orthopaedic surgeons may be asked to produce a report on the patient's initial treatment while in the accident unit. They may be asked to comment at a later stage, when the patient has returned home, or may see the patient in a follow-up clinic and be asked to produce a report for the insurance company. The doctor's report is of course up to the individual conscience and competence of the particular doctor, but reports dealing with the more complicated aspects of spinal injury such as post-traumatic syringomyelia, life expectancy and pressure sores are best dealt with by the appropriate spinal, urological or neurosurgical consultant. It does happen that general reports from an orthopaedic surgeon are submitted in the absence of these specialist reports and when the hearing is imminent and the case is being evaluated, there is a great flurry of activity and only then are reports requested from the relevant experts. These are produced at great expense and lead to irritation on the part of the patient who will already have been examined by innumerable consultants.

If you give a report you must be prepared to go to court and substantiate the findings. As this can be a very time-wasting exercise, involving sitting around for days in the corridors of uncomfortable courts, many consultants cannot afford the time away from their clinical practice and decline to give reports. This problem is compounded by the fact that the solicitors ask consultants to be available for up to a week to give evidence and then, at the last minute, postpone or cancel the case. These cases may well take place at courts some distance from the consultant's practice and necessitate stays overnight; this is to be deplored and the reluctance of consultants to appear is understandable. This has given rise to a great deal of friction between the medical and legal professions with regard to cancellation fees; to such a degree that the matter has been dealt with in the high court.

In an article in the British Medical Association News Review (1986), Judge Bingham stressed that each case for payment must be judged on its own merits. However he made it clear that there were limits on what could be demanded of witnesses in the name of public duty. In the case under discussion the cancellation had been made 24 hours before the hearing was due. It was unreasonable to expect that the witnesses would not lose income as a result, said the judge. He added:

> The court is undoubtedly very much assisted by the expert evidence of medical and other witnesses at the peak of their professions. If such men are to respond to invitations to give expert evidence in court and to keep time free for that purpose, it is right that they should not run the risk of a last minute cancellation which would leave them substantially out of pocket. It would, therefore, be very unfortunate if witnesses such as these were deterred from making their services available, and if the court were dependent on the evidence of those who had no very pressing demands on their time.

Current practice accepted in Great Britain and Northern Ireland is:

Cancellation of court hearing with notice of 48 hours or less — full fee payable.
Cancellation of court hearing with notice of 48 hours to 1 week — half fee payable.

Obviously the size of the fee is a matter for negotiation but if you give a report it is essential to settle the terms before agreeing to appear in court.

CONCLUSION

Spinal injury cases are amongst the most expensive of those that come to court. As such, many different disciplines are involved in the formulation of the final claim — orthopaedic surgeons, neurosurgeons, urological surgeons, psychologists, nurses and housing experts. Individuals providing reports should restrict themselves to the areas where they have specific expertise. The orthopaedic surgeon should regard himself in this light and the purpose of this chapter has been to outline the complexities of such cases. The orthopaedic surgeon should understand that his report will be considered as one amongst many.

REFERENCES

British Medical Association News Review 1986. Doctors win fight over court fees. Vol 12, no. 7, July, p 11

Cornes P F 1987 Rehabilitation and return to work of personal injury claimants. Rehabilitation Studies Unit, University of Edinburgh

Lee R H, Aitken R C B 1984 Prediction of fracture patients' rehabilitation problems by orthopaedic surgeons. Health Bulletin 42: 174–186

18. Head injury

B. Jennett

INTRODUCTION

Considerable confusion often arises when doctors and lawyers discuss the consequences of head injury. There are several reasons for this. One is that, unlike injuries to other parts of the body where the severity of damage is usually maximum at the moment of injury, a relatively mild injury to the head can lead to serious complications. These may be temporarily life-threatening, yet if they are competently treated there may be complete recovery. But there is the paradox that severe permanent disability can be the outcome of an injury that initially was not serious but that resulted in secondary brain damage.

Another problem is that the most disabling sequelae are often the psychosocial rather than physical, and these may not be obvious when the patient is examined for a medicolegal report. Defining their nature and severity depends on skilled interpretation of accounts of the patient's behaviour by others. The opinion of a psychologist and/or psychiatrist experienced in this particular field can be useful, sometimes essential.

Yet another difficulty is the development of complications months or years after injury (e.g. epilepsy, meningitis), when the patient has already made a good recovery. There may then be arguments about establishing the causal relationship between previous injury and a long delayed complication.

EARLY COMPLICATIONS

These can develop within the first few hours or days after injury and can cause secondary brain damage which far exceeds that sustained in the original accident.

Intracranial complications

These include swelling of the brain, infection and the development of haematoma (blood clot) that may either be on the surface of the brain

431

(extradural or subdural) or within its substance (intracerebral). Intracranial haematoma often poses a threat to life and rapid surgical intervention to remove the clot is then required. Even when this is done there is considerable early mortality and many survivors have persisting deficits or a high risk of developing late traumatic epilepsy, or both. Early traumatic epilepsy, defined as fits developing during the first week after injury, is more frequent in children; it can occur after quite mild injury. Adults have early fits only when there has been substantial brain damage, as evidenced by depressed fracture, intracranial haematoma or coma. Repeated early fits or status epilepticus may aggravate the brain damage. The late consequences of early epilepsy are discussed later.

Extracranial complications

About a third of head-injured patients also have major extracranial injuries and complications related to these can cause or aggravate secondary brain damage. Extracranial complications which combine to damage the brain include low blood pressure or shock, inadequate respiration and loss of blood due to haemorrhage. Their effect is to reduce the oxygen supply to the brain.

Secondary brain damage

In some cases it is obvious that secondary brain damage is dominant, in that the patient was clearly not severely affected soon after injury, but then developed complications. In other cases it is a matter of conjecture how much of the eventual brain damage resulted from primary as distinct from secondary factors. A matter raised in some cases is the extent to which secondary complications might have been avoided and the secondary brain damage might have been less if medical management had been more appropriate. When neurosurgical services are regionalized, as they are in Europe, delay in referral to a neurosurgeon can occur. Sometimes the delay is simply a function of distance, but more often it is because the risks of certain complications were underestimated or the early signs of their development were not recognized. Initial assessment and observation in the first few hours and days after injury are therefore concerned with discovering factors which increase the risk or likelihood of complications, and with detecting the early signs when these do develop.

SIGNIFICANCE OF SKULL FRACTURES

It is brain damage that matters after head injury but damage to the scalp, the skull and the face bears witness to the head having been subjected to a certain degree of violence. Thousands of patients who attend accident departments with lacerations or bruising of the face or scalp have sustained no brain damage. More than half of these mild injuries occur in children, many of them with scalp laceration. Unless a fracture of the skull vault or base indicates the possibility that secondary intracranial complications may develop, these patients can usually be sent home without risk.

Only 1 or 2% of those who attend accident departments after head injury have a skull fracture. Because severe brain damage can occur without a skull fracture, and a skull fracture can occur without brain damage or complications, there has been continuing controversy about the significance of discovering a fracture, and therefore about the indications for taking a skull X-ray (Jennett 1987a). A distinction must be made between a linear fracture of the vault of the skull, a compound depressed fracture of the vault of the skull and a fracture of the base of the skull. The latter two fractures indicate a breach in the integrity of the coverings of the brain and each is associated with a risk of intracranial infection. Their significance is therefore not in doubt.

Compound depressed fracture of the vault

A compound depressed fracture of the vault of the skull underlying a scalp laceration usually causes some local brain damage but unless the brain as a whole has been subjected to damage there will have been no loss of consciousness. At least a quarter of patients with compound depressed fractures are fully conscious when first seen, have had no alteration of consciousness and have no abnormal neurological signs. In a patient who is fully conscious it is easy to overlook a depressed fracture unless there is obvious penetration of the brain, as evidenced by brain and cerebrospinal fluid coming out of the laceration. A compound injury is even more likely to be missed if the brain has been penetrated by a sharp object which has been withdrawn, leaving only a small puncture wound. Examples are when a child falls against a knitting needle or the axle of a toy wheel, or when an assault has been carried out at any age with a sharp instrument such as a screwdriver. If a scalp laceration or puncture wound overlying a penetrating injury wound is treated by simple suture without proper debridement there is a risk of meningitis or brain abscess.

Fracture of the base of the skull

Meningitis is also a risk after a fracture of the base of the skull involving the air sinuses or the middle ear cavity. This kind of injury is usually associated with some initial impairment of consciousness. The clue may be the development of bilateral black eyes several hours after injury, or the leakage of blood and cerebrospinal fluid from the nose or one or both of the ears. In the event of there also being facial injuries these sinister signs may easily be overlooked. Meningitis may be delayed for months or years after a fracture of the base of the skull. Some such patients have continuing cerebrospinal fluid rhinorrhoea or otorrhoea, but when the leak is trivial or intermittent the fistula is often not recognized although the risk of meningitis remains.

Linear fracture

A linear fracture of the skull does not in itself call for any immediate treatment. For this reason its detection has been considered to be unimportant by radiologists who are concerned about the large number of patients with mild injuries who are X-rayed in accident departments. When such a fracture is associated with clinically severe head injury there is no call for an immediate X-ray because such patients will obviously be admitted and radiological examination can be carried out from the ward. There may be no fracture of the skull in some serious (even fatal) head injuries where acceleration/deceleration forces have led to deep unconsciousness.

A linear fracture is of greatest importance in the patient who is walking and talking on arrival at the accident department and who could safely be sent home if it were known that he did not have a skull fracture. In such mildly injured patients a skull fracture increases the likelihood of the development of an acute intracranial haematoma several hundred times (Mendelow et al 1983, Teasdale et al 1989). This is a potentially lethal complication and its successful treatment depends on early recognition followed by expeditious surgery. It is therefore considered wise to admit such patients to hospital for observation rather than to risk their developing this complication at home, when some delay in appropriate management would be inevitable. That is the rationale for advising that a skull radiograph should be taken when a fracture is possible, rather than likely.

Apart from deciding which mild injuries should be kept under observation rather than sent home, a fracture is also important in patients who are confused or in a coma because in these cases it also indicates an increased risk of intracranial haematoma. This is important when it comes to deciding which patients should have a computerized tomography (CT) scan and which should be transferred to a regional neurosurgical unit. In the USA there are 7 times more neurosurgeons and 10 times as many scanners as in the UK and these decisions are not therefore crucial, so it is no surprise that skull X-rays should be regarded as much less important than in the UK. Unfortunately some radiologists in the UK seem not to realize the implications of this difference in provision. Also they seem not to recognize how useful it can be to know whether a mildly injured patient has a skull fracture, because of its importance as a risk factor for complications. Guidelines have been published for identifying which adult patients should have an X-ray, be admitted, have a CT scan and be referred to neurosurgeons (A group of neurosurgeons 1984).

SEVERITY OF BRAIN DAMAGE

Apart from the small minority of patients who have a penetrating injury, evidence of brain damage depends largely on observed or reported alteration of consciousness, and much less often on the presence of focal neurological signs. All but 5% of head-injured patients are fully conscious by the time they arrive at the accident department, although witnesses may testify to some of them having been briefly unconscious or dazed. The most direct evidence of this altered consciousness is whether the patient himself remembers the accident and events subsequent to it, such as roadside conversations or being transported to hospital. The duration of post-traumatic amnesia is the most reliable clue to minor brain damage.

Glasgow coma scale

If a patient is confused or in a coma then the extent and duration of this is usually recorded at the time by the Glasgow coma scale (Table 18.1; Teasdale & Jennett 1974). This also makes it possible to define coma more clearly and to distinguish it from other states of reduced consciousness or responsiveness. Coma is defined as not opening the eyes, not obeying commands and not uttering any recognizable words. Many doctors, however, still use the word loosely and may qualify it as light or deep coma, although there are no agreed definitions for these terms. The advantage of using the Glasgow coma scale is that overall severity may be

Table 18.1 Glasgow coma scale

Variable	Score
Eye-opening	
Spontaneous	E 4
To speech	3
To pain	2
Nil	1
Best motor response	
Obeys	M 6
Localizes	5
Withdraws	4
Abnormal flexion	3
Extensor response	2
Nil	1
Verbal response	
Oriented	V 5
Confused conversation	4
Inappropriate words	3
Incomprehensible sounds	2
Nil	1
Coma score (E + M + V) = 3–15	

Table 18.2   Distribution of severity of 1919 admissions (Derived from Miller & Jones 1985)

Glasgow coma scale*	Severe <8	Moderate 9–12	Mild 13–15
All admissions	5%	11%	84%
Computerized tomography scans	40%	21%	29%
Intracerebral haematoma	59%	23%	18%
Hospital > 1 month	50%	25%	25%
Vegetative or severe at 1 month	28%	28%	44%

*On their 14-point scale <7, 8–12, 13 or 14 — here adjusted for full scale.

expressed by the total score on the scale. This scale was used to classify a large series of head injuries into three grades of severity (Table 18.2). This study showed that severe injuries are relatively infrequent and that most patients who developed haematomas and most who required surgery had been classified as mild or moderate on admission.

Another advantage of using this scale when observing the patient in the early hours or days after injury is that it enables any deterioration in conscious level to be rapidly recognized. Such a change is the earliest and most consistent sign that intracranial complications are developing — in particular an intracranial haematoma.

Post-traumatic amnesia

The best guide to the severity of brain damage that is available to the doctor who is called on months later to submit a legal report is the duration of the post-traumatic amnesia. Its advantage is that it can be ascertained by asking the patient when he himself realized where he was. It is usually possible to distinguish this from what he was told by friends and relatives or by nurses about when they believed he first woke or spoke. The duration of the post-traumatic amnesia is always much longer than the time when witnesses report such evidence of the recovery of consciousness. Only an approximate estimate of post-traumatic amnesia is needed in order to categorize the severity of injury according to this scale:

<5 minutes: very mild
5 minutes–1 hour: mild
1–24 hours: moderate
1–13 days: severe
>14 days: very severe

In assessing severity it is important to distinguish the severity of the initial injury to the skull and to the brain from the subsequent brain damage due to complications. An apparently mild injury may be potentially serious, because complications could develop. An initially serious injury or a life-threatening complication may be followed by a good recovery, but that does not mean that the damage was not severe. Similarly serious sequelae (or death) can follow a relatively mild injury, because of complications. Assessment of severity of injury should therefore not be based on outcome.

SEQUELAE OF UNCOMPLICATED MILD INJURIES

Most patients after head injury complain for a time of headache and dizziness, and sometimes of poor concentration and memory, fatigue and irritability. These symptoms comprise the post-concussional syndrome and because they commonly occur in patients who have had only a few minutes of post-traumatic amnesia, or none at all, it was believed that they were psychological in origin and not related to organic dysfunction of the brain. That has now been disproved, because for some 2–3 weeks after such a mild injury it can be shown that all patients have some impaired processing of information when formal psychological tests are carried out. There may also be disorders of the vestibular apparatus controlling balance, and an increased sensitivity to noise (hyperacusis). If these various subjective complaints are ignored by doctors, instead of the patient being reassured that they are likely to be temporary and are not evidence of serious damage, the symptoms may become a source of anxiety to the patient and this may make matters worse. These symptoms may also be exaggerated or prolonged if the patient returns to work too soon, particularly if this involves paper work and intellectual effort. Normally these complaints do not persist for more than a month but there are a few patients who, for reasons that are often not obvious, continue to complain for months and a few who find it difficult to adjust to normal life again. This has been termed an accident neurosis and if this is suspected then a skilled psychiatric opinion should be obtained. In view of the clear organic background to these symptoms in the early stages, it is unwise to assume that the patient is malingering or exaggerating.

Some patients who have had compound depressed fracture or an intracranial haematoma on the surface of the brain that was expeditiously removed make a rapid recovery and return to school or work within a few weeks. It is all too easy in such circumstances to dismiss the injury itself as having been mild when in fact it had been associated with considerable immediate risk. Moreover both these types of injury carry a substantial risk of late epilepsy (see later).

SEQUELAE OF MORE SEVERE INJURIES

Glasgow outcome scale

The development of the Glasgow outcome scale (Jennett & Bond 1975) has made it easier to place brain-damaged patients into broad categories

Table 18.3 Glasgow outcome scale (from Jennett & Bond 1975)

Outcome	Patient's social capacity
Dead	
Vegetative	Eyes open, not sentient
Severely disabled	Conscious but dependent
Moderately disabled	Independent but disabled
Good recovery	Normal activities

and to define the timescale of recovery. The scale refers to the patient's social capacity rather than to neurological deficits, and it does so on a simple scale of 4 for survivors (Table 18.3).

A good recovery is recorded if the patient has either assumed all normal activities or is judged capable of doing so, although he may have some minor deficits. A moderate recovery describes a patient who has a clearcut deficit — it may be weakness in a limb, defective vision or hearing, or paralysis of one or more cranial nerves. However, the patient is fully independent, able to travel by public transport and capable of fending for himself. He may have returned to his own work but that does not mean that he is not to some extent disabled. It is important not to regard failure to return to work as evidence of deficit, or return to work as evidence that there is no deficit.

Patients are classified as severely disabled if they are conscious but dependent, in the sense of requiring another person for some activity every day. That dependence can vary from being bedridden to needing help only with going out of doors or perhaps with some particular task during each day. Dependence may be required because of purely physical defects, such as paralysis or loss of speech, but some patients who have no physical deficit may be wholly dependent. This is because they are so seriously impaired mentally that they are unable to be left alone in the house or to fend for themselves. This mental deficit may not always be immediately obvious, and careful enquiry needs to be made of friends and relatives.

Formal assessment by a psychologist and psychiatrist should be carried out in order to establish the nature of the deficit; sometimes undue dependence is developed when there is greater capability than there appears — however, there is usually no doubt about the patient's severe disability.

Vegetative state

The vegetative state (Jennett & Plum 1972) refers to the patient who has lost all function in the cerebral cortex. After head injury this is usually the result of severe initial diffuse axonal injury in the white matter of the cerebral hemispheres and brain stem. When this is the case the patient has always been deeply unconscious from the outset. There is often no skull fracture and CT scan may show only small abnormalities, although these are of significance when interpreted by a skilled neuroradiologist. They include small haemorrhagic contusions in the corpus callosum and superior cerebellar peduncle and often some blood in the third ventricle. At post-mortem the brain often looks normal to the naked eye but a skilled neuropathologist can detect the tell-tale signs of diffuse axonal injury. Occasionally this condition results from secondary hypoxic brain damage, especially if there has been an episode of cardiac arrest.

Patients in the vegetative state are awake but not aware. That is, they have long periods of eye-opening (with sleep–wake rhythm) but they show no signs of psychologically meaningful response. Because the brain stem is relatively intact they breathe on their own, can swallow and have a wide range of reflex activities, moving their spastic limbs in response to painful stimuli; they can follow a visual stimulus or turn towards a loud noise. They never utter a word but can groan or cry out. These physiologically decerebrate patients are sometimes said to be in a permanent coma but that is a misleading term for someone whose eyes are open. They are of course quite different from patients who are brain dead, whose brain stem no longer functions and who are ventilator-dependent.

Provided that they are tube-fed and have basic nursing care these patients can live for many years and can extract very large sums in compensation. Many observers have described this as a state worse than death and in the USA there have been a number of court decisions giving permission to discontinue giving food and water, on the grounds that this is futile treatment bringing no benefit to the patient. The American Medical Association has endorsed this view from a medical standpoint and this legal and ethical issue is now under discussion in the UK (Jennett 1987b).

Neurophysical deficits

These are best classified as those affecting cranial nerves and vision, those affecting language function and those affecting the limbs. The commonest cranial nerve deficit is loss of sense of smell or anosmia. This frequently occurs with fractures of the base but it can also occur after a relatively mild concussion; it is usually a permanent deficit. It can be of considerable significance in certain jobs and it also deprives the patient of warning smells, such as fire or escaping gas. Apart from that there is the loss of pleasure because the aroma of food, which is part of the taste, is affected.

Visual symptoms may consist of a squint, double vision, loss of part of the visual field or even loss of all sight in one or both eyes.

Loss of hearing in one ear is quite common due to damage to the nerve to the inner ear.

Facial paralysis is likewise due to a fracture of the base of the skull but is less common; it may be permanent although partial recovery is usual.

Disorder of language function most commonly affects the patient's ability to speak fluently even though he may be able to think of the words to say — so-called expressive dysphasia. More subtle forms involve the ability to read, to understand the spoken word or to write. This most commonly occurs with damage to the left side of the brain but in some left-handed persons it may result from damage to the right side.

Damage to the controlling mechanisms of one or more of the limbs can result in hemiplegia, resembling a stroke, or to problems affecting one limb or all four. Some patients suffer severe ataxia and loss of balance as a result of damage in the cerebellum and brain stem. The frequency of these features after severe injury is shown in Tables 18.4 and 18.5 (Jennett et al 1981).

Table 18.4   Neurophysical sequelae at 6 months after injury (from Jennett et al 1981)

	All cases ($n=150$)	After intracranial haematoma ($n=77$)	No intracranial haematoma ($n=73$)
Any cerebral hemisphere dysfunction	65%	62%	67%
Cranial nerve palsy			
All cases	37%	38%	36%
As the only sign	13%	10%	15%
Ataxia	9%	4%	14%

Table 18.5   Sequelae of cerebral hemisphere damage at 6 months after injury (from Jennett et al 1981)

	All cases ($n=150$)	After intracranial haematoma ($n=77$)	No initial haematoma ($n=73$)
Hemiparesis			
All cases	49%	56%	62%
As the only hemisphere sign	24%	14%	34%
Dysphasia			
All cases	29%	32%	26%
As the only sign	7%	10%	4%
Hemiparesis and dysphasia	21%	17%	26%
Hemianopia			
All cases	5%	5%	5%
As the only sign	1%	1%	1%
Epilepsy			
All cases	17%	25%	8%
As the only sign	8%	12%	1%

Mental dysfunction

This includes disorders of behaviour, changes in personality and impaired cognitive performance (Brooks 1984). There are many neuropsychological tests for measuring different aspects of cognition — attention, vigilance, memory, complex information processing, problem-solving and learning new tasks. It is such tests of performance rather than verbal IQ tests that show deficits after head injury. However, the scores of some patients are well within the normal range of the population as a whole, yet they may be performing well below their pre-traumatic levels as estimated from their educational or occupational attainments. The patterns of impairment can vary widely between patients with seemingly similarly severe brain damage. No doubt this is because of the widespread and varied nature of the lesions, differing pre-traumatic psychosocial status and the effects on cognitive function of other consequences of the injury for both the patient and his family.

Personality changes and altered behaviour are common in patients with definite cognitive deficits, but also in those whose test results show little abnormality. Again the patient may not seem beyond the range of normal, but may none the less be greatly changed according to his family. Reduced drive and depression are common and these combine to frustrate attempts at rehabilitation or re-employment and may also result in lack of insight by the patient about his deficits. Lack of social restraint, tactlessness, irritability and impulsive behaviour characterize some patients. These behavioural problems and the stress and burden they cause to the family tend to get worse rather than better after the first few months and may last for years. This may be because the tolerance and optimism of the family during the early post-traumatic period are difficult to sustain as they realize that the changes are permanent.

TIMESCALE OF RECOVERY

This is important for managing the patient medically, for advising him socially and for knowing when it is time to settle a legal case. Most substantial recovery occurs within the 6–12 months after injury. It is unusual for a person to move from one category on the Glasgow outcome scale to the next better one after 1 year. But that is not to deny that there may be considerable improvements within the categories of moderately or severely disabled. Such recovery more often reflects adaptation or acceptance of disability rather than actual return of function.

Even in the severest cases it is therefore usually possible within a year of injury to state with confidence that the patient is likely always to have a severe degree of disability and to be dependent, and this should usually be enough to consider the settlement of the case. Sometimes false hopes of substantial late recovery are held out to the patient or his family but it is now generally recognized that careful assessment a year or 18 months after injury will usually enable a confident prognosis to be given.

POST-TRAUMATIC EPILEPSY

This is the only common late complication, and it can develop in patients who have made a good recovery. About 5% of patients admitted to hospital after head injury develop late epilepsy (after the first week) but the incidence is very much higher after certain types of injury. These are when there has been an acute intracranial haematoma evacuated within 2 weeks of injury, when there has been a compound depressed fracture or when there has been a fit during the first week after injury (early epilepsy). The risk after depressed fracture ranges from less than 3% to more than 60% according to combinations of four factors — post-traumatic amnesia of greater than 24 hours, tearing of the dura, focal signs and early epilepsy. In patients without intracranial haematoma or depressed fracture the risk of epilepsy is low unless there has been an early fit; this applies whether post-traumatic amnesia is more or less than 24 hours (Jennett 1987c).

Once a late fit does occur the tendency for fits to recur continues and this has serious implications for the patient, particularly in limiting eligibility to drive. Patients who have suffered a high-risk type of injury will normally not be eligible to drive a private car for a year after injury; those whose job depends on driving heavy goods vehicles or public service vehicles may find themselves debarred for longer, perhaps permanently (Jennett 1985, Jennett 1983).

SUMMARY

1. The best guide to the severity of brain damage available to the doctor called upon to submit a medicolegal report months after head injury is the duration of the post-traumatic amnesia.
2. The commonest cranial nerve deficit following severe head injury is anosmia. It occurs particularly after basal skull fractures.
3. The most substantial recovery after severe head injury occurs within 6–12 months after injury. A confident prognosis can usually be given 12–18 months after injury.
4. About 5% of patients admitted to hospital with head injuries develop late epilepsy (after the first week).
5. Whether a head injury has initially been mild or severe, many sequelae are possible. The relationships between the sequelae, the severity of the injury, the complications and the management are often complex. Those not experienced in this field should be cautious about expressing opinions which may be challenged by an expert.

REFERENCES

A group of neurosurgeons 1984 Guidelines for the initial management of head injury in adults. British Medical Journal 288: 983–985

Brooks D N 1984 Psychological, social and family consequences of closed head injury. Oxford University Press, Oxford

Jennett B 1983 Anticonvulsant drugs and advice about driving after head injury and intracranial surgery. British Medical Journal 627–628

Jennett B 1985 Epilepsy after head injury and carniotomy. In: Medical aspects of fitness to drive. P A B Raffle (ed), Medical Commission on Accident Prevention

Jennett B 1987a Skull X-rays after mild head injuries. Archives of Emergency Medicine 4: 133–135

Jennett B 1987b Decisions to limit treatment. Lancet 2: 787–789

Jennett B 1987c Epilepsy after head injury and intracranial surgery. In: Epilepsy. A Hopkins (ed), Chapman and Hall, London, pp 401–416

Jennett B, Bond M 1975 Assessment of outcome after severe brain damage. Lancet i: 480–484

Jennett B, Plum F 1972 Persistent vegetative state after brain damage. Lancet i: 734–737

Jennett B, Snoek J, Bond M R et al 1981 Disability after severe head injury; observations on the use of the Glasgow outcome scale. Journal of Neurology, Neurosurgery and Psychiatry 44: 285–293

Mendelow A D, Teasdale G, Jennett B et al 1983 Risks of intracranial haematoma in head injured adults. British Medical Journal 288: 983–985

Miller J D, Jones P A 1985 Lancet i: 1141–1144

Teasdale G, Jennett B 1974 Assessment of coma and impaired consciousness: a practical scale. Lancet ii: 81–84

Teasdale G, Murray G, Anderson E et al 1989 Risks of an intracranial haematoma in children and adults: implications for the management of head injuries (in preparation)

FURTHER READING

Jennett B, Galbraith S 1983 Introduction to neurosurgery, 4th edn. Heinemann, London

Jennett B, Teasdale G 1981 Management of head injuries. F A Davis, Philadelpia

Miscellaneous topics

19. Repetitive stress injury

J. P. Jackson

INTRODUCTION

Repetitive stress injury (RSI) has now become, as Semple (1986) put it, a catch-all phrase for a range of conditions which give rise to pain and discomfort in the upper limb. Many of these patients are suffering from well recognized complaints with an established pathology. Over-use problems such as rotator cuff tendinitis, tennis elbow, golfer's elbow, ulnar neuritis, abductor pollicis longus bursitis, de Quervain's tenosynovitis, median nerve compression and many more are all clearly distinguishable and will respond to appropriate treatment. When the diagnosis is in doubt and the symptoms are vague the condition may be labelled RSI. Appropriate treatment is not easily prescribed. Alternatively, once the patient has been diagnosed as suffering from RSI an underlying problem may be missed. Ireland (1988) cited as an example a 21-year-old music student with pain in the wrist of 10 months' duration who was labelled as suffering from RSI. Subsequently, it was found that the cause of his pain was an un-united fracture of the scaphoid.

On the other hand the General, Municipal, Boilermakers and Allied Trade Union (GMBATU 1986), in its pamphlet entitled Tackling Teno, stated that of 19 patients treated by means of surgical decompression for carpal tunnel syndrome, only 1 claimed that the operation was successful, while 13 maintained that they were permanently crippled by the operation. These would be most surprising results, if indeed the diagnosis was correct, since the operation is simple to perform and almost universally successful. It must be highly improbable that even 1 patient would be harmed by it, let alone 13 being crippled.

The most common source of error in this saga appears to be an initial diagnosis of tenosynovitis. The Health and Safety Executive in their advisory booklet MS10 (Health and Safety Executive 1977) described this as the second commonest prescribed industrial disease in the UK, occurring among factory workers and others carrying out repetitive tasks. The source of this information is derived from certificates signed by general practitioners. In some cases the initial diagnosis may be correct.

447

Tenosynovitis characteristically resolves within a few days or weeks and it would be difficult to account for patients being signed off work for months as suffering from tenosynovitis or 'teno' unless some other factor had entered the equation. Since tenosynovitis or tendinitis are the conditions which are most frequently confused under the heading of RSI, it seems sensible to discuss them in some detail before considering the problem of RSI.

Tenosynovitis

This is a well defined condition related to the tendon mucous sheaths. The cause is still a matter of some conjecture, but in all probability it is related to the performance of rapid repetitive movements. Other factors also thought to be of importance are unaccustomed use or resumption of work following absence, as occurs after periods away for sickness and holiday (Thompson et al 1951; Kelly & Jacobson 1964). In addition, in a number of cases, local trauma seems to have been the precipitating cause. As Kurppa et al (1979) pointed out, there seemed to be no studies on aetiology with an adequate control group or indeed with any control group at all. These authors went on to note that the hypothesis of the work-relatedness of peritendinitis or tenosynovitis had not been scientifically tested. There remains, therefore, some doubt about the causation of this condition.

The symptoms are quite easily recognizable. There is pain and swelling localized to the area of the tendon sheath. Sometimes there may be crepitus. In the most commonly affected area around the wrist, the tendon sheaths are well defined. Those on the dorsal and volar aspects of the wrist are shown in Figures 19.1 and 19.2. There is tenderness over the area of the sheath and pain may also be precipitated by stretching the affected muscle–tendon units or activating them against resistance. Occasionally, crepitus may be felt or, less commonly, heard over the affected area.

Stenosing tenosynovitis

Following the initial inflammatory process, a stenosis of the tendon sheath sometimes takes place as increasing fibrosis occurs. Related to this, there may be localized thickening of the tendon and as a result a trigger effect is produced. This often occurs in the finger flexors. Not uncommonly the short extensor and the long abductor of the thumb may be affected by stenosis. This was the case in 58% of patients examined by Rais (1961). This particular condition was first described by de Quervain (1895) who was of the opinion that it was due to excessive wrist movements. It was often thought to be associated with the wringing of clothing and gained the name of washerwoman's thumb.

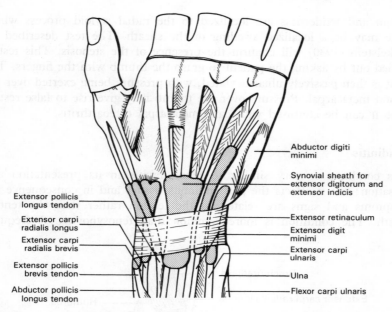

Fig. 19.1   Tendons and tendon sheaths, on the dorsal surface of the wrist (adapted from Gray's Anatomy)

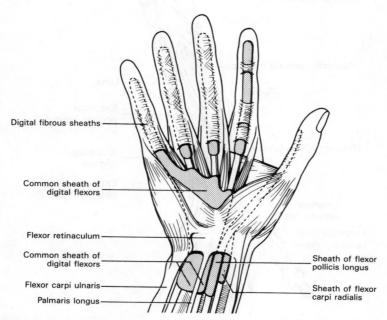

Fig. 19.2   Tendons and tendon sheaths on the volar surface of the wrist (adapted from Gray's Anatomy)

Pain and tenderness are localized to the radial styloid process where there may be a localized swelling of the sheath. The test described by Finkelstein (1930) will confirm the presence of the stenosis. This test is carried out by asking the patient to grasp the thumb with the fingers. The wrist is then passively ulnar-deviated, with pressure being exerted over the second metacarpal. Pressure over the thumb may give rise to false results since it can be confused with carpometacarpal osteoarthritis.

Tendinitis

This condition is very similar to tenosynovitis in its presentation and causation, but it affects the peritendinous tissues and in consequence the symptoms and signs are related to the tendon rather than the tendon sheath. The condition is more common than tenosynovitis. A frequent

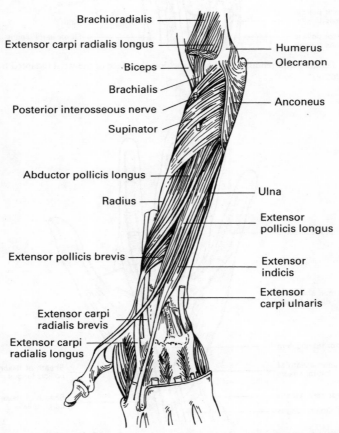

Fig. 19.3 Muscles and tendons on the dorsal surface of the forearm (adapted from Gray's Anatomy)

site is at the point where the abductor pollicis longus and extensor pollicis brevis muscles cross obliquely over the radial wrist extensors. This point lies about 4–8 cm proximal to Lister's tubercle (Fig. 19.3). Crepitus is commonly found and for this reason the condition is often referred to as peritendinitis crepitans.

The course of tenosynovitis and tendinitis is fairly short and indeed it is largely self-limiting. In most cases, rest is prescribed though this does not appear to be absolutely necessary. In the series reported by Thompson et al (1951), many were allowed to continue to work, though some had the addition of splinting and physiotherapy. Indeed, Thompson et al stated that cessation from work was neither desirable nor necessary, though they believed that the type of work might need to be altered. From this it is clear that if the complaints are prolonged beyond a matter of days or a few weeks, then the diagnosis needs to be seriously questioned. The exception to this are those cases in which stenosis has followed the inflammatory condition. Surgery may then be necessary.

Finally, it should be noted that there is quite a definite pathology associated with both tenosynovitis and tendinitis. There is exudation either in the sheath or in the peritendinous tissues, and this may be followed by a deposit of fibrin. Macroscopically the sheaths become thickened, lose their lustre and occasionally adhesions may form.

REPETITIVE STRESS INJURY

It is against the background of causes of upper limb discomfort and pain that the diagnosis is made.

Numerous claims for compensation have resulted from RSI worldwide — serious enough to add greatly to industrial costs. In Japan and Australia the number of cases has assumed epidemic proportions and it is now threatening to do the same in the UK. In New South Wales, Australia there was a 220% increase in the 1979–1980 period over the 1970–1971 period. The classification these appeared under was synovitis, bursitis and tenosynovitis (Browne et al 1984).

In current practice the diagnosis of RSI is usually made on the following basis:

1. A genuine entity arising de novo.
2. An attack of an identifiable condition causing upper limb pain which fails to respond to treatment and is followed by continuing and more widespread symptoms for which there is no obvious pathology. A diagnosis of RSI is therefore made.
3. The common aches and discomfort of normal use may be magnified by the patient and/or his advisers, so that there are continuing complaints with no demonstrable abnormality and a diagnosis of RSI is made.

RSI has been described by Fry (1986) as occurring in five different grades:

1. Pain in one site on causal activity.
2. Pain in multiple sites on causal activity.
3. Pain with some other uses of the hand; tender structures demonstrable. There may be pain at rest or loss of muscle function.
4. Pain with all uses of the hand, tenderness and loss of motor function.
5. Continuous pain with gross physical signs.

Although physical signs have been described, it should be pointed out that at no time has anything objective been noted. Tenderness and pain are, of course, entirely subjective phenomena, although Fry (1986) described them as semi-subjective. Ireland (1988), in a review article, stated that the pain of which the patient complains is often consistent in a given patient. It is not, however, consistent between patients and does not conform to any known neurological pathway, anatomical structure or physiological pattern. There are no primary objective physical findings in the upper limb. Persistent tenderness is frequently of equal severity at any randomly selected point on the limb. Clinical investigations, including biochemistry, radiography, electromyography and nerve conduction studies, radioisotope bone scanning, thermography and haematology, are all negative in the assessment of this condition (Ireland 1988).

In a medical context the term 'injury' implies damage to tissues and at no time has this been demonstrated in RSI. Clelland (1987) pointed out that the diffuse nature of the pain complained of by the patient with this condition differs from that which is usually experienced as a result of damage to a defined anatomical structure. He pointed out that sufferers often present with their affected limb in a position of sustained flexion at the elbow and wrist — a posture that healthy subjects find uncomfortable.

There is no evidence, even in the long term, that patients who are complaining of this pain will suffer any tissue damage. This, of course, contrasts with the ordinary function of pain, which is a means of protecting damaged tissues or warning that a stimulus is potentially damaging. Clelland (1987) also pointed out that, paradoxically, any injury that may have occurred required far longer to heal than would be anticipated if any demonstrable physical damage had been inflicted.

The Australian literature, which is full of references to this condition, has been very largely influenced by the epidemic which started in the late 1970s and early 1980s. The epidemic is perhaps best exemplified by the description given by Hocking (1987) of the course taken by this condition as it affected Telecom Australia. Figure 19.4 shows that this was first reported as long ago as 1981 and rose to a peak in mid 1984 but had very largely subsided by 1987.

The aetiology of this complaint remains obscure. There was an attempt to associate the increase in RSI with the frequency of movements carried out by the patient. The introduction of new electronic equipment

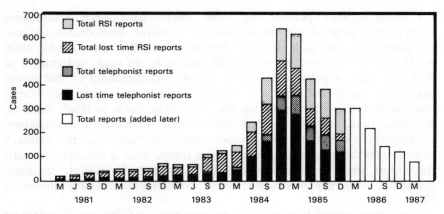

Fig. 19.4 Course of epidemic of RSI in Telecom Australia (from Hocking 1987, copyright 1987, The Medical Journal of Australia, reprinted with permission)

requiring much greater rates of movement compared to older mechanical or even electrical devices has been cited as a cause. Study of the key-stroke rate in Telecom Australia failed to bear this out and, indeed, argued rather convincingly against it. Amongst approximately 500 telegraphists whose work involved 12 000 key-strokes per hour, there were only 17 reports of RSI over 5 years. The telephonists, however, who have a very much slower key-stroke rate of a few hundred an hour, showed a far greater incidence of RSI — 343 cases from 1000 keyboard staff membes over a period of 5 years.

Key-stroke rates are frequently cited throughout the literature as being a cause. Ireland (1988) pointed out that the oft-quoted fatigue-inducing number of 15 000 key-strokes per hour should be translated into the equivalent of typing at the rate of 50 words per minute, an accepted office secretarial typing rate. Furthermore, most secretaries believe that the introduction of firstly electric typewriters and secondly electronic typewriters has made their job easier rather than the reverse, and no typist who has been converted to using electronic typewriters would willingly return to the original mechanical machine.

Hocking (1987) also noted that women in younger age groups were proportionately more involved with claims for RSI compensation. He suggested that biological degeneration with age is not a major contributing factor to RSI, which might have been expected if this condition had a pathological basis. Furthermore, there was no relationship between the duration of employment and the prevalence of symptoms in the survey of telephonists.

Observation of the epidemic in Japan suggested that in the telephone and telegraph system the decline of the epidemic has been due to the introduction of light-weight headsets. However, this apparatus had been in use in Telecom Australia before the epidemic started there, suggesting that new technology or its ergonomics probably did not cause RSI.

Clelland (1987) pointed out that there have been educational programmes emphasizing the seriousness of upper limb discomfort and the potentially damaging effects of manual tasks. The suggestion has been made that if an employee has been affected as in the suggested grade 1 of RSI (i.e. pain in one site on causal activity), continuation of that action may well result in chronic disability and even render the worker unemployable for the rest of his life. This may result in many workers, suffering from perfectly normal discomforts, resorting to absenteeism. Furthermore, therapists who diagnose injury further focus the patient's attention on the uncomfortable part. As a result, what is otherwise a trivial discomfort may be transformed into a protracted, painful, disabling condition. This may preclude effective work and degrade the quality of life.

The effects of RSI have been further emphasized by literature published by the trade unions. Office Secretary of June 1986 has an article which starts, quite reasonably, by showing the various tendon sites that may be affected by tendonitis and tenosynovitis. The journal then goes on to quote cases of workers who have lost their jobs as a result. No objective evidence to establish the diagnosis or causation of their complaints is given. The article stated that the standard typewriter keyboard puts 60% of the work-load on the left hand, especially the middle and index fingers. Despite this both of the cases reported by Office Secretary were affected bilaterally. Further statements are made that the right middle finger is isolated and, as a result, less oxygen gets to the muscles as the blood vessels are constricted. This appears to be a rather contentious statement, since there are no muscle bellies present in the middle finger.

Landworker in August 1982 described tenosynovitis and tendinitis satisfactorily but went on to suggest that symptoms such as weak wrists and weak arms were of great significance. GMBATU in their pamphlet Tackling Teno, distributed in the 1980s, quoted the same two secretaries, reproducing photographs that had appeared in Office Secretary. Once more there are quite reasonable descriptions of tenosynovitis and tendinitis, but the pamphlet also includes various other diagnoses, such as tennis elbow, carpal tunnel syndrome, etc. as types of RSI. The reader may also be worried by suggestions that the condition is irreversible if there is any delay in making the diagnosis and stopping work. The pamphlet further states: 'Don't delay! You may be permanently crippled if you do'. Against this background of advice it would be surprising if the average worker were not seriously worried. The pamphlet states quite unequivocally that the only treatment is rest, although Thompson et al (1951) clearly showed that this is not so for tenosynovitis and tendinitis.

CONCLUSIONS

Following the increase in literature detailing the diagnosis of and problems related to RSI, there have been several thoughtful and analytical articles on the subject. Ferguson (1987) considered that this condition could now be seen as a complex psychosocial phenomenon. He believed that elements of mass hysteria existed, based upon a background of widespread discomfort, fatigue and morbidity. He believed that the term RSI implied injury and cause where neither may exist. Patients have equated discomfort with injury; compensation for work-related injury is seen as an inalienable right, as it is financed by a third party.

Hadler (1985) stated that at any given time 10% of adults experience some discomfort in the neck with or without arm pain and 35% of adults can recall such an episode.

Ireland (1988) was of the opinion that muscle fatigue, when used in the unscientific lay sense, was a common and ubiquitous symptom seen after unaccustomed muscular activity and was usually described by the patient as muscle ache or tiredness. The pain or discomfort usually subsided within 48 hours of stopping work and was certainly not known to persist years after discontinuing the activity, as often occurred with RSI. He believed that recommencing the unaccustomed activity usually speeded up the recovery process and prevented the pain recurring.

For a condition that has been described as 'musculotendinous injuries caused by overload' (Browne et al 1984), it is surprising that treatment is so disappointing. Browne et al stated: 'In advanced RSI the only treatment is symptomatic, but usually does not hasten recovery or enable employees to return to their previous work' — this, in a condition caused by injury, but injury so imperceptible that no evidence of abnormal pathology can be found.

There is undoubtedly a need for fruitful research into the aetiology of pain and discomfort secondary to musculoskeletal activity. Indeed, work in this field is currently being carried out. None the less, caution must be exercised in prescribing rest and other treatment for patients who have a condition for which there is no apparent need for these palliatives. Arm pain is a ubiquitous recurring experience in all workers, and is responsible for mild to modest transitory nuisance. Evidence that it presages the onset of a serious and crippling condition is, to say the least, flimsy.

It may be more useful to conceptualize the discomfort of RSI as a form of fatigue resulting from differences in biomechanics and performance. The data available are consistent with this alternative hypothesis. If this was explained to patients, the impact of discomfort on their sense of well-being might be greatly reduced. Furthermore, the worker could campaign to provide a more comfortable workplace without viewing himself as ill or injured. There is no doubt that ergonomists may be able to design more satisfactory work furniture and equipment.

As Ireland (1988) pointed out, such an improvement in the work environment has not been shown to coincide with any increased medical awareness of the psychological aspects of RSI. He also classified the condition as a sociopolitical phenomenon rather than a medical condition and believed that the responsibility for its prevention did not rest with the medical profession, but with those authorities capable of changing the milieu which is conducive to it.

Medical responsibility lies in differentiating between RSI and those clearly defined physical conditions which require and will almost certainly respond to the appropriate physical treatment.

Ireland (1988) was of the opinion that the majority of RSI patients did experience the symptoms of which they complained, but were innocent victims of circumstance rather than seekers of secondary gain. This, however, is open to question: certainly the probability is that employers are only negligent in few, if any, of the cases and it is likely that in a high proportion of cases the spur of financial gain has a significant effect on the level of symptoms.

REFERENCES

Browne C D, Nolan B M, Faithfull D K 1984 Occupational repetitive strain injuries. Guidelines for diagnosis and management. Medical Journal of Australia 140: 329–332
Clelland L G 1987 RSI: a model of social iatrogenesis. Medical Journal of Australia 147: 236–239
Comerford P 1986 RSI — occupational hazard of the office. Office Secretary, June
De Quervain F 1895 Euber, Eine, Form Von Cronischer Tendovaginitis Cor. — Bl.f. Schweiz Aerzte, Basel 25: 389–394
Ferguson D A 1987 RSI: putting the epidemic to rest. Medical Journal of Australia 147: 213–214
Finkelstein H 1930 Stenosing tenosynovitis at the radial styloid process. Journal of Bone and Joint Surgery 12: 509
Fry H J H 1986 Overuse syndrome, alias tenosynovitis/tendinitis. The terminological hoax. Plastic and Reconstructive Surgery 414–417
General, Municipal, Boilermakers and Allied Trade Unions. 1986 Tackling teno. GMBATU
Hadler N M 1985 Illness in the workplace: the challenge of musculo-skeletal symptoms. Journal of Hand Surgery 10A: 451–456
Health and Safety Executive. 1977 Guidance note MS10. Her Majesty's Stationery Office, London
Hocking B 1987 Epidemiological aspects of 'repetitive strain injury' in Telecom. Medical Journal of Australia 147: 218–222
Ireland D L R 1988 Psychological and physical aspects of occupational arm pain. Journal of Hand Surgery 13B: 5–10
Kelly A P, Jacobson H S 1964 Hand disability due to tenosynovitis. Industrial Medicine and Surgery 570–574
Kurppa K, Waris P, Rokkanen P 1979 Peritendinitis and tenosynovitis: a review. Scandinavian Journal of Work Environment and Health 5: (suppl 3): 19–24
Landworker, 1982, August, Tenosynovitis — the poultry worker's enemy
Rais D 1961 Heparin treatment of peritenomyosis (peritendinitis) crepitans acuta. Acta Clinica Scandinavica 268: (suppl.): 1–88
Semple C 1986 Editorial: Tenosynovitis. Journal of Hand Surgery 11B: 155–156
Thompson A R, Plewes L W, Shaw E G 1951 Peritendinitis crepitans and simple tenosynovitis: a clinical study of 544 cases in industry. British Journal of Industrial Medicine 8: 150–155

20. The psychological effects of trauma

R. N. Bloor

INTRODUCTION

The psychological effects of trauma may present as persistent and inexplicable somatic symptoms with no demonstrable physical basis (Tarsh & Royston 1985), as psychological symptoms such as depression and anxiety (Parker 1977) or as a mixture of organic and psychological symptoms (Woodyard 1982). The complexity of the reactions seen is reflected in the range of diagnostic labels attached to these symptoms, such as post-concussional syndrome (Taylor 1967) and accident neurosis (Miller 1961). More recently the concept of post-traumatic stress disorder was introduced (Walker 1981). Woodyard (1982) described a model of three varieties of compensation syndrome — exaggeration, compensation neurosis and malingering. Parker (1977) preferred the term accident neurosis as this carried no unwarranted implications concerning aetiology. Trimble (1984) used post-traumatic neurosis as a general term for the symptom complex.

The adoption of neurosis as part of the terminology in this area is best avoided, as the range of psychological reactions reported includes psychotic disturbance (White et al 1987); the use of compensation or litigation in the terminology ignores the large number of patients who develop symptoms when no legal action is involved (White 1981). The use of a general term such as post-traumatic state allows discussion of the range of responses seen following trauma without implying aetiological or specific psychopathological classifications. However, it needs to be combined with a more specific formulation of the patient's condition. Hoffman (1986) discussed possible models for such formulations.

INCIDENCE

The incidence of psychological problems following trauma is very difficult to assess (Weighill 1981). This is because of the poor standard of classification in the literature and the highly selective case groups which have been studied. Many studies describe patients selected because they are claiming compensation. This is a small proportion of total accident cases; Harris

457

(1981) estimated that only 12% of all accident victims become involved in compensation claims.

Studies of groups which are not selected by litigation indicate that there is a high incidence of psychological problems following trauma. White (1981) studied 163 unselected accident victims; psychological sequelae were seen 1 year after the accident in 75% of the group and some 25% were classified as suffering moderate to severe problems. Braverman (1976), in a study of ski-related trauma where no litigation or compensation was involved, interviewed 21 subjects: 11 had a definite psychiatric reaction and of these 11, 3 had a post-traumatic stress disorder.

Fowlie & Aveline (1985) studied aircrew following ejection from aircraft. No compensation was involved. Self-report measures showed that 71% of the group suffered psychological problems following ejection; 40% reported that these problems were unresolved.

Studies of litigant groups are poorly standardized in terms of classification of symptoms and they are of course pre-selected, therefore comparison between studies is difficult. Woodyard (1980) in a study of 600 unselected compensation cases identified 16% of the subjects as suffering from a compensation syndrome. This included 8% whom he defined as exaggerating their symptoms. Parker (1977) in a study of 750 unselected accident litigants identified 13% as exaggerating or deceiving. Parker also showed an incidence of 39% of neurotic problems in the groups after excluding patients with head injury, bereavement reactions or other obvious aetiological factors. When subjects have sustained a head injury then the incidence of neurotic symptoms is 67–75% (Kelly 1972).

There is closer agreement on the frequency of occurrence of more clearly defined patterns of stress reaction. Post-traumatic stress disorder was seen in 12% of subjects reported by Parker (1977) and 10% of subjects studied by Hoffman (1986). Post-traumatic psychosis is rare; it occurred in 2% of subjects in Parker's study. The aetiology of compensation psychosis is undecided (White et al 1987).

SYMPTOMS

Neurosis

Studies of patients with post-traumatic neurosis report a wide range of symptoms. Parker (1977) in his study of 750 consecutive accident victims listed the most common complaints in a subgroup of 296 neurotic patients. The most common symptom was tension headache; he described this as differing from organic headache in that it was described in colourful language with hand gestures showing bearing-down or band-like sensations. Analgesics gave little or no relief, yet were taken in considerable quantities and for prolonged periods. In the same patient group the second most common symptom was irritability. Parker described the combination of headache and irritability as common in the neurotic group but headache without irritability was seen more often in the patients who grossly exaggerated their symptoms.

Trimble (1984) described the neurotic symptoms as anxiety and depression with associated symptoms such as palpitations, sleeplessness, panic attacks, breathlessness and phobias. He claimed that the presence of these symptoms, whether or not associated with apparent physical illness, favoured a diagnosis of neurosis and rendered malingering unlikely. Kelly (1981) described the primary symptoms of post-traumatic syndrome as headache, vertigo, poor concentration, unreliable memory, sleeplessness, depression manifested by fatigue, impotence, lack of libido, and unreasonable resentment. Hodge (1971) described symptoms of anxiety, insomnia, recurrent dreams of the accident, emotional instability, fear of driving, a preoccupation with symptoms and hostility combined with 'righteous indignation'.

Thompson (1965), in a study of 500 cases which were the subject of litigation, reported that the most common symptom complex was of anxiety and its physical manifestations, with symptoms referable to the cardiovascular, gastrointestinal and respiratory systems. Panic attacks, emotional tension, psychoneurotic depression, hyperventilation, phobias and repetitive dreams were also observed.

Post-traumatic stress disorder

This is a DSM-III classification (American Psychiatric Association 1980). It is characterized by a variety of symptoms and may be identified by using a set of diagnostic criteria.

DSM-III diagnostic criteria for post-traumatic stress disorder are:

1. Existence of a recognizable stressor that would evoke significant symptoms in almost anyone.
2. Re-experiencing of the trauma as evidenced by at least *one* of the following:
   a. recurrent and intrusive recollections of the event.
   b. recurrent dreams of the event.
   c. suddenly acting or feeling as if the traumatic event were recurring because of an association with environmental or ideational stimulus.
3. Numbing of responsiveness to, or reduced involvement with, the external world, beginning some time after the trauma as shown by at least *one* of the following:
   a. markedly diminished interest in one or more significant activities.
   b. feeling of detachment or estrangement from others.
   c. constricted affect.

4. At least *two* of the following symptoms that were not present before the trauma:
   a. hyperalertness or exaggerated startle response.
   b. sleep disturbance.
   c. guilt about surviving when others have not, or about behaviour required for survival.
   d. memory impairment or trouble with concentration.
   e. avoidance of activities that arouse recollection of the traumatic event.
   f. intensification of symptoms by exposure to events that symbolize or resemble the traumatic event.

Symptoms may arise soon after the accident or may present after a latent interval (Walker 1981); the symptoms may resolve or continue for many years (Tennant et al 1986).

In a study of post-traumatic stress disorder after car accidents, Kuch et al (1985) described 30 patients who met the DSM-III criteria. Only 4 of the 6 symptoms in group 4 above occurred in more than 40% of the patients. They were intrusive recollections, feeling of recurrence, disturbed sleep and intensification of symptoms by re-exposure.

Phobic symptoms

Phobia following trauma has been described. Thompson (1965) found 21% in his series of 500 accident patients. The phobias were not of a classical form and were in the main related to the injury, such as fear of driving following a car crash or fear of heights following a fall. In the 2 cases where there was evidence of a classical claustrophobia, there was a history of pre-existing neurosis.

The phobia pattern following trauma may be directly derived from the circumstances of the injury (Hodge 1971). Patients will demonstrate avoidance or reduction of the activity related to the trauma (Kuch et al 1985).

Hysterical symptoms

Woodyard (1982) believed 'compensation neurosis' to be characterized by symptoms including tension headache, depression, irritability, aggression and loss of libido. Pain out of proportion to the severity or site of the injury was present, and showed only a transient response to conventional methods of treatment. Dissociation or conversion symptoms were described as frequent. Woodyard also described patchy, variable hyperaesthesia unrelated to dermatomes or peripheral nerves.

Tarsh & Royston (1985) studied a group of 35 accident victims selected for gross somatization and symptoms with no adequate organic cause. They classified 10 of the subjects as suffering from illness of a hysterical or hypochondriachal type which would have legitimately been referred to a psychiatrist. Of these patients, 5 had hysterical disuse of the upper limb; 2 involved the fingers only, while 3 involved either hand or hand and arm. Two of the 10 had severe hysterical gait disorder and the remaining 3 had profound, totally disabling hypochondriasis.

Thompson (1965) classified 73 of his 500 cases as suffering from hysterical neurosis. In 96% of these cases the symptom was located at the site of injury; 92% displayed *belle indifférence* and 21% had a mixed anxiety/hysterical neurosis. Hysterical symptoms were most common in the industrial injury cases — a finding also reported by Parker (1977).

Psychosis

Psychosis may develop as an acute reaction following head injury. As the acute phase resolves the patient may recover completely or may be left with continuing problems (Lishman 1978). Achte et al (1967) described psychosis developing as a delayed feature of head injury; they observed schizophrenia, paranoid psychosis, depressive psychosis and hypomanic psychosis in a series of 3552 soldiers with head injury. Bracken (1987) reported that a search of the literature revealed 20 cases of manic psychosis following head injury. Lishman (1978) concluded that the generally accepted view was that psychosis following head injury should be seen as indicating a constitutional predisposition in the majority of cases, with the injury serving as a trigger for the appearance of the symptoms.

Malingering

Malingering is defined as the conscious simulation of symptoms or of disability (Enelow 1971), or the deliberate imitation of disease or disability for gain (Woodyard 1982). The diagnosis of malingering may only be made with any degree of certainty when the patient is observed outside the clinical setting performing an act that he claimed to be impossible.

Woodyard (1982) suggested that symptoms which were clearly absurd were an indicator of malingering; he cited as an example loss of memory following a back injury.

Trimble (1984) pointed out that malingering must be diagnosed on positive criteria, but noted that there was a lack of experimental evidence which would allow such criteria to be defined. Hurst (1940) set two diagnostic criteria which give a positive diagnosis of malingering:

1. The patient is observed to perform an act he claims he is not able to do.
2. The patient admits to malingering.

Miller & Cartilige (1972), reviewing earlier studies, stated that when symptoms were entirely subjective, the distinction between malingering and neurosis rested in the last resort on the credibility of a witness.

ASSESSMENT

The accident

Hoffman (1986) discussed the importance of a detailed investigation of the history of the accident when assessing a patient who has suffered a personal injury. Pilowsky (1985) pointed out that the patient may suppress the more horrific aspects of the accident unless closely questioned. He also emphasized the importance of obtaining the patient's perception of the danger involved in the trauma; even trivial accidents may be perceived as life-threatening by the patient, and this perception often dictates the psychological response to the trauma. These cases of cryptotrauma are often missed without careful history-taking.

Injury type

Whiplash injury

Whiplash or hyperextension injury of the neck carries a high risk of post-traumatic neurotic symptoms; 50% may develop psychoneurotic illness (Gay & Abbott 1968). Hodge (1971) stated that the type of accident which produced a whiplash injury is also the type which produces the traumatic neuroses. In a study of 100 cases of whiplash injury after settlement of compensation, Gotten (1956) reported that 54 patients showed no appreciable symptoms, 34 had minor discomfort and 12 had severe symptoms. This would support McNab (1973) who stated that out of a group of 266 whiplash injury patients, after settlement 45% still had symptoms despite satisfactory settlement of the court action.

Head injury

Post-concussional syndrome may follow closed or penetrating head injury. Trimble (1984) in a review of the literature suggested that this is related to organic injury. Lishman (1968) in a study of 670 patients showed that the degree of psychiatric disability correlated with the length of post-traumatic amnesia; this was confirmed by Guthkelch (1980) in a prospective study of 398 head injury patients. Kelly (1972) noted an incidence of 65–75% neurotic symptoms in a prospective study of 152 head injuries.

Trimble (1984) reported that many studies showed considerable psychiatric morbidity following head injury, and that no studies have shown neurotic symptoms to be influenced by compensation in head injury cases. The prognosis of neurosis following head injury is poor if the patient has not returned to work by the time the settlement has occurred (Kelly & Smith 1981).

Back injury

Krusen & Ford (1958), in a study of 509 patients with low back injury, showed that only 56% of compensation cases improved compared with 89% of non-compensation cases. The compensation cases were however referred for treatment much later than the non-compensation group.

Woodyard (1982) in his study of 52 cases of neurosis/malingering found that spinal injury carried a greater risk of residual symptoms than other injuries. Fifteen of the 19 patients with residual symptoms had suffered lumbar or cervical injury. This is supported by Balla & Moraitis (1970) in a study of 82 Greek patients with back or neck injuries.

Other factors

Studies of patients with post-traumatic disorders have commented on two main sets of factors which may influence the presentation and course of the reaction — pre-existing illness and ethnic and cultural factors.

Pre-existing illness

Parker (1977) found that 20% of his patients had obvious neurotic symptoms prior to the accident and 24% had clear obsessional traits. Modlin (1967), in a study of psychosocial aspects of post-accident anxiety, noted the presence of rigid personality in a group within his study. Studies of patients with low back pain (Leavitt 1985) have shown that patients with low back pain but no organic findings have scores on the Minnesota Multiphasic Personality Inventory which show significant elevation of hypochondriasis and hysteria scales. Pheasant et al (1979) showed that these elevated scores were good prognostic indicators of poor response to surgery in low back problems.

Assessment of pre-trauma personality, based as it is on retrospective data, is often not reliable. This may account in part for the great variations in proportions of patients who were reported to have pre-existing problems. Thompson (1965) reported that 87% of his group of post-traumatic neurosis patients had pre-existing neurotic traits. Culpan & Taylor (1973) found that previous personality seemed to be of no particular significance in the majority of post-traumatic neurotics.

Ethnic and cultural factors

Tarsh & Royston (1985) confirmed the findings of Balla & Moraitis (1970) that immigrant status may be important in the prognosis of post-traumatic disorders with back and other injuries. Tarsh & Royston discussed the role of the family in the maintenance of illness after trauma and pointed out the importance of identifying family over-protectiveness. There may be role changes resulting from the illness which are difficult to reverse. These factors require consideration when assessing the patient's reaction to trauma.

PROGNOSIS

The prognosis in cases of psychological reactions to trauma has been the subject of much discussion. Miller (1961), in a study which had undue influence on contemporary views, argued that virtually all post-accident neurosis cases recover after the settlement of litigation. This study of 50 highly selected cases from a series of 500 litigants was of an unrepresentative neurotic group. The conclusions have not been supported by other workers.

Kelly & Smith (1981) in a study of 43 cases of post-traumatic syndrome showed that 17 of the patients had returned to work prior to settlement. Failure to return to work by settlement day indicated a poor prognosis. Such patients rarely returned to work at all.

Mendelson (1982) confirmed that in an unselected series of 101 patients involved in litigation following trauma, only 35 resumed work prior to settlement. Of the rest, 53 were followed up, 9 had returned to work following settlement and 44 were not working at an average of 15 months after settlement. This study agreed with Kelly & Smith (1981) that the older the patient, the less likely the possibility of return to work.

Woodyard (1982) in a study of 52 cases of compensation neurosis found that in 41 cases where return to work could be assessed, only 27% were at work in less than 6 months and 61% were out of work for at least a year. Of these 41 patients, only 6 returned to their previous employment and 18 never returned to work.

In a study of 35 litigants with gross somatic symptoms of no demonstrable organic pathology, Tarsh & Royston (1985) found that return to work was unusual and full recovery rare. The authors concluded that in this selected group the prognosis for recovery was as bad as if the illness had a physical basis. Balla & Moraitis (1970) studied 82 patients of Greek origin after industrial or traffic injuries. They acknowledged that legal proceedings were a complicating factor which might adversely affect the prognosis. They showed that a settlement of legal matters had little or no influence on most patients; their symptom pattern remained unaltered.

Krusen & Ford (1958) in a study of 509 patients with low back injury discussed the role of compensation in dictating outcome. The group studied included 54% who were eligible for compensation while the remainder were not seeking compensation. Of the compensation group, 56% improved compared with 89% of the non-compensation group. There was a correlation between duration of symptoms before treatment and lack of improvement. This finding has been confirmed by Kelly (1981) in cases of post-traumatic syndrome. Mendelson (1982), in a review of the effect of legal settlement on compensation claims, concluded that compensation and financial gain are only part of a complex of factors, such as psychological impact of the accident, cultural and ethnic variables and family dynamic changes, which all determine prognosis and outcome.

MEDICOLEGAL REPORTS

Guidance for compiling a psychiatric report for litigation following personal injury is available. Hoffman (1986) suggested the following outline:

Source of information
History of the accident
Post-accident course
Past history
Family medical and psychiatric history
Personal history and life events
Mental status
Independent information
Summary
Prognosis

More general guidance on involvement with the courts is given by Grounds (1985) and Gibbens (1974). These articles deal solely with the psychiatrist in court.

CONCLUSIONS

1. Psychological reaction to trauma arises in a variety of clinical forms. There is no evidence to suggest a single response; the differential diagnosis of the response involves careful psychiatric investigation, and in some cases detailed psychological testing.
2. Compensation and financial gain have not been seen to be the major determining factor in the development of post-traumatic states. There is no evidence to suggest that symptoms disappear with settlement of litigation.
3. Treatment of post-traumatic states is possible but this is best done in the early stages if treatment is to have maximum benefit.
4. The prognosis of post-traumatic states is variable but is affected by a variety of factors including litigation, pre-existing neurosis, ethnic variables and family dynamics, physical injury and general background stressors such as unemployment and financial problems.
5. The role of the orthopaedic surgeon in the management of post-traumatic psychological reactions is in the main to be aware of the problem, to identify cases where a reaction is present and to initiate early referral for further assessment and treatment.

REFERENCES

Achte K A, Hillbom E, Aalberg V 1967 Post-traumatic psychoses following war brain injuries. Reports from the Rehabilitation Institute for Brain-injured Veterans in Finland, vol I, Helsinki

American Psychiatric Association 1980 Diagnostic and statistical manual of mental disorders III. American Psychiatric Association, Washington

Balla J I, Moraitis S 1970 Knights in armour: a follow-up study of injuries after legal settlement. Medical Journal of Australia 2: 355–361

Bracken P 1987 Mania following head injury. British Journal of Psychiatry 150: 681–682

Braverman M 1976 Validity of psychosomatic reactions. Journal of Forensic Sciences 22: 654–662

Culpan R, Taylor C 1973 Psychiatric disorders following road traffic and industrial injuries. Australia and New Zealand Journal of Psychiatry 7: 32–39

Enelow A J 1971 Compensation in psychiatric disability and rehabilitation. Thomas, Springfield

Fowlie D G, Aveline M O 1985 The emotional consequences of ejection, rescue and rehabilitation in RAF aircrew. British Journal of Psychiatry 146: 609–613

Gay J R, Abbott K H 1968 Common whiplash injuries of the neck. Journal of the American Medical Association 152

Gibbens T C N 1974 Preparing psychiatric court reports. British Journal of Hospital Medicine 12: 278–284

Gotten N 1956 Survey of 100 cases of whiplash injury after settlement litigation. Journal of the American Medical Association 162: 865

Grounds A 1985 The psychiatrist in court. British Journal of Hospital Medicine 34(1)/: 55–58

Guthkelch A N 1980 Post traumatic amnesia, post concussional symptoms and accident neurosis. European Neurology 19: 91–102

Harris D 1981 Financial needs: an academic viewpoint. Naidex 1981 conference, Warwickshire, October pp 231–233

Hodge J R 1971 The whiplash neurosis. Psychosomatics 12: 245–250

Hoffman B F 1986 How to write a psychiatric report for litigation following personal injury. American Journal of Psychiatry 143: 164–169

Hurst A F 1940 Medical diseases of war. Edward Arnold, London

Kelly R E 1972 The post-traumatic syndrome. Pahlevi Medical Journal 3: 530

Kelly R 1981 The post-traumatic syndrome. Journal of the Royal Society of Medicine 74: 242–245

Kelly R, Smith B N 1981 Post-traumatic syndrome: another myth discredited. Journal of the Royal Society of Medicine 74: 275–277

Krusen E M, Ford D E 1958 Compensation factor in low back injuries. Journal of the American Medical Association 166: 1128–1133

Kuch K, Swinson R P, Kirby M 1985 Post-traumatic stress disorder after car accidents. Canadian Journal of Psychiatry 30: 426–427

Leavitt F 1985 The value of the MMPI conversion V in the assessment of psychogenic pain. Journal of Psychosomatic Research 29: 125–131

Lishman W A 1968 Brain damage in relation to psychiatric disability after head injury. British Journal of Psychiatry 114: 373

Lishman W A 1978 Organic psychiatry. Blackwell, Oxford

McNab I 1973 The whiplash syndrome. Clinical Neurosurgery 20: 232–241

Mendelson G 1982 Not cured by verdict: effect of legal settlement on compensation claimants. Medical Journal of Australia 2: 132–134

Miller H 1961 Accident neurosis. British Medical Journal 1: 919–925, 992–1228

Miller H, Cartilige H 1972 Simulation and malingering after injuries to the brain and spinal cord. Lancet, i, 580–585

Modlin H C 1967 The post accident anxiety syndrome: psychosocial aspects. American Journal of Psychiatry 123: 1008

Parker N 1977 Accident litigants with neurotic symptoms. Medical Journal of Australia 2: 318–322

Pheasant H C, Gilbert D, Goldfarb J, Herron L 1979 The MMPI as a predictor of outcome in low back surgery. Spine 4: 78–84

Pilowsky I 1985 Cryptotrauma and accident neurosis. British Journal of Psychiatry 147: 310–311

Tarsh M J, Royston C 1985 A follow-up study of accident neurosis. British Journal of Psychiatry 146: 18–25

Taylor A R 1967 Post-concussional sequelae. British Medical Journal 2: 67

Tennant C C, Goulston K J, Dent O F 1986 The psychological effects of being prisoner of war: 40 years after release. American Journal of Psychiatry 143: 618–621

Thompson G N 1965 Post-traumatic psychoneurosis — a statistical survey. American Journal of Psychiatry 121: 1043–1048

Trimble M R 1984 Post-traumatic neurosis. Wiley, Chichester

Walker J I 1981 Post-traumatic stress disorder after a car accident. Postgraduate Medicine 69: 82–86

Weighill V E 1981 Compensation neurosis: a review of the literature. Journal of Psychosomatic Research 27: 97–104

White A 1981 Psychiatric study of patients with severe burn injuries. British Medical Journal 284: 465–467

White A C, Armstrong D, Rowan D 1987 Compensation psychosis. British Journal of Psychiatry 150: 692–694

Woodyard J E 1980 Compensation claims and prognosis. Journal of Social and Occupational Medicine 30: 2–5

Woodyard J E 1982 Diagnosis and prognosis in compensation claims. Annals of the Royal College of Surgeons of England 64: 191–194

21. The metabolic consequences of polytrauma

D. A. White

INTRODUCTION

Much of our understanding of polytrauma and advances in its treatment has come from efforts to deal with casualties of military conflicts.

Developments in immediate resuscitation, by control of the airway and adequate volume replacement, and rapid evacuation, frequently by helicopter, have improved the initial survival of multiply injured patients. As a result, many who would previously have died are now undergoing aggressive surgery and reaching intensive care units. Following multiple trauma, shock and massive transfusion, failure of one or more organ systems is common and patients often succumb to the later problem of multisystem organ failure (MSOF). With improved immediate care the emphasis has shifted away from the initial trauma towards the complications of these injuries, the treatment of secondary insults and the response to trauma and infection, all of which contribute to mortality and morbidity.

Critically ill and malnourished patients have a compromised immune response and lowered resistance to infection. These are both important aetiological factors in the development of MSOF. Sepsis is still the commonest cause of late death after multiple injury, and it is the primary or a contributory cause in 75% of deaths following burns (Polk 1979). Similarly, 78% of deaths from non-neurological causes after trauma were caused by sepsis (Miller et al 1982).

Treatment of MSOF is essentially supportive, but because of the high mortality there is a need to identify those patients at risk and to institute measures to prevent the development of MSOF.

THE STRESS RESPONSE

Trauma induces a series of circulatory, endocrine, metabolic and immunological changes known as the stress response. Although recognized for some years, the stress response was first investigated by Cuthbertson (1932) in patients with limb fractures. Physicians and surgeons have become increasingly concerned with this response since it was realized that patients lost weight and muscle bulk even after only moderate degrees of trauma.

It is now appreciated that as well as the local effects of injury and sepsis, there are also general effects — the response to trauma being multisystemic.

Recent work by Burke et al (1979) in burn injury patients has contributed to our understanding and improved their survival. However, some aspects still remain unclear since the relationship between endocrine and metabolic responses is extremely complex, although of the utmost importance to recovery.

In contrast to the response to starvation, where there is utilization of fat stores and conservation of lean body mass, critically ill and injured patients are unable to make this metabolic adaptation. The net effect of this neurohumoral stress response is to stimulate catabolic processes resulting in glycolysis, gluconeogenesis, hyperglycaemia and increased nitrogen excretion. Protein, particularly muscle, is mobilized and enters an amino acid pool in the liver where it is used for production of acute-phase proteins or conversion to glucose. In addition aldosterone and antidiuretic hormone activity result in sodium and water retention and the loss of potassium. These metabolic changes are proportional to the severity of injury, and are prolonged by hypotension and sepsis. This, together with their elevated basal metabolic rate i.e., +10% in uncomplicated surgery, +20–50% after major trauma or sepsis, +50–125% after burns, leads to a negative nitrogen balance, with nitrogen losses of up to 35 g per day.

Nutritional significance of the stress response

In 1936 Studley first drew attention to the relationship between an increased surgical mortality and preoperative malnutrition. Most physicians now recognize that pre- and post-operative nutritional states and post-injury support are important factors in patients' survival and recovery.

The morbidity and mortality of malnourished patients undergoing major surgery are higher than would be expected from infective processes alone.

Modification of the stress response

The neuroendocrine response to trauma appears to have evolved to assist survival in a primitive environment by maintaining blood flow to vital organs and increasing delivery of appropriate substrates to them. But in modern medical practice, however severe physiological derangements can be treated rapidly and suitable substrates are available, the benefits of this stress response can be questioned — and it may even be deleterious.

Understanding the underlying response to injury makes it possible to modify or suppress these metabolic effects, thus minimizing the loss of energy stores and protein with their attendant complications.

Afferent stimuli from injury, pain, emotional factors (fear and apprehension), hypoxia, hypercarbia, fluid loss and hypothermia all contribute to the magnitude of the response. The initial priorities must thus be to correct hypoxia, hypercarbia and hypovolaemia, and establish an adequate circulation to deliver oxygen and nutrients to the tissues.

Efforts can then be made to reduce the magnitude of the stress response by early stabilization of fractures, surgical debridement, amputation of crushed limbs or early grafting of burns. Sepsis in particular should be aggressively treated by drainage of abscess cavities and the rational use of antibiotics.

Nursing patients with fractures of the long bones in a thermoneutral environment (30°C) has been shown to reduce their urinary nitrogen losses and prevent depression of albumin synthesis. Similarly, burn injury patients nursed in a thermoneutral environment have lower resting energy expenditure than those subjected to the stress of hypothermia.

High-dose opiates (fentanyl or morphine) have been shown to depress but not abolish the stress response in surgical patients. However, they are associated with profound respiratory depression.

To date, the most effective way to block afferent stimuli from the damaged tissue is with epidural analgesia, using a combination of local anaesthetic agent and opioid by continuous infusion.

Prevention of infection by asepsis and minimal invasive monitoring commensurate with patient safety are more important than reliance on prophylactic antibiotics.

NUTRITIONAL SUPPORT

Most patients do not require any special nutritional treatment. They recover from their injury and gain weight, but a minority continue to make poor progress and require nutritional support. Those who lose more than 15% of their ideal body weight have a higher morbidity, and those losing more than 30% have a high mortality (Abbott 1976).

Unfortunately the role of nutritional support following injury is not as well documented as that for elective surgery. However, trauma, burns, major surgery and sepsis all initiate the stress response and render patients hypercatabolic so that many patients in a previously normal nutritional state become malnourished as a result of their injury or sepsis. Normal adult patients lose up to 8% of body weight within 2 weeks of elective surgery, but this figure increases up to 18% during a 3-week period following multiple trauma if there is no nutritional support.

Buzby et al (1980) noted that the incidence of post-surgical complications was up to 6 times higher in severely malnourished patients compared with those who were well-nourished. Heatley et al (1979) and Bojanowicz (1977) showed that preoperative nutritional support significantly reduced the incidence of post-operative wound infection, and Sagar et al (1979) noted that the duration of hospital stay was significantly reduced by early post-operative feeding.

Becker et al (1977) pointed out that many head-injured patients die from the effects of widespread infection, possibly as a consequence of malnutrition. In a prospective randomized trial following isolated, closed head injury, Rapp et al (1983) demonstrated that patients who received parenteral nutrition within 72 hours of admission had improved survival compared with patients receiving enteral nutrition after a delay of 6 days. They also showed that parenterally fed patients had higher albumin levels and nitrogen balances than those fed enterally. Head-injured patients frequently have very high resting metabolic rates, despite the small size of their wound.

Patients initiate a hypercatabolic response to injury, but the magnitude of these changes is not fully appreciated. Hill et al (1977) noted evidence of deterioration of nutritional status during hospital stay that was both unrecognized and, in many cases, untreated. Hessov (1977) noted that in an acute orthopaedic ward the daily energy intake was less than the basal metabolic requirement in 55% of patients and in 85% was less than the standard for bedridden patients, as described by Randall (1971), i.e. basal metabolism +30%.

Those who have sustained multiple trauma lose a minimum of 20 g of nitrogen per day (equivalent to 600 g of skeletal muscle). Nutritional support is thus indicated in catabolic patients and those with reduced intake to prevent the onset of protein-energy malnutrition.

The aim of nutritional support is to minimize protein loss during the early stages of injury and maximize lean tissue synthesis during convalescence. Nutritional support has inherent risks and limitations, and should therefore be applied with reference to the other priorities in critically ill patients.

Irrespective of the calorie input, incapacity leads to the rapid onset of muscle wasting, especially in critically ill or septic patients who require intensive physiotherapy to stem this muscle loss.

Post-injury weakness and mental fatigue often follow and may last for many months despite apparent physical healing. However, the extent to which patients are affected and the duration are very variable.

MULTIPLE SYSTEM ORGAN FAILURE

It is perhaps rather naive to think in terms of solitary organ dysfunction in patients with multiple injuries. For many years it has been recognized that diseases and toxins could affect multiple organ systems (lungs, kidneys, coagulation, heart and liver). Tilney et al (1973) first described a syndrome of sequential organ failure in surgical patients, and the term multiple system organ failure (MSOF) was coined by Borzotta & Polk (1983). Although not a new syndrome, it has been increasingly recognized as a result of improved resuscitation, surgery and advances in life support which enable critically injured patients to survive their initial injuries.

Multiple organ dysfunction and failure are extremely common in the multiply injured patient, especially in the presence of sepsis. Any organ or group of organs may be involved. The true incidence is unknown, although it is related to the diligence with which organ dysfunction is sought.

Faist et al (1983) noted that its onset can be precipitous or insidious, and there appear to be two distinct patterns of onset of MSOF in patients suffering polytrauma:

1. A rapid single-phase MSOF caused by trauma and shock, usually occurring within 72 hours of injury. The common pattern is of adult respiratory distress syndrome (ARDS), followed by acute renal failure, coagulopathy and hepatic failure. The mortality is approximately 50%.
2. A delayed two-phase MSOF beginning after 7–10 days, due to trauma, shock or sepsis. There is an insidious onset of ARDS with mild renal failure and coagulopathy from which patients improve, only to develop intra-abdominal abscesses or pneumonia. The mortality approaches 70%.

The sequence of organ failure is variable and difficult to predict. In patients with polytrauma, Faist et al (1983) noted that the lung, clotting system, kidney and liver were involved, whereas Fry et al (1980) noted that patients undergoing emergency surgery for both trauma and non-trauma had lung, liver, gastric mucosa and kidney involvement. However, no organ system is protected from potential failure in severely ill patients.

Baue (1975) noted that pre-injury and preoperative organ dysfunction may initiate, compound or accelerate the sequence of MSOF.

Causes of MSOF

1. Sepsis
2. Massive trauma.
3. Shock
4. Hypoxaemia
5. Extensive burns
6. Major surgery
7. Massive blood transfusion

There is ample evidence that infection is the commonest cause of MSOF. But sepsis is often not suspected, let alone diagnosed, in the critically injured or ill patient until it is well established. These patients are anergic with blunted febrile and total white blood cell response to infection. The polymorphonuclear 'shift to the left' is usually still present and is a good indicator of infection. The anergic phase is characteristically transient after polytrauma or severe injury, but if sepsis intervenes this anergic state persists until the source of infection can be eliminated by surgical debridement, drainage and the use of chemotherapy.

The fact that the onset of MSOF may also indicate the presence of hitherto undetected infection in postoperative trauma patients was pointed out by Polk & Shield (1977). In their cases the infections were intra-abdominal abscesses which, if left undrained, produced a mortality approaching 100%.

In one study of patients with ARDS it was noted that MSOF developed more commonly in infected (93%) than non-infected (47%) patients (Bell et al 1983). All bacteraemic patients with a clinically identifiable source of infection survived, whereas those without a clinically identifiable source died. Autopsies showed that all the latter had sources of infection which could have been surgically drained.

Mortality

Mortality in MSOF is related to the number of organ systems involved, the duration of organ failure and the presence and degree of lactic acidosis, which is a poor prognostic sign.

Failure of one organ system for more than 24 hours carries a 40% mortality; failure of two organ systems for more than 24 hours carries a 60% mortality, while failure of three organ systems for more than 72 hours carries a 98% mortality.

Prevention

As the ultimate prognosis for MSOF is very poor, prevention is extremely important. This includes:

1. Adequate resuscitation — preventing prolonged hypoxia or hypotension.
2. The prevention of sepsis by:
   a. strict aseptic techniques.
   b. avoiding unnecessary invasive procedures.
   c. avoiding prophylactic antibiotics.
3. Thorough search for and treatment of sepsis.

PULMONARY CONTUSION

Blair et al (1969) noted that major chest injury was present in 75% of deaths caused by trauma (it was the primary cause in 25% of cases and was associated with a further 50% of deaths).

Pulmonary contusion is a common finding (32–75%) in patients sustaining blunt chest injury. Mortality from pulmonary contusion alone ranges from 14 to 39%, but it plays a major role in 25% of deaths from chest injuries caused by road traffic accidents (Kirsch 1984).

The clinical effects of a flail chest depend upon the size of the segment and the underlying lung injury. Mortality increases markedly as the size of the flail segment increases from 100 to 200 cm^2 (Wiener & Barrett 1986).

Death due to chest injury alone is rare (4–8%). It is usually related to extrathoracic injury; increasing to 15% if another region is involved and to 30–35% if two or more regions are involved. Old age or pre-existing chest disease also increase mortality. Sankaran & Wilson (1970) reviewed 100 patients with flail chest and noted a significant increase in mortality related to:

1. Shock, with three or more associated injuries.
2. Associated head injury.
3. Injury producing seven or more fractured ribs.
4. Age over 30.

More recently, James & Moore (1983) noted that the overall mortality for patients suffering chest trauma was 5% but rose to 23% for those requiring mechanical ventilation and 37% for patients older than 60 years with respiratory failure. The commonest causes of death were respiratory tract infection (36%), severe head injury (34%) and exsanguination (19%).

Post-traumatic empyema occurs in 5–6% of patients with chest trauma despite the use of antibiotics, pulmonary toilet and chest drains. It occurs after penetrating injuries, however bacterial contamination may also arise from within the injured lung, from prolonged respiratory support or secondary to intra-abdominal sepsis. Aron et al (1977) showed that early decortication in the presence of fever, malaise and leucocytosis combined with evidence of residual pleural haematoma allowed complete re-expansion of the underlying lung and avoided the need for pulmonary resection.

FAT EMBOLISM SYNDROME

Up to 90% of patients who die after major trauma, including bony injury, can be shown at autopsy to have fat droplet deposits in their lungs and elsewhere. Subclinical hypoxaemia can be detected in 50% of patients suffering major trauma (Sevitt 1973). The majority of these patients are asymptomatic and true fat embolism syndrome is much less common (5–10%). It was originally described by Zenker in 1862 as a triad of respiratory insufficiency, cerebral dysfunction and petechial haemorrhages. It is most commonly seen in young adults and is particularly associated with fractures of long bones. Fat droplets greater than 8 μm give rise to clinical problems; plasma lipase converts natural fat to free fatty acids which damage endothelial and alveolar cells.

Classically, symptoms appear within 72 hours of long bone fractures, but can also occur with minor fractures or trauma involving adipose tissue. Breathlessness, irritating cough and occasionally haemoptysis are common pulmonary signs. Generalized cerebral involvement produces confusion, restlessness, coma and epileptiform seizures, although focal signs (hemiplegia or paraplegia) can also occur. Early development of neurological signs distinguishes fat embolism syndrome from ARDS.

There is a high incidence of acute gastric erosions, caused either by gastric mucosal infarction or hypothalamic infarction which stimulates gastric acid secretion. Thrombocytopenia is seen in 50% of patients and hypocalcaemia is common. The haemoglobin may fall and occasionally disseminated intravascular coagulation may occur. Renal function is rarely impaired.

The severity of fat embolism syndrome is related to the extent of the injury and some orthopaedic procedures have a high risk of mortality — such as open reduction and fixation of subcapital femoral neck fracture (Sevitt 1973).

Fat embolism syndrome is a significant cause of mortality in polytrauma patients. Respiratory failure is the most frequent cause of death. Mortality has fallen from 50 to 5–15% since its recognition, due to the advent of arterial gas monitoring and provision of oxygen therapy. The prognosis is unpredictable. Neurological sequelae have a good prognosis for functional recovery although patients with focal signs or paraplegia have a much less predictable prognosis. Patients who die usually have very florid neurological disease. The disease is usually self-limiting and therefore treatment is essentially supportive.

Use of prophylactic oxygen to prevent hypoxaemia will reduce the severity of the disease. Riska et al (1976) noted that proper immobilization of fractures prior to transport and early operative fixation of fractured long bones reduced the incidence of fat embolism syndrome.

ADULT RESPIRATORY DISTRESS SYNDROME

Just over 20 years ago Ashbaugh et al (1967) described a syndrome of life-threatening respiratory distress as a consequence of non-pulmonary trauma, similar to the respiratory distress seen in premature babies. This has now been labelled adult respiratory distress syndrome (ARDS) and is characterized by severe dyspnoea, tachypnoea, refractory hypoxaemia, loss of lung compliance and diffuse alveolar infiltrates on X-ray.

It is a non-specific reaction of the lungs to a wide range of insults, particularly shock, septicaemia, trauma and burns. Originally it was thought to be a separate entity but is now recognized as a part of the spectrum of MSOF.

The lung is frequently the first organ affected in MSOF, probably because it has such a large surface area and mechanically filters all the cardiac output. It also acts as a metabolic organ in its own right, deactivating serotonin and producing prostacyclin.

Definition

Despite the lack of a universally accepted definition of ARDS, the diagnosis is based on five prerequisites:

1. Respiratory distress.
2. Arterial hypoxaemia.
3. Bilateral diffuse infiltrates on chest X-ray.
4. Low total respiratory compliance.
5. Low pulmonary capillary wedge pressure (less than 16 mmHg).

Treatment

Treatment is based on organ support and the treatment of the underlying cause.

Greenspan et al (1985) showed a significant increase in the incidence of ARDS associated with delay in the operative stabilization of major fractures in patients with multiple orthopaedic injuries (at least two long bone fractures and an injury severity score (ISS) greater than 18). This was particularly true for the more seriously injured patients with an ISS in excess of 40.

Johnson et al (1985) observed that an aggressive approach to early operative stabilization of fractures in patients with multiple musculoskeletal injury improved the long-term survival and reduced the overall morbidity. Those patients who were immobilized because of fractures of the spine, pelvis or femur had a higher morbidity due to respiratory failure, sepsis or MSOF.

Mortality

Patients at risk of developing ARDS include those with multiple trauma, sepsis and disseminated intravascular coagulation.

Death usually results from renal, hepatic or cardiac failure associated with systemic sepsis. Mortality is approximately 50%, rising to 90% in septicaemic patients. This mortality has not changed appreciably over the past 20 years, despite a better understanding of the condition, more advanced monitoring and more sophisticated methods of pulmonary support. Septicaemic shock has emerged as the major cause of ARDS, with sepsis syndrome being the commonest cause of death.

Many non-septicaemic patients who develop ARDS subsequently

become infected during the course of their illness, and secondary pulmonary infection is common because of altered host defence mechanisms within the lung.

Prognosis

Factors which worsen the prognosis include:

1. Age.
2. Severity — patients with higher airway pressures have a worse prognosis.
3. Degree of hypoxaemia.
4. Infection — bacterial infection is associated with a much poorer prognosis.
5. Failure of other organs — mortality increases with the number of organs affected.
6. Delay in stabilization of fractures has been shown to increase the incidence of ARDS and worsen the morbidity and mortality.
7. Pre-existing disease.

Smith & Gordon (1986) produced a ventilator index which allowed a quantitative assessment of severity of the lung lesion and ease of weaning from the ventilator and was a reliable predictor of irreversible damage. Patients with a ventilator index above a critical value of 80 were unlikely to survive.

Survivors

Boggis & Greene (1983) stated that abnormal pulmonary function was seen in approximately 40% of survivors 6 months after recovery from ARDS. They observed reduced lung volumes, carbon dioxide diffusing capacity and exercise PaO_2. Improvement in these parameters continued during the first year.

ACUTE RENAL FAILURE

Maintenance of normal renal function is crucial to the survival of trauma victims. Despite advances in the care and support of patients with acute renal failure, the survival of trauma patients who develop renal failure has not improved appreciably. Thus prevention of renal dysfunction must be one of the major priorities during care of trauma patients.

Following trauma numerous stimuli may provoke renal failure. Hypovolaemia results in inadequate renal blood flow causing acute renal ischaemia. Acute renal failure develops in two phases:

1. *Initiating phase*: Hypotension induces a powerful vasoconstrictor reflex which diverts blood flow to more critical organs. There

follows a marked reduction in renal blood flow which itself precipitates vasoconstriction and selectively reduces cortical blood flow.

2. *Perpetuating phase*: Renal perfusion remains low even after correction of hypovolaemia, due to persistent vasoconstriction of renal afferent arterioles, or occlusion of small vessels by swelling of ischaemic tubular cells or casts, and only returns to normal some time later. Renal tubules remain collapsed despite restoration of renal perfusion, probably due to a defect in glomerular filtration. This was previously termed acute tubular necrosis; however, the terms acute tubular dysfunction or vasomotor nephropathy are preferable since the condition is reversible and tubular cell death is not a major feature, unless ischaemia is profound when acute cortical necrosis occurs.

Release of pigments, myoglobin and haemoglobin from acute injury may also provoke a renal failure.

Drugs, especially aminoglycoside antibiotics and contrast media, can initiate and potentiate further damage in already compromised kidneys.

Late renal failure occurring 4 or more days after injury is most frequently related to sepsis and endotoxaemia. Systemic sepsis causes maldistribution of renal blood flow with relative cortical ischaemia.

Complications of acute renal failure may be classified as early or late.

Early complications

Care must be taken to prevent hyperkalaemia, acidosis and pulmonary oedema in early renal failure.

Late complications

There is an increased susceptibility to infection because of impaired leucocyte function, antibody production and cellular immune responses. (A leucocytosis of $15-20 \times 10^3/l$ is often seen in renal failure and does not necessarily imply infection.)

McMurray et al (1978) showed that infection occurs in approximately 74% of patients with acute tubular necrosis and is responsible for 54% of deaths. Septicaemia is the most serious, but peritonitis, urinary tract and respiratory infections are all common.

Pulmonary infections are a particular problem in patients on ventilators, and the combination of acute renal failure and pulmonary failure carries a high mortality.

Disseminated intravascular coagulation is frequent and is often precipitated by infection.

Stress ulcers and uraemic enterocolitis can be reduced by maintaining gastric pH at 4.0–4.5 with antacids (magnesium trisilicate mixture) and H_2 antagonists. Gastrointestinal bleeding is also reduced by dialysis and enteral feeding.

Diuretic phase

Urine output increases over a period of days, but renal function is much slower to improve. Deaths can still occur, usually from infection or fluid and electrolyte imbalance.

Mortality

The overall mortality is still high, ranging from 20 to 70%. Most deaths in acute renal failure occur during the first 14 days, but 20% still occur during recovery (Kennedy et al 1973) and care must be taken to prevent a secondary renal insult during this period. Mortality is not related to age.

Acute renal failure in surgical intensive care unit patients with ventilatory failure is still associated with a mortality of 90%. If there is superimposed hepatic failure, the mortality approaches 100%. Trauma patients who develop renal failure have a poor prognosis, which is related to their injuries and sepsis.

Prognosis

Prognosis is adversely affected by:

1. Severity of initiating insult.
2. Duration and degree of hypotension.
3. Presence of respiratory failure.
4. Liver damage with jaundice. Wilkinson et al (1974) noted that 80% of patients with hepatic coma grade III or IV had evidence of renal dysfunction.
5. Presence of untreated sepsis, especially intra-abdominal.
6. Presence of oliguria. Finn (1983) stated that patients with non-oliguric failure had a better prognosis.

The mortality rate in the immediate post-operative period for non-oliguric renal failure (27%) is half that of oliguric failure.

Kopsa et al (1979) noted very occasional recovery of renal function after prolonged periods of anuria (2 or more months). However, anuria lasting more than 6 weeks suggests the development of irreversible cortical necrosis.

Conversion of oliguric to non-oliguric renal failure simplifies patient management; dialysis is required less frequently, there are fewer complications, recovery is faster and mortality is lower.

In patients who recover there is usually no residual renal impairment. Function returns to 80% of normal by 1 year (Hinds 1987). Residual defects include a slight reduction in glomerular filtration rate and the inability to acidify and concentrate urine properly. Severe renal impairment remains in a small minority of patients who eventually require chronic dialysis or transplantation after a period of months or years. These patients often show focal glomerular hyalinization and thickening, persistent tubular damage and interstitial scarring on renal biopsy (Thompson & Mansell 1985).

GASTROINTESTINAL FAILURE

Blunt or penetrating abdominal trauma and spinal injuries frequently result in paralytic ileus which responds well to conservative treatment.

Pneumoperitoneum, associated with pneumothorax, pneumo-mediastinum and subcutaneous emphysema, may occur as a result of barotrauma in ventilated patients, and rarely may be caused by delayed gastric or colonic perforation.

Stress bleeding from the gastrointestinal tract is particularly common after severe injury, and has been well recognized in patients following burns (Curling's ulcers) and head injuries (Cushing's ulcers). It is almost invariable in patients suffering other types of major injury, shock and sepsis. Lucas et al (1971) noted a 100% incidence of erosive gastritis in such patients examined endoscopically.

Stress ulcers are often multiple, situated in the fundus and the first part of the duodenum, and appear to be small with well defined borders and little surrounding oedema. The main dangers are the risk of haemorrhage and, less commonly, perforation. Acute gastrointestinal bleeding is potentially lethal — continuous or recurrent bleeding from peptic ulceration carries a 10% mortality, whilst massive colonic bleeding in the elderly has a 15% mortality.

Diagnosis is made following frank haematemesis, melaena or aspiration of blood from a nasogastric tube. Fibreoptic endoscopy is then indicated to establish the exact site and nature of the bleeding, which may be from previous peptic ulcer disease.

Bleeding stops spontaneously in 80%, but if it is uncontrolled or becomes persistent definitive surgery is required, although there is no ideal surgical procedure in these circumstances. Total gastrectomy prevents further bleeding but carries a very high operative mortality in critically ill patients. Vagotomy and pyloroplasty or antrectomy carry a lower mortality but have a much higher incidence of recurrent bleeding. Subtotal gastrectomy is probably the best compromise in terms of mortality versus further bleeding.

Recently endoscopic haemostasis by chemical or thermal (diathermy or laser) means has been used in the treatment of bleeding peptic ulcers and it may become a suitable option in stress ulceration.

Prevention

Pingleton & Hadzima (1983) noted that enteral nutrition protects against gastrointestinal bleeding. Hastings et al (1978) and McAlhany et al (1976) have shown reduction in stress bleeding by the hourly administration of antacids by nasogastric tube to maintain gastric pH above 4.0.

The use of H_2 antagonists in preventing acute gastrointestinal bleeding has been disappointing. Groll et al (1986) noted that the incidence of haemorrhage (8%) in general intensive care unit patients was not reduced by cimetidine prophylaxis. This view was supported by Priebe et al (1980) who suggested that it was less effective than conventional antacids in the prevention of gastrointestinal bleeding. Greene & Bollinger (1984) have also noted no improvement with combination therapy (anatacid and H_2 antagonists). Prospective studies by Hastings et al (1978) in critically ill patients showed no benefit in mortality despite the effectiveness of these drugs in reducing bleeding.

There is no information regarding the long-term morbidity in patients who develop acute gastrointestinal bleeding following trauma.

MASSIVE TRANSFUSION AND COAGULOPATHY

Biochemical abnormalities are invariably seen following massive transfusion. Stored blood may contain up to 25 mmol/l of potassium, producing hyperkalaemia in 12% of patients. Acidosis may occur after rapid transfusion of stored blood (pH 6.9) and may require correction with sodium bicarbonate if the base deficit exceeds 7. Hypocalcaemia is a frequent finding on the first day after a massive transfusion but seldom causes problems unless transfusion exceeds 100 ml/min; in these circumstances calcium supplements are required.

Haemostatic failure is common in critically ill patients. It may present as inappropriate bleeding from the skin and mucous membranes, continued oozing from wounds, concealed haemorrhage or may be discovered on routine testing. Circulating clotting factors and platelets are lost during massive haemorrhage but the development of coagulopathy depends upon the fluids used during resuscitation.

Counts et al (1979) noted that dilutional thrombocytopenia was a more frequent cause of bleeding than disseminated intravascular coagulation, and recommended the use of platelet concentrates if the platelet count fell below 50 000/mm ^{3}.

Soon after major trauma, platelets respond to the release of catecholamines and tissue thromboplastin, leading to enhanced coagulation. Disseminated intravascular coagulation may be initiated by hypotension, trauma (particularly polytrauma) or sepsis. It is characterized by consumption of platelets and clotting factors as well as occlusion of the microcirculation leading to gangrene of the tips of the fingers, toes and ears. This consumption coagulopathy is accentuated by secondary fibrinolysis.

Disseminated intravascular coagulation is most commonly seen in shocked patients whose restoration of blood volume has been delayed. Clinical presentation is variable and often associated with shock and acidosis, as well as ARDS or renal failure following trauma. Diagnosis may be particularly difficult in patients with severe dilutional coagulopathy. The hallmarks of disseminated intravascular coagulation are reduction in platelets and fibrinogen level (less than 100 mg/dl), increased fibrin degradation products and clot lysis.

HEPATIC FAILURE

Flint (1982) noted that hepatic failure after injury frequently presented as cholestatic jaundice.

Early elevation of serum bilirubin within 3 days of trauma or surgery may be the result of resorption of haematomas or transfusion reaction, and usually resolves within 5 days. Onset of jaundice after this period is most frequently a result of sepsis, particularly pneumonia or intra-abdominal collections of pus, and it may be an indication for abdominal exploration (Fry et al 1980). This late-onset hepatic failure may be heralded by elevation of serum glutamic pyruvic transaminase, serum glutamic oxaloacetic transaminase and alkaline phosphatase levels (reflecting cellular injury) before jaundice (reflecting functional impairment) becomes apparent.

Hepatic failure usually follows pulmonary, renal and clotting failure as part of MSOF, and is often a terminal event.

Correction of the primary cause of liver dysfunction (hypotension, hypoxia) is essential in traumatized patients with hepatic dysfunction.

REFERENCES

Abbott M W 1976 In: Fischer J E (ed) Total parenteral nutrition. Little, Brown & Co., Boston, p. 3
Aron K V, Grover F L, Richardson J D, Trinkle J K 1977 Post traumatic empyema. Annals of Thoracic Surgery 23: 254–258
Ashbaugh D G, Bigelow D B, Petty T L, Levine B E 1967. Acute respiratory distress in adults. Lancet ii: 319
Baue A E 1975 Multiple, progressive or sequential system failure. Archives of Surgery 110: 779
Becker D P, Miller J D, Ward J D et al 1977 The outcome from severe head injury with early diagnosis and intensive management. Journal of Neurosurgery 47: 491
Bell R C, Coalson J J, Smith J D, Johannson W G 1983, Multiple system organ failure and infection in adult respiratory distress syndrome. Annals of Internal Medicine 99: 293
Blair E, Topuzlu C, Deane R S 1969 Major blunt chest trauma. Current problems in Surgery, May
Boggis C R M, Greene R 1983 Adult respiratory distress syndrome. British Journal of Hospital Medicine 29: 167
Bojanowicz K 1977 Zeitschrift für Ernaehrungswissenschaft. Journal of Nutritional Science (suppl) 20: 14
Borzotta A P, Polk H C 1983 Multiple system organ failure. Surgical Clinics of North America 61: 315
Burke J F, Wolfe R R, Mullay C J et al 1979 Glucose requirements during burn injury. Annals of Surgery 190: 274

Buzby G P, Mullen J L, Matthews D C, Hobbs C L, Rosato E F 1980 Prognostic nutritional index in gastrointestinal surgery. American Journal of Surgery 139: 160–166

Counts R B, Haisch C, Simon T L et al 1979 Haemostasis in massively transfused trauma patients. Annals of Surgery 190: 91–99

Cuthbertson D P 1932 Observations on the disturbances of metabolism produced by injury to the limbs. Quarterly Journal of Medicine 1: 233

Faist E, Baue A E R, Dittmer H, Herbere G 1983 Multiple system organ failure in polytrauma patients. Journal of Trauma 23: 775

Finn W F 1983 Recovery from acute renal failure. In: Brenner B M, Lazarus J M (eds) Acute renal failure. W B Saunders, Philadelphia, pp 753–774

Flint L M 1982 Liver failure. Surgical Clinics of North America 62: 157–165

Fry D E, Pearlstein L, Fulton R L, Polk H C 1980 Multiple system organ failure: the role of uncontrolled infection. Archives of Surgery 115: 136–140

Greene W L, Bollinger B R 1984. Cimetidine for stress-ulcer prophylaxis. Critical Care Medicine 12: 571–575

Greenspan L, McLellan B A, Greig H 1985 Abbreviated injury severity score. A scoring chart. Journal of Trauma 25: 60–64

Groll A, Simon J B, Wigle R D et al 1986 Cimetidine prophylaxis for gastrointestinal bleeding in an intensive care unit. Gut 27: 135–140

Hastings P R, Skillman J J, Bushell I S, Silen W 1978 Antacid prophylaxis of bleeding in the critically ill. New England Journal of Medicine 298: 1041–1045

Heatley R V, Williams R H P, Lewis H M 1979 Preoperative intravenous feeding — a controlled trial. Postgraduate Medical Journal 55: 541–545

Hessov I B 1977 Energy and protein intake in elderly patients in an orthopaedic surgical ward. Acta Chirurgica Scandinavica 143: 145–149

Hill G L, Pickford I, Young G A et al 1977 Malnutrition in surgical patients: an unrecognized problem. Lancet i: 689

Hinds C J 1987 Acute renal failure. In: Intensive care. A concise textbook. Baillière Tindall, London pp 309–326

James O F, Moore P G 1983 Causes of death after blunt chest injury. Australian and New Zealand Journal of Surgery 53: 37–42

Johnson K D, Cadambi G B, Seibert G B 1985 Incidence of adult respiratory distress in patients with multiple skeletal injury: effect of early operative stabilization of fractures. Journal of Trauma 25: 375–384

Kennedy A C, Burton J A Luke R G et al 1973. Factors affecting the prognosis in acute renal failure. A survey of 251 cases. Quarterly Journal of Medicine 42: 73–86

Kirsch M M 1984 In: The multiply injured patient with complex fractures. Lea & Febiger, Philadelphia, pp 18–32

Kopsa H, Schmidt P, Zazgornik J, Pils P, Bache P 1979 Recovery of kidney function following prolonged acute renal failure. Proceedings of the European Dialysis and Transplant Association 16: 495–499

Lucas C E, Sugawa C, Riddle J et al 1971 The natural history and surgical dilemma of stress gastric bleeding. Archives of Surgery 102: 226

McAlhany J C, Czaja A J, Pruit B A 1976 Antacid control of complications from acute gastroduodenal disease after burns. Journal of Trauma 16: 645–649

McMurray S D, Luft F C, Maxwell D R et al 1978 Prevailing patterns and predictor variables in patients with acute tubular necrosis. Archives of Internal Medicine 138: 950–955

Miller S E, Miller C L, Trunkey D D 1982 The immune consequences of trauma. Surgical Clinics of North America 62: 167–181

Pingleton S K, Hadzima S K 1983 Enternal alimentation and gastrointestinal bleeding in mechanically ventilated patients. Critical Care Medicine 11: 13–16

Polk H C 1979 Consensus summary on infection. Journal of Trauma 19: 894–896

Polk H C, Shield C L 1977 Remote organ failure: a valid sign of occult intra-abdominal infection. Surgery 81: 310

Priebe J H, Skillman J J, Bushnel L S, Long P C, Silen W 1980 Antacid versus cimetidine in preventing acute gastrointestinal bleeding. New England Journal of Medicine 302: 426–430

Randall H T 1971 Surgical nutrition. Parenteral and oral. In: Kinney J M (ed) Manual of preoperative and postoperative care. Saunders, Philadelphia, pp 75–94

Rapp R P, Young B, Twyman D et al 1983 The favourable effect of early parenteral feeding on survival in head-injured patients. Journal of Neurosurgery 58: 906

Riska E B, von Bonsdorf H, Hakkinen S et al 1976 Prevention of fat embolization by early fixation of fractures in patients with multiple injuries. Injury 8: 110–116

Sagar S, Harland P, Sheilds R 1979 Early postoperative feeding with elemental diet. British Medical Journal 1: 263–265

Sankaran S, Wilson R F 1970 Factors affecting prognosis in patients with flail chest. Journal of Thoracic and Cardiovascular Surgery 60: 407–410

Sevitt S 1973 The significance of fat embolization syndrome. British Journal of Hospital Medicine 9: 784–788

Smith P, Gordon I J 1986 An index to predict outcome in adult respiratory distress syndrome. Intensive Care Medicine 12: 86

Studley H O 1936 Percentage weight loss: a basic indicator of surgical risk in patients with chronic peptic ulcer. Journal of the American Medical Association 106: 458

Thompson F D, Mansell M A 1985 Renal failure. In: Dobb G (ed) Clinics in anaesthesiology, vol 3. W B Saunders, Philadelphia, pp 955–972

Tilney N L, Bailey G L, Morgan A P 1973 Sequential system failure after rupture of abdominal aortic aneurysms. Annals of Surgery 178: 117

Wiener S L, Barrett J 1986 Multiple organ failure after trauma. In: Trauma management for civilian and military physicians. W B Saunders, Philadelphia, pp 343–353

Wilkinson S P, Blendis L M, Williams R 1974 Frequency and type of renal and electrolyte disorders in fulminant hepatic failure. British Medical Journal 1: 186

Zenker F A 1862 Beitrage zur anatomie der lungen. In G. Shonfeld Buchlandlung, Dresden

22. Post-traumatic reflex sympathetic dystrophy

M. W. Ward

INTRODUCTION

Mitchell et al (1864) are credited with the first description of a painful syndrome which may occur following injury. The term 'causalgia' was later given to this syndrome which, over the next century, became known under a large variety of names. The International Association for the Study of Pain (1986) listed 67 different terms in the English, French and German literature. The term 'reflex sympathetic dystrophy' (RSD) has been widely used to describe this syndrome over the past two decades, whereas previously it appeared only intermittently in papers by Evans (1946), Toumey (1948) and Drucker et al (1959). Terms which have been used to refer to the condition, now generally accepted as reflex sympathetic dystrophy in the English language literature, include the following:

algodystrophy; Sudeck's atrophy; shoulder–hand syndrome; reflex neurovascular dystrophy; causalgia; post-traumatic dystrophy; post-traumatic pain syndrome; algoneurodystrophy; painful osteoporosis; reflex hyperaemic deossification; reflex dystrophy of the extremities; reflex trophoneurosis; post-traumatic acute bone atrophy; traumatic angiospasm.

The condition is rare and is estimated to occur only once in 2000 accidents involving an extremity (Plewes 1956).

PATHOGENESIS

RSD represents an exaggerated response to a painful event affecting an extremity. Trauma is by far the most common painful stimulus which precipitates the development of RSD, but it can also be initiated by other painful conditions such as myocardial infarction, cerebrovascular disease, herpes zoster infection and cervical osteoarthritis. Lankford & Thompson (1977) believed that a certain type of patient was particularly susceptible to the syndrome and such patients were described as being emotionally labile with a low tolerance to cold and pain.

Current opinion concerning the mechanism by which the pathological changes are brought about implicates the sympathetic nervous system. Livingston (1943) postulated the formation of a self-sustaining cycle in which chronic irritation of a peripheral sensory nerve as a result of trauma and soft tissue damage produced increased afferent input and an abnormal level of activity in the internuncial neuronal pool of the spinal cord. This leads to the continuous stimulation of sympathetic and motor efferent nerve fibres. Others, such as Doupe et al (1944), postulated a mechanism which involved the development of an artificial synapse between sensory afferents and sympathetic efferents, allowing a direct cross-stimulation and formation of the pain cycle. This artificial synapse is called an ephase.

The gate control theory of pain transmission further developed the concept of a fine-tuning mechanism activated by cells in the substantia gelatinosa of the dorsal horn of the spinal cord (Melzak & Wall 1965). These cells can modulate the afferent impulses which are carried by small C-fibres and large A-fibres so that selective activation of the C-fibres inhibits the cells of the substantia gelatinosa and 'opens the gate' to pain transmission. A-fibre activity can stimulate the substantia gelatinosa to increase its inhibitory effect on pain transmission and 'close the gate'.

The clinical experience that a wide variety of treatment methods may be effective lends support to the conclusion that the pathogenesis of the syndrome is likely to be concerned with both peripheral and central pathways.

CLINICAL FEATURES

RSD is, above all, a painful condition, and pain dominates all three stages of the syndrome which are classically described. The condition may occur at any age, including childhood, although most reported series seem to have a peak incidence in the third and fourth decades. Most series also report a preponderance of females in a 2:1 ratio and a similar lower limb to upper limb ratio.

Sufferers of the RSD syndrome usually complain bitterly of pain in the hand or foot of the injured limb. In some patients this pain extends proximally in the limb to cover a wider area. The pain is invariably distressing and is variously described as an excruciating, burning pain with other dramatic adjectives used to amplify the nature of the pain such as throbbing, knife-like, shooting or crushing.

The severity of the pain experienced is characteristically out of proportion to the severity of the initiating injury and is often accentuated by emotional factors such as surprise and anger and by environmental disturbances.

The pain of RSD is rarely limited to a defined dermatomal distribution, except in the early stages in individuals who have sustained direct injury to a peripheral nerve. This non-dermatomal picture is in keeping with sympathetic efferent distribution in the limbs, which likewise follows a non-dermatomal pattern.

Seemingly bizarre features are not uncommon in respect of the immediate environs of the affected limb; individuals may have a strong preference for touching and being touched by moist objects rather than dry ones. Even more bizarre is the need to place water into the shoes to avoid pain when walking, even though the affected part is in the upper limb.

In summary, patients often present as pain-wracked individuals who guard the affected extremity with the utmost care. Other clinical features, such as loss of motion, swelling, vasomotor instability and trophic changes, usually occur but are variable.

Stage 1

Pain is usually severe and may occur immediately following injury or be delayed for some weeks. Movement of the affected part is curtailed and there is frequently soft tissue oedema, increased blood supply to the skin with increased skin temperature and redness. Marked hyperaesthesia is common and trophic changes such as decreased nail and hair growth plus hyperhidrosis occur. This stage lasts for about 6 weeks.

Stage 2

The pain continues, characteristically at a severe level, and becomes more diffuse. Movement of the affected part becomes further restricted and the oedema becomes hard and non-pitting and extends over a wider area. Nail and hair growth diminish and the skin becomes cool, tight and may appear cyanotic. Hyperhidrosis continues during this stage, which lasts for 2 to 3 months.

Stage 3

The pain is now intractable and has spread to affect the entire limb. Dermal blood flow is decreased so that the skin appears pale, cool and atrophic. Nails become grooved and fissured and joint movements are severely restricted with the development of joint contractures. These physical changes are considered irreversible (Drucker et al 1959, Lankford & Thompson 1977).

RSD usually involves an entire limb or a complete hand or foot. Segmental RSD has been described in which only two digits were affected by the syndrome (Helms et al 1980).

RSD IN CHILDREN

Prior to 1978, few individual cases of RSD occurring in children had been reported. In that year, a paper by Bernstein et al described the syndrome in 23 children between the ages of 9 and 16 years with a mean age of 12.4 years.

The conclusions of these authors drew attention to differences between the syndrome occurring in children and in adults, which in part were substantiated by Ruggeri et al (1982). Children do not develop the severe disabling pain experienced by adults and trophic changes are rare.

The characteristic radiographic changes seen in adults do not occur and a much milder diffuse osteopenia is the usual finding in children.

Children are seemingly much easier to treat than adults and invariably respond to simple physical therapy methods. A high proportion of the children in Bernstein et al's (1978) series had a history of overt parental conflict (10 out of 12); a tendency to accept responsibility beyond their years was recognized in 11 of 13 children and all of the 12 children had what was felt to be a marked indifference to the implications of their illness for future functioning.

INVESTIGATIONS

Radiographic changes

Patients with RSD develop a localized high-turnover osteoporosis due to increased osteoclastic resorption. This is partly stimulated by immobilization and is dependent on the presence of an intact thyroid and parathyroid (McKay et al 1977). The osteoporosis may be generalized but an X-ray appearance of small rounded areas of translucency up to 10 mm in diameter and superimposed on the generalized reduction in bone density is more distinctive.

Genant et al (1975) described five types of bone resorption which may occur in RSD:

1. Irregular resorption of trabecular bone in the metaphysis creating the patchy or spotty osteoporosis.
2. Subperiosteal bone resorption.
3. Intracortical bone resorption.
4. Endosteal bone resorption.
5. Surface erosions of subchondral and juxta-articular bone.

Soft tissue swelling may be seen on radiographs and there may be radiological evidence of joint effusion (Gamble & Yale 1966).

Scintigraphic changes

Kozin et al (1981) used 99m Tc methylene diphosphonate and 99m Tc ethane-1-hydroxyl-1-1-diphosphonate to obtain flow studies and static images. The flow studies showed a high incidence of asymmetrical blood flow in the affected extremity and increased peri-articular uptake in the involved extremity on the static images.

The majority of the flow studies showed an increased activity on the affected side although a few demonstrated decreased activity.

Scintigraphic studies seem to be more useful in the early detection of RSD and changes are detected before the onset of radiographic changes. These findings are supported by the earlier work of Genant et al (1975) and Greyson & Tipperman (1984).

Other investigations

Thermography may help in the diagnosis of RSD, as documented by Uematsu et al (1981). All patients with RSD affecting the knee reported by Katz & Hungerford (1987) showed more than 1°C decreases in cutaneous temperature around the affected knee.

Synovial biopsy has been performed most recently by Ogilvie-Harris & Roscoe (1987) and consistent findings of non-specific subsynovial fibrosis with synovial proliferation were obtained. There were no inflammatory changes and the degree of subsynovial fibrosis was more pronounced in later cases.

Bone biopsy studies in RSD were reported by Basle et al (1983) following light and electron microscopic examination. Vascular modification in the medullary spaces of bone occur with reduced arteriolar flow, interstitial oedema and stasis. Degeneration of osteocytes and demineralization of lamellar bone trabeculae follow.

Endosteal resting cells are thought to differentiate into osteoblasts which form new irregular bone trabeculae. Remodelling of dead and newly formed trableculae occurs later as a result of osteoclast resorption.

Blood tests of haematological and biochemical indices seem to be characterized by normality in RSD.

Sympathetic blockade has been regarded as an essential diagnostic investigation by a number of authors (Toumey 1948, Patman et al 1973, Katz & Hungerford 1987). Regional sympathetic blockade of the stellate ganglion (upper limb) and lumbar sympathetic chain (lower limb) should produce relief of pain, albeit temporary, in patients with RSD. The results of such sympathetic blockade using local anaesthetic also have direct prognostic implications in respect of certain treatment methods which may be offered in cases which have been resistant to physiotherapeutic methods of treatment.

RESULTS OF TREATMENT

As a preventive measure, the importance of early mobilization of an injured extremity has long been emphasized but, as pointed out by Schutzer & Gossling (1984), no properly controlled trial has been conducted to test this principle. The treatment of established cases of RSD is controversial in the extreme.

Physical methods

Physical methods are believed to play an important part in the management of all stages of the RSD syndrome. Such methods must be used with care, however, as it is possible to make existing symptoms worse by the use of extremes of heat and cold or by passive exercises conducted by an over-enthusiastic therapist. Increased afferent transmission may, under these somewhat extreme treatment regimens, exacerbate the condition.

Early active range of motion exercises of the involved part and its contralateral counterpart should be the goal of physical therapy. Splinting of the hand has been used to resist the development of contractures in the hand.

Mild analgesics should be used as required in conjunction with these physical methods.

The results of such treatment in promptly diagnosed cases of RSD is believed to be good.

Electroacupuncture

Chan & Chow (1981) reported on 20 patients who had the features of RSD and whose injury had occurred between 1 and 6 months prior to the commencement of acupuncture with electrical stimulation. All patients had failed to respond to at least a month of conventional physiotherapy plus analgesics. Physiotherapy was continued throughout the course of electroacupuncture.

The results of this small group of patients showed that 70% had a marked improvement in respect of pain relief and a further 20% had some improvement. However, only 30% of the 10 patients in whom movements were measured achieved any improvement in range of movement.

All of these patients who were reassessed between 3 and 22 months after their electroacupuncture course (17 patients) either retained or improved their initial level of pain relief.

Regional local anaesthetic block with methylprednisolone

Poplawski et al (1983) reported the results of 27 patients (28 extremities) who had resistant RSD syndrome. They were treated by a method of regional local anaesthetic blockade using 1% Xylocaine plus 80 mg methylprednisolone. These substances were injected intravenously into the affected limb after exsanguination and the block was restricted to the affected limb for 20–30 minutes by an arterial tourniquet. During this time, manipulation of stiff joints and massage of indurated soft tissue were carried out. Conventional physiotherapy was continued after the block and repeat blocks were carried out for recurrence of pain or stiffness or for loss of previously gained movement.

Individual patients in the group received between 1 and 5 blocks.

The results of this treatment method showed that 21 out of the 28 extremities were significantly improved. The 7 extremities which did not achieve improvement all occurred in patients whose RSD syndrome had existed for longer than 9 months. Of the significantly improved group, only 2 patients who had had the syndrome for longer than a year were improved.

Sympathetic blockade

Prior to 1930, many patients with RSD who did not respond to conventional physiotherapy techniques suffered a life of misery, including drug addiction, mental deterioration and chronic invalidism. Suicide was not an uncommon event.

Spurling in 1930 reported the first cure of a patient with causalgia following a cervicothoracic sympathectomy. His report marked a turning point in the outlook for patients with the more resistant forms of RSD; a number of methods of achieving interruption of the abnormal sympathetic reflex have been developed since then.

Schutzer & Gossling (1984) described how a curative effect can be obtained from a single regional block of the stellate ganglion (upper limb) or lumbar sympathetic chain (lower limb). This is most likely to be achieved in early cases and it is more usual to require a number of such blocks in order to obtain pain control. In practice, 3 or 4 such local anaesthetic blocks are usually followed by a surgical sympathectomy.

Following these principles, Katz & Hungerford (1987) achieved 65% good and 35% fair, early results in a group of patients with symptoms of RSD of the knee, over a period of from 2 months to 11 years. Once again, this study stressed the importance of early therapeutic intervention if good results are to be obtained; a period of 6 months from onset of RSD symptoms limits the early case.

Regional sympathetic blockade using guanethidine was originally described by Hannington-Kiff in 1974. Guanethidine acts as a false transmitter, displacing noradrenaline from its storage sites. The technique of blockade is similar to that described already in the local anaesthetic/corticosteroid infusion technique of Poplawski et al of 1983 and blockade for 3–4 days can be achieved. In 1977, Hannington-Kiff published the results of 17 consecutive cases treated by the intravenous guanethidine method. Symptoms had been present for 1–7 months. Seven patients had a response to treatment that was 'great and maintained' in respect of the improvement obtained following one treatment.

Nine patients had a second treatment some 3–4 weeks after the initial treatment, having only achieved a 'moderate' improvement initially. Five of these patients had an upper limb RSD and all had an improved response to the second guanethidine injection. Three patients who had RSD affecting the ankle or foot did not benefit from the second injection and it would seem that the response to this treatment method is considerably better in the affected upper limb than in the lower limbs.

Systemic corticosteroids

Prednisolone has been the most commonly administered corticosteroid in a number of uncontrolled trials over the past 15 years and results which compare with those of sympathetic interruption have been achieved in the region of 80% good response.

The mechanism by which corticosteroids act in RSD is unknown and their use remains empirical.

Propranolol

Propranolol has been used in high oral doses (Simson 1974) in the RSD syndrome and some favourable results have been obtained. Its use has not gained any great popularity but it does remain in the armamentarium for the treatment of resistant cases.

PSYCHOLOGICAL ASPECTS

Many authors over the years have drawn attention to abnormalities of personality of RSD sufferers but this aspect has not received scientifically based support. Patients have been described as being dependent, over-reactive, and often hostile to the physician.

A strong placebo response has clouded the results in many cases and this has been seen in as many as 20% of patients in some trials of treatment.

Poplawski et al (1983) probably gave the best advice on managing these patients when they stated that communication with the patient, reassurance and treatment of anxiety are important aspects of therapy in the management of this syndrome.

CONCLUSIONS

The RSD syndrome is becoming increasingly recognized as a potent cause of disability following injury of any sort to any part of an extremity. Management in the early stages is dependent on early recognition of the developing syndrome and when treatment is instituted early the results are very favourable.

Unfortunately the index of suspicion is not yet high enough and there are many patients who are not diagnosed until the later stages of the syndrome's development. Prior to the recognition of the syndrome many patients undoubtedly receive injudicious physical methods of treatment as part of the general rehabilitation offered routinely after injury.

Although advances have been made in the management of the more resistant cases, many of the treatment methods are empirical and there seems to be much scope for research in this field.

REFERENCES

Basle M F, Rebel A, Renier J C 1983 Bone tissue in reflex sympathetic dystrophy
syndrome. Sudeck's atrophy. Structural and ultrastructural studies. Metabolic Bone
Disease and Related Research 4: 305–311
Bernstein B H, Singsen B H, Kent J T et al 1978 Reflex neurovascular dystrophy in
childhood. Journal of Paediatrics 93: 211–215
Chan C S, Chow S P 1981 Electroacupuncture in the treatment of post-traumatic
sympathetic dystrophy (Sudeck's atrophy). British Journal of Anaesthesia 53: 899–901
Doupe J, Cullen C H, Chance G Q 1944 Post-traumatic pain and the causalgic syndrome.
Journal of Neurology. Neurosurgery and Psychiatry 7: 33–48
Drucker W R, Hubay C A, Holden W D, Bukovnic J A 1959 Pathogenesis of post-
traumatic sympathetic dystrophy. American Journal of Surgery 97: 454–465
Evans J A 1946 Reflex sympathetic dystrophy. Surgery, Gynaecology and Obstetrics
82: 36–43
Gamble F O, Yale I 1966 Clinical foot roentgenology. Williams & Wilkins, Baltimore
Genant H, Kozin F, Bekerman C, McCarty D, Sims J 1975 The reflex sympathetic
dystrophy syndrome. Radiology 117: 21–32
Greyson N, Tipperman P 1984 Three-phase bone studies in hemiplegia with reflex
sympathetic dystrophy and the effect of disuse. Journal of Nuclear Medicine 25:
423–429
Hannington-Kiff J G 1974 Intravenous regional sympathetic block with guanethidine.
Lancet i: 1019–1020
Hannington-Kiff J G 1977 Relief of Sudeck's atrophy by regional intravenous guanethidine.
Lancet i: 1132–1133
Helms C, O'Brien E, Katzberg R 1980 Segmented reflex sympathetic dystrophy syndrome.
Radiology 135: 67–68
International Association for the Study of Pain 1986 Sub committee on taxonomy.
Classification of chronic pain. Pain (suppl 3): 529
Katz M M, Hungerford D S 1987 Reflex sympathetic dystrophy affecting the knee. Journal
of Bone and Joint Surgery 69B: 797–803
Kozin F, Soin J S, Ryan L M, Carerra G F, Wortmann R L 1981 Bone scintigraphy in the
reflex sympathetic dystrophy syndrome. Radiology 138: 437–443
Lankford L L, Thompson J E 1977 Reflex sympathetic dystrophy, upper and lower
extremity. Diagnosis and management. C V Mosby, St Louis, pp 163–178
Livingston W K 1943 Pain mechanisms. A physiologic interpretation of causalgia and its
related states. Macmillan, New York, p 212
McKay N N S, Woodhouse N J Y, Clarke A K 1977 Post-traumatic reflex sympathetic
dystrophy syndrome (Sudeck's atrophy): effects of regional guanethidine infusion and
salmon calcitonin. British Medical Journal 1: 1575–1576
Melzak R, Wall P D 1965 Pain mechanisms. A new theory. Science 150: 971–979
Mitchell S W, Morehouse C R, Keen W W 1864 Gunshot wounds and other injuries of
nerves. J B Lippincott, Philadelphia
Ogilvie-Harris D J, Roscoe M 1987 Reflex sympathetic dystrophy of the knee. Journal of
Bone and Joint Surgery 69B: 804–806
Patman R D, Thompson J E, Persson A V 1973 Management of post-traumatic pain
syndrome — report of 113 cases. Annals of Surgery 177: 780–787
Plewes L W 1956 Sudeck's atrophy in the hand. Journal of Bone and Joint Surgery
38B: 195–203
Poplawski Z J, Wiley A M, Murray J F 1983 Post-traumatic dystrophy of the extremities.
A clinical review and trial of treatment. Journal of Bone and Joint Surgery 65A: 642–655
Ruggeri S B, Athreya B H, Doughty R, Gregg J R, Das M M 1982 Reflex sympathetic
dystrophy in children. Clinical Orthopaedics and Related Research 163: 225–230
Schutzer S P, Gossling H R 1984 The treatment of reflex sympathetic dystrophy syndrome.
Journal of Bone and Joint Surgery 66A: 625–629
Simson G 1974 Propranolol for causalgia and Sudeck atrophy. Journal of the American
Medical Association 227: 327
Spurling R G 1930 Causalgia of the upper extremity. Treatment by dorsal sympathetic
ganglionectomy. Archives of Neurology and Psychiatry 23: 784–788

Toumey J W 1948 Occurrence and management of reflex sympathetic dystrophy (causalgia of the extremities). Journal of Bone and Joint Surgery 30: 883–894

Uematsu S, Hendler N, Hungerford D S, Long D, Ono N 1981 Thermography and electromyography in the differential diagnosis of chronic pain syndromes and reflex sympathetic dystrophy. Electromyography and Clinical Neurophysiology 21: 165–182

Appendix: specimen format for a medicolegal report

N.B: This is not the only format for a medicolegal report. It is introduced more as an *aide-mémoire* for those who may be unfamiliar with the information required by the legal profession.

TITLE PAGE

Name, address, telephone number of reporting surgeon.

Medical report on:	
Name	Mr John Smith
Address	23 South Street Westford
Date of birth	8 December 1952
Date of report	3 March 1989
Status	Married
Date of injury	6 May 1988
Occupation at time of injury	Lorry driver
Present occupation	Unemployed
Time lost from work as a result of injury	Six months
Report requested by and confidential to	Jones, Brown and Fox Solicitors 11 High Street Eastford
Your ref.	XY2/P3 dated 3 January 1989
Our ref.	ABC/DJF
Documents available	1. Southern General Hospital notes 2. Medical Report from Mr A. B. Lee

SUGGESTED FURTHER HEADINGS

History of injury

Brief details of the patient's recollection of the incident. If a road traffic accident, was the patient wearing a seat belt or crash helmet?

497

Treatment to date

This will give an account of the management of the problem up to the present time from:

1. The patient's account.
2. The hospital notes.

This section will include a precise account of the injuries recorded at the time of admission to or attendance at hospital.

Present condition

This will detail the patient's current symptoms and signs and discuss X-rays:

1. Symptoms
   Pain
   Stiffness
   Sleep loss
   Marital or social problems
   Functional impairment
2. Signs
   Deformity
   Loss of joint movement
   Description of scars
   Shortening
   Wasting, weakness
   (Consider use of clinical photographs)
3. X-rays, if appropriate

Effect of accident on occupation

Effect of accident on social activities

How have the patient's social and sporting activities been affected by the accident/injury? What is he unable to do now that he could do before the accident/injury?

Opinion and prognosis

An opinion as to whether the injuries sustained are compatible with the mechanism described is useful.

The prognosis is particularly important and should consider:

1. Is further treatment required? (If *yes*, describe its nature, duration and gravity.)

2. Is further time off from work expected?
3. What is the likelihood of complications developing?
4. If there is a cosmetic abnormality, is it likely to improve or to deteriorate?
5. Is there any reduction in the patient's life expectancy?
6. Describe the psychological state of the patient.
7. Does the patient have any special needs? If so, are they on-going?

CONCLUSIONS

In some cases a brief summary and concluding paragraph may be helpful.

SIGNATURE BLOCK

It is important to record your qualifications and position so that the origin and standing of the provider of the report are clear to whoever is reading it.

Index

Abscesses, intra-abdominal, 473, 474
Accident neurosis, 437, 457
Acetabular fractures, 237–243, 285
  complications of surgical treatment,
    241–242
  incidence of osteoarthritis, 240
  prognostic factors, 237–239
  return to work and leisure activities, 241
  timing of medicolegal reports, 240
Acromial fractures, 46
Acromioclavicular joint, 33–39
  acute superior dislocation, 34–38
    complications, 37–38
    conservative versus operative treatment,
      35–36
    operative treatment, 36–37
  anterior dislocation, 38
  dislocations associated with coracoid
    process fractures, 47
  grade 1 and 2 injuries, 33, 34
  inferior dislocation of distal end of
    clavicle, 38
  posterior dislocation, 38
Activities of daily living, impairment of, 7
Adhesive capsulitis, 93, 94
Adolescents
  clavicular fractures, 44
  spinal fractures, 414
Age of patient
  acetabular fractures, 239
  ankle fractures, 346
  calcaneal fractures, 361
  Colles' fractures, 165
  femoral head and neck fractures, 250,
    254–256
  nerve injuries and, 226
  recurrent anterior dislocation of shoulder,
    56, 57
Alcoholism, 352
Amenity, loss of, 18
Amnesia, post-traumatic, 436–437, 462
Amputations, 8
  foot, traumatic partial, 376–377
  hand, 230–231

Anal reflex, 421
Ankle, 339–354
  fractures, 339, 340–349
    children, 352–354
    classification, 340–343
    factors influencing development of
      osteoarthritis, 344–346
    incidence of osteoarthritis, 343–344
    non-union, 348
    social/occupational factors, 347–348
    time taken for osteoarthritis to develop,
      346–347
  ligament injuries, 339–340
  stiffness after tibial fractures, 327,
    333–334
  tibial plafond/pilon fractures, 349–352
Anosmia, 439
Anterior cruciate ligament injuries, 292,
  293, 294, 295–302
  anatomy, 295–296
  anterolateral rotatory instability, 300–302
  children, 303
  diagnosis, 296–297
  function, 296
  isolated, 298–300
  natural history, 297
Anterior interosseus nerve lesions, 152–153,
  154
Anuria, 480
Anxiety, post-traumatic, 459
Arcuate complex injury, 293, 295
Arcuate ligament injury, 292
ARDS *see* Respiratory distress syndrome,
  adult
Arterial injuries, 8, 128, 229
  see also Ischaemic contractures; *Specific*
    arteries
Arthritis, post-traumatic, 9–10
  ankle injuries, 339–340, 343–347
  elbow injuries, 116, 118, 121, 122,
    123–125, 128, 131
  femoral fractures, 276–277, 280–281
  foot injuries, 360, 365, 366, 369, 374
  hip injuries, 240, 244, 245–246

501

Arthritis *cont.*
 knee injuries, 310, 316–317
 shoulder injuries, 34, 37–38, 67–68
 wrist injuries, 172–173, 176, 183, 203
Arthrodesis
 carpal instability, 207, 208
 Kienböck's disease, 190
Arthroplasty
 replacement *see* Prostheses, replacement
 soft tissue interposition, scaphoid
  fractures, 185
Ataxia, 440
Atlanto-occipital dislocations, 411
Avascular necrosis
 carpal lunate, 187–188, 201, 204
 carpal scaphoid, 181, 182, 202
 carpal trapezoid, 194
 femoral head
  femoral neck fractures, 250, 252, 254,
   255, 258, 259, 260, 261
  femoral shaft fractures, 285
  hip dislocations, 244, 245, 247, 248,
   262, 263
 humeral neck, 71, 73, 74
 radial head, 120, 133
 talus, 363–364, 366, 369, 378–379
Axillary artery damage, 61
Axillary nerve injury, 46, 60, 66

Back injuries *see* Spinal injuries
Bankart procedure, 63
Barton's fractures, 161, 175–176
Baumann's angle, 129–130
Behavioural problems after head injury, 441
Biceps brachii muscle
 distal tendon avulsions, 49–50
 distal tendonitis, 109
 rupture, 48–50
Bipolar fixation with pins and casts, Colles'
  fractures, 169–170
Birth injuries, 32, 44, 68, 103
Bladder
 dysfunction, 6, 11, 421–422
 injuries, 398, 399, 404
Blood transfusions, massive, 482–483
Bone biopsy, 491
Bone grafts, 43, 95–96, 146, 183–184, 185
Bowel function, 6
Braces, humeral, 87, 89–90
Brachial artery injuries, 102, 103
Brachial plexus injuries, 31, 43, 45, 60
Brain damage
 assessment of severity, 435–437
 categorization of residual, 437–441
 secondary, 432
Bristow procedure, 63
Burns, hands, 231

Calcaneal fractures, 357–362
 children, 378

 extra-articular, 358–359
 intra-articular, 359–360
 prognostic factors, 360–361
 residual symptoms and timing of reports,
  360
Calcaneofibular abutment, 360
Calcification *see* Ossification
Capitate injuries, 195–196
Capitolunate instability, 209
Capitular epiphyseal injuries, 125–128
 baseball players, 114
 classification, 125–126
 complications, 111–112, 126–128
Care, provision of, spinal cord injured
  patients, 423
Carpal bones
 dislocations and fracture dislocations,
  198–205
  classification, 198, 199
  greater arc, 199, 201–203
  lunate and perilunate dislocations,
   198–201
  radiocarpal dislocations, 199, 204–205
  variants, 199, 203–204
 isolated injuries, 179–198
Carpal instability, post-traumatic, 173, 183,
  198–200, 205–210
 classification, 205–206
 dorsiflexed intercalated segment instability
  (DISI), 205, 207, 208, 209
 lateral, 206–207
 medial, 207–208
 proximal, 208–209
 volar palmar flexed intercalated segment
  instability (VISI), 205, 207, 208
Carpal translocation
 dorsal, 208–209
 palmar, 209
Carpal tunnel syndrome, 226–227, 447
Carpectomy, proximal row, 185, 201
Carrying angle, elbow, 108
Cartilage, articular, surgical replacement, 10
Causalgia *see* Reflex sympathetic dystrophy
Cervical spine injuries, 407–415
 children, 411
 fractures, 407–408
 hyperextension (whiplash) injuries, 12,
  409–410, 462
 soft tissue injuries, 408–411
 strains, 410–411
Chest injury, major, 474–475
Children
 ankle fractures, 352–354
 assessment of prognosis, 10–11
 cervical spine injuries, 411
 clavicular fractures, 44
 elbow development, 107–108
 elbow injuries *see* Elbow, childhood
  injuries
 femoral fractures, 281–285

Children *cont.*
  femoral neck fractures, 257–262
  foot injuries, 378–381
  forearm fractures, 141–145
  Galeazzi fracture dislocation, 154–155
  humeral shaft fractures, 103
  knee ligament disruption, 303
  Monteggia fracture dislocation, 151–152
  pelvic fractures, 403–404
  reflex sympathetic dystrophy, 489–490
  scaphoid fractures, 185–186
  shoulder dislocation, 68
  sternoclavicular joint injuries, 32
  thoracolumbar spine injuries, 414
  tibial fractures, 335–337
  see also Epiphyseal injuries
Chondropathy, elbow, 114
Chylothorax, 43
Claim, statement of, 19
Claudication, 8, 229
Clavicle
  congenital pseudoarthrosis, 44
  inferior dislocation of distal, 38
  osteolysis of distal, 38
  prominent lateral end, 35, 36
  thickening of medial end, 32
  traumatic floating, 32
Clavicular fractures, 39–45
  children and adolescents, 44
  classification, 39
  complications, 43
  conservative treatment, 40–41
  non-union, 42–43
  primary internal fixation, 41–42
Coagulation, disseminated intravascular,
    479, 482–483
Coagulopathy, 473, 482–483
Coccygeal fractures. 402–403
Cognitive impairment, 441
Cold intolerance, hands, 226, 229, 230
Colles' fractures, 161–175
  complications, 171–173
  conservative treatment, 162–169
    factors affecting functional results,
      165–169
    residual subjective symptoms, 162–165
  operative treatment, 169–171
  tears of triangular fibrocartilage complex
    with, 178
Compartment syndrome, tibial fractures,
    333
Compensation, 3
  composition of damages, 16–18, 418–419
  role in post-traumatic psychological
    problems, 457–458, 464
Compensation psychosis, 458
Compensation syndrome, 457, 458
Computerized tomography (CT scanning)
  pelvic injuries, 391
  skull fractures, 434

Conscious level, assessment of, 435–436
Consent, 5
Contractures
  Dupuytren's, 173
  hands, 223, 231
  ischaemic, 111, 130, 131, 333
Coracoclavicular ligament, calcification of,
    35, 36, 37
Coracoid process fractures, 46–47
Corticosteroids, 492–493, 494
Court, giving evidence in, 23–25, 428–429
Coxa valga, 283
Coxa vara, 258, 259, 260, 262
Cranial nerve palsies, head injury, 439, 440
Cross-examination, 24
Cross-union complicating forearm fractures,
    147
Cubital tunnel, 112
  external compression syndrome, 112–114
Cubitus valgus, 111, 112, 121, 127–128,
    133
Cubitus varus (gunstock deformity), 130,
    132
Cultural factors, post-traumatic
    psychological problems, 463
Cystic degeneration of spinal cord (post-
    traumatic syringomyelia), 426

Damages, assessment and composition,
    16–18, 418–419
De Quervain's tenosynovitis, 448
Dead arm syndrome, 64
Deltoid muscle paralysis, 46
Depression: post-traumatic, 459
Discs, intervertebral
  cervical spine injuries, 410
  degenerative changes, 413
  injuries in children, 414
  thoracolumbar injuries, 413–414
Driving eligibility, 442
Dupuytren's contracture, 173
Dysphasia, 440

Earning capacity, loss of, 18
Earnings, loss of, 17
Elbow, 107–133
  adult injuries, 109–123
    chondropathy and surface articular
      fractures, 114
    dislocation, 122–123
    insertion tendonopathy, 109–110
    lower humeral fractures, 114–116
    Monteggia fracture dislocation,
      121–122, 148–153
    neurological trauma, 110–114
    olecranon fractures, 116–118
    radial head and neck fractures,
      118–121
  anatomy, 108
  childhood injuries, 11, 125–133

Elbow *cont.*
　dislocation, 128–129
　epiphyseal injuries, 125–128, 132–133
　supracondylar fracture, 129–132
development, 107–108
loose bodies, 114, 124
measurement of motion, 108–109
post-traumatic arthritis *see* Arthritis, post-
　traumatic, elbow injuries
recurrent or habitual dislocation, 123,
　129
Electrical stimulation, 146, 184–185
Electroacupuncture, reflex sympathetic
　dystrophy, 492
Employers, reports to, 5
Employment, loss of, 7, 17
　foot injuries, 366, 374
　head injuries, 438
　pelvic fractures, 396
　psychological reactions and, 464
　see also Occupation; Work, time lost from
Empyema, post-traumatic, 475
Enteral nutrition, 481–482
Enterocolitis, uraemic, 479
Enthesopathies, elbow, 109–110
Epicondylitis
　lateral (tennis elbow), 109–110
　medial (golfer's elbow), 109–110
Epidural analgesia, 471
Epilepsy
　early traumatic, 432
　post-traumatic, 440, 442
Epiphyseal injuries
　clavicle, 44
　distal femur, 284
　distal radius and ulna, 176–178
　distal tibia and fibula, 352–354
　elbow, 125–128, 132–133
　femoral shaft fractures and, 283
　proximal femur, 258, 259–260, 261
　proximal humerus, 76–77
　proximal tibia, 335
　sternoclavicular joint, 30
Ethnic factors, post-traumatic psychological
　problems and, 463
Examination, physical, 7–8
Expert witnesses, 23–25, 428–429
Extensor tendon injuries, hands and wrists,
　147, 172, 176, 227–229, 448–450

Facial paralysis, 439
Fat embolism syndrome, 475–476
Fees, expert witnesses, 24, 429
Femoral epiphyseal injuries
　distal, 284
　proximal, 258, 259–260, 261
Femoral head, avascular necrosis *see*
　Avascular necrosis, femoral head
Femoral head and neck fractures, 249–257
　adults under 50 years, 254–256
　associated injuries, 239, 247–248, 285

children, 257–262
　basal cervicotrochanteric, 259–260
　complications, 260–262
　intertrochanteric, 260
　transcervical, 258
　transphyseal, 257–258
classification, 249–250
extracapsular (trochanteric), 253–254
intracapsular, 250–253
　Garden stage I/II, 251
　Garden stage III/IV, 251–253
Femoral shaft fractures, 271–279
　angular deformities, 276
　associated ipsilateral injuries, 285–287
　children, 282–283
　delayed union, 272–273
　femoral shortening, 275, 282
　knee function, 277
　non-union, 274
　refracture, 274
　rotational deformities, 275, 276–277
　social and occupational factors, 277–278
Femoral shortening, 269, 271, 275, 282
Femoral subtrochanteric fractures, 267–271
　children, 281–282
　classification in relation to prognosis,
　　267–269
　conservative treatment, 269
　problems of predicting prognosis,
　　270–271
　surgical treatment, 269–270
Femoral supracondylar/intercondylar
　　fractures, 279–281
Femur, 267–287
Fibular epiphyseal fractures, distal,
　352–354
Fibular fractures, 325–326
　see also Ankle fractures
Fingernail deformity, 230
Fingers
　amputation, 230–231
　stiffness after Colles' fractures, 164
　vibration white, 229, 232–233
Flexor tendon injuries, hands and wrists,
　172, 185, 197, 201, 227–229,
　448–450
Foot, 357–381
　calcaneal fractures, 357–362, 378
　childhood injuries, 378–381
　interphalangeal dislocations, 376
　metatarsal fractures, 374–375, 380
　metatarsophalangeal injuries, 376
　mid-tarsal fracture dislocations, 370–371,
　　380
　phalangeal fractures, 376
　sesamoid fractures, 376
　talar fractures and dislocations, 362–370,
　　378–379
　tarsometatarsal fracture dislocations,
　　372–374, 380
　traumatic partial amputations, 376–377

Forearm fractures, 137–155
  adults, 137–141
    conservative treatment, 137–138
    intramedullary fixation, 138–139
    plate fixation, 139–140
  children, 141–145
    conservative treatment, 141–143
    internal fixation, 143
    malunion, 143–144
    plastic deformation, 144
  complications, 146–148
    nerve and tendon lesions, 146–147
    non-union, 146
    refracture after plate removal, 147–148
    synostosis, 147
  see also Galeazzi fracture dislocation;
    Monteggia fracture dislocation;
    Radial fractures; Ulnar fractures

Galeazzi fracture dislocation, 153–155
  adults, 154
  children, 154–155
Gastrectomy, 481
Gastrointestinal bleeding, 479, 480, 482
Gastrointestinal failure, 481–482
Glasgow coma scale, 435–436
Glasgow outcome scale, 437–438
Glenohumeral joint see Shoulder joint
Glenoid fractures, 58–59, 66
Golfer's elbow (medial epicondylitis),
    109–110
Greenstick fractures, forearm, 142
Grip strength, 163–164, 222
Guanethidine intravenous regional
    sympathetic blockade, 493
Gunstock deformity (cubitus varus), 130,
    132
Guyon's canal, ulnar nerve compression,
    226, 227

Haematoma, intracranial, 431–432, 436, 442
Haematuria, 398
Haemothorax, 31, 43
Hamate
  dislocation, 197–198
  fractures, 196–197
Hand injuries, 221–233
  amputations, 230–231
  blood vessels, 229
  burns, 231
  fractures, 229–230
  injection injuries, 232
  ligaments, 229
  medicolegal reporting, 222–223
  nerve compression syndromes, 226–227
  nerves, 223–226
  scheme for estimation of residual
    disability, 225
  skin, 223
  tendons, 227–229
  vibration white finger, 232–233

Hanging cast, 87, 88–89
Hawkin's sign, 363–364
Head injury, 431–442
  associated with spinal cord injury, 421
  early complications, 431–432
  nutritional state, 472
  post-traumatic epilepsy, 440, 442
  psychological problems, 437, 458, 461,
    462
  sequelae of more severe injuries, 437–441
  sequelae of uncomplicated mild injuries,
    437
  severity of brain damage, 435–437
  skull fractures associated with, 432–434
  timescale of recovery, 441–442
Headaches, post-traumatic, 458–459
Hearing, loss of, 439
Heel broadening, 360, 361
Heel pad atrophy, 361
Hemiplegia, 440
Hepatic failure, 473, 483
Heteropic ossification, acetabular fractures,
    242
High Court actions, 19
Hip, 237–264
  acetabular fractures, 237–243
  dislocations, 243–249, 285
    anterior, 243–244
    children, 262–263
    posterior, 244–248
    time from injury to reduction, 248
    timing of medicolegal reports, 248
  femoral head and neck fractures see
    Femoral head and neck fractures
  fractures in children, 257–262
Holstein-Lewis fracture, 99, 101
Housing provision, spinal cord injured
    patients, 422–423, 424–425
Humeral neck
  anatomical fractures, 69, 70, 71
  avascular necrosis, 71, 73, 74
  surgical fractures, 69, 70, 71–72
Humeral shaft fractures, 87–104
  children, 103
  conservative management, 87–92
    anatomical site and, 91
    compound injuries, 90–91
    hanging cast, 88–89
    radiological alignment and functional
      results, 91–92
    splints or braces, 89–90
    thoracobrachial cast, 90
    traction, 90
  delayed or non-union, 95–97
  primary operative management, 92–95
    external fixation, 95
    indications, 93
    intramedullary fixation, 93–94
    plate fixation, 94–95
  radial nerve injury see Radial nerve palsy,
    humeral shaft fractures

Humerus
  distal fractures, 114–116
  greater tuberosity fractures, 58, 69, 70,
    72
  head defects, 58
  lateral condylar epiphyseal injuries see
    Capitular epiphyseal injuries
  lateral epicondylar fractures, 125
  lesser tuberosity fractures, 69, 70, 72
  lower epiphyseal separation, 125
  medial epicondylar fractures, 125
  proximal fractures, 66, 69–78
    epiphyseal, 76–77
    four-part, 69, 74
    fracture dislocations, 69, 70, 74–75
    incidence and classification, 69–70
    minimally displaced, 70–71
    non-union, 76
    replacement arthroplasty, 75–76
    three-part, 69, 72–73
    two-part, 69, 71–72
  supracondylar fractures in children, 111,
    129–132
  supracondyloid process fractures, 103–104
Hyperextension (whiplash) injuries of
    cervical spine, 12, 409–410, 462
Hypochondriacal symptoms, 461
Hysterical symptoms, 460–461

Ileus, paralytic, 481
Iliac crest avulsion fractures, 391–392
Iliac spine, anterior superior, avulsion
    fractures, 391–392
Iliac wing fractures, 393, 403–404
Impotence, 398–400
Incontinence of urine, 397, 399, 422
Infections see Sepsis/infections
Injection injuries, hands, 232
Insertion tendonopathy, elbow, 109–110
Insurance companies, 3, 12
Interphalangeal dislocations, 376
Intracranial haematoma, 431–432, 436, 442
Irritability, post-traumatic, 458–459
Ischaemic contractures, 111, 130, 131, 333
Ischial tuberosity avulsion fractures,
    391–392

Jaundice, 480, 483
Jones fracture, 375

Kienböck's disease, 187–191
  aetiology, 187–188
  treatment, 188–190
Knee, 291–318
  dislocation, 303–304
  ligament injuries, 292–304
    anterior cruciate ligament see Anterior
      cruciate ligament injuries
    children, 303
    classification, 292–293

    lateral compartment instability,
      294–295
    medial collateral structures, 293–294
    posterior cruciate ligament, 302–303
    with tibial plateau fractures, 314
  meniscal injuries, 305–307
  patellar injuries, 307–311
  tibial plateau fractures, 311–318
Knee instability
  anterolateral rotatory, 293, 295, 300–302
  anteromedial rotatory, 292–294, 297
  children, 303
  classification, 292–293
  isolated anterior cruciate, 298–300
  post-traumatic arthritis, 317
  posterolateral rotatory, 293, 295
  straight, 292
  with tibial plateau fractures, 314
Knee stiffness
  femoral fractures, 269, 277
  tibial fractures, 327, 333–334

Language function disorders, 440
Lateral capsular ligament injury, knee, 293
Lateral compartment instability of knee,
    292, 294–295
Leg length discrepency
  ankle fractures, 353, 354
  femoral fractures, 269, 271, 275, 282–283
  pelvic fractures, 402
  tibial fractures, 332–333
Life expectancy
  estimation of, 11–12, 17, 22
  spinal cord injury, 427
Limbs, loss of, 8
  see also Amputations
Literature, scientific, reliance on, 13, 22–23
Livingstone v. Reywards Coal Co. [1880], 16
Local anaesthetic block, reflex sympathetic
    dystrophy, 492–493
Loose bodies, elbow joint, 114, 124
Lunate
  avascular necrosis, 187–188, 201, 204
  dislocations, 203–204
  excision and prosthetic replacement, 189
  fractures, 187–188
  Kienböck's disease, 187–191
  and perilunate dislocations, 198–201
Luxatioerecta, 68

Malgaigne fractures, 390–391, 395–397
Malingering, 9, 461
Malnutrition, trauma and, 470, 471–472
Mammary vessel injuries, 31
Medial collateral ligament injury, knee, 292,
    293–294, 314
Median nerve injuries
  carpal fracture dislocations, 201, 202
  Colles' fractures, 171–172
  forearm fractures, 146–147
  hamate fractures, 197

Median nerves injuries *cont.*
  hands, 224
  humeral fractures, 102, 103, 111, 131
Medical expenses, compensation for, 16–17
Medical records, 5, 19
Medicolegal reports *see* Reports, medicolegal
Meningitis, base of skull fractures, 433–434
Meniscal injuries, 305–307
  degenerative tears, 307
  with tibial plateau fractures, 314
Meniscectomy, 305–307
  anterolateral rotatory instability, 300–301
  anteromedial rotatory instability, 294
  open, 306–307
  partial arthroscopic, 307
Mental dysfunction, head injury, 438, 441
Metatarsal fractures, 374–375, 380
Metatarsophalangeal injuries, 376
Methylprednisolone, regional local
  anaesthetic block with, 492–493
Mid-carpal instability, 209
Mid-tarsal fracture dislocations, 370–371,
  380
Monteggia fracture dislocation, 121–122,
  148–153
  adults, 149–151
  children, 151–152
  complications, 152–153
  incidence and classification, 148–149
Motor power assessment, 8, 421
Multiple system organ failure (MSOF), 469,
  472–474
  causes, 473–474
  mortality, 474
  prevention, 474
Multiple trauma *see* Polytrauma
Myositis ossificans, 128–129, 244, 392

Navicular fractures, 371
  Naylor v. *Preston Area Health
    Authority et al* [1987], 22
Negligence
  medical, 3, 12
  by reporting clinician, 9
Nerve injuries
  assessment, 8
  Colles' fractures, 171–172
  elbow, 110–114, 128, 131
  forearm fractures, 146–147
  hands, 223–227
  Monteggia fracture dislocation, 152–153
  pelvic fractures, 397
  shoulder dislocation, 60
  see also Specific nerves
Neurological disorders, head injury, 439–440
Neuromas, 226
Neurosis, post-traumatic, 457, 458–459
Neurotic traits, pre-existing, 463
Nutritional support, 471–472, 481–482

Obstetric problems

pelvic fractures, 11, 394, 402
spinal cord injury, 422
Occupation
  change of, 10, 278, 366, 374
  hand injuries and, 225–226
  see also Employment, loss of; Work, time
    lost from
Occupational injuries
  carpal tunnel syndrome, 226–227
  repetitive stress injuries, 447–456
  vibration white finger, 232–233
Olecranon epiphyseal injuries, 125
Olecranon fractures, 116–118
Opiates, high-dose, 471
Ossification
  coracoclavicular ligament, 35, 36, 37
  heteropic, acetabular fractures, 242
  see also Myositis ossificans
Osteoarthritis, post-traumatic *see* Arthritis,
    post-traumatic
Osteolysis, distal clavicle, 38
Osteophytosis, acetabular, 240
Osteoporosis
  femoral neck fractures, 254
  reflex sympathetic dystrophy, 490

Pain
  assessment of, 6, 21
  damages for, 18, 418
Paralytic ileus, 481
Patellar dislocation, 310–311
Patellar fractures, 307–310
  femoral shaft fracture with, 285–286
  prognosis, 308–310
Patellectomy, 309–310
Patellofemoral joint arthritis, 280–281
Pelvic fractures, 387–404
  anteroposterior compression, 389, 393–394
  associated acetabular fractures, 239
  avulsion fractures, 391–392
  children, 403–404
  classification, 387–388
  complications, 397–402
    malunion, 402
    neurological, 397
    non-union and delayed union, 400–401
    obstetric problems, 11, 394, 402
    urological injury and impotence,
      398–400
  iliac wing, 393, 403–404
  isolated four-rami fractures (butterfly or
    straddle), 388, 389
  lateral compression, 389–390, 394–395
  open-book disruption, 388, 389
  pubic rami, 392–393, 404
  rotationally stable/vertically unstable,
    393–395
  rotationally and vertically unstable
    (Malgaigne), 390–391, 395–397
  stable, 391–393
  vertical shear, 390–391

Perilunate dislocation, 198–201
Peritalar dislocation, 368–369
Peritendinitis crepitans, 451
Peroneal nerve injuries, 304, 315, 317
Peroneal tendinitis, 360
Personality
    changes after head injury, 441
    pre-traumatic, 463
    reflex sympathetic dystrophy and, 494
Phalangeal fractures, 376
Phobic symptoms, post-traumatic, 460
Physical examination, 7–8
Physical therapy, reflex sympathetic
        dystrophy, 492
Pisiform injuries, 192
Pivot shift instability, 291, 300
Plantar fasciitis, 360
Pneumoperitoneum, 481
Pneumothorax, 43, 45
Polytrauma, 469–483
    acute renal failure, 478–481
    adult respiratory distress syndrome,
        476–478
    fat embolism syndrome, 475–476
    gastrointestinal failure, 481–482
    hepatic failure, 483
    massive transfusion and coagulopathy,
        482–483
    multiple system organ failure, 469,
        472–474
    nutritional support, 471–472
    pulmonary contusion, 474–475
    stress response, 469–471
Popliteal artery injuries, 304, 315
Post-concussional syndrome, 437, 457, 462
Post-phlebitic syndrome, tibial fractures,
        334
Posterior cruciate ligament injury, 292,
        301–303
Posterior interosseus nerve injuries, 152, 153
Posterior oblique ligament injury, knee, 292
Pregnancy
    pelvic fractures and, 11, 394, 402
    spinal cord injured patients, 422
Pressure sores, spinal cord injury, 421, 426,
        427
Prognosis, assessment of, 9–12, 21–22
    see also Life expectancy
Prostheses, replacement
    elbow joint, 124–125
    femoral head, 252–253
    Kienböck's disease, 189
    proximal humerus, 75–76
    radial head, 120–121
Psychological problems, 21, 457–465
    assessment and investigation, 462–463
    head injury, 437, 458, 461, 462
    incidence, 457–458
    medicolegal reports, 465
    prognosis, 464
    reflex sympathetic dystrophy and, 494

spinal cord injury, 422–423
symptoms, 458–461
Psychosis
    compensation, 458
    post-traumatic, 458, 461
Pubic rami fractures, 392–393, 404
Published literature, reliance on, 13, 22–23
Pulmonary contusion, 474–475
Pulmonary infections, 473, 478, 479

Radial epiphyseal injuries
    distal, 176–178
    proximal, 132–133
Radial fractures
    distal, 161–176
        with dorsal displacement see Colles'
            fracture
        marginal articular (Barton's fractures),
            161, 175–176
        with palmar displacement (Smith's
            fracture), 161, 175–176
        undisplaced, 161
    Galeazzi fracture dislocation, 153–155
    head and neck, 118–121
        classification, 118–119
        complications, 120–121
        conservative management, 119
        operative management, 119–120
    Monteggia fracture dislocation with, 149,
        150–151
    see also Forearm fractures
Radial head dislocation, 149
    see also Monteggia fracture dislocation
Radial head excision, 120–121
Radial nerve palsy
    acute posterior dislocation of shoulder, 66
    external compression neuropathy, 111
    forearm fractures, 146–147
    humeral shaft fractures, 94, 95, 96,
        97–103
        children, 103
        incidence, 97–99
        recovery rates, 99–103
    Monteggia fracture dislocation, 152
    supracondylar humeral fractures, 131
Radial shortening, post-traumatic, 168
Radial shortening procedures, Kienböck's
        disease, 190
Radiocarpal joint
    dislocations, 199, 204
    instabilities, 208–209
Radiological examinations, 8
Radioulnar joint, distal
    disruption, Galeazzi fracture dislocations,
        153–155
    involvement in Colles' fractures, 166–168
    isolated dislocation, 178
    subluxation complicating radial head
        excision, 120
    tears of triangular fibrocartilage complex
        (TFC), 178–179

Records, medical, 5, 19
Recreation, loss of facility in, 7
Reflex sympathetic dystrophy (RSD), 487–494
  children, 489–490
  clinical features, 488–489
  investigations, 490–491
  pathogenesis, 487–488
  psychological factors, 494
  results of treatment, 491–494
Refractures
  femoral shaft fractures, 274
  forearm fractures, 147–148
  tibial fractures, 334
Renal disease, spinal cord injury, 422, 426
Renal failure, acute, 473, 478–481
  complications, 479
  mortality, 480
  prognosis, 480–481
Repetitive stress injuries (RSI), 109–110, 447–456
  aetiology, 452–453
  diagnosis, 451
  grades, 452
  Kienböck's disease, 187
Replacement prostheses see Prostheses, replacement
Reports, medicolegal, 3–13, 15–25
  commissioning, 18–19
  disclosure to other party, 4, 23
  form and content, 5–12, 20–23
    assessment of present condition, 8–9, 21
    history, 5–7
    physical examination, 7–8
    prognosis, 9–12, 21–22
    radiological and other examination, 8
  giving evidence in court, 23–25, 428–429
  independence, 4, 15
  legal procedures, 19–20
  medical negligence and, 12
  psychiatric, 465
  purpose, 16–18
  specimen format, 497–499
  use of published works and statistics, 13, 22–23
Respiratory distress syndrome, adult (ARDS), 473, 474, 476–478
  definition, 477
  mortality, 477–478
  prognosis, 478
  survivors, 478
  treatment, 477
Respiratory infections, 473, 478, 479
Respiratory problems, spinal cord injury, 426, 427
Restituto integrum, 16
Road traffic accidents, 5–6
Rotator cuff pseudorupture, 46
Rotator cuff tears, 50–53
  acute, 51

  associated with anterior dislocation of shoulder, 59–60
  chronic, 51–53

Sacral fractures, 402–403
Sacroiliac dislocations, 395, 396
Saturday night palsy, 111
Scanograms, 275
Scaphocapitate syndrome, 195–196
Scaphoid dislocations, 203–204
Scaphoid fractures, 179–187, 202
  children, 185–186
  conservative treatment, 180–182
  non-union, 182–185
  operative treatment, 182
  tendon rupture complicating, 185
Scapholunate dissociation, 173, 183, 200, 206–207
Scaphotrapezium-trapezoid instability, 207
Scapular fractures, 45–48
  apophysis (type II), 46–47
  body (type I), 45–46
  superior lateral angle (type III), 47–48
Scapular spine fractures, 46
Scar contractures, hands, 223
Schooling, loss of, 7
Sciatic nerve palsy, 241–242
Scintigraphic changes, reflex sympathetic dystrophy, 490–491
Sensory loss, assessment of, 8, 224, 421
Sepsis/infections
  intracranial, 433–434
  multiple trauma, 469, 473–474, 477–478, 479, 483
  tibial fractures, 326
Septicaemic shock, 477
Sesamoid fractures, 376
Sex chromosome anomalies, 108
Sex of patient
  ankle fractures, 346
  avascular necrosis of femoral head and, 252
  recurrent anterior dislocation of shoulder and, 58
Sexual problems, 6, 398–400, 422
Shoulder, 29–78
  acromioclavicular joint injuries, 33–39
  biceps brachii rupture, 48–50
  clavicular fractures, 39–45
  glenohumeral joint injuries see Shoulder joint
  proximal humeral fractures, 69–78
  rotator cuff tears, 50–53
  scapular fractures, 45–48
  sternoclavicular joint injuries, 29–33
Shoulder joint (glenohumeral joint), 53–69
  anterior dislocations and subluxations, 53–62
  chronic anterior dislocation, 64–65
  dislocation in children, 68
  posterior dislocation, 65–69
    acute, 66

Shoulder joint *cont.*
    arthritis after, 67–68
    chronic, 66–67
    habitual, 66
    incidence and classification, 65–66
    recurrent (dislocation and subluxation),
        67
    primary anterior dislocation, 54–62
    factors associated with recurrence,
        55–59
    nerve injury complicating, 60
    rotator cuff tears associated with,
        59–60
    vascular injury complicating, 61
    recurrent anterior dislocation, 62–64
    recurrent anterior subluxation, 64
    subglenoid dislocation associated with
        fracture of coracoid process, 47
Silicone synovitis, 189
Skin grafts, 231
Skin injuries, hands, 223
Skull fractures, 432–434
    compound depressed, 433, 442
    linear, 434
    skull base, 433–434
Smell, loss of sense of, 439
Smith's fractures, 161, 175–176
Social problems, spinal cord injury,
    422–423
Spinal cord injuries, 6, 417–429
    bladder function, 421–422
    clinician providing the report, 427–429
    compensation guidelines, 418–419
    content of medicolegal reports, 419–427
    general medical examination, 420–421
    prognosis and life expectancy, 11,
        423–427
    provision and facilities for care, 423
    sexual function, 422
    social and psychological problems,
        422–423
Spinal injuries, 407–415, 462–463
    cervical, 407–411
    thoracolumbar, 411–415, 462–463, 464
Splints, humeral, 87, 89–90
Sternoclavicular joint, 29–33
    anterior dislocation (grade III), 30–31
    childhood injuries, 32
    recurrent anterior dislocation, 30–31
    retrosternal dislocation (grade III),
        31–32
    sprains and subluxations (grades I and
        II), 29–302Stress disorder, post-
        traumatic, 457, 458, 459–460
Stress fractures
    humeral shaft, 103
    pubic rami, 392–393
Stress injuries, repetitive *see* Repetitive
    stress injuries

Stress response, 469–471
Stress ulcers, 479, 481
Subclavian vessel injuries, 31, 43, 45
Subpoenas, 24–25
Subtalar dislocation, 368–369
Subtalar joint
    fractures involving, 357, 359–360
    stiffness, 327, 333–334, 360
Suffering, 18, 418
Supracondyloid process of humerus,
    fractures of, 103–104
Sympathetic blockade, 491, 493
Sympathetic dystrophy, reflex *see* Reflex
    sympathetic dystrophy
Synostosis complicating forearm fractures,
    147
Synovial biopsy, 491
Synovitis, silicone, 189
Syringomyelia, post-traumatic, 426

Talocrural angle, 346, 347
Talus, 362–370
    dislocations about, 368–370
    fractures of the body, 366
    fractures in children, 378–379
    neck fractures, 362–366
        clinical results, 365–366
        complications, 362–365
    osteochondral fractures of the dome,
        368
    peripheral fractures, 366–367
        head, 366–367
        lateral process, 367
        posterior process, 367
Tarsometatarsal fracture dislocations,
    372–373, 380
Tendinitis, 450–451
    peroneal, 360
Tendon injuries
    biceps brachii, 49–50
    Colles' fractures, 172
    forearm fractures, 146–147
    hands, 227–229
    scaphoid non-union, 185
Tendonopathy, insertion, elbow, 109–110
Tennis elbow (lateral epicondylitis),
    109–110
Tenosynovitis, 447–448, 451
    de Quervain's, 448
    stenosing, 448–450
Thermography, reflex sympathetic
    dystrophy, 491
Thermoneutral environment, 471
Third party expenses, 17
Thoracic duct injury, 31, 43
Thoracobrachial casts, 87, 90
Thoracolumbar spinal injuries, 411–415
    burst fractures, 412

Thoracolumbar spinal injuries *cont.*
  children, 414
  psychological factors affecting outcome, 462–463, 464
  soft tissue injuries, 413–414
  stable fractures, 411–412
  unstable fractures, 412
Thrombocytopenia, dilutional, 482
Tibial epiphyseal injuries
  distal, 352–354
  proximal, 283, 335
Tibial fractures, 323–337
  children, 335–337
  complications, 330–335
    compartment syndrome/ischaemic contractures, 333
    delayed union/non-union, 330–331
    joint stiffness, 333–334
    malunion, 331–333
    post-phlebitic syndrome, 334
    refracture, 334
  conservative versus operative treatment, 327–330
  femoral shaft fractures with, 286–287
  functional bracing with early weight bearing, 329
  operative treatment, 329–330
  plaster immobilization, 327–328
  prognostic factors, 323, 324–327
  see also Ankle fractures
Tibial plafond/pilon fractures, 349–352
  classification, 349
  prognostic indicators, 350–352
Tibial plateau fractures, 311–318
  classification, 311, 312
  complications of surgery, 317–318
  grading of results, 311, 313
  long-term results, 314–316
  post-traumatic osteoarthritis, 316–317
  prognostic factors, 312–314
Tibiofemoral joint arthritis, 280
Tracheal injury, 31
Traction
  femoral subtrochanteric fractures, 269
  humeral fractures, 87, 90
  supracondylar fractures of the humerus, 129
  whiplash injuries, 410
Trans-scaphoid perilunar fracture dislocation, 199, 201–203
Transfusion, massive, 482–483
Trapezium
  dislocation, 193–194
  fractures, 192–193
Trapezoid fractures, 194–195
Triangular fibrocartilage complex (TFC) of wrist, tears of, 178–179
Triquetral injuries, 191–192
Triquetrohamate instability, 207–208

Triquetrolunate instability, 207, 208
Turner's syndrome, 108

Ulna
  distal epiphyseal injuries, 176–178
  lengthening procedures, Kienböck's disease, 190
Ulnar fractures, isolated, 145–146
  see also Forearm fractures; Monteggia fracture dislocation
Ulnar-minus variant, 187–188, 190
Ulnar nerve injuries
  Colles' fractures, 171, 172
  compression in Guyon's canal, 226, 227
  cubital tunnel external compression syndrome, 112–1142 distal humeral fractures, 115–116
  elbow dislocation in children, 128
  forearm fractures, 146–147
  Galeazzi fracture dislocation, 154
  hamate fractures, 197
  hands, 224
  humeral shaft fractures, 102
  medial humeral epicondylar fractures, 125
  Monteggia fracture dislocation, 153
  osteoarthritic change causing, 124
  pisiform fractures, 192
  proximal radial epiphyseal injuries, 133
  radial head excision, 121
  supracondylar fractures of the humerus, 111, 131
  tardy ulnar palsy, 111–112, 128, 197
Ulnar translocation, 208
Uraemic enterocolitis, 479
Urethral injuries, 398–400, 404
Urinary incontinence, 397, 399, 422
Urinary tract infections, spinal cord injury, 426
Urological injuries, 398–400

Vascular injuries, 8, 128, 229
  see also Arterial injuries; Ischaemic contractures
Vegetative state, 438–439
Venous damage, 8
Ventilator index, 478
Vibration white finger, 229, 232–233
Visual problems, head injury, 439, 440
Volkmann's ischaemic contracture, 111, 130

Whiplash injuries, 12, 409–410, 462
Whitehouse v. *Jordan* [1981], 15, 20
Witnesses, expert, 23–25, 428–429
Work, time lost from
  ankle fractures, 347–348
  femoral shaft fractures, 278
  foot injuries, 358
  hip injuries, 241

Work, time lost from *cont.*
  pelvic fractures, 395
  see also Employment, loss of; Occupation
Wrist, 161–210
  carpal dislocations and fracture
    dislocations, 198–205
  distal radial fractures, 161–176
  epiphyseal fractures of distal radius and
    ulna, 176–178

  isolated carpal bone injuries, 191–198
  isolated distal radioulnar joint injuries,
    178–179
  lunate fractures and Kienböck's disease,
    187–191
  post-traumatic carpal instability, 205–210
  scaphoid fractures, 179–187
  tenosynovitis, 448, 449
Writs, 19